Y0-BZE-580

ESH
EUROPEAN
SCHOOL OF
HAEMATOLOGY

2012
Revised Edition

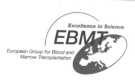

Excellence in Science
EBMT
European Group for Blood and
Marrow Transplantation

Haematopoietic Stem Cell Transplantation

Editors: J. Apperley, E. Carreras, E. Gluckman, T. Masszi

ESH and the editors wish to thank
Dr Diana Samson for her essential contribution
to the production of this handbook

Supported by an educational grant from

CHUGAI
sanofi aventis

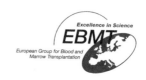

Welcome to the 6th edition of the ESH-EBMT Handbook. It is now more than ten years since our original idea to create a Pocket book to accompany the annual training course and we could not have imagined how popular this small contribution to the transplant literature was to become. Fifty thousand copies of the 5th edition were printed and distributed free of charge by our partner, CHUGAI Sanofi-Aventis.

Over the years, the book has undoubtedly got bigger and hopefully better as feedback from our contributors and readers have suggested ways to improve the content. For this edition, all chapters have been completely rewritten and all references updated. To reflect changes in practice we also commissioned some new sections to address for example, JACIE, indications for transplant and post-transplant immunotherapy.

We have also expanded the disease-specific chapters and included the regenerative disorders. In addition we introduced new chapters on statistics, methodology of clinical trials and ethics. All chapters included MCQs to test the newly acquired knowledge.

As always we are grateful for comments (good and bad!) from our readers as this is the only way that we can constantly improve the Handbook.

This new edition will be first edited on paper and later on will be accessible on-line.

As with the previous editions it will be distributed free of charge through orders through the ESH website.

We extend our many thanks to all our contributors who worked so hard to meet our deadlines and to the staff at ESH who had the unenviable task of reminding the authors and section editors of these deadlines, so necessary to ensure that the book would be ready for distribution at the EBMT annual meeting. Very special mention must be made of Diana Samson, responsible for the final editing process, who was so accommodating of late arrivals and so meticulous in her work. Without all these individuals we could not have hoped to be ready on time. We hope you enjoy and make use of the product of their efforts!

Jane Apperley   Enric Carreras   Eliane Gluckman   Tamás Masszi

ESH
EUROPEAN
SCHOOL OF
HAEMATOLOGY

Dear Readers,

ESH is proud to present this 6th revised edition of the ESH-EBMT Handbook on Haematopoietic Stem Cell Transplantation.

ESH and EBMT have worked together for many years to make high-level training and tools for continuing education freely available to junior and senior scientists, physicians, nurses and data managers with interest in the field.

Today, the need for education is greater than ever: new transplant centres continue to open throughout Europe and the world; the number of haematopoietic stem cell transplants continues to increase; our understanding of transplant biology is improving and new transplant procedures and techniques are being implemented. For all of these reasons, freely accessible education and educational tools are of increasing importance to transplant specialists worldwide.

ESH is also engaged in EUROCORD-ED, as the partner for educational activities and tools, including the regular conference on the biology and clinical application of cord blood stem cells (*www.eurocord-ed.org*).

We invite you to visit the ESH website (*www.esh.org*) to find information on ESH activities and freely accessible educational tools, including the PowerPoint presentations of the ESH-EBMT Training Courses and other conferences.

We would like to warmly thank the editors and authors of this Handbook. They have once again generously donated their time and expertise to further education in this field.

CHUGAI Sanofi-Aventis has been the corporate partner of the ESH-EBMT Handbook since its first edition. This partnership has been provided through educational grants and with exemplary respect for the scientific independence of the editors and authors.

ESH aims to provide you with the educational tools that meet your professional needs. We welcome your comments and suggestions for improvement and we invite you to contact us at: *didi.jasmin@univ-paris-diderot.fr*.

Eliane Gluckman
ESH President

Bob Löwenberg
*ESH Chair of
the Scientific Committee*

Didi Jasmin
ESH Executive Director

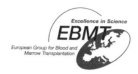

Excellence in Science

EBMT

European Group for Blood and
Marrow Transplantation

Dear Friends,

On behalf of the EBMT Board and all the contributors, it is with great pleasure that I introduce this new edition of the ESH-EBMT Handbook on Haematopoietic Stem Cell Transplantation. The first edition of the Handbook appeared in 1998, when Professor Alois Gratwohl, a former President of EBMT, wrote *"the present EBMT manual is a draft of a handbook which will hopefully one day become a standard tool in the daily management of patients undergoing blood or marrow stem cell transplantation"*. There is no doubt that his vision has been fulfilled beyond expectation.

The EBMT Handbook has become the manual of choice for many doctors and practitioners involved in haematopoietic stem cell transplantation (HSCT). As a result of the outstanding efforts of the Editorial Board and the contributors, this current Handbook is a complete update of all aspects of HSCT. Within its twenty-four chapters, there is a comprehensive review of the current state-of-the-art in this difficult and challenging field. There is no doubt that during the past years significant contributions have helped to improve the outcome of HSCT and our deeper understanding of HLA-matching and other immunogenetic factors involved in donor selection has led to an increase in the number of unrelated bone marrow donors, which has reached nearly 20 million worldwide. We have also seen a significant increase in the use of peripheral haematopoietic stem cells instead of bone marrow, the increased use of cord blood transplantation with an increase in the number of cord blood banks, and an increase in the use of HSCT in older patients. We now have a deeper understanding of the knowledge of the management of graft-versus-host disease, post-transplant infections and late-effects. Similarly, the field is changing with the development of new drugs either to support stem cell transplantation or to replace HSCT in the treatment of some conditions. However, despite all these developments, HSCT is still a procedure with a high mortality risk, and if this could be reduced significantly, HSCT could be of benefit in many other conditions. We have already begun to see the development of the application of stem cell transplantation in regenerative medicine and I am optimistic that this will become a main indication for stem cell transplantation. Therefore, I am convinced that the use of this Handbook on a daily basis will benefit not only doctors, but many patients as well.

The EBMT Board are extremely grateful to ESH, the Editorial Board, the contributors and to CHUGAI Sanofi-Aventis for an educational grant, which will permit the free distribution of this Handbook.

I wish all of you the best use of this Handbook and I am very grateful to you for making HSCT a safer procedure for many patients not just in Europe, but worldwide.

Professor Alejandro Madrigal
President EBMT

Contributors

Chapter 1

Eliane Gluckman — Eurocord, Hôpital Saint Louis, Paris, France

Chapter 2

Alejandro Madrigal — Anthony Nolan Research Institute, Royal Free Hospital, London, United Kingdom

Anna Sureda — Addenbrooke's Hospital, Cambridge, United Kingdom

Chapter 3

Christian Chabannon — Department of Haematology, Institut Paoli Calmettes, Marseille, France

Eoin McGrath — JACIE Accreditation, EBMT Executive Office, Barcelona, Spain

Chapter 4

Aleksandra Wodnar-Filipowicz — Stem Cell Competence Center, University of Basel, Basel, Switzerland

Chapter 5

Bronwen E. Shaw — Anthony Nolan Research Institute, London, United Kingdom

Alejandro Madrigal — Anthony Nolan Research Institute, Royal Free Hospital, London, United Kingdom

Chapter 6

Eliane Gluckman — Eurocord, Hôpital Saint Louis, Paris, France

Chapter 7

Carlheinz Mueller — Zentrales Knochenmarkspender-Register für Deutschland, Ulm, Germany

Sergio Querol — Anthony Nolan Research Institute and UCL Medical School, Royal Free Campus, London, United Kingdom

Chapter 8

Alois Gratwohl	Basel University Hospital, Basel, Switzerland
Enric Carreras	Fundacion International Josep Carreras, Barcelona, Spain

Chapter 9

Rachel Pawson	NHS Blood and Transplant Bristol Centre, Bristol, United Kingdom
Derwood Pamphilon	NHS Blood and Transplant Bristol Centre, Bristol, United Kingdom

Chapter 10

Tamás Masszi	Department of Internal Medicine, Semmelweis University, Budapest, Hungary
Arno Mank	Academic Medical Centre, Amsterdam, The Netherlands

Chapter 11

Enric Carreras	Fundacion International Josep Carreras, Barcelona, Spain

Chapter 12

Montserrat Rovira	Department of Haematology, Hospital Clinic of Barcelona, Barcelona, Spain
Josep Mensa	Department of Infectious Diseases, Hospital Clinic of Barcelona, Barcelona, Spain
Enric Carreras	Fundacion International Josep Carreras, Barcelona, Spain

Chapter 13

Jane Apperley	Department of Haematology, Imperial College, London, United Kingdom
Tamás Masszi	Department of Internal Medicine, Semmelweis University, Budapest, Hungary

Chapter 14

Antoine Toubert	INSERM UMR940 and Laboratoire d'Immunologie et d'Histocompatibilité, Hôpital Saint-Louis, Paris, France

Chapter 15

André Tichelli — Department of Haematology, University Hospital Basel, Basel, Switzerland

Gérard Socié — Service d'hématologie et de greffes de moelle osseuse, Hôpital Saint-Louis, Paris, France

Chapter 16.1

Jean-Michel Cayuela — Laboratoire Central d'Hématologie, Hôpital Saint-Louis, Paris, France

Chapter 16.2

Thomas Lion — Labdia Labordiagnostik GmbH, Children's Cancer Research Institute, Vienna, Austria

Chapter 17

Inge Jedema — Department of Hematology, Leiden University Medical Centre, Leiden, The Netherlands

J.H. Frederik Falkenburg — Department of Hematology, Leiden University Medical Centre, Leiden, The Netherlands

Chapter 18

Alois Gratwohl — Basel University Hospital, Basel, Switzerland

Helen Baldomero — Basel University Hospital, Basel, Switzerland

Anna Sureda — Addenbrooke's Hospital, Cambridge, United Kingdom

Chapter 19.1

Mohamad Mohty — Acute Leukemia Working Party of EBMT, Paris, France

Chapter 19.2

Mohamad Mohty — Acute Leukemia Working Party of EBMT, Paris, France

Chapter 19.3

Nicolaus Kröger — Department of Stem Cell Transplantation, University Medical Center Hamburg, Hamburg, Germany

Chapter 19.4

Jiri Pavlu — Imperial College at Hammersmith Hospital, London, United Kingdom

Jane Apperley — Department of Haematology, Imperial College, London, United Kingdom

Chapter 19.5

Peter Dreger — Abteilung Innere Medizin V, Universitätsklinikum Heidelberg, Heidelberg, Germany

Johannes Schetelig — Medizinische Klinik und Poliklinik I, Universitätsklinikum Carl Gustav Carus, Dresden, Germany

Chapter 19.6

Jesús San-Miguel — Servicio de Hematologia. Hospital Universitario de Salamanca, Salamanca, Spain

José A. Pérez-Simón — Servicio de Hematologia Hospital Virgen del Rocio, Sevilla, Spain

M. Victoria Mateos — Servicio de Hematologia. Hospital Universitario de Salamanca, Salamanca, Spain

Chapter 19.7

M. Teresa Cibeira — Department of Haematology, Institut d'Investigacions Mèdiques August Pi i Sunyer, Hospital Clínic, Barcelona, Spain

Jordi Esteve — Department of Haematology, Institut d'Investigacions Mèdiques August Pi i Sunyer, Hospital Clínic, Barcelona, Spain

Chapter 19.8

Harry C. Schouten — University Hospital Maastricht, Maastricht, The Netherlands

Anna Sureda — Addenbrooke's Hospital, Cambridge, United Kingdom

Chapter 19.9

Anna Sureda — Addenbrooke's Hospital, Cambridge, United Kingdom

Harry C. Schouten — University Hospital Maastricht, Maastricht, The Netherlands

Chapter 19.10

Marco Bregni — Department of Haematology, San Raffaele Scientific Institute, Milan, Italy

Chapter 19.11

John A. Snowden — Department of Haematology, Sheffield Teaching Hospitals NHS Foundation Trust, and Department of Oncology University of Sheffield, Sheffield, United Kingdom

Riccardo Saccardi — Department of Haematology, Careggi University Hospital, Florence, Italy

Dominique Farge — Service de Médecine Interne et Pathologie Vasculaire and INSERM U697, Hôpital Saint-Louis, Paris, France

Chapter 19.12

Judith Marsh — Department of Haematological Medicine, King's College Hospital, London, United Kingdom

Carlo Dufour — Haematology Unit, Istituto Giannina Gaslini, Genoa, Italy

Chapter 20.1

Giorgio Dini — Department of Haemato-Oncology, Giannina Gaslini Children's Hospital, Genoa, Italy

Stefano Giardino — Department of Haemato-Oncology, Giannina Gaslini Children's Hospital, Genoa, Italy

Chapter 20.2

Christina Peters — St. Anna Children's Hospital, Vienna, Austria

Chapter 20.3

Franco Locatelli — Department of Paediatric Haematology-Oncology, IRCCS Ospedale Bambino Gesù, Rome - University of Pavia, Pavia, Italy

Alice Bertaina — Department of Paediatric Haematology-Oncology, IRCCS Ospedale Bambino Gesù, Rome - University of Pavia, Pavia, Italy

Giuseppe Palumbo — Department of Paediatric Haematology-Oncology, IRCCS Ospedale Bambino Gesù, Rome - University of Pavia, Pavia, Italy

Chapter 20.4

Franco Locatelli — Department of Paediatric Haematology-Oncology, IRCCS Ospedale Bambino Gesù, Rome - University of Pavia, Pavia, Italy

Charlotte M. Niemeyer — Division of Pediatric Hematology and Oncology, Department of Pediatrics and Adolescent Medicine, University of Freiburg, Freiburg, Germany

Chapter 20.5

Alexander Claviez — Department of Paediatrics and Bone Marrow Transplant Unit, Medical, Kiel, Germany

Chapter 20.6

Paul Veys — Department of Blood and Marrow Transplantation, Great Ormond Street Hospital for Children NHS Trust, London, United Kingdom

H. Bobby Gaspar — Molecular Immunology Unit, UCL Institute of Child Health, London, United Kingdom

Chapter 20.7

Jaap J. Boelens — Department of Pediatrics: Blood and Marrow Transplantation Program, UMC Utrecht, Utrecht, The Netherlands

Marc Bierings — Department of Pediatrics: Blood and Marrow Transplantation Program, UMC Utrecht, Utrecht, The Netherlands

Robert Wynn — Blood and Marrow Transplant Unit, Royal Manchester Children's Hospital, Manchester, United Kingdom

Chapter 20.8

Eliane Gluckman — Eurocord, Hôpital Saint Louis, Paris, France

Chapter 20.9

Emanuele Angelucci — Unità Operativa di Ematologia e Centro Trapianti di Midollo

	Osseo Ospedale Oncologico di Riferimento Regionale "Armando Businco", Cagliari, Italy
Donatella Baronciani	Unità Operativa di Ematologia e Centro Trapianti di Midollo Osseo Ospedale Oncologico di Riferimento Regionale "Armando Businco", Cagliari, Italy

Chapter 20.10

Ruth Ladenstein	St. Anna Children's Hospital and St. Anna Kinderkrebsforschung, Vienna, Austria
Ulrike Pötschger	St. Anna Kinderkrebsforschung, Vienna, Austria

Chapter 21

Richard M. Szydlo	Centre for Haematology, Department of Medicine, Imperial College, London, United Kingdom

Chapter 22

Mohamad Mohty	Acute Leukemia Working Party of EBMT, Paris, France

Chapter 23

Eliane Gluckman	Eurocord, Hôpital Saint Louis, Paris, France
Marie Caroline Le Bousse-Kerdilès	INSERM U972, Institut André Lwoff, Université Paris XI - Hôpital Paul Brousse, Villejuif, France

Chapter 24

Cliff Chaplin	St. Bartholomew School of Nursing and Midwifery, London, United Kingdom

* CONTENTS

* CHAPTER 1

A brief history of HSCT

Eliane Gluckman

1. How haematopoietic stem cell transplant was born: From the threat of atomic irradiation to animal models and to humans

After the atomic bomb explosion in Japan, ending WW2, many scientists began to explore ways of protecting humans from irradiation. The first experiments were performed in mice and later in dogs by E.D. Thomas (1). As early as 1956, the idea that bone marrow transplant might exert a therapeutic effect against malignancies was proposed by Barnes and Loutit who observed an anti-leukaemic effect of transplanted spleen cells in experimental murine models (2). They also observed that animals that had been given allogeneic rather syngeneic marrow cells died of "wasting disease", which would now be recognised as being graft-versus-host disease (GvHD). E.D. Thomas carried out the first transplants in dogs using high dose irradiation (3) and J. Van Bekkum established a transplant model in monkeys (4). In 1959, the first human bone marrow transplants gave a proof of concept that infusing bone marrow could provide haematological reconstitution in lethally irradiated patients with acute leukaemia (5). E.D. Thomas transplanted 2 patients with advanced acute lymphoblastic leukaemia with a syngeneic graft after high dose total body irradiation; the patients engrafted but died a few months later of relapse. G. Mathé gave allogeneic bone marrow for treatment of several patients who had suffered accidental irradiation exposure, most survived with autologous reconstitution (6). In 1965 Mathé was the first to describe long-term engraftment of a sibling bone marrow demonstrating chimerism, tolerance and an anti-leukaemic effect (7). Although the transplant itself was successful, the patient eventually died of varicella with chronic GvHD. In 1970, M. Bortin reported 203 transplants performed between 1958 and 1968 with only 3 patients alive at time of the report. The major causes of death were graft failure, GvHD and relapse. Following these disappointing results, few centres persisted and the number of transplants declined sharply. Major progress came from the discovery of the HLA system by J. Dausset (9) and J.J. Van Rood (10). Selection of HLA identical siblings as bone marrow donors diminished the risk of rejection and GvHD. Using animal models, R. Storb and E.D. Thomas developed the model of total body irradiation for conditioning (in dogs) and the use of methotrexate for GvH prevention (11), and in mice G. Santos showed that the use of cyclophosphamide could add immune suppression to the myelo-ablation of TBI (12). He was also the first to use busulfan instead of TBI (13).

2. From 1970 to the present time

Following this pioneer work major progress has been achieved and nowadays haematopoietic stem cell transplant has saved the life of many patients worldwide.

The major landmarks have been:
- The use of cyclosporin for GvHD prevention: cyclosporin is a cyclic oligopeptide immunosuppressant which is an inhibitor of T-cell activation. It is produced by a fungus and was discovered in the early 1970s. It was initially used in organ transplants, where the side effect of nephrotoxicity was noted, which was solved by adjusting the dose according to pharmacokinetic measurements (14, 15). Compared to methotrexate alone, the combination of cyclosporin and short methotrexate is still the gold standard for GvH prevention (16).
- Better management of early complications: This included isolation in laminar air flow rooms, gut decontamination and development of new broad-spectrum antibiotics. Toxicity was reduced by fractionation of TBI and better hydration was found to prevent cyclophosphamide-induced haemorrhagic cystitis.
- Better treatment of infectious complications with new antiviral, antibacterial and antifungal drugs, including treatment of *Herpes simplex virus* infection with acyclovir and the introduction of ganciclovir for treatment of CMV infection. Fungal infections with *Candida sp* and *Aspergillus* which were the most common causes of death were actively treated and prevented by amphotericin B and new azoles (the first used was ketoconazole).
- Development of bone marrow registries for treating patients without an HLA identical sibling donor. The first unrelated bone marrow registry was established in London, in 1973, by Shirley Nolan whose son was diagnosed with Wiskott Aldrich syndrome. Following this first donor recruitment drive, the number of bone marrow and peripheral haematopoietic stem cell donors has increased all over the world with more than 18 million donors now registered, including 500.000 cord blood donors.
- Improved methods of high resolution HLA typing.
- Use of new sources of haematopoietic stem cells: G-CSF mobilised peripheral blood stem cells (17), cryopreserved umbilical cord blood (18), haploidentical related haematopoietic stem cells (19).
- Autologous haematopoietic stem cell transplantation (20).
- New methods of GvHD prevention: T-cell depletion, *in vivo* monoclonal anti T-cell antibodies.
- Use of donor lymphocyte infusions to treat relapse (21).
- New methods of reduced intensity conditioning to decrease early transplant related mortality (22).

3. International cooperation

International collaboration through a number of non-profit organisations has been a key factor for the development of haematopoietic stem cell transplantation.

Thanks to the dedication and far-sighted view of a few pioneers, it was realised that it was essential to work together in order to facilitate the development of haematopoietic stem cell transplant, help new centres and laboratory facilities to be established, provide guidelines, develop accreditation through JACIE and promote the development of new research protocols.

EBMT (European Group for Blood and Marrow Transplantation) was born in 1974 when the number of bone marrow transplants was very small and results quite disappointing. The first meeting was held in Saint Moritz at the initiative of J.J. Van Rood and B. Speck. Three teams were present, the Leiden group with J. Vossen and J.J. van Rood, the Basel group with B. Speck and the Paris group with E. Gluckman. This was a very small meeting with not more than 10 participants; the idea was to meet in a nice place where we could both work and exercise our skills in skiing. Both qualifications were and remained for a long time a prerequisite to be member of the group. Over many years the group met in different ski locations including Saint Moritz in Switzerland and Courchevel in France and slowly the meeting attracted more and more haematologists from all over Europe interested in bone marrow transplantation.

CIBMTR (Center for International Blood and Marrow Transplant Research) was founded in 1972 by M. Bortin in Milwaukee. In 1972, just four years after the first successful haematopoietic stem cell transplantation (HSCT), pioneers in the field realised the significance of what they were undertaking. Several of the pioneers in this evolving science also understood the importance of collaborating in order to better understand the data being generated at individual centres. Dr. Mortimer M. Bortin and several colleagues established the IBMTR at the Medical College of Wisconsin to do just that. Physicians in the field agreed to voluntarily contribute their patient data to this outcomes registry. At the time, there were only about 12 transplant centres and fewer than 50 patients per year worldwide receiving a transplant. M. Horowitz the current director has developed the database and this worldwide database now includes data on 350,000 autologous, related and unrelated donor transplant recipients. CIBMTR is also performing both observational and prospective research.

NMDP (National Marrow Donor Program) was founded in 1986 and the first NMDP-facilitated transplant took place in December 1987. Today the registry is called Be the Match Registry and has grown to 9 million donors and nearly 145.000 umbilical cord blood units.

WMDA (World Marrow Donor Association). On March 10th 1988 an *ad hoc* committee was formed to discuss international collaboration for identification of matched unrelated donors, initially started as the Cooperative Marrow Donor Programme. The founders of this group were: Prof. J.J. van Rood, Prof. J. Goldman and Prof. E.D. Thomas. Prof. J. Goldman proposed a change in the name of the organisation from

Cooperative Marrow Donor Programme to World Marrow Donor Association (WMDA). The WMDA is a voluntary organisation of representatives of bone marrow donor registries, cord blood banks, other organisations and individuals, with an interest in haematopoietic stem cell transplantation. It provides a forum for mutual discussion of all issues regarding the clinical use of haematopoietic stem cells from unrelated donors across international boundaries. These discussions, which take place in working groups, make it possible to formulate guidelines on logistics, quality control, accreditation, ethics, finances and registry accreditation. It works in close association with BMDW (Bone Marrow Donors Worldwide). BMDW is continuing the effort to collect the HLA phenotypes and other relevant data of volunteer stem cell donors and cord blood units. The current number of donors is 17,596,872 and cord blood units 482,451.

Eurocord is a registry of cord blood transplants which works in close collaboration with cord blood banks (members of Netcord) to analyse results of cord blood transplant and provide quality standards and accreditation to the unrelated cord blood banks. It has collected more than 7,000 cord blood transplant from 483 centres, 50 countries and 54 cord blood banks.

4. Main EBMT Landmarks

The main EBMT Landmarks have been:
- The evaluation of progress in allogeneic and autologous bone marrow transplantation.
- The establishment of a European bone marrow transplant registry with the publication of current indications for transplant, categorised as validated, experimental or not recommended.
- Publication of a yearly survey of haematopoietic stem cell transplantation in Europe.
- The definition of JACIE standards for establishment and accreditation of a bone marrow transplant unit.
- The organisation of an annual meeting, a ESH-EBMT training course and a ESH-EBMT handbook.
- The organisation of working parties with elected chairs.
- The creation of the EBMT nurses group.

5. Conclusion

Since the first transplant to the present time, enormous progress has been made and many patients survive a lethal disease thanks to the efforts of a few pioneers and also to the immense dedication of all the participants in this drive to cure more patients. This has been made possible by the early recognition that we had to work together through close and frank collaboration, and by realising that a bone marrow transplant unit is a result of a team effort including physicians from different specialties, scientists, nurses, laboratory technicians, radiotherapists, blood banks, and data managers.

References

1. Thomas ED, Blume KG. Historical markers in the development of allogeneic hematopoietic cell transplantation. Biol Blood and Marrow Transplant 1999; 5: 341–346.
2. Barnes DWH, Loutit JP. Treatment of murine leukemia with X-rays and homologous bone marrow. Brit Med J 1956; 2: 626–627.
3. Thomas ED, Collins JA, Herman EC, Ferrebee JW. Marrow transplants in lethally irradiated dogs given methotrexate. Blood 1962; 19: 217–228.
4. Van Bekkum DW, de Vries MJ. Radiation chimeras. New York Academic Press 1967.
5. Thomas ED, Lochte HL, LU WC, Ferrebee JW. Intravenous infusion of bone marrow in patients receiving radiation and chemotherapy. New Engl J Med 1957; 257: 491–496.
6. Mathé G, Jammet H, Pendic B et al. Transfusion and grafts of homologous bone marrow in humans accidentally irradiated to high dose. Rev Franc Etudes Clin Biol 1959; 4: 226–229.
7. Mathé G, Amiel H, Schwarzenberg L et al. Adoptive immunotherapy of acute leukemia: experimental and clinical results. Cancer Res 1965:25:1525-31.
8. Bortin MM. A compendium of reported human bone marrow transplants. Transplantation 1970; 9: 571–587.
9. Dausset J. Iso-leuko-antibodies. Acta Haematol 1958; 20: 156–166.
10. Van Rood JJ. The detection of transplantation antigens in leukocytes. Semin Hematol 1968; 2: 187–214.
11. Storb R, Raff RF, Appelbaum FR et al. Comparison of fractionated to single dose total body irradiation in conditioning canine littermates for DLA identical marrow grafts. Blood 1989; 74: 1139–1143.
12. Santos GW, Owens AH. Allogeneic marrow transplants in Cyclophosphamide treated mice. Transplant Proc 1969; 1: 44–46.
13. Santos GW, Tutschka PJ. Marrow transplantation in the busulfan treated rat preclinical model of aplastic anemia. J Natl Cancer Inst 1974; 53: 1781–1785.
14. Powles RL, Barrett AJ, Clink H et al. Cyclosporin A for the treatment of graft versus host disease in man. Lancet 1978; 2: 1327–1331.
15. Gluckman E, Devergie A, Lokiec F et al. Nephrotoxicity of cyclosporin in bone marrow transplantation. Lancet 1981; ii: 144–145.
16. Storb R, Deeg JH, Whitehead J et al. Methotrexate and cyclosporine compared with cyclosporine alone for prophylaxis of acute graft versus host disease after marrow transplantation for leukemia. N Engl J Med 1986; 314: 729–735.
17. Korbling M, Freireich EJ. Twenty-five years of peripheral blood stem cell transplantation. Blood 2011; 117: 6411-6416.

18. Gluckman E. History of cord blood transplantation. Bone Marrow Transplant 2009; 44: 621–626.
19. Aversa F, Tabilio A, Velardi A et al. Treatment of high-risk acute leukemia with T-cell depleted stem cells from related donors with one fully mismatched HLA haplotype. N Engl J Med 1998; 339: 1186–1193.
20. Dicke KA, Zander A, Spitzer G et al. Autologous bone marrow transplantation in relapsed adult acute leukemia. Lancet 1979; i: 514–517.
21. Kolb HJ, Mittermtiller J, Clemm CH et al. Donor leukocyte transfusions for treatment of recurrent chronic myelogenous leukemia in marrow transplant patients. Blood 1990; 76: 2462–2465.
22. Baron F, Baker JE, Storb R et al. Kinetics of engraftment in patients with hematologic malignancies given allogeneic hematopoietic cell transplantation after non myeloablative conditioning. Blood 2004; 104: 2254–2262.

NOTES

*CHAPTER 2

The European Group for Blood and Marrow Transplantation: Present and future

Alejandro Madrigal, Anna Sureda

1. Introduction

The European Group for Blood and Marrow Transplantation (EBMT) is a non-profit organisation, established in 1974 in order to allow scientists and physicians involved in clinical bone marrow transplantation to share experience and develop co-operative studies. Over the last 36 years the EBMT has developed into the leading scientific society in Europe and is at the cutting edge in the field of stem cell transplantation.

The mission of EBMT is to "foster excellence in science in order to further improve the outcomes of stem cell transplantation and inform all concerned, including patients and their families, about developments in the field".

To this end, the Society works to the highest standards to promote all aspects associated with the transplantation of haematopoietic stem cells from all donor sources and donor types, including basic and clinical research, education, standardisation, quality control and accreditation for transplant procedures.

The EBMT plays a key role in:
• Measuring trends in transplant activity
• Collection and analysis of patient transplant data in Europe
• Classifying indications for stem cell transplantation for both neoplastic and non-neoplastic disorders in adults and children
• Initiating pioneering prospective studies employing new ideas and techniques within the field of HSCT and cellular therapy
• Networking and education of professionals
• Communications, lobbying and alliance building
• Setting strict quality standards
• Improving patient self-care through education and communication.

2. The EBMT today

2.1 EBMT as a scientific society - Developments in HSCT and cell therapy fields

The EBMT is supported by 3612 members, based in 536 transplant centres in 57 countries worldwide. The success of EBMT vastly depends on the capacity of the society to motivate and commit the member centres to contribute to the goals of EBMT through submitting transplant data to the central registry and enrolling patients in both retrospective, non-interventional observational trials and prospective clinical trials.

HSCT activity in Europe has significantly increased over recent years. The average number of HSCT performed within the EU is 293 per 10M inhabitants and 60% of the transplant teams associated with EBMT perform both autologous and allogeneic HSCT.

It is clear that the field of HSCT is a quickly growing one. Nevertheless, HSCT is currently facing multiple challenges. New drugs have recently appeared on the market. The new EU directive for prospective clinical trials has imposed major bureaucratic constraints which have significantly affected the development of clinical trials in Europe. Finally, and more recently, stem cells have been used for other purposes than haematopoietic rescue after high-dose therapy. EBMT as a transplant organisation has to face the clear need to find its own niche, focusing its scientific and research activities on diseases and indications where the advantage of having a large number of affiliated transplant centres overcomes the inherent difficulties of economic issues, and the geographical barriers of powerful and well-developed national scientific groups.

2.2 Scientific activities of the EBMT - The key players

The EBMT scientific activities are largely coordinated through the Working Party (WP) structure, which has grown over the years. The nature of the 11 current WPs is varied; the majority of them are disease-based WPs (acute leukaemia, aplastic anaemia, autoimmune diseases, chronic leukaemias, inborn errors, lymphomas and solid tumours) but others constitute the so-called "transversal" WPs with scientific activities extending across varied diseases (immunobiology, infectious diseases, late effects and paediatrics).

Over the last two decades HSCT nursing has grown rapidly and has acknowledged the care needs of the patients, their families and donors. HSCT nurses are involved in the decision-making process about treatment options for their patients. The EBMT Nurses Group started in January 1985 and is involved in the care of the HSCT patient. Finally, other scientific activities of the EBMT are nowadays coordinated through different Committees: Education, Nuclear Accident, Prospective Clinical Trials, Developmental, Outreach, Quality Assessment of the Grafts and Statistical.

2.3 Scientific activities of the EBMT - The tools

2.3.1 The Registry. The role of retrospective analyses

The HSCT Registry is one of the major treasures of EBMT. Data are entered and maintained in a central database with internet access. Each EBMT centre is represented in this database and users from a centre can view, modify, obtain reports and download their own data. In addition, all centres can obtain general overviews of the complete EBMT data. The database is run on a system called ProMiSe (Project Manager Internet Server). The national registries operating have become part of the EBMT data flow by mutual consent and are using the same central database. Most national registries enter data for those centres in their country which do not wish to access the central database directly. For countries without national registries, the EBMT Data Office in Paris fulfills the same role.

The EBMT Registry holds data on 350,888 transplants. Over two years ago the Board recognised the need to invest resources to improve our principal tool. EBMT needs to build a flexible and robust data management system that meets evolving needs and provides an integrated infrastructure to maximise the research potential in Europe in collaboration with members and partners.

The publication of retrospective analyses represents the major part of the scientific output of the EBMT. Last year 46 retrospective analyses from 150 studies were published in major peer-reviewed journals giving a total impact factor for 2009 of 140 and a ratio impact factor/number of publications of 8. A special mention must be made of the "Indications and Recommendations Manuscript" that the EBMT Board regularly publishes in the journal *Bone Marrow Transplantation*. The most recent version of the recommendations, published in 2010, are more comprehensive and detailed and are extensively used, not only by centres or individuals, but also by national health authorities and health insurance companies looking for economical and reimbursement issues.

2.3.2 The Increasing EBMT activity in non-interventional observational clinical trials
EBMT has significantly increased the number of on-going and ready-to-start non-interventional observational studies (NIS). Nowadays the EBMT trial portfolio includes 15 studies. Although NIS are not designed to modify treatment strategies in a given population of patients they aim to prospectively collect data on clinical practice issues and responses to a homogeneous treatment procedure.

Prospective Clinical Trials. The Prospective Clinical Trials Committee. EBMT has recently faced the difficulties inherent in the development of the 2001 EU Directive on Prospective Clinical Trials, significantly exacerbated because of the European nature of the organisation itself. A very active approach was undertaken by the Prospective Clinical Trials Office with the objective to review the status of the different on-going prospective clinical trials and meanwhile the initiation of new EBMT Sponsored Clinical Trials was put on hold. An Action Plan has recently been approved by the EBMT Board which will address the issues facing the Clinical Trials Office.

2.4 The increasing commitment of EBMT to education
EBMT's mission is "to foster excellence in science in order to further improve the outcomes of HSCT and inform all concerned, including patients and their families, about developments in the field". The EBMT Education Committee is undertaking a strategic review of the educational side of the organisation with the aim of

consolidating and improving the educational opportunities offered to EBMT members. Elements that fall under the "EBMT Education" umbrella include the EBMT Handbook and Annual Training Course, both organised in conjunction with the European School of Haematology. In addition, a number of specialist courses and sessions are organised on an annual basis through the various WPs and Committees.

2.5 EBMT in the context of the European Union

The EBMT is an active member of the Committee for Advanced Therapies (CAT) of the European Medicines Agency (EMA). It is a multidisciplinary committee, gathering together some of the best available experts in Europe to assess the quality, safety and efficacy of advanced therapy medicinal products (ATMPs), and to follow scientific developments in the field. In this context, EBMT participated as an external expert in the EUSTITE Project (European Union Standards and Training in the Inspection of Tissue Establishments). In addition, EBMT itself and several WPs of the EBMT have participated in EU-funded projects such as the European Leukaemia Net (ELN), AlloStem, Eurocord-Ed, SOHOV&S Project and the CLINT Project (facilitation of international prospective clinical trials in stem cell transplantation).

2.6 Regulatory environment and JACIE Accreditation

The Joint Accreditation Committee-ISCT (Europe) and EBMT is a non-profit body established in 1998 for the purposes of assessment and accreditation in the field of HSCT. JACIE's primary aim is to promote high quality patient care and laboratory performance in haematopoietic stem cell collection, processing and transplantation centres through an internationally recognised system of accreditation. There are currently 224 registered centres, 75 inspections in preparation (including re-accreditations), 198 completed inspections, 104 facilities accredited and 34 re-accreditations in progress. Seventeen countries in Europe have already adopted the JACIE model.

2.7 EBMT budget and income sources

The EBMT budget allocated to all of these activities is close to 2,5M€ and the organisation supports salaries for around 35 FTEs in 4 main offices (Barcelona, London, Paris and Leiden-Rotterdam). The financial structure is based on three main sources of income (EBMT Membership, Corporate Sponsors and the profits of the Annual Congress).

3. The EBMT in the future

Throughout its existence the EBMT has been evolving as an organisation, but an important stage has now been reached where fundamental change is required in order to respond to present and future challenges. The opportunity to make such changes occurs only occasionally and it is important to use this time creatively. In April 2010 the EBMT found itself in a position where creative changes could be made. This was afforded by the arrival of a new President ready to govern a Board made-up of equal numbers of experienced and new Board Members, combined with the creation of a new Executive Director position, backed by the knowledge and motivation of the Operations Team. Recognition is also due to the outgoing Board who left the organisation in a favourable financial situation.

Against this background the EBMT Board has taken on the crucial task of developing a 3-year Strategic Plan to cover the period 2011–2013. This process commenced in May 2010 with the development of a Vision document elaborated by the President and developed in discussion with the Board. The Vision document encompasses 4 key areas: Excelling in Science, Advancing Clinical Practice, Improving Governance and Maximising Resources. Transparent and participative consultation with stakeholders (volunteers, members, staff, collaborative partners, industry, etc.) has been fundamental to the process of identifying the principal needs and the steps required to meet them.

Working Groups consisting of representatives of the Board, Committee Chairs, guests and staff were established to work on these 3 areas in preparation for the Strategy Meeting held in October 2010. Each Working Group reviewed the current situation and produced a SWOT analysis related to the areas under review. These documents formed the basis for discussion of the Strategic Objectives and the actions required to achieve them. In relation to the area of Resources, IT consultants Birchman Group were contracted to carry out a review of EBMT's Information Systems and to produce an IT Plan for 2011–2014.

In parallel, a Membership Survey was conducted to evaluate the needs and wishes of the membership base. The survey was completed by 506 members, from 345 centres in 45 countries, which represents approx. 65% of member centres. The results of the survey were presented at the outset of the strategy meeting to inform the discussions and will be further evaluated as part of the strategy. An analysis and overview of the scientific output of the EBMT was also presented as a benchmarking exercise. This analysis will be refined to take into account the output of relevant EBMT Committees, reviews and editorials and will be adjusted for factors in the Citation Index.

3.1 Excelling in science and advancing clinical practice

In the current resource-limited climate where competition on a scientific level is increasingly tough, a major priority for the EBMT is to establish a well-formulated Scientific Policy to steer the research direction and future investment of the

Society. Despite leading the field of stem cell transplantation in Europe, in a context of changing indications and regulations, as well as continuous evolution, it is essential to evaluate the current situation in order to remain relevant and forward looking. In this context a review and restructuring of EBMT Working Parties and Committees will be conducted with a view to defining priorities, improving synergies and exploiting the EBMT's research potential to a maximum. One aim will be to establish a strong presence in the Cell Therapy field – as the production of cell-based therapeutic products is a unique feature of EBMT activities, with strong implications for product harmonisation as well as human safety - and fostering closer links with the International Society for Cellular Therapy (ISCT) and others.

Building effective partnerships at a central, national and international level is fundamental to the strategy. The EBMT is privileged to have leaders of "groups of excellence" within its membership and would like to stimulate further innovative research through identifying groups working on translational research, mostly - although not exclusively - in the two main relevant fields to its activities: immune recognition of tumour and infectious targets and stem cell biology, and facilitating forums to explore new synergies and ways of working together: EBMT may choose to focus its attention on translational research, while partnering with other scientific societies that promote more basic approaches. Similarly, there is strong potential for productive collaborations with national societies and study groups on the European level, and to facilitate activities of members globally through joint initiatives with international partners.

The EBMT Registry represents a key tool for the scientific research and regulatory activities of the Society and its partners. Another major strand of the strategy plan is to update the Registry System with state-of-the-art software designed to meet future data collection and retrieval needs. By creating a consortium of partners including national and donor registries, ascertaining needs and what each party can contribute, the goal is to share resources and create a system of maximum utility. The overall aim is to significantly improve the research infrastructure in Europe whilst promoting standardised data collection and international harmonisation. While data collection must be improved and harmonised, organising sample collection to complement the registry activities is of utmost importance, in view of the growing needs to assess increasing numbers of biological parameters in the context of daily care as well as during the conduct of biomedical research. In relation to developing data reporting and maximising scientific research potential, the European Union, Pharma Industry and Biotech Companies are vital partners. The EBMT will seek to capitalise on these relationships by adopting a win-win approach, developing platforms for effective interaction, and modelling different elements in order to synergise with key decision-makers.

Building on a strong Registry base, retrospective and non interventional studies will remain the cornerstone of the EBMT and efforts will be dedicated over the next 3 years to optimising study coordination and conduct. A Study Office structure will be created to oversee all EBMT studies and personnel, and processes for inviting member centres to participate in studies will be streamlined.

In spite of the well-documented challenges of conducting trans-national clinical trials in the academic setting and the difficulties experienced in this regard over the last four years, EBMT remains committed to performing prospective clinical trials. Academic clinical trials aimed at acquiring scientific knowledge form the basis for continuously improving patient care. Improved vision, strategy and governance will be critical for the effective management of clinical trials. Following an in-depth review of EBMT clinical trials, a new clinical trials committee is to be established to provide more effective leadership. The number of trials will be limited for manageability and the challenge lies in identifying niche studies that only the EBMT can perform, as well as creating opportunities for cooperation with national study groups.

The beneficiaries of EBMT's scientific research are ultimately the patients, which makes advancing clinical practice through education and training a fundamental element of the strategy. To date, education initiatives within the EBMT have evolved organically without a strategic overview or planning. In order to draw the diverse strands together, the Education strategy entails a focus on three key areas: scope, organisation and financing. The aim is to build a balanced, high quality educational programme covering the needs of the EBMT Community. The organisation will be based on a mixed model, building a strong and streamlined organisational structure which encourages local initiative within established parameters, supported by robust central co-ordination and overview. Nurses and allied health professionals are at the heart of patient care and in view of this it is aimed to dedicate resources to increasing the level of research, training and education for nurses. The EBMT Nurses Group will review Nursing Strategy.

3.2 Improving governance

Good governance is the bedrock for effective, efficient and accountable implementation of the EBMT mission. The EBMT has already begun a process of professionalisation, resulting in the appointment of an Executive Director in January 2010. The Board recognises the need for responsible governance and intends to consolidate these advances by devising a system of governance in which Science, Education and Quality are well represented, and aims to promote effective decision-making through the following measure:

- Review structure of current Board and develop it into a Scientific Board with a remit for the scientific direction.

- Review structure and mandate of the Executive Committee and develop a representative body which is empowered to take decisions for the efficient and effective management of the organisation.
- Review current Working Party/Committee structure and decide how to reorganise them to meet the current scientific and other needs of the Society.

It will be important to reinforce the role of the Executive Director and the Management Team in the Operational arena and introduce a system of Business Planning to improve decision-making and accountability (strategic plan, annual plans, annual review, etc.) and to increase efficiency within the EBMT Offices through common management policies and a clear definition of responsibilities of each office. Strong internal and external communications are important aspects of accountability and dissemination. To these ends, strategies will be aimed at increasing the level of Board communications, lobbying and alliances:

- To develop a more professional organisational structure: The Board, Working Parties, Committees and the Executive Director/Management Team
- To increase the level of Board communications, lobbying and alliances
- To increase efficiency within the EBMT Offices.

3.3 Maximising resources
Last, but not least, is the maximisation of resources. There is a clear need for integrated information systems across the organisation to improve the management of finances, communications, databases and studies. Improving the EBMT's web presence and the creation of an online communications infrastructure is an important element of the communication strategy. Not only is there a need to improve the resources at the disposal of the EBMT and its members, but also to increase the level of resources to fund core activities. The Annual Congress is an important scientific, educational and networking event, as well as a major source of income for the Society. In this regard it is important to develop the congress to remain competitive, whilst refining the venue selection process in order to minimise risk and maximise profit. It is also essential to develop the relationship with Industry and official Donors and to implement new fundraising strategies aimed at diversifying and developing the funding base of the Society. The EBMT will also continue to promote JACIE as the global standard and system of accreditation, as well as the watchdog for regulatory changes in Europe and worldwide.

4. Conclusions
The success of this long process will be based on the commitment and a comprehensive and shared vision among all members of the organisation. We need

to work together towards introducing a new model of organisation based on a clear mandate and vision, which will foster excellence in science in order to further improve the outcome of SCT and inform all concerned, including patients and their families.

Acknowledgements

The authors would like to thank Mélanie Chaboissier, EBMT Communications Coordinator and Andreu Gusi Puig, EBMT Executive Director, for their important contributions to this chapter.

References

1.   EBMT Strategic Plan 2011–2013.
2.   My Vision of EBMT. Alejandro Madrigal, 2010.

Multiple Choice Questionnaire

To find the correct answer, go to http://www.esh.org/online-training/handbook/

1. **Please identify which of the one does not represent a key role for EBMT:**
   a) Measuring trends in stem cell transplantation activity ☐
   b) Pioneering prospective clinical trials in the transplantation field ☐
   c) Networking and education of professionals ☐
   d) Paying a percentage of the transplant budget of each patient to the relevant country ☐

2. **With respect to the organisational characteristics of the EBMT, please indicate the correct answer:**
   a) The EBMT is supported by 3612 members, based in 536 transplant centres in 57 countries around the world ☐
   b) The EBMT scientific activities are largely conducted through the Working Party Structure. There are 13 Working Parties in total ☐
   c) The Executive Committee of the EBMT is constituted by the President, the Secretary and the Treasurer ☐
   d) Both a and c are correct ☐

3. **Please, indicate which of the following represents a challenge for EBMT:**
   a) The new EU directive in relation to prospective clinical trials............☐
   b) The development of new drugs that are challenging the role of stem cell transplantation in some indications.................................☐
   c) The fact that stem cells are being used for additional purposes other than haematopoietic stem cell transplantation..........................☐
   d) All of the above..☐

NOTES

* CHAPTER 3

JACIE & quality management in HSCT

Christian Chabannon, Eoin McGrath

1. Introduction and overview

JACIE (Joint Accreditation Committee – ISCT & EBMT) (1) is a non-profit body established for the purposes of assessment and accreditation in the field of haematopoietic stem cell transplantation (HSCT). The Committee was founded in 1998 by the European Group for Blood and Marrow Transplantation (EBMT) and the European branch of the International Society for Cellular Therapy (ISCT), the two leading scientific organisations involved with HSCT in Europe (2). JACIE modelled itself on the US-based Foundation for the Accreditation of Cellular Therapy (FACT) (3, 4), established in 1996 by the ISCT and the American Society for Blood and Marrow Transplantation (ASBMT). JACIE actively collaborates with FACT in establishing standards for the provision of quality medical and laboratory practice in HSCT; the two organisations now issue joint FACT-JACIE standards, which are applicable internationally (5).

The primary aim of JACIE is to improve the quality of HSCT in Europe by providing a means whereby transplant centres, collection and processing facilities can demonstrate high quality practice. The need to reinforce quality management (QM) in the practice of highly sophisticated medical procedures such as HSCT was identified partly because of past observations that incidents and adverse events can occur even in experienced transplant centres. It also stems from the increasing use of unrelated donors and international exchanges of cell products, necessitating measures to ensure consistent quality control procedures for these products (6). Improving quality of HSCT is achieved through external inspection of facilities to ensure compliance with the FACT-JACIE standards. An additional and wider aim is to ensure harmonisation between FACT-JACIE standards and other national/international standards, including the EU Tissues & Cells Directive (Directive 2004/23/EC) and the related Commission Directives 2006/17/EC and 2006/86/EC (7–9).

JACIE accreditation provides a means whereby transplant facilities can demonstrate that they are working within a QM system covering all aspects of the transplantation process, and thus show compliance with the requirements of national and international regulatory authorities. While JACIE accreditation was initially established as a voluntary process, an increasing number of countries and competent authorities have now included JACIE accreditation as a requisite for authorisation of transplant programmes or for reimbursement of treatment costs by healthcare insurance. These include The Netherlands, Switzerland, France and Italy.

The current organisation of JACIE ensures wide consultation, with over 20 European countries now represented on the Board in addition to nursing, paediatrics and cord-blood representatives. Officers in the executive committee run day-to-day operations, and together with the President, vice-President, past-President, Medical Director and

Chair of the Accreditation Committee plan and oversee annual operations, and report to the JACIE board and the EBMT board. The Accreditation Committee reviews all inspection reports and advises the JACIE Board.

2. The FACT-JACIE standards

The FACT-JACIE standards (5) cover all aspects of clinical transplant programmes, collection facilities (bone marrow (BM) collection and apheresis collection) and processing of collected cell products. The standards also apply to the use of therapeutic cells (TC) derived from blood or marrow, including donor lymphocytes and mesenchymal stem cells; discussion is ongoing to decide to which extent future versions of the standards should cover the delivery of various form of cell therapies in medical disciplines beyond haematology and oncology (regenerative medicine). Current standards cover the clinical use of Cord Blood Units (CBU) by clinical programmes but not the collection or banking of CBU which are covered by the related Netcord-FACT standards and inspected/accredited by FACT-Netcord (3, 10).

Within each subsection of the standards are detailed lists of specific requirements; for example, the standard on donor evaluation and selection contains specific items relating to clinical evaluation, laboratory testing, informed consent etc. The current edition of the standards is the 4th edition, dated 2008 (5). The 5th edition is expected to be released in March 2012.

The standards are accompanied by a manual which contains the standards together with detailed guidance on the interpretation and measures required to demonstrate compliance. Each standard is followed by specific questions relating to that standard; these questions form the basis of the inspection checklist, which must be completed prior to inspection by the applicant centre and verified by the inspector during the inspection.

The complete standards and the accompanying guidance manual are available on the JACIE website, together with other useful information relating to JACIE organisation, inspection and accreditation (1).

2.1 General aspects of the standards

Although the standards are very specific in certain areas, some essential principles apply throughout. The first of these is a requirement for documentation of policies, procedures, actions, requests and so on. This applies to the need to have written policies and procedures, and extends to all aspects of transplant activity. For example, the initial diagnosis of a patient must be documented by source material or reports. A request from the clinical unit to the laboratory for issue of cells must be made in writing. A potential donor must not only be properly evaluated for eligibility, but the programme must have clear written criteria for what constitutes an eligible donor and must clearly document whether the donor meets these criteria.

The second is a requirement that personnel must not only be appropriately qualified, they must be trained in the procedures they regularly perform and their competency to perform the task after training must be assessed and documented.

Similarly there is a requirement for validation of all equipment and procedures. Validation is a term used to describe the activity required to prove that any procedure, process, equipment, material, activity or system actually leads to the expected results. For example a new apheresis machine must be shown to produce the expected results in terms of cell yields.

Also important is the requirement for close cooperation and interaction between the different parts of the programme, especially important where a clinical programme may use a distant collection and/or processing facility. Mechanisms for transfer of information must be clearly established.

2.2 Quality management (QM)

An active quality management programme (QMP) is essential to ensure that all aspects of the programme run effectively. A QMP is a mechanism to ensure that procedures are being carried out by all staff members in line with agreed standards. In a transplant programme, this ensures that the clinical, collection and laboratory units are all working together to achieve good communication, effective common work practices and increased guarantees for patients. It is a means of rapidly identifying errors or accidents and resolving them so that the possibility of repetition is minimised. It assists in training and clearly identifies the roles and responsibilities of all staff. Once the required level of quality has been achieved, the remaining challenge is to maintain this standard of practice. With a working QMP in place and adequate resources, the fundamental elements necessary to sustain the programme are continued staff commitment and vigilance.

The culture and systems for QM are well-established in laboratories but are relatively new in clinical units; many programmes have experienced difficulty setting up a QMP to cover the clinical programme and collection facility.

It is recommended that a programme should have a dedicated quality manager, ideally with specific training in QM, not only to develop the QMP and meet the initial requirements for accreditation but to ensure continued adherence to standards. To assist centres in developing a QMP JACIE has published "A practical guide to implementing quality management in a stem cell transplantation (SCT) programme" (1).

Within a programme there can be one QM system covering all areas, i.e. clinical, collection and processing, or the laboratory may have a separate system, and other combinations are possible. When there is more than one system, there should be a clear mechanism for interaction between them.

2.3 Policies and procedures
There are specific requirements for how policies and procedures should be written, to ensure that all essential aspects are covered. Procedures necessary to perform a given procedure should be easily available to staff. Electronic access is acceptable but there must be at least one hard copy available at all times and staff must know where to access this.

For each section – clinical, collection and processing – there is a list of specific policies and procedures that must be covered. All Standard Operating Procedures (SOPs) must be reviewed no more than every two years or earlier if changes are introduced in a procedure between the scheduled review dates.

2.4 Clinical programme, collection facility and processing facility standards
The following paragraphs will comment on some particular aspects of the standards, but for full details the reader should refer to the standards and manual.

2.4.1 Definition of a programme
The standards define a Clinical Transplantation Programme as an integrated medical team housed in geographically contiguous or proximate space with a single Programme Director and common staff training programs, protocols, and QMP. Programmes that include non-contiguous institutions in the same area must share common protocols, staff training procedures, QMP, and review of clinical results and evidence of regular interaction. This means that two separate units should not combine together for the purposes of JACIE accreditation unless they are truly working together in everyday practice. Where two separate clinical transplantation units are working together, they must be within one hour travelling time to ensure close and regular interaction. Centres may apply for accreditation as complete programmes comprising clinical programme, collection facility and a processing laboratory or as a single collection or processing facility which may serve a number of clinical programmes. Clinical units must be using collection and processing facilities that meet the FACT-JACIE standards.

2.4.2 Clinical programme activity
To ensure continuing proficiency in a transplant programme, a minimum volume of patients must be treated per year. The current minimum activity requirements for each 12-month period are as follows:

- For allogeneic transplantation: At least 10 new patients
- For autologous transplantation only: At least 5 new patients
- For centres performing both allogeneic and autologous transplantation there is no minimum requirement for autograft numbers, provided that the minimum number of allografts is met
- For combined adult and paediatric programmes, a minimum of 5 new adult patients and 5 new paediatric patients
- For programs utilising more than one clinical site for transplantation, a minimum of 5 new patients must be transplanted at each site.

2.4.3 Donor evaluation

This section covers information, consent, and requirements for evaluation including medical history and testing for infectious disease markers.

The medical history for allogeneic donors must include a number of specific items relating to possible transmission of infections and non-infections disease. The use of a standard donor history questionnaire is recommended.

Testing for infectious diseases must conform to national and international regulations. The complete list of mandatory markers differs for autologous and allogenic transplantation. A positive result may result in the definitive rejection of a donor (i.e HIV), or in the decision to proceed with the use of a positive donor, following a careful risk-benefit evaluation and possibly specific measures for the recipient; such deviations must be notified to and accepted by the recipient. In some instances such as West Nile Virus and *Trypanosoma Cruzi* risk assessment should be performed in accordance with governmental regulations. The tests must be performed within 30 days prior to collection of cells. If more than one collection is performed the tests will need to be repeated if they are out of this time period.

Other required tests include at least: ABO group and Rh type and pregnancy assessment for all female donors of childbearing potential. For allogeneic donors HLA-A, -B, -DR typing must be performed and HLA-C testing for unrelated donors and related donors other than siblings, in all cases by an EFI-accredited laboratory.

2.4.4 Data collection

The programme must collect all the data necessary to complete in the EBMT MED-A forms. Prior to inspection the team must submit records of this data for 10 consecutive patients and on the day of inspection the inspectors verify the data against the source material. It is important to have records of the tests used to confirm the original diagnosis as well as of all the peri-transplant data.

2.4.5 Bone marrow collection

If a programme regularly uses BM, this must be collected in a facility that meets the FACT-JACIE standards. This means that the BM collection facility must also be inspected and accredited. The minimum activity required to apply for accreditation is an average of 1 collection in the year preceding application for accreditation, and has been decreased as a consequence of the reduced activity in this field by most adult transplant programmes. Even where only one harvest is performed per year, all requirements of the standards must be met, e.g. relevant SOPs must be in place and regularly reviewed, with evidence of continued training of staff and review of procedures.

2.4.6 Apheresis collection

The minimum activity requirement for an apheresis collection facility (CF) is an average of 10 procedures per year during each accreditation cycle. A CF must have a Director and a Medical Director. These can be the same person, but the Director does not have to be medically qualified.

2.4.7 Processing facility standards

A processing facility must have a Director and a Medical Director. These can be the same person, but the Director does not have to be medically qualified. There must be appropriate and validated assays and test procedures for the evaluation of cellular therapy products. Procedures must be demonstrated to result in acceptable target cell viability and recovery. Where processing includes exposure to the environment this must take place in an environment with specified air quality and cleanliness, as established through appropriate validation and testing. The FACT-JACIE standards do not specify any defined level of air quality. However in EU member states the laboratory must comply with the requirements of the EU Directive on air quality.

3. The inspection and accreditation process

3.1 Initial application

The centre implements measures as described in the JACIE accreditation manual, then applies for inspection by submitting the application form containing basic information about the programme/facility and a number of supporting documents including a self-assessment checklist. The application information and checklist must be submitted in English but all other documentation, including SOPs is accepted in the language of the centre where the inspectors assigned are able to read and speak the language of the centre.

3.2 Inspection

An on-site visit is carried out by a team of trained inspectors, usually one per facility (clinical/collection/processing). Inspectors are medical, scientific or other professional persons working in HSCT, with specific qualifications and experience for inspecting clinical, collection and/or processing facilities (1). Inspectors must attend a JACIE-sponsored training course and pass an examination. Where a clinical programme performs adult and paediatric transplants, an adult and a paediatric inspector will attend. Inspectors may also be from another country but should be either native or fluent speakers of the relevant language. In countries where it is not possible to assign an inspector who speaks the language, a local expert is requested to assist with translation of interviews and documents as necessary.

An inspection visit generally lasts between 1 and 2 days and involves meeting with staff during their work, review of documents/records and completion of a detailed checklist relating to the standards. The inspectors prepare their report in English, noting any areas of non-compliance with the standards. The report is reviewed by the Inspection Report Assessors and presented to the Accreditation Committee for discussion and recommendations for actions.

3.3 Report and correction phase

Based on the inspectors' findings, a summary report is prepared making specific recommendations for corrections and improvements. Between 3 and 9 months is allowed for the centre to correct deficiencies, depending on the amount of work required.

The centre must indicate acceptance of the findings and then in due course submit documentary evidence to confirm corrections or amendments. The original inspectors review the documentation. In some cases a limited revisit may be the best way to show that deficiencies have been remedied. The inspectors confirm to JACIE that all necessary corrections have been made or indicate that there are still outstanding areas for completion.

3.4 Accreditation

The Accreditation Committee reviews all the reports and relevant documentation and if satisfied that all previous deficiencies have been corrected, awards accreditation, subject to an annual report from the centre noting any significant changes in personnel or procedures and including annual activity figures. At the end of year 2 of accreditation, a short interim audit is performed to ensure that the programme has maintained its quality management system functioning.

Reaccreditation follows the same process as the initial accreditation.

4. Outcome of inspections

4.1 Inspections to date

To date, 235 facilities have formally applied for accreditation at least once. Of these, 135 centres applied for accreditation for a combination of clinical, collection and processing facilities; 16 centres applied for clinical and collection only; 18 centres applied for collection and processing only; 37 for the clinical programme only; 2 for clinical and processing only; 1 for BM collection only; 8 for apheresis collection only and 18 for processing only.

Since 2000, 223 inspections have been performed. Of these, 177 were first-time inspections and 46 were reaccreditation inspections.

Almost all centres were found to be functioning at a high level of excellence (11). However some deficiencies in compliance were found in all programmes inspected so far, varying from minor non-compliances, e.g. in formatting of SOPs, to major deficiencies e.g. lack of reliable alarm systems for products stored in liquid nitrogen. In almost all cases correction of deficiencies was verified by submission of documentation by the centre. The median time taken for correction of deficiencies is just over 5 months. In a very small number of cases a limited re-inspection was required to demonstrate correction of deficiencies.

At the time of writing, 145 inspected centres have achieved accreditation at least once and 32 centres have achieved re-accreditation. These centres are listed on the JACIE website (1).

4.2 Common deficiencies

The four most common deficiencies are in QMP, documentation, labelling and donor management (11, 12). This is consistent with the experience of the FACT accreditation programme in the United States (13).

Deficiencies in QMP were by far the most common cause of failure of compliance with the standards, including problems with policies and procedures (SOPs). They can only be corrected by maintaining resource and efforts over several accreditation cycles, thus contributing to improving the knowledge of QM by all professionals participating in the programme. Similarly building and maintaining comprehensive documentation that covers all aspects of the activity requires a long-standing commitment of the entire team. Documentation of key aspects of patient and donor management must be improved for an accurate evaluation of the risk-benefit ratio of the proposed transplantation.

JACIE standards for labelling of components require that essential information is shown including a unique alphanumeric identifier, name of the product and the recipient's name. The label must be securely attached, of a size that allows the contents of the pack to be inspected and clearly labelled using indelible ink. In the majority of centres it was found that labelling of products during collection and processing was not compliant with the standards in a variety of ways, and a common problem in designing JACIE-compliant labels was identified. This has been addressed by an international collaboration – the Cellular Therapy Coding and Labelling Advisory Group (CTCLAG) – which has designed HSC and TC component labels and standardised terminology based on the ISBT 128 system for stem cell component identification (14, 15). Adoption of ISBT 128 labels must be en route in the 4th and 5th edition of the standards, and it is expected that complete implementation will be requested by the 6th edition. Further information is available at: *http://www.iccbba.org/subject-area/cellular-therapy*.

4.3 Experience of centres implementing JACIE

It was anticipated that implementation of the JACIE standards would pose some difficulties for applicant centres, particularly in relation to establishing a QMP. It was also anticipated that there would be resource implications in terms of staff time because of the amount of detailed documentation that is required to demonstrate compliance with the standards.

The most difficult part of preparation was implementing the QM system, adverse event reporting system and other documentation. Lack of a culture of QM has been cited as an important problem; there is an important need for training of clinical staff (doctors and nurses) in QM. Where extra personnel were required, these were frequently quality managers and data managers; many programmes testified that part of the challenge was to maintain these individuals in the programme, once JACIE accreditation was granted.

In ongoing surveys, centres indicated that they had benefited from implementing the JACIE standards. The areas of greatest perceived benefit are in procedures and practices, staff motivation, control of adverse events, and co-ordination between different areas of the programme. Significant benefits have also been perceived in facilities, patient care and safety and training of new and existing staff. Improvements clearly depend on the level of existing services, so that failure to demonstrate improvement may reflect good pre-existing resources. In other areas procedures were only set up as part of implementing JACIE, so that it is difficult to monitor improvements without an established baseline for comparison. Indeed implementation of JACIE may have the paradoxical effect of seeming to increase adverse events because these were not previously adequately reported.

More importantly, EBMT recently conducted a retrospective registry analysis on more than 100.000 transplants, looking to see whether preparation and obtaining of JACIE accreditation may contribute to improve HSCT outcome. The statistical analysis took into account confounding criteria related to both transplanted patients and transplant programme/centre characteristics, such as the year HSCT was performed, centre size, gross national income for the country in which HSCT was performed, the EBMT risk score for patients who underwent HSCT and other factors, and concluded that there is stepwise improvement in the outcome of HSCT performed in a centre that engaged in preparing and eventually obtaining JACIE accreditation (16). Although this will need further and careful evaluation, this is nevertheless initial evidence that introduction of a QMP can improve the results of a medical procedure, together with the introduction of new drugs and regimens, and other organisational aspects of HSCT activities (17–19). This is also an incentive for hospitals and clinics to devote the necessary resource for obtaining and maintaining JACIE accreditation (20), in addition to obtaining the mandatory authorisations for their activities in this field.

5. Conclusion

The JACIE accreditation system is now firmly established in Europe and the experience of centres that have been inspected is that implementation of the JACIE standards has led to significant improvements in different aspects of their transplant programmes. Key points are shown below. JACIE has further assisted with a number of training courses and tools for preparing centres for accreditation. JACIE has also developed a close working relationship with other organisations involved in cellular therapy, which will form the basis for a new global approach to harmonisation of standards and accreditation systems worldwide. This collaboration represents an innovative and proactive approach to solving the problems of international exchange of tissues and cells.

The future of JACIE will depend on how globally the system can develop. Most accredited centres are located in Western Europe, while transplant programmes located in Eastern Europe have so far only minimally engaged in the process. Recently, a few Eastern Mediterranean transplant programmes have expressed interest in JACIE, and indeed the first one of these centres was granted accreditation in 2010. In addition to the well-established partnership with FACT, JACIE maintains contacts with investigators in the Asian-Pacific area. The future of JACIE will also depend on major changes arising in the regulatory field; JACIE has been conceived for programmes that use grafts produced in mostly academic facilities, and these are differently regulated than pharmaceutical companies; the recently released European regulation on Advanced Therapy Medicinal Products (ATMPs) (21) is not currently applicable to "historical" HSCT, but will undoubtedly affect our practices in the mid- and long-term; JACIE will have to consider its role and mission in this evolving context.

Key points

Promoting excellence in haematopoietic stem cell transplantation

Promoting harmonisation in haematopoietic stem cell transplantation

Standards

Definition of a programme for haematopoietic stem cell transplantation

On-site inspection

Implementation of quality management

Documentation of deviations

Training of personnel

Donor screening and validation

ISBT 128 labeling system

Acknowledgements
The authors wish to express their appreciation to Derwood Pamphilon currently serving as Medical Director, Alessandro Rambaldi currently serving as vice-President, Jane Apperley currently serving as past-President, Christiane Vermylen currently Chair of the Accreditation Committee, and to all past and present members of the executive office, the accreditation committee, the board, as well as to all inspectors and all personnel involved in preparing or obtaining JACIE accreditation for their centres, for their invaluable help in establishing JACIE as a key component in improving safety and quality of care for patients who undergo HSCT at European centres.

References
1. JACIE. www.jacie.org.
2. Kvalheim G, Berli M. EBMT and ISHAGE-Europe create a foundation for inspection and accreditation in Europe. Cytotherapy 1999; 1: 363–364.
3. FACT. www.factwebsite.org
4. Warkentin PI. Voluntary accreditation of cellular therapies: Foundation for the Accreditation of Cellular Therapy (FACT). Cytotherapy 2003; 5: 299–305.
5. FACT-JACIE. FACT-JACIE International Standards For Cellular Therapy Product Collection, Processing, and Administration. 4th edition, 2008.
6. Gratwohl A, Baldomero H. Trends of hematopoietic stem cell transplantation in the third millennium. Curr Opin Hematol 2009; 16: 420–426.
7. Directive 2004/23/EC of the European Parliament and of the Council of 31 march 2004 on setting standards of quality and safety for the donation, procurement, testing,

processing, preservation, storage and distribution of human tissues and cells.

8. Commission Directive 2006/17/EC implementing Directive 2004/23/EC of the European Parliament and of the Council as regards certain technical requirements for the donation, procurement and testing of human tissues and cells.

9. Commission Directive 2006/86/EC implementing Directive 2004/23/EC of the European Parliament and of the Council as regards traceability requirements, notification of serious adverse reactions and events and certain technical requirements for the coding, processing, preservation, storage and distribution of human tissues and cells.

10. Netcord. www.Netcord.org.

11. Samson D, Slaper-Cortenbach I, Pamphilon D et al. Current status of JACIE accreditation in Europe: A special report from the Joint Accreditation Committee of the ISCT and the EBMT (JACIE). Bone Marrow Transplant 2007; 39: 133–141.

12. Pamphilon D, Apperley JF, Samson D et al. JACIE Accreditation in 2008: Demonstrating excellence in stem cell transplantation. Hematol Oncol Stem Cell Ther 2009; 2: 311–319.

13. Warkentin PI, Nick L, Shpall EJ. FAHCT accreditation: Common deficiencies during on-site inspections. Cytotherapy 2000; 2: 213–220.

14. Ashford P, Distler P, Gee A et al. Terminology and labeling of cellular products: 1. Standards. Bone Marrow Transplant 2007; 40: 1075–1083.

15. Slaper-Cortenbach I. ISBT 128 coding and labeling for cellular therapy products. Cell Tissue Bank 2010; 11: 375–378.

16. Gratwohl A, Brand R, Niederwieser D et al. Introduction of a quality management system and outcome after hematopoietic stem-cell transplantation. J Clin Oncol 2011; 29: 1980–1986.

17. Loberiza FR Jr., Zhang MJ, Lee SJ et al. Association of transplant center and physician factors on mortality after hematopoietic stem cell transplantation in the United States. Blood 2005; 105: 2979–2987.

18. Horan JT, Logan BR, Agovi-Johnson MA et al. Reducing the risk for transplantation-related mortality after allogeneic hematopoietic cell transplantation: How much progress has been made? J Clin Oncol 2010; 29: 805–813.

19. Gooley TA, Chien JW, Pergam SA et al. Reduced mortality after allogeneic hematopoietic-cell transplantation. N Engl J Med 363: 2091–2101.

20. Apperley J. Just another cost increasing exercise (JACIE)? Bone Marrow Transplant 2004; 34: 835–838.

21. Regulation (EC) No 1394/2007 of the European Parliament and of the Council of 13 November 2007 on advanced therapy medicinal products and amending Directive 2001/83/EC and Regulation (EC) No 726/2004.

Multiple Choice Questionnaire

To find the correct answer, go to http://www.esh.org/online-training/handbook/

1. **Which of the following statements about JACIE accreditation is correct:**

a) The 3rd version of FACT-JACIE standards is in use................................ ☐
b) JACIE accreditation is mandatory in all European member states........ ☐
c) Transplantation of related CBU does not fall in the scope of JACIE...... ☐
d) Inspectors are professionals in the field of stem cell transplantation,
   collection or processing, who have received prior training for
   inspection... ☐

2. **Which of the following statements about quality management is correct:**
   a) Quality management is the last step to achieve, once all medical and
      technical issues have been dealt with... ☐
   b) Deficiencies related to quality management are among the most
      frequent noted during document reviews and on-site inspections .... ☐
   c) Personnel training is necessary only in programs that perform either
      paediatric transplantations, or innovative forms of stem cell
      transplantation that are evaluated in the context of clinical research.... ☐
   d) Document control is necessary only when requested by national
      regulations, which is usually the case for collection and processing...... ☐

3. **Which of the following statements about clinical activity is correct:**
   a) Access to an ICU must be secured in advance, in case transplanted
      patients develop complications and need to be transferred .... ☐
   b) Quality management is not mandatory for the clinical activity, but
      only for collection and processing activities.................................. ☐
   c) Consent must be obtained from donor and recipient, only when they
      are solicited to participate in a clinical research study in the context
      of stem cell transplantation .... ☐
   d) A program performing only autologous transplantation in children
      cannot receive JACIE accreditation .... ☐

4. **Which of the following statements about JACIE accreditation is correct:**
   a) At the end of the inspection, the inspector team leader will decide
      whether or not to accredit the applicant program.......................... ☐
   b) Accreditation is valid for four years.. ☐

c) The main objective of JACIE is to ensure that all transplant performed in Europe comply with European directives on cell and tissue procurement . . . . □

d) ISBT 128 is a system that allow for the exchange of information relating to donor consent . . . . □

---

5. **Which of the following statements about donor evaluation is correct:**

a) JACIE has accurately defined and regularly updates which testing is to be performed on donors for transmittable diseases. JACIE prescriptions prevail over national or international regulations . . . . □

b) Criteria for donor evaluation must be flexible, in order to adapt for the variable and more or less urgent need of transplantation in recipients diagnosed with different diseases . . . . □

c) In case of donor positive or incomplete testing for transmittable disease, the recipient physician must be informed . . . . □

d) A biohazard label must be affixed to all collected, processed and distributed cell products because these contain cells of human origin . . . □

NOTES

*CHAPTER 4

Biological properties of haematopoietic stem cells

Aleksandra Wodnar-Filipowicz

1. Introduction

Over the past 50 years, stem cells have captured the imagination of scientists, clinicians and the lay public alike with the promise of providing a remedy for major degenerative diseases of our civilisation and even dysfunctions associated with normal ageing. The blood-forming system serves as a paradigm for understanding stem cells, their biology and clinical applications. Haematopoietic stem cells (HSCs) reside in small numbers in the bone marrow of adult mammals and are required throughout life to replenish the short-lived mature blood cells belonging to individual haematopoietic lineages. The remarkable regenerative potential of human HSCs is best illustrated by the successful stem cell transplantations in patients with a variety of genetic disorders, acquired states of bone marrow failure and cancers.

This review discusses the current knowledge in the stem cell field. The central place will be taken by HSCs, being the first-discovered, the best-understood and, at present, the only clinically-applicable population of stem cells. I will summarise the contemporary methods to analyse HSCs, describe the properties of these cells, the interactions within the microenvironment in which they reside, and the mechanisms regulating their functions. I will also present current concepts regarding leukaemic stem cells (LSCs), as a population responsible for the initiation and persistence of haematologic tumours. Finally, I will discuss embryonic stem (ES) cells and induced pluripotent stem (iPS) cells and the therapeutic relevance emerging from basic research findings on the differentiation of these cell types into specialised human tissues.

2. Stem cell definition

Stem cells are defined as undifferentiated cells capable to divide for indefinite periods, to self-renew and to generate functional progeny of highly specialised cells. This common definition includes cells present in different physical locations and having fundamentally different proliferative properties and functions (Figure 1).

A fertilised egg (zygote) represents a totipotent stem cell, a cell with unrestricted differentiation potential, indeed, the only cell with the capacity to give rise to all cells necessary for the development of foetal and adult organs. ES cells, forming a cluster inside the blastocyst, are pluripotent stem cells, capable to generate a variety of specialised cell types, but limited in their differentiation potential since unable to develop into a foetus. Further developmental processes lead to generation of multipotent stem cells residing in adult somatic tissues. Their physiological functions are to maintain tissue homeostasis by replenishing mature cell populations of the given tissue or organ, and to respond to stress by repairing damaged tissue. The progress in technologies to detect and enumerate stem cells has led to the discovery of stem cells that reside in most, likely all, mammalian tissues. HSCs are

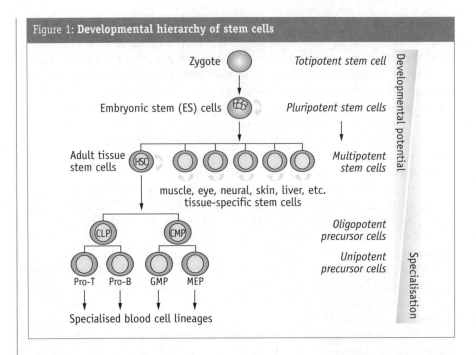

Figure 1: **Developmental hierarchy of stem cells**

Zygote — *Totipotent stem cell*

Embryonic stem (ES) cells — *Pluripotent stem cells*

Adult tissue stem cells (HSC) — *Multipotent stem cells*

muscle, eye, neural, skin, liver, etc.
tissue-specific stem cells

CLP   CMP — *Oligopotent precursor cells*

Pro-T   Pro-B   GMP   MEP — *Unipotent precursor cells*

Specialised blood cell lineages

Developmental potential

Specialisation

the prototype of multipotent adult tissue stem cells (1). In a step-wise differentiation process, HSCs give rise to the committed oligopotent progeny of the lymphoid and myeloid lineages and, further downstream, to the lineage-restricted unipotent precursors of mature blood cells.

3. Methods to analyse HSCs

In humans, bone marrow is the only organ harbouring HSCs and pursuing active multilineage haematopoiesis. Upon birth, HSCs are also present in the cord blood as a result of stem cell migratory properties during foetal development. Fifty years of research on bone marrow-derived stem cells, initiated in the early 1960's by Till and McCulloch, has led to an ever-increasing improvement in methods to quantitate and isolate these cells (2). The haematopoietic system is among the best-defined differentiation cascades in mammalian tissues, since the bone marrow is relatively easy to access and precursor cells of all individual blood lineages have distinct morphological features.

Historically, *in vitro* assays for clonogenic precursors of the myeloerythroid lineages were the first techniques that provided evidence for the existence of multipotent progenitors in the bone marrow. These *in vitro* assays defined the populations of primitive, long-term culture-initiating cells (LTC-ICs) and committed, colony-forming units (CFUs). The introduction of a model of immunocompromised non-obese diabetic/severe combined immunodeficiency (NOD/SCID) mice, by the laboratory of John Dick, was essential in providing a model for studies on the repopulation ability of human HSCs *in vivo* (3). This was followed by establishment of the Rag2$^{-/-}$γc$^{-/-}$ model of recipient mice that are highly permissive for human haematopoiesis, and also use of serial transplants to document the existence of long-term bone marrow-repopulating cells. Limiting dilution assay allows an estimation of the frequency of HSCs among the bulk haematopoietic cells. Although xenogeneic transplantation systems cannot fully reflect the physiology of the interactions in the human bone marrow, they provide the only experimental approach to study human haematopoiesis *in vivo*.

The use of functional assays was paralleled by progress in the phenotypic characterisation of haematopoietic cells by flow-cytometry, using monoclonal antibodies recognising cell surface molecules specific for cell lineages and their differentiation state (Figure 2). These distinct phenotypic properties are also the

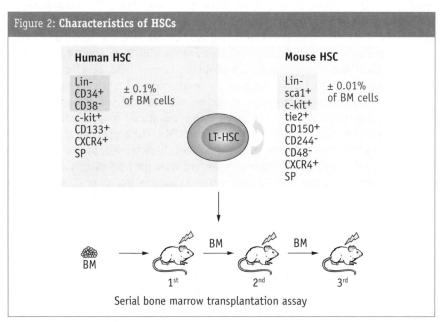

Figure 2: **Characteristics of HSCs**

Human HSC

Lin-
CD34+
CD38-   ± 0.1%
c-kit+   of BM cells
CD133+
CXCR4+
SP

Mouse HSC

Lin-
sca1+
c-kit+   ± 0.01%
tie2+   of BM cells
CD150+
CD244-
CD48-
CXCR4+
SP

LT-HSC

BM

BM   BM

1st   2nd   3rd

Serial bone marrow transplantation assay

LT-HSC: long term-repopulating HSC; BM: bone marrow

basis for the purification of HSCs and their progeny by immunomagnetic bead-based methods and flow cytometry-based sorting. The laboratory of Irving Weissman did fundamental work in precisely defining murine bone marrow-derived HSCs as cells devoid of lineage markers (lin-) and expressing the stem cell antigen (sca1) and the receptor c-kit. The murine lin-sca1+c-kit+ (LSK) cell population, constituting ± 0.01% of bone marrow cells, has self-renewing and long-term repopulating activity *in vivo* (1, 4). Recently, SLAM receptors were introduced as phenotypic markers of murine haematopoiesis, with CD150+CD244-CD48- cells identified as highly enriched in HSCs. Other cell surface markers defining the HSC compartment include the tie2 and flt3 receptors. These, together with c-kit, function as receptors for early-acting haematopoietic growth factors: stem cell factor, angiopoietin-1 and flt3 ligand, which act as key positive regulators of haematopoiesis. Cell surface expression of CXCR4, the chemokine receptor for CXCL-12, is essential for homing to, and retention of HSCs in the bone marrow.

The most primitive human HSCs express CD34 and lack CD38 cell surface antigens and have the capacity to reconstitute sublethally irradiated NOD/SCID or Rag2-/-γc-/- hosts. The CD34+CD38- cells reside in the HSC compartment, constituting ± 0.1% of bone marrow cells, which is heterogeneous and also contains c-kit-, flt3-, and CD133- expressing cells. Both mouse and human HSCs are present among the side population (SP) cells that express the drug transporter protein Abcg2, conferring on them the ability to actively efflux the DNA-intercalating dye Hoechst 33342 or the mitochondrial-binding dye Rhodamine 123. Based on results using the NOD/SCID reconstitution assay, the CD34+CD38-Rho^{low} cell population harbours human HSCs at a frequency of approximately 1 in 30 (1, 4). Despite the availability of methods that greatly facilitate and enhance the precision of studies with well-defined cell populations, genuine human HSCs have not yet been either quantified or purified, and thus remain at present less well defined than murine HSCs. The properties of stem cells from tissues other than bone marrow are even less characterised, primarily because it has been difficult to isolate them in sufficient numbers from skin, muscle, brain or liver. Nevertheless, the flow cytometry-based characterisation of these rare and not easily-accessible somatic tissue stem cells indicates that several cell surface markers are shared with HSCs, including CD34, c-kit, sca1, or CD133, underlying common features of multipotent adult stem cell populations.

4. Properties of HSCs
In order to maintain a supply of mature blood cells throughout the lifetime of an individual, without exhausting the HSC pool, HSCs are predominantly in a quiescent, non-dividing, G_0 state and enter the cell cycle in small numbers (5, 6). HSC

quiescence under steady-state haematopoiesis is critical for long-term maintenance of the stem cell compartment, conferring protection of their genomic integrity by minimising the accumulation of replication-associated mutations and by providing a shield against myelotoxic insults. However, HSCs do exit quiescence and rapidly expand and differentiate in order to regenerate haematopoiesis in response to stress conditions, such as blood loss, infections, or treatment-induced pancytopenias.

Recent studies in the laboratory of Andreas Trumpp, using a combination of flow-cytometric cell sorting and a label-retaining assay based on uptake and long-term retention of BrdU by quiescent HSCs, have subdivided the murine HSC compartment into subpopulations of highly dormant and activated HSCs (7). Dormant cells, with the phenotype of lin$^-$sca1$^+$ckit$^+$CD150$^+$CD48$^-$CD34$^-$, divide rarely, about 5 times in the lifetime of a mouse, and represent a silent reservoir of the most primitive and potent HSCs. These can be activated to undergo self-renewal in response to stress following bone marrow injury by toxic compounds, including chemotherapeutics, mobilisation with G-CSF, or treatment with interferon (IFN)-α. Remarkably, the activated HSCs can return to dormancy upon re-establishment of homeostasis in the system (Figure 3). This reversible switch between dormancy and self-renewal

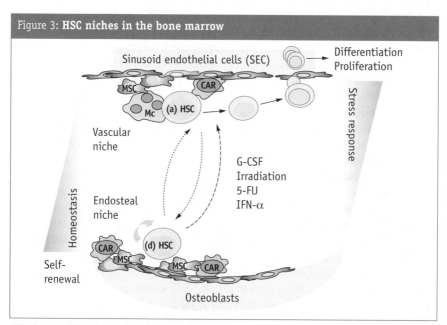

Figure 3: HSC niches in the bone marrow

(d): dormant HSCs, (a): activated HSCs; MSC: mesenchymal stem cells; CAR: CXCL12-expressing reticular cells; Mc: monocytes/macrophages

followed by differentiation, is a powerful safeguard mechanism allowing repair without depletion of the HSC pool, thus preserving the bone marrow reconstituting capacity of HSCs. The fine-tuning of HSCs properties takes place in a specialised microenvironment in the bone marrow, termed the HSC niche (Figure 3).

5. The bone marrow HSC niche

The concept of a stem cell niche defines a microenvironment that provides the HSCs and their descendants with regulatory signals that are essential for their quiescence, self-renewal, proliferation and differentiation, in order to produce appropriate numbers of mature cells throughout life (8–11). Important cell-cell interactions, mediated by adhesion molecules and their ligands, by cytokines and chemokines and their corresponding receptors, control the fate of HSCs and their progeny. Methodological progress in immunohistochemical analysis of the bone marrow and recent introduction of *in vivo* imaging with confocal microscopy, have enabled insights into the bone marrow tissue *in situ* and provided a functional definition of the niche (12–14). The trabecular endosteum harbours quiescent HSCs. Osteoblastic cells, lining the inner surface of the bone, are critical components of the endosteal niche, sustaining the quiescence or self-renewal of HSCs, the properties essential for long-term haematopoiesis. HSCs have also been found in association with endothelium of the sinusoids distal to endosteum. The vascular niche is thought to be the site where actively dividing HSCs and their progeny are located, and where trafficking into and out of the bone marrow occurs. Most likely, the vascular niche plays a dominant role in stress response, by regulating HSC activation and a balanced lineage-specific differentiation, in response to G-CSF or myeloablative treatments.

Haematopoiesis occurs in close physical contact with the stroma lining the bone marrow niches. The cellular composition of stroma remains incompletely characterised, largely due to paucicity of phenotypic markers that unambiguously discriminate between the distinct stromal cell sub-populations. The essential component of endosteal niches are bone-lining osteoblasts, cells that express high levels of N-cadherin, an adhesion molecule mediating cell-cell contact with HSCs. Osteopontin serves as a marker to visualise the spindle-shaped osteoblasts by immunohistochemistry. Vascular niches for HSCs are formed by a complex system of sinusoid capillaries branching throughout the bone marrow cavity. The vasculature, expressing the pan-endothelial marker CD31, comprises heterogeneous cellular compartments. Perivascular sinusoid endothelial cells expressing VEGF-receptors are the essential functional component of the niche. They are surrounded by reticular cells, termed CAR cells, abundantly expressing the CXCL12 chemokine for the CXCR4 receptor expressed by HSCs. CAR cells are also major producers of stem cell factor, the ligand for c-kit receptor, thus providing the HSCs and progenitor cells with key regulatory factors. A likely human counterpart of murine CAR cells, is the population of sub-endothelial cells expressing the CD146 marker. Recently, much attention has been focused on a stromal cell population of fibroblast-like cells, termed mesenchymal stem cells (MSCs). This abundant nestin-expressing cell population was shown to have a multilineage potential, giving rise to numerous tissue types, including cartilage, bone, fat, and muscle, suggesting that bone marrow MSCs have the potential to repair bone and cartilage. This indicates that both haematopoietic and non-haematopoietic stem cell populations of bone marrow have a therapeutic value for tissue regeneration.

6. Regulatory mechanisms in HSC niches

In steady-state haematopoiesis, a complex interplay between the cell-extrinsic cues and the cell-intrinsic regulatory pathways regulate the fate of HSCs, defining the homeostatic balance between the quiescent state or cycling and differentiation (Figure 4). The extrinsic mechanisms are dictated by the environment of stromal and osteoblastic cells (8, 15). The intrinsic mechanisms involve the downstream

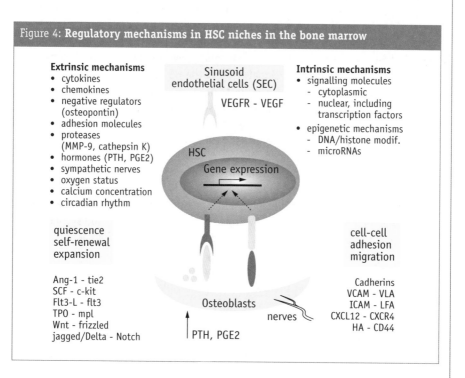

Figure 4: **Regulatory mechanisms in HSC niches in the bone marrow**

signalling molecules, including the transcription factors, and epigenetic regulators acting through chromatin remodelling.

Chemokines, most prominently CXCL12 produced by CAR cells, are responsible for HSC homing into the niche. Direct physical interactions between HSCs and niche cells are mediated by adhesion molecules, such as integrins and cadherins. The membrane-bound and locally secreted cytokines define the HSC fate by initiating specific intracellular signalling pathways. The most prominent examples are stem cell factor, flt3 ligand, angiopoietin-1, Notch ligands and wnt ligands, which act synergistically as positive regulators of stem and progenitor cells. HSC quiescence is also dependent on negative regulators: osteopontin and TGF-β. Despite progress in our understanding of the growth factors involved in HSC self-renewal, the *ex vivo* expansion of HSC numbers has not brought clinically-relevant effects, arguing for the complexity of humoural and cellular components in regulating haematopoiesis *in vivo*. According to recent findings, the extrinsic environmental cues in the HSC niche include also hormonal regulators, such as parathyroid hormone, and the sympathetic nerves, both systems signalling through the osteoblastic niche components. The oxidative conditions in the niche are another important regulator of HSCs. The endosteal niches, close to the bone and far from the capillaries, are hypoxic zones that harbour cells with a profound long-term repopulating potential. Hypoxia favours low Hoechst dye uptake and slow metabolism, the hallmarks of quiescent HSCs. These external signals trigger the HSC-intrinsic molecular networks that are the regulators of cell-cycle arrest or entry, cell proliferation or apoptotic death. Of major importance is the PI3-kinase-dependent pathway that integrates numerous signals delivered by growth factors, nutrients, and oxygen status. The PI3K negative regulator PTEN phosphatase, the cytoplasmic kinase Akt, and the transcription factor FoxO are major players regulating the signal strength delivered by PI3K. The hyperactivation of this enzyme may lead to HSC exhaustion, while hypoactivation preserves the quiescence.

The information on the structure and cellular composition of the niches has largely been deciphered in the mouse. Unravelling the regulation of HSC quiescence in the human system is of great importance for understanding the physiology of HSCs, and equally importantly, the pathophysiology of diseases originating from HSC abnormalities. This will provide the basis for progress in treatment of haematopoietic disorders and for advancing the bone marrow transplantation.

7. Leukaemic stem cells

The stem cell model of cancer envisages the existence of a sub-population, within a heterogenous cancer cell mass, possessing the hallmarks of cancer cells and representing the origin of the neoplasm (16). Leukaemia is the first malignancy in which the leukaemia-initiating stem cells have been experimentally demonstrated in a xenograft transplantation model. According to current understanding, leukaemia is a stem cell disease, in which the self-renewal mechanisms are preserved but the tight proliferation control is lost due to malignant transformation. Leukaemic stem cells (LSCs) reside within a hierarchy of haematopoiesis; they are derived from the most primitive HSCs but also committed progenitors that acquired the self-renewal properties due to oncogenic events, such as point mutations or chromosomal translocations. As a consequence of the transforming event, LSCs are capable of limitless self-renewal resulting in uncontrolled expansion of malignant blasts. The phenotypic features specific for LSCs are not well defined, although abnormal expression levels of a number of cell surface antigens, including CD47, CD90, CD96, or CD123, have been reported in primary human leukaemias. LSCs are thought to reside within the CD34$^+$CD38$^-$/CD38$^+$ cell populations, which contain transplantable cells giving rise to human leukaemia in NOD/SCID mice. Many molecular mechanisms that regulate the function of normal HSCs are shared by LSCs. HSC-characteristic adhesion molecules, such as integrins or CD44, are also involved in LSC interactions with the stroma. Differences between normal and leukaemic cells have their origin in genetic alterations affecting the intracellular signal transduction pathways. As an example, oncogenic lesions in the cytokine receptors c-kit and flt3 are responsible for constitutive activation of downstream signaling in cells at the earliest stages of haematopoietic differentiation, resulting in HSC to LSC transition.

As with normal HSCs, quiescence is also closely associated with protection from myelotoxic insults in leukaemia. It is thought that quiescent LSCs are resistant to both conventional chemotherapy and targeted therapies; importantly, they remain intact and contribute to relapse following discontinuation of therapy (Figure 5A). Niches harbouring LSCs facilitate the resistance by providing protection, and also by adapting to the needs of transformed cells through altered cell and cytokine milieu. At present, numerous approaches to therapeutically target quiescent LSCs as well as interactions of abnormal stem cells with the niche are being developed (17). The novel treatment concepts include interference with cancer cell adhesion in the niche, by use of the of anti-CD44 antibodies, induction of quiescent LSCs to enter the cell-cycle, by the use of IFN-α, or interference with bone marrow chemotactic properties, by the use of agents mobilising LSCs out of niches into circulation. Based on increasing molecular understanding of LSC properties, these approaches, possibly used in combination with conventional therapies and/or specific small molecular inhibitors, may lead to a substantial improvement in leukaemia cure rate (Figure 5B).

Figure 5: Therapeutic relevance of LSCs

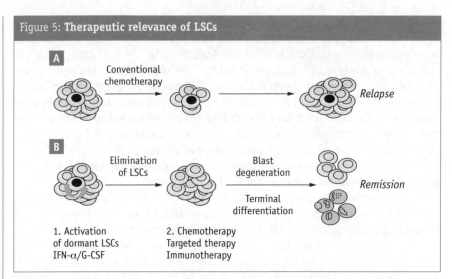

Leukaemic blasts are depicted as yellow cells, LSCs are depicted as black cells, differentiated peripheral blood cells are depicted as blue cells

8. Embryonic stem cells

Human ES cells can be isolated from the preimplantation embryo 4–5 days after fertilisation, and cultured *in vitro* giving rise to immortalised cell lines (18). This technique, initiated in 1998 by the laboratory of James Thomson, is based on isolation of the inner cell mass from a blastocyst at the 30-cell stage and further culture over a layer of supporting stromal cells. Depending on culture conditions, differentiation of ES lines to cells bearing characteristics of various somatic tissue types can be achieved, including haematopoietic, neural, muscle and other tissues (Figure 6A). ES cells are being intensely studied, with a major aim being to understand the molecular basis of "stemness", and to explore their therapeutic potential. The ability of ES cell lines to differentiate *in vitro* to myeloerythroid lineages suggests, that they may be useful for derivation of blood products for transfusions. The exciting perspective for ES cell-based replacement therapies of damaged tissue, the possibility to follow tissue growth and differentiation *in vitro* in studies on human developmental biology, or their use as tools for drug screening, are all the potential values of cultured human ES cells. The controversial aspect of ES-related research is associated with the origin of these cells, being derived from a donated surplus human blastocyst from *in vitro* fertilisation procedures. Destruction of human embryos in order to obtain the ES cells has been of serious

Figure 6: ES and iPS cells

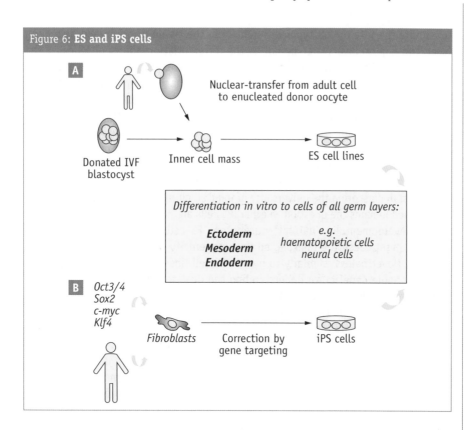

ethical concern. Novel work describes the derivation of human ES cell lines from single blastomers at the 8-cell stage, without embryo destruction. In parallel, cellular techniques have been developed which allow manipulations, such as nuclear transfer, from a somatic cell to the enucleated oocyte, and further generation of ES cell lines bearing genetic information defined by the donated nucleus. The cloning of the sheep "Dolly" and other mammals from adult cells showed that the genome of even fully specialised cells remains genetically totipotent. The possibility to obtain ES-derived cells with genetic information of the patient by nuclear transfer, is an approach which - in the future - might yield transplantable tissue of a full immunological compatibility (Figure 6A).

9. Induced pluripotent stem cells and cell reprogramming

The term "adult stem cell plasticity" defines the ability of tissue-specific stem cells to acquire the fate of cell types different from the tissue of origin and belonging to all three germ layers, i.e. similar to the differentiation ability of ES cells. The generation of iPS cells from mouse and human somatic cells in the laboratories of Shinya Yamanaka and James Thomson in 2007, has demonstrated that adult mammalian cells can be reprogrammed to a pluripotent state by the enforced expression of a few defined transcription factors: Oct4, Sox2, Klf4 and c-myc (19). Derivation of human iPS cells is ethically and legally less problematic than generation of ES cell lines, since it is not associated with the use of fertilised zygotes (Figure 6B). The technical feasibility of the reprogramming approach resulted in generation of iPS cells from numerous species, with numerous somatic cell types as targets, underscoring the universality of induced pluripotency and reprogramming. Unanswered remains the question whether iPS cells are indeed biologically equivalent to the developmentally "natural" pluripotent ES cells. For example, epigenetic changes might cause the unexpected immunogenicity of transplanted autologous iPS cells. Nevertheless, similarly to human ES cell lines, the iPS technology offers unquestionable benefits for understanding the disease mechanisms, for providing a platform for drug discovery and testing, and also for development of novel approaches to therapy (20). Disease-specific iPS cells have been generated from somatic cells from patients with numerous genetic disorders; these serve as valuable disease models for further studies (Figure 6B). Haematopoietic and mesenchymal bone marrow progenitors, both normal and bearing genetic defects, can be reprogrammed to the pluripotent state. Importantly, iPS technology combined with correction of a genetic defect by gene transfer, has allowed the successful treatment of sickle cell anaemia in a mouse model with iPS cells generated from autologous skin. The haematopoietic progenitors from Fanconi anaemia were the source of the first human patient-specific corrected and reprogrammed iPS cells, which resumed normal mitomycin-insensitive properties. Of concern for *in vivo* application of iPS cells, as well as of ES cells, is the formation of teratoma tissue upon transplantation, raising the danger of cancerous transformation of pluripotent cells. A novel finding on a direct conversion of human dermal fibroblasts to multilineage blood progenitors by ectopic expression of a transcription factor Oct4, demonstrated a reprogramming which bypassed the pluripotency state. The direct restoration of multipotency may offer the possibility of autologous cell replacement therapy as an alternative approach that avoids the potential dangers associated with the use of human ES or iPS cells.

10. Conclusions and future perspectives

The ultimate goal for regenerative medicine is to channel the multipotent and/or pluripotent stem cells with high proliferative capacity into specified differentiation programs within the body for a multitude of therapeutic uses. The key characteristics of the different types of stem cells are shown in Key points. Transplantation of HSCs is the proof-of-principle of a curative effect of cellular therapies. Recent major technical advancements in isolation, expansion and controlled differentiation of human ES cells and iPS cells reprogrammed from adult stem cells and, additionally, the establishment of nuclear transfer technology opened a number of potential new therapeutic approaches for the restoration of damaged or diseased tissue. The principle of self-renewal and lineage-making decisions of stem cells of different tissue-origin requires understanding in molecular terms. Determining how epigenetic features relate to the transcriptional signatures of various types of adult stem cells, as well as ES and iPS cells, is a key challenge for the future. The new challenge in stem cell biology is related to identifying the molecular and the functional programmes of malignant versus normal stem cells. Further understanding of the stem cell niche is essential for advancing the approaches to control developmental pathways by both cell-autonomous and microenvironmental cues. All this information will be used to guide the future work towards specific targeting the fate of normal and malignant stem cells in clinical settings.

Key points

Hierarchy of stem cells

Totipotent	Zygote	Unrestricted differentiation potential
Pluripotent	ES cells	Derived from blastocyts at 30-cell stage
	iPS cells	Reprogrammed from adult somatic cells: normal/diseased
Multipotent	Adult somatic stem cells, e.g. HSCs	Differentiation limited to specific tissues

HSC characteristics

Mouse HSCs	lin⁻sca1⁺c-kit⁺CD150⁺Rho^{low}
	Long-term syngeneic bone marrow repopulation in mice
Human HSCs	lin⁻CD34⁺CD38⁻Rho^{low}
	Long-term xenogeneic bone marrow repopulation in NOD/SCID mice
Quiescent HSCs	Support haematopoietic homeostasis
Activated HSCs	Support haematopoietic response to stress conditions: bleeding, infection, toxicity, cell-cycle induction, mobilisation

HSC niche in the bone marrow

Endosteal niche	Harbours quiescent (dormant) HSCs
	Main cellular components: osteoblasts, nestin+ mesenchymal stem cells (MSCs), CXCL12 secreting CAR cells
Vascular niche	Harbours activated HSCs
	Main cellular components: sinusoid endothelial cells, CXCL12 secreting CAR cells, nestin+ MSCs, monocytes/macrophages
Regulatory mechanisms	Extrinsic: cytokines, chemokines, adhesion molecules, hormones, calcium, oxygen, sympathetic nerves, etc.
	Intrinsic: cytoplastic signalling molecules, transcription factors, microRNAs, epigenetic status

LSCs

Leukaemia-initiating cells	Uncontrolled self-renewal capacity of malignant HSCs and progenitor cells resistant to conventional chemotherapy and targeted therapy
	Responsible for relapse and fatal outcome
LSC-targeting approaches	Induction of cell-cycling: with IFN-α and G-CSF
	Decrease adhesion to niche cells: with anti-CD44 antibodies
	Prevent immune evasion: with anti-CD47 antibodies

Acknowledgements
This work has been supported by the Swiss National Science Foundation grant 3100-110511.

References

1. Bryder D, Rossi DJ, Weissman IL. Hematopoietic stem cells: The paradigmatic tissue-specific stem cell. Am J Pathol 2006; 169: 338–346.
2. Purton LE, Scadden DT. Limiting factors in murine hematopoietic stem cell assays. Cell Stem Cell 2007; 1: 263–270.
3. Dick JE, Bhatia M, Gan O et al. Assay of human stem cells by repopulation of NOD/SCID mice. Stem Cells 1997; 15: 199–203.
4. Warr MR, Pietras EM, Passegué E. Mechanisms controlling hematopoietic stem cell functions during normal hematopoiesis and haematological malignancies. Wiley Interdiscip Rev Syst Biol Med 2011; Mar 15. doi: 10.1002/wsbm.145.
5. Arai F, Suda T. Maintenance of quiescent hematopoietic stem cells in the osteoblastic niche. Ann N Y Acad Sci 2007; 1106: 41–53.

6. Li J. Quiescence regulators for hematopoietic stem cell. Exp Hematol 2011; 39: 511–520.
7. Trumpp A, Essers M, Wilson A. Awakening dormant haematopoietic stem cells. Nat Rev Immunol 2010; 10: 201–209.
8. Wilson A, Trumpp A. Bone-marrow haematopoietic-stem-cell niches. Nat Rev Immunol 2006; 6: 93–106.
9. Nagasawa T, Omatsu Y, Sugiyama T. Control of hematopoietic stem cells by the bone marrow stromal niche: The role of reticular cells. Trends Immunol 2011; 32: 315–320.
10. Ehninger A, Trumpp A. The bone marrow stem cell niche grows up: Mesenchymal stem cells and macrophages move in. J Exp Med 2011; 208: 421–428.
11. Anjios-Afonso F, Bonnet D. Prospective identification and isolation of murine bone marrow derived multipotent mesenchymal progenitor cells. Best Pract Res Clin Haematol 2011; 24: 13–24.
12. Scadden DT. The stem-cell niche as an entity of action. Nature 2006; 441: 1075–1079.
13. Butler JM, Kobayashi H, Rafii S. Instructive role of the vascular niche in promoting tissue growth and tissue repair by angiocrine factors. Nature Reviews 2010; 10: 138–146.
14. Burness ML, Sipkins DA. The stem cell niche in health and malignancy. Semin Cancer Biol 2010; 20: 107–115.
15. Rizo A, Vellenga E, de Haan G, Schuringa JJ. Signaling pathways in self-renewing hematopoietic and leukemic stem cells: Do all stem cells need a niche? Hum Mol Genet 2006; 15: 210–219.
16. Lane SW, Gilliland DG. Leukemia stem cells. Semin Cancer Biol 2009; 20: 71–76.
17. Becker MW, Jordan CT. Leukemia stem cells in 2010: Current understanding and future directions. Blood Rev 2011; 25: 75–81.
18. Ludwig TE, Levenstein ME, Jones JM et al. Derivation of human embryonic stem cells in defined conditions. Nat Biotechnol 2006; 24: 185–187.
19. Yamanaka S, Blau HM. Nuclear reprogramming to a pluripotent state by three approaches. Nature 2010; 465: 704–712.
20. Stadtfeld M, Hochedlinger K. Induced pluripotency: History, mechanisms, and applications. Genes Dev 2010; 24: 2239–2263.

Multiple Choice Questionnaire

To find the correct answer, go to http://www.esh.org/online-training/handbook/

1. Haematopoietic stem cells are defined as:
a) Totipotent stem cells .... ☐
b) Pluripotent stem cells .... ☐
c) Multipotent stem cells .... ☐
d) Committed stem cells .... ☐

2. **Human adult haematopoiesis normally takes place in the following organs:**
    a) Bone marrow ☐
    b) Peripheral blood ☐
    c) Spleen ☐
    d) Liver ☐

3. **The osteoblastic niche in the bone marrow is important for regulation of:**
    a) Haematopoietic stem cell trafficking through bone marrow sinusoids ☐
    b) Haematopoietic stem cell quiescence and self-renewal ☐
    c) Cell-cycling and differentiation of haematopoietic stem cells ☐
    d) Active metabolism of haematopoietic stem cells ☐

4. **Leukaemic stem cells have the following characteristics:**
    a) Can be easily defined according to their cell surface markers ☐
    b) Contain acquired genetic alterations at the level of stem cells and committed progenitors ☐
    c) Reside exclusively in vascular niches in the bone marrow ☐
    d) Are devoid of adhesion molecules specific for osteoblastic niches ☐

5. **Embryonic stem cells are characterised by:**
    a) Totipotent differentiation potential ☐
    b) Differentiation potential reprogrammed by gene transfer ☐
    c) Pluripotency to generate a variety of specialised cell types ☐
    d) Ability to form a blastocyst ☐

NOTES

* CHAPTER 5

Immunogenetics of allogeneic HSCT

Bronwen E. Shaw, Alejandro Madrigal

1. Introduction

The primary role of HLA molecules is to present peptide to T-cells, enabling them to recognise and eliminate "foreign" particles present in an individual, and also to prevent the recognition of "self" as foreign. These natural functions need to be overcome (or manipulated) in order to allow grafts between HLA non-identical individuals to be accepted. The HLA system displays extensive polymorphism, most likely due to the need for the immune system to keep up with and control infectious pathogens (evolutionary pressure). Despite this massive diversity in the HLA system we are able to identify compatible donors due to the Mendelian inheritance of HLA and the presence of well defined haplotypes and linkage dysequilibrium. Our knowledge of donor selection strategies has been enhanced considerably over the last decade by the publication of studies analysing the outcome in very large groups of transplant patients, all with high resolution tissue typing results. There is a large degree of consensus in the literature regarding the selection of the optimal donor. Many questions, however, remain, such as the impact of non-classical HLA loci or non-HLA genetics on clinical outcome.

2. The Major Histocompatibility Complex

The Major Histocompatibility Complex (MHC) was discovered in mice by Peter Gorer and George Snell (1). They uncovered an antigen which was involved in the rejection of a tumour, and subsequently showed that similar antigens in other strains of mice were probable alleles of the same "tumour resistance" gene. The identification of such antigens in humans followed the description of anti-leukocyte antisera, detectable by agglutination assays, in the sera of patients who had received multiple blood transfusions.

2.1 Genetic organisation

The MHC contains more than 200 genes, most of which have functions related to immunity, and is contained within 4.2 Mbp of DNA on the short arm of chromosome 6 at 6p21.3. It is divided into three main regions: the HLA Class I region (containing HLA-A, -B and -C genes), the HLA Class II region (containing HLA-DR, -DQ and -DP) and lying between these, the Class III region (densely packed with genes including those encoding complement factors and tumour necrosis factor, TNF).

2.2 Structure and function of HLA molecules

The overall structure of the HLA Class I and Class II molecules is similar, with most of the polymorphism located in the peptide binding groove (PBG) (1). HLA molecules are expressed on the cell surface where they present peptides to T-cells as antigens on the cell surface. While each MHC allele can present thousands of different peptides, the T-cell receptor recognises the peptide only if it is presented by the same MHC molecule as encountered during priming, a concept known as MHC restriction (1).

Class I molecules are found on most nucleated cells and platelets and consist of an α chain which is associated with and stabilised by β_2 microglobulin (β_2m) (a non polymorphic protein encoded on chromosome 15). Bound peptides are classically 8-10 amino acids long and interact with the Class I molecule through pockets in the PBG. The exposed portion of the peptide, and the upper faces of the two α-helices of the Class I molecule interact with the CD8 T-cell receptor.

The Class II molecules are generally restricted to cells of the immune system (e.g. B cells, dendritic cells), but can be induced on other cell types during the immune response, and consists of two transmembrane glycoproteins, the α and β chains. The PBG of the Class II molecules has open ends which allow the peptide to extend beyond the groove at both ends, and therefore to be longer (12–24 amino acids). The peptide is presented to CD4 T-cells.

2.3 Polymorphism

The HLA region is the most polymorphic currently known in the human genome (*http://www.ebi.ac.uk/imgt/hla/stats.html*) (Table 1). In Class I molecules the α chain is highly polymorphic. In Class II molecules the β chain is highly polymorphic while limited polymorphism is exhibited in the α chains. The polymorphism is concentrated in the areas which encode the peptide-binding groove and the sites of interaction with the T-cell receptor.

2.4 Nomenclature and tissue typing

In view of the enormous degree of polymorphism, it became clear more than 20 years ago that serological typing techniques were completely inadequate to uncover the

Table 1: **The number of HLA alleles currently named at each locus (April 2011)**

HLA locus	Number of Class I alleles	HLA locus	Number of Class II alleles
HLA-A	1601	HLA-DRB	1027
HLA-B	2125	HLA-DQA1	44
HLA-C	1102	HLA-DQB1	153
		HLA-DPA1	32
		HLA-DPB1	149

level of diversity present in the HLA system. Advances in DNA-based tissue typing techniques have moved the field forward dramatically and DNA typing can result in low, medium or high resolution results (Table 2). HLA nomenclature has been reviewed to accommodate these changes. Each HLA allele name is unique and follows strict nomenclature conventions, where a number corresponding to up to four sets of digits separated by colons is assigned. The first digits (before the first colon) describe the allele group, which often corresponds to the serological antigen e.g. A*24 (the asterisk denotes DNA-based typing). This is the level obtained by low resolution typing techniques. Low resolution typing (or serology) may be appropriate in certain circumstances (e.g. screening of potential sibling donors), however is generally insufficient for selecting unrelated donors. The second set of digits (after the first colon) are used to list the subtypes, different numbers denoting one or more nucleotide substitution that changes the amino acid sequence of the encoded protein e.g. A*24:02 or A*24:05. Medium resolution tissue typing techniques (e.g. SSO, SSP) can define specific allele groups and subtypes, although often as a "string" of possible alleles within a particular allele group. The use of National Marrow Donor Program (NMDP) codes can be hepful in this setting (*http://bioinformatics.nmdp.org/HLA/hla_res_idx.html*). High resolution typing methods are employed to resolve the tissue type to allele level, with no ambiguity. In practice, these first two sets of digits are required in order to refer to a type as high resolution and it is recommended that selection of an unrelated donor is based on such results. The allele name can, however, extend by several more divisions, representing firstly synonymous mutations, and then intronic (or other non-coding) variants, although these are currently not considered when selecting donors or scoring HLA matches. The addition of an optional letter at the end of a sequence indicates a major alteration in its expression (e.g. an "N" for a null allele).

2.5 Linkage disequilibrium and haplotypes
Linkage disequilibrium (LD) means that certain alleles occur together with a greater

Table 2: **An example of HLA nomenclature and its relation to tissue typing techniques**

Typing method	Nomenclature
Serological	A1
DNA-based: Low resolution	A*01
DNA-based: Medium resolution	A*01:01/01:04N
DNA-based: High resolution	A*01:01

frequency than would be expected by chance (non-random gametic association). A haplotype describes a group of genes which are inherited together. Certain HLA haplotypes are common in particular ethnic groups. In general, LD is more frequently observed between loci that are in close proximity. Strong LD is displayed between the α and β subunit of each of the HLA Class II molecules and explains why tissue typing involves only the highly polymorphic β subunits. HLA-B and HLA-C display strong LD, however, more than one HLA-C allele may be in LD with a particular HLA-B allele (e.g. >95% of Caucasoid individuals who have HLA-B*07:02 will have HLA-C*07:02, while those who express B*18:01 may express either C*07:01, C*12:03 or C*05:01). Thus, allele prediction based on LD studies is not completely accurate, particularly in ethnic groups whose HLA types has not yet been well studied. High resolution typing pre-transplant in these circumstances is mandatory to avoid mismatches.

In many cases LD may extend across the entire Class I and II regions (haplotype), however identity for all the HLA loci does not necessarily predict for identity for the intervening genes. Recombination events are known to occur with increased frequency at certain points within the MHC (1). One example is between HLA-DP and the other Class II loci, explaining the difficulty in finding a donor matched for HLA-DPB1 in addition to the other HLA loci. Another involves the TNF region in Class III.

2.6 Structural/functional aspects of HLA

Antigenic mismatches are characterised by amino acid substitutions in both peptide binding and T-cell recognition regions, whereas allelic mismatches are characterised by amino acid substitution only in the peptide binding regions. Both limited and extensive polymorphic differences may result in functional immunogenicity. This is because limited polymorphisms are not functionally null. It is recognised that small differences between MHC molecules influence T-cell recognition. Indeed, prior to DNA sequencing, serologically defined groups of related HLA variants were sub-divided on the basis of their differential reactivity with alloreactive T-cells. It has been suggested that limited differences may induce stronger alloresponses than numerous differences (2) because the foreign MHC molecule closely resembles self-MHC and is therefore more likely to cross-react with self-educated T-cells. Originally donor selection included functional studies (mixed lymphocyte cultures (MLC) or cytotoxic T-lymphocyte precursor frequency, CTLp) between patient and donor in an attempt to directly demonstrate the degree of allogenicity between a pair. These have subsequently largely been replaced by DNA typing methods (due to speed and ease), however they are still performed in some laboratories in certain circumstances. In order to "mimic" functional tests, attempts have been made to create scoring systems which will electronically predict the likelihood of allogenicity, based on functional and the structural difference between two HLA alleles. Currently these are not in routine practice.

The concept of "permissive" (not resulting in clinical consequences) and "non-permissive" HLA mismatching has been explored in solid organ transplantation (3). The minimal structural unit that is recognised by the T-cell receptor is an epitope and this type of analysis takes into account amino acid sequence polymorphisms as critical components of immunogenic epitopes that can elicit alloantibodies or T-cell responses. This type of analysis is less well characterised in HCT, however evidence for "permissive" mismatching does exist (see below).

3. Donor search and probability of finding a donor

3.1 Probability of finding a donor

The probability and speed of finding a well matched unrelated donor (UD) is significantly improved if high resolution typing is available for the patient prior to the search being done. Typing must ideally, therefore, be done by DNA methods to avoid "hidden" mismatches particularly in the case of antigenically "silent" alleles, and include at least HLA-A, -B -C and -DRB1. Many labs or transplant centres consider HLA-DQB1 typing to be desirable and HLA-DPB1 to be optional.

The probability to identify an unrelated donor can be estimated using various surrogate markers, such as: the patient haplotype, the presence of rare alleles or unusual HLA associations (B/C, DRB1/DQB1) and the numbers of potential donors identified at search. A search should not be continued beyond a set agreed time period (based on factors such as the disease and stage), as studies have shown that the probability of finding a donor diminishes significantly over time and there is evidence to show that the outcome in patients is worse as the time between diagnosis and transplant is lengthened. In addition, alternative teatment strategies can be addressed early in patients where the chance of finding an unrelated donor appears low.

Two studies have directly addressed this issue. Tiercy et al. (4) developed a probability estimate of the chances of identifying a 10/10 HLA allele-matched donor through the Swiss Blood Stem Cells Foundation. Based on allele and haplotype frequencies, the probability of finding a donor in 305 consecutive searches was classed as high (>95% chance to identify a 10/10 matched donor), intermediate or low (<5% chance). The probability estimate was found to be correct in 96, 56 and 88% of high, intermediate and low probability cases, respectively. In the 144 patients in the low risk group, 127 could not find a 10/10 matched donor (as predicted when the search was initiated), suggesting other strategies should be pursued early on for these patients.

Hirv et al. (5) performed a similar study analysing the outcomes of 549 UD searches. Patients were divided into four groups based on their HLA-DRB1 and -DQB1 type and haplotype (comparing these to frequencies on the national register). In the group with a high probability to find a 10/10 matched donor (n=318), 78% were successful, this was 50% in the medium group (n=157), 18% in the low group (n=56) and 4% in the very low group. In addition, they report a median search time of 22 days (range: 2–2870 days). Median search times were 20, 27, 45 and 477 days in each of the four groups (high to very low respectively).

3.2 Interpreting the search report

The search may be performed by the transplant centre (TC) directly or by their associated H&I (histocompatibility and immunogenetics) laboratory/donor centre or registry. Unrelated donor (and cord blood unit) search reports can be difficult to interpret due to a wide variability in the quality and resolution of the tissue typing available for each individual donor, based on the era in which they joined the registry and the tissue typing techniques which were available at the time. In order to select appropriate donors for confirmatory typing (CT), in a time efficient manner, it is critical for the person interpreting the search report to have a good knowledge of HLA haplotypes and LD, as well as knowledge of NMDP codes and HLA nomenclature. It is also important to recognise that the "best" donor may not be the first one listed on the search report. In practice this will usually mean close collaboration between the TC and the H&I laboratory/registry. Models to facilitate this process include the use of computer generated haplotype prediction models (e.g. haplogic used by the NMDP and optimatch used by the Zentrale Knochenmarkspender-Register für die Bundesrepublik Deutschland, ZKRD) where the program delivers a probability score in the report, and graft identification and advisory services (e.g. GIAS used by Anthony Nolan) where the entire search and CT request procedure is devolved to the H&I lab according to a set of pre-agreed algorithms.

4. Clinical impact of HLA matching

4.1 Interpreting studies

It is clear that discrepancies are found between different studies reporting on the impact of HLA matching and caution should be excercised when comparing or interpreting the results. Diverse factors such as: the year of transplantation, patient demographic profile and ethnicity (homogeneity of HLA in the population), conditioning type, stem cell source and T-cell depletion, amongst other factors, are likely to impact on the results and should be taken into account.

4.2 HLA allele level matching

The best donor remains an HLA-identical sibling donor, suggesting that - despite numerous other donor factors (e.g. age, gender) playing a role - genetic factors are the most important donor determinant of patient outcome. It should be recalled, however, that recombination events may result in a mismatch at HLA-loci in siblings, particularly for HLA-DPB1.

The best unrelated donor has been shown to be one who is matched, at high resolution, for the major polymorphic HLA loci. HLA-A, -B, -C, -DRB1 (8/8) are all considered critical and many would consider an 8/8 matched donor as the gold standard. Some controversy remains about the need to include HLA-DQB1 in donor selection strategies (10/10), however, in practice many TCs routinely type for this locus and consider a 10/10 matched donor as the gold standard.

HLA-DPB1 is not routinely included in all donor selection strategies, however, is often considered in certain circumstances.

4.3 HLA-A, -B, -C, -DRB1

Recent large studies from the NMDP/Center for International Blood and Marrow Transplant Research (CIBMTR) have investigated the impact of HLA mismatching in recipients of myeloablative conditioned transplants (6–8). All three showed a significant survival disadvantage with any degree of HLA mismatching at HLA-A, -B, -C, -DRB1 (8/8), such that outcome with a 6/8 match is worse than a 7/8 match, which is worse than an 8/8 match. Two of the studies showed no difference in the risk of mortality between a single class I versus a single DRB1 mismatch (6, 8). In the Lee study the impact on overall survival (OS) from an HLA-A or -DRB1 mismatch was more marked than a mismatch at HLA-B or -C (7). The earlier NMDP study had suggested that low resolution mismatches at HLA-A, -B, -C or -DRB1, were associated with a more adverse outcome than the effects seen with high resolution mismatches (6), while the later study showed no significant differences in survival dependant on whether the mismatch was allelic or antigenic, except at HLA-C where an antigenic mismatch increased transplant risks while an allelic mismatch did not (7).

4.4 Individual locus mismatches

Data from the International Histocompatibility Working Group (IHWG) in Hematopoietic Cell Transplantation (9) showed that a single mismatch for HLA-A, -B and -C was significantly associated with a worse overall survival, while mismatches for single HLA-DRB1 or -DQB1 allele did not confer a significant survival detriment. Data from the JMDP (10) showed a worse overall survival in those with HLA-A or -B mismatches, while HLA-C, -DRB1 and DQB1 mismatches did not impact significantly on OS. A later study by the same group (11), showed mismatches for HLA-A, -B and -DQB1 to be independent risk factors for mortality with a trend to a worse mortality in HLA-C mismatched recipients, but no impact of HLA-DRB1. One CIBMTR study (12) has reported on patients who received reduced intensity conditioning (RIC) using peripheral blood stem cells (PBSC). Their data showed that HLA-C antigenic mismatches were the only mismatches to impact on OS.

4.4.1 HLA-DQB1
While some studies have not shown any survival disadvantage associated with a single HLA-DQB1 mismatch (6, 7), others have found that, although there is no independent influence on survival of a single HLA-DQB1 mismatch, there is a significantly worse survival if an HLA-DQB1 mismatch was found in addition to a Class I mismatch (8, 13).

4.4.2 HLA-DPB1
Several studies have shown that matching of HLA-DPB1 results in a reduction in graft-versus-host disease (GvHD). In addition, a strong association has been reported between DPB1 matching and an increased relapse risk (14). Despite these statistically significant effects on transplant complication, not all studies have shown a survival detriment associated with DPB1 matching status, however, at least one study has shown an interaction with disease stage (a significant survival advantage in DPB1 matched patients with early stage leukaemia, compared with a survival disadvantage with DPB1 matching in late stage leukaemia) (15).

4.5 Clinical evidence for tolerated HLA mismatches
In certain circumstances the use of an HLA mismatched donor has been shown to be associated with an outcome similar to that when using an HLA matched donor. Several studies have shown that single, or even multiple, mismatches may be tolerated in the setting of high risk/late stage disease (7, 13) and in at least one study have remarked that more advanced disease has a greater impact on patient outcomes than increasing degrees of HLA mismatching. Thus, as mentioned above, care should be taken not to prolong the search unnecessarily, if an "acceptable" HLA mismatched donor is available. Another setting in which mismatches appear to be tolerated is in transplants using T-cell depletion in the conditioning. Recipients of T-cell depleted transplantation protocols using alemtuzumab (15, 16), or other methods of TCD (17), have shown that a single HLA mismatch is tolerated in these settings.

4.5.1 Clinical evidence for permissive and non-permissive mismatches
It is clear from transplant outcome studies that not all HLA mismatches result in

a deleterious clinical outcome. As discussed above, a mismatch would generally be expected to produce a worse outcome, but there are situations where it does not (e.g. multiple mismatches in an advanced stage leukaemia); this is termed a tolerated mismatch. The term "permissive" or "non-permissive" refers to a mismatch within a particular locus which results in a different outcome (e.g. Class I position 116 mismatches increased transplant complications, while mismatches at another amino acid position do not). As mentioned previously, changes at an amino acid or epitope level may be more significant triggers of an allogeneic response than allelic mismatches, with the result that certain mismatches may be "permissive" (i.e. not associated with worse clinical outcomes than a match), while others may be "non-permissive" (i.e. associated with worse clinical outcomes than either a match or a "permissive" mismatch).

Uncovering such mismatches is incredibly complex, due to the polymorphic nature of HLA, and compounded by the clinical heterogeneity of transplant study populations. Several groups have attempted to address this question. The JMDP have found specific allele mismatch combinations at both Class I and II loci to be associated with protection from relapse and OS (18). Comparisons between Japanese and Caucasian patients have found that different allelic mismatches are tolerated differently in these populations (19). Other groups have investigated this question taking into account differences at the amino acid or epitope level. Mismatches for position 116 in the Class I heavy chain (20) and other positions across both Class I and II loci (11) have been implicated.

Currently the most mature evidence for a clinical impact of epitope matching can be found for the HLA-DPB1 locus. The fact that HLA-DPB1 is frequently mismatched in patient/donor pairs, allows for anaysis of specific mismatches in a way that would be difficult at other loci. In addition, the polymorphism in DPB1 is limited to six hypervariable regions (HVR), A-F, which are shuffled between alleles. Zino et al. developed a functional "epitope-based" algorithm, in which they classified different DPB1 mismatches into permissive or non-permissive based on immunogenicity to a shared T-cell epitope (21, 22). The highly immunogenic molecules in this model (DPB1*09:01, *10:01, *17:01) share HVRs A, B, D and F, while those in the intermediate group (DPB1*03:01, *14:01, *45:01) have substitutions in HVR D as well as A or C. They and others have subsequently shown that scoring patient and donor mismatches in this way is significantly predictive of transplant outcomes (22, 23).

Combining these approaches further refines donor selection. The outcome in patients matched for DPB1 at an allelic level were similar to those with an allele level mismatch, but permissive epitope mismatch. Conversely, the presence of non-permissive mismatches resulted in a significantly worse overall survival.

4.6 Other HLA loci
There is currently little clinical evidence suggesting an important clinical impact for matching for the HLA Class II α-chains or for DRB3, 4, 5.

5. Non-HLA genetic factors
Even when the HLA loci are identical between the donor and the recipient (in both unrelated donor and sibling transplantation), GvHD and graft rejection may still occur. Thus, it is recognised that other genetic factors exist which may mediate transplant complications through various mechanisms. It is beyond the scope of this chapter to investigate this topic in details, and comprehensive reviews are recommended (24–27).

5.1 Killer immunoglobulin-like receptors
Natural killer (NK) cells form part of the innate immune system and are known to play a major role in control of viral infections and tumour surveillance. NK cells express a variety of receptors, both inhibitory and activating, including killer-cell immunoglobulin-like receptors (KIR), NKG2D and DNAM-1. The ligands for KIR are MHC class I molecules, with ligands for the other receptors including MIC-A and CD155, but not all ligands are known. Interaction of an inhibitory KIR with its specific MHC class I ligand can result in inhibition of activation of the NK cell. If the ligand is "missing" (as in a mismatched transplant setting) the NK cell can become activated and lyse the target cell. It now seems likely that licensing (education) is required for NK cells to leave their anergic state.
Several studies in transplantation have shown the importance of NK cells, in particular KIR, in mediating transplant outcome through a number of postulated mechanisms. KIR incompatibility at both the phenotypic and genotypic level has been associated with transplant outcome using several models, including: the ligand-ligand model and the receptor-ligand model. The presence or absence of certain receptors (and haplotypes), as well as the overall number of receptors or haplotypes present, has also been shown in some studies to impact transplant outcomes. Further studies are likely to help to uncover the complexity of these genes and to enhance our knowledge about the value in selecting donors in different transplant settings.

5.2 Cytokine, chemokine and immune response gene polymorphisms
The proinflammatory cytokines, their receptors and related inhibitors have been implicated in a large number of immunological diseases, including GvHD following allogeneic HSCT. There are thousands of single nucleotide polymorphisms (SNPs) found in the regions of DNA encoding the cytokine genes and their promoter regions. These may be important for a number of reasons, but especially if they result in a

variation in the functional level or activity of the cytokine produced. Polymorphic cytokine genes studied in the transplant context include tumour necrosis genes (TNF), interleukin (IL)-10, the IL-1 gene family, IL-2, IL-6, interferon (IFN)-γ, TGF-β1 and TGF-β1 receptors. Chemokine gene polymorphisms (e.g. CCR5, CCR9) have recently been subject to increased investigation and may have particular relevance to post transplant infectious complications.

Several genes related to the innate immune system, particularly those involved in the recognition of pathogens, have recently been studied in the HSCT setting. The NOD- like receptors (NOD2/CARD15) and the Toll-like receptors (TLR) have been shown to impact on transplant complications including disese relapse, GvHD and susceptibility to infections. Other genes of interest include the oestrogen and vitamin D receptors, myeloperoxidase, mannose binding lectin and Fc receptors.

5.3 Minor histocompatibility antigens
Minor histocompatibility antigens (mHags) are immunogenic peptides derived from polymorphic cellular proteins. These peptides bind to HLA antigens (many in an HLA restricted manner) and can be recognised by allogeneic T-cells. They are only of clinical importance if they are immunogenic and occur at a moderately frequent distribution in the population. Best studies are the HA and H-Y systems and specific CTLs against both have been detected early post transplant. An important factor is whether they are expressed only on cells derived from the haematopoietic precursors (e.g. HA-1 and -2), or occur on haematopoietic and non-haematopoietic cells (e.g. H-Y antigens). A therapeutic role in enhancing the GvL effect (without increasing GvHD) has been shown to be possible, particularly into those with expression limited to haematopoietic cells.

5.4 Donor selection based on non-HLA immunogenetic factors
Although a few multi-centre/collaborative studies reporting the impact of these factors on HSCT outcome are now available, the majority of studies report results from a single centre. Unfortunately the study populations often differ, and in many reports the clinical impact of the factor investigated conflicts with results from other reports. For these, and other, reasons the non-HLA immunogenetic factors have yet to enter routine practice in the stem cell transplantation field and are only considered in particular patient subgroups or treatment protocols.

6. Conclusion
Genetic disparity, in particular at the HLA loci, between patient and donor is a critical factor influencing transplantation outcome. Comprehensive efforts by the HLA community to developed nomenclature and tissue typing techniques which allow

for a standardised interpretation of results from transplant studies as resulted in some clear recommendation for donor selection to be made. Nevertheless, several issues remain to be explored, such as the impact of stem cell source and conditioning, T-cell depletion, non-HLA genetic factors, other donor factors (age, CMV status, gender), delays in accessing the donor (i.e. the time to transplantation) and the impact of HLA matching on cord blood transplant outcome. The importance of large collaborative studies should be emphasised.

Key points

Immunogentic factors, in particular HLA, are critical to the outcome of HSCT

HLA is the most polymorphic gene system in humans, thus high resolution typing techniques to uncover diversity are recommended before donor search and selection

Close collaboration between the TC and registry, as well as HLA matching prediction algorithms, are critical

An unrelated donor matched for HLA-A, -B, -C, -DRB1 (+/- -DQB1) is the gold standard

In mismatched donors, evidence for selection of a particular locus or an allelic compared to antigenic mismatch is conflicting

An HLA mismatch may be well-tolerated in certain clinical settings

References

1. Marsh SGE, Parham P, Barber LD. The HLA FactsBook. London: Academic Press; 2000.
2. Lechler RI, Lombardi G, Batchelor JR et al. The molecular basis of alloreactivity. Immunol Today 1990; 11: 83–88.
3. van Rood JJ, Lagaaij EL et al. Permissible mismatches, acceptable mismatches, and tolerance: New trends in decision making. Clin Transpl 1993: 285–292.
4. Tiercy JM, Nicoloso G, Passweg J et al. The probability of identifying a 10/10 HLA allele-matched unrelated donor is highly predictable. Bone Marrow Transplant 2007; 40: 515–522.
5. Hirv K, Bloch K, Fischer M et al. Prediction of duration and success rate of unrelated hematopoietic stem cell donor searches based on the patient's HLA-DRB1 allele and DRB1-DQB1 haplotype frequencies. Bone Marrow Transplant 2009; 44: 433–440.
6. Flomenberg N, Baxter-Lowe LA, Confer D, et al. Impact of HLA class I and class II high-resolution matching on outcomes of unrelated donor bone marrow transplantation: HLA-C mismatching is associated with a strong adverse effect on transplantation outcome. Blood 2004; 104: 1923–1930.

7. Lee SJ, Klein J, Haagenson M et al. High-resolution donor-recipient HLA matching contributes to the success of unrelated donor marrow transplantation. Blood 2007; 110: 4576–4583.
8. Arora M, Weisdorf DJ, Spellman SR et al. HLA-identical sibling compared with 8/8 matched and mismatched unrelated donor bone marrow transplant for chronic phase chronic myeloid leukemia. J Clin Oncol 2009; 27: 1644–1652.
9. Petersdorf EW, Gooley T, Malkki M, Horowitz M. Clinical significance of donor-recipient HLA matching on survival after myeloablative hematopoietic cell transplantation from unrelated donors. Tissue Antigens 2007; 69 (Suppl 1): 25–30.
10. Morishima Y, Sasazuki T, Inoko H et al. The clinical significance of human leukocyte antigen (HLA) allele compatibility in patients receiving a marrow transplant from serologically HLA-A, HLA-B, and HLA-DR matched unrelated donors. Blood 2002; 99: 4200–4206.
11. Kawase T, Morishima Y, Matsuo K et al. High-risk HLA allele mismatch combinations responsible for severe acute graft-versus-host disease and implication for its molecular mechanism. Blood 2007; 110: 2235–2341.
12. Woolfrey A, Klein JP, Haagenson M et al. HLA-C Antigen mismatch is associated with worse outcome in unrelated donor peripheral blood stem cell transplantation. Biol Blood Marrow Transplant 2011; 17: 885–892.
13. Petersdorf EW, Anasetti C, Martin PJ et al. Limits of HLA mismatching in unrelated hematopoietic cell transplantation. Blood 2004; 104: 2976–2980.
14. Shaw BE, Arguello R, Garcia-Sepulveda CA, Madrigal JA. The impact of HLA genotyping on survival following unrelated donor haematopoietic stem cell transplantation. Br J Haematol 2010; 150: 251–258.
15. Shaw BE, Mayor NP, Russell NH et al. Diverging effects of HLA-DPB1 matching status on outcome following unrelated donor transplantation depending on disease stage and the degree of matching for other HLA alleles. Leukemia 2010; 24: 58–65.
16. Shaw BE, Russell NH, Devereux S et al. The impact of donor factors on primary non-engraftment in recipients of reduced intensity conditioned transplants from unrelated donors. Haematologica 2005; 90: 1562–1569.
17. Tiercy JM, Passweg J, van Biezen A et al. Isolated HLA-C mismatches in unrelated donor transplantation for CML. Bone Marrow Transplant 2004; 34: 249–255.
18. Kawase T, Matsuo K, Kashiwase K et al. HLA mismatch combinations associated with decreased risk of relapse: Implications for the molecular mechanism. Blood 2009; 113: 2851–2858.
19. Morishima Y, Kawase T, Malkki M, Petersdorf EW. Effect of HLA-A2 allele disparity on clinical outcome in hematopoietic cell transplantation from unrelated donors. Tissue Antigens 2007; 69 (Suppl 1): 31–35.
20. Ferrara GB, Bacigalupo A, Lamparelli T et al. Bone marrow transplantation from unrelated donors: The impact of mismatches with substitutions at position 116 of the human leukocyte antigen class I heavy chain. Blood 2001; 98: 3150–3155.
21. Fleischhauer K, Zino E, Mazzi B et al. Peripheral blood stem cell allograft rejection mediated by CD4(+) T lymphocytes recognizing a single mismatch at HLA-DP beta 1*0901. Blood 2001; 98: 1122–1126.

22. Zino E, Frumento G, Marktel S et al. A T-cell epitope encoded by a subset of HLA-DPB1 alleles determines nonpermissive mismatches for hematologic stem cell transplantation. Blood 2004; 103: 1417–1424.

23. Crocchiolo R, Zino E, Vago L et al. Nonpermissive HLA-DPB1 disparity is a significant independent risk factor for mortality after unrelated hematopoietic stem cell transplantation. Blood 2009; 114: 1437–1444.

24. Pegram HJ, Ritchie DS, Smyth MJ et al. Alloreactive natural killer cells in hematopoietic stem cell transplantation. Leuk Res 2011; 35: 14–21.

25. Dickinson AM. Non-HLA genetics and predicting outcome in HSCT. Int J Immunogenet 2008; 35: 375–380.

26. Spaapen R, Mutis T. Targeting haematopoietic-specific minor histocompatibility antigens to distinguish graft-versus-tumour effects from graft-versus-host disease. Best Pract Res Clin Haematol 2008; 21: 543–557.

27. Penack O, Holler E, van den Brink MR. Graft-versus-host disease: Regulation by microbe-associated molecules and innate immune receptors. Blood 2010; 115: 1865–1872.

Multiple Choice Questionnaire

To find the correct answer, go to http://www.esh.org/online-training/handbook/

1. HLA Class II molecules are found on the following cell types:
a) All nucleated cells ☐
b) B-cells ☐
c) Immune cells ☐
d) T-cells ☐

2. The phenomenon where certain alleles occur together more frequently than would be expected by chance is termed:
a) Haplotype ☐
b) Linkage disequilibrium ☐
c) Phenotype ☐
d) Stochastic recombination ☐

3. A "permissive" mismatch means that:
a) The mismatch causes fewer clinical problems than expected ☐
b) The mismatch is antigenic ☐
c) The mismatch can only be recognised by high-resolution typing techniques ☐

d) The mismatch is non-functional... ☐

---

4. **The HLA locus with the least clinic evidence for the importance of matching on clinical outcome is:**
   a) HLA-A.. ☐
   b) HLA-C.. ☐
   c) HLA-DRB1 .... ☐
   d) HLA-DQB1 .... ☐

---

5. **Mismatching for the following locus has been associated with a reduction in disease relapse:**
   a) HLA-A.. ☐
   b) HLA-B.. ☐
   c) HLA-DRB1 .... ☐
   d) HLA-DPB1 .... ☐

✳ CHAPTER 6

Choice of the donor according to HLA typing and stem cell source

Eliane Gluckman

1. Introduction

Allogeneic haematopoietic stem cell transplantation (allo-HSCT) is widely used to treat patients with malignant and non-malignant haematological disorders. Initially, the principal source of HSCs was bone marrow (BM) from an HLA-identical sibling for transplantation in children and young adults. Subsequently, the choice of donors and the sources of HSCs have enlarged, extending transplant indications to more patients, especially adults. Today, transplant physicians must choose among stem cell sources between bone marrow, granulocyte colony-stimulating factor (G-CSF)-mobilised peripheral blood stem cells (PBSC), or umbilical cord blood (UCB). The donor can be an HLA identical sibling, an matched unrelated donor (MUD), a haploidentical family peripheral blood stem cell (PBSC) or bone marrow donor or, an HLA-mismatched unrelated UCB donor.

2. Use of different cell sources for HSCT in Europe

Baldomero et al. performed an EBMT survey of HSCT activity in 2009 and analysed the trends over the previous 5 years (1, 2). They collected reports of 31,322 HSCT from 624 centres from 43 countries of which 28,033 were first transplants (41% allogeneic and 59% autologous). The main indications were leukaemias (31%; 92% allogeneic), lymphomas (58%; 12% allogeneic), solid tumours (5%; 6% allogeneic) and non-malignant disorders (6%; 88% allogeneic). For allogeneic HSCT there were more unrelated than HLA-identical sibling donors (51% vs 43%). The proportion of peripheral blood as stem cell source was 99% for autologous and 71% for allogeneic HSCT. Unrelated cord blood was used in 756 cases (7%). For further details, see the EBMT activity survey at *www.ebmt.org*. Figure 1 shows World Marrow Donor Association (WMDA) data on the use of different stem cell sources worldwide.

3. Choice of the stem cell source

Traditionally, haematopoietic stem cells were harvested from the posterior iliac crests under general anaesthesia. More recently, mobilised peripheral blood stem cells (PBSC) have been increasingly used in both auto- and allo-HSCT. Mobilisation of haematopoietic stem cells to the peripheral blood in sufficient numbers can be achieved by the classical administration of growth factors such as G-CSF (allo-HSCT) and/or myelosuppressive chemotherapy (auto-HSCT). Unmanipulated cord blood (CB) cells collected and cryopreserved at birth have been used both in related and unrelated HLA-matched and mismatched allogeneic transplants in children, and more recently in adults. Comparison of the yield of various cell sources is given in Table 1.

In all cases, safety of the donor is the major concern meaning that the pre-collection work-up should be particularly meticulous, and should be performed by

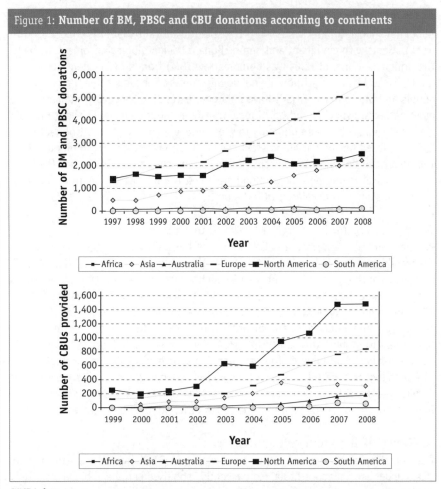

Figure 1: **Number of BM, PBSC and CBU donations according to continents**

WMDA data

a trained experienced doctor. Informed consent must be fully and deeply explained, and all the risks must be discussed. In some countries, this medical examination is performed by a different medical team (e.g. anaesthetists). All possible medical contraindications must be looked for and no risk should be taken however great is the need of the patient. In some countries a special procedure is applied for child donors. It is a requirement to establish a central reporting system to collect adverse events and long-term follow-up of the donors (3, 4).

Table 1: **Number of cells according to stem cell source**				
	Volume collected	Med CD34 content	Med CD3 content	Target cell dose
Bone marrow	10–20 mL/kg	$2-3 \times 10^6$/kg*	25×10^6/kg	$>2 \times 10^8$ TNC/kg
Peripheral blood	150–400 mL	8×10^6/kg	250×10^6/kg	$5-10 \times 10^6$ CD34+/kg
Umbilical cord blood	80–160 mL	0.2×10^6/kg	2.5×10^6/kg	$>3 \times 10^7$ TNC/kg

per kg recipient body weight

3.1 HLA identical sibling bone marrow transplant
When available, this is the preferred source of HSCs; typically bone marrow cells are harvested under general anaesthesia in the posterior iliac crest. There are no contraindications related to age; collections have been performed at all ages from a few months to elderly adults. As long as general anaesthesia can be given. The yield is better in young children and adults and decreases with age. The volume of collection must be adjusted to the donor and recipient weight but should not exceed 10–20 mL/kg donor body weight. Collection teams should not aspirate a volume more than 5 mL for each aspiration to avoid dilution of the bone marrow with blood. After collection, the bone marrow is filtered and volume reduced and is then infused iv directly to the patient.

3.2 Peripheral blood stem cell transplant
G-CSF mobilised PBSC have been recently used more frequently for HLA identical sibling transplants. The indications for using PBSC rather than BM are not really standardised, but many factors are involved: availability of operating room, lack of personnel to perform bone marrow aspiration, contraindication to general anaesthesia and choice of the donor. Most teams avoid collecting PBSCs in young children because of possible side effects of G-CSF or problems of venous access. According to NMDP, 76% of adult unrelated donors donated G-CSF mobilised PBSC. Severe but rare adverse effects have been observed including splenic rupture and sickle cell crisis. There are no definitive conclusions regarding the long-term effects of G-CSF treatment on healthy donors (4). More recently plerixafor, a novel small molecule antagonist, which reversibly inhibits the interaction of SDF1 and CXCR4, has been used in poor mobilisers with or without G-CSF. It has not been tested in healthy donors (5). Recently biosimilars of G-CSF appeared in the market. In view of the absence of long-term studies their use is not recommended in healthy normal donors (6).

3.3 Haplo-identical related HSCT donors
The number of related haplo-identical donors is increasing, but there are very few large comparative or randomised studies (7, 8).

Historically, the first haplo-identical transplants pioneered by the Perugia group utilised G-CSF mobilised T-cell depleted CD34+ cells. More recently, interesting preliminary data have been reported with new protocols using unmanipulated bone marrow cells or marrow harvested after *in vivo* G-CSF, together with high dose immunosuppression or cyclophosphamide (9–12).

3.4 Matched unrelated HSCT donors

The number of matched unrelated donor transplants has been increasing worldwide, with more than 18 million adult donors registered in Bone Marrow Donor Worldwide (BMDW; *www.bmdw.org*). This collection of HLA phenotypes from bone marrow donor registries and cord blood banks give the opportunity to transplant physicians from around the world to perform preliminary searches through the internet for a preliminary view of the availability of potential suitable donors (Figure 1 and Figure 2).

The annual report of the WMDA (*www.wmda.org*) is a product of the Donor Registries

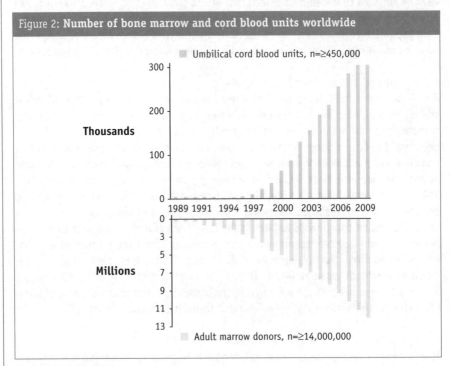

Figure 2: **Number of bone marrow and cord blood units worldwide**

From WMDA and BMDW

Working Group whose mission is to develop guidelines for donor recruitment and maintenance of donor confidentiality, track the efficiency of donor searches and develop consensus standards for the logistics of transporting stem cell products across international borders (13, 14). The standards by which stem cell products are collected and transported result from the collaborative efforts of several organisations represented within the Worldwide Network for Blood and Marrow Transplantation (*www.wbmt.org*). Most often the donors are chosen on the basis of high resolution allelic typing for HLA-A, -B, -C, -DRB1, -DQB1, -DPB1. The best choice is a 9/10 or 10/10 donor. In the case of several potential donors, it is better to recruit a donor who is male, young, ABO matched and CMV negative if the recipient is negative or CMV positive if the recipient is positive. The choice between bone marrow and PBSC depends on donor choice, centre preference and indication for HSCT. It is known that using PBSC gives more GvHD which is favourable in malignant diseases where increasing GvHD decreases the risk of relapse while in non-malignant diseases, especially in aplastic anaemia, it decreases survival (15).

3.5 Cord blood

3.5.1 Cord blood bank organisation

Since the first human cord blood transplant, performed in 1988, cord blood banks have been established worldwide for collection and cryopreservation of cord blood for allogeneic haematopoietic stem cell transplant (16). Today, a global network of cord blood banks and transplant centres has been established and provides a common inventory. Several studies have shown that the number of cells is the most important factor for engraftment, while some degree of HLA mismatch is acceptable (16, 17). The absence of ethical concern and the unlimited supply of cells explains the increasing interest in using cord blood for developing regenerative medicine. Since the first UCBT, more than 20,000 CBT have been reported worldwide and more than 600,000 cord blood units have been stored in more than 100 cord blood banks (*www.bmdw.org, www.nmdp.org*) (18).

The main practical advantages of using cord blood as an alternative source of stem cells are the relative ease of procurement, the absence of risk for mothers and donors, the reduced likelihood of transmitting infections, particularly CMV, and the ability to store fully tested and HLA typed potential transplants in the frozen state, available for immediate use.

Eurocord was established in 1995; its principal objectives were to collect outcomes data provided by cord blood banks and transplant centres. Eurocord has collected, from 1988 to October 2010, 6736 UCBT from Europe and transplant centres in other countries. Five hundred and ninety-six transplants have been reported using related donors (majority HLA identical sibling donors), mainly for children with malignant and non-malignant disorders and 6140 have been performed in the unrelated transplant setting for children (n=3287) and adults (n=2770). In order to promote education and information, Eurocord has launched a new European program entitled: *an On-line CME program in cord blood technology and transplantation* for providing a learning tool on the scientific, technical, clinical, regulatory aspects of cord blood, easily accessible at a time and language convenient for users (*www.eurocord-ed.org*). Based on this international cooperation Eurocord has published crucial reports which have been the basis of the rapid development of cord blood transplant.

Netcord (*www.netcord.org*) was created in 1998 to establish good practices in umbilical cord blood storage, facilitate donor search, improve the quality of the grafts, standardise excellence criteria on an international scale and importantly establish procedures for bank accreditation. The inventory of Netcord, the cooperative network of large experienced UCB banks, currently has more than 300,000 cryopreserved UCB units ready for clinical use for unrelated recipients and more than 8,624 grafts shipped. In the USA, the National Marrow Donor Program (NMDP) has established a similar cord blood bank network. Collaborations between Netcord-Eurocord and NMDP have been established with the goal to provide the most appropriate and high quality cord blood unit for a specific patient. A summary of cord blood banks activity is available at *www.wmda.org* (18). National regulatory agencies and transplant centres are aware of the need of international standards whose major objectives are to promote quality throughout all phases of cord blood banking with the goal to achieve consistent production of high quality placental and umbilical cord blood units for transplantation. All these aspects are detailed in the last version of the Netcord-FACT Standards (*www.factwebsite.org*). As the number of cord blood units is increasing, it appeared that it was necessary to improve the quality of the units for cost-efficient management of the banks. The optimal number of cord blood units is not really known but should approach 9 *per* 10,000 inhabitants. Most banks prefer to bank only the largest units of more than 70 mL in order to obtain at least 3×10^7 nucleated cells/kg recipient bodyweight.

3.5.2 Criteria for cord blood donor choice

In several studies including Eurocord, neutrophil and platelet recovery were associated with the degree of HLA mismatch, the number of total nucleated cells (TNC) collected and infused and the use of G-CSF after transplant. Coexistence of HLA class I and II disparities and high CD34+ cell dose in the graft were associated with only with more severe GvHD grade III-IV. Disease relapse was higher in matched transplants, showing a graft versus leukaemia effect (17–20).

General considerations:

- Current HLA definition in cord blood banks is based on HLA serological typing for -A and -B and allelic typing for HLA-DRB1. Avoid cord blood units with 3 or 4 HLA disparities.
- At selection, diagnosis and presence of patient HLA antibodies against the HLA antigens of the cord blood unit should be considered. HLA compatibility appears to be more important for patients with non-malignant disorders than for those with malignant disorders.
- If the criterion for the minimum number of cells for a single UCB transplantation is not achieved, a double cord blood transplantation should be considered.
- CFU-GM and viability are generally not used for donor selection.
- Cell dose requirements must increase with the number of HLA mismatches.

Cord blood units with 6/6 or 5/6 HLA match. HLA-A or HLA-B mismatches are preferable to DRB1 mismatches.
In malignant disorders:
- Nucleated cell dose:
  - at freezing, the cell dose should be >2.5 to 3.0 x 10^7/kg
  - after thawing, the cell dose should be >2.0 to 2.5 x 10^7/kg.
- CD34+ cell dose: at freezing or after thawing, the dose should be approximately 1.2 to 1.7 x 10^5/kg.
- Based on Eurocord unpublished and preliminary data, it seems likely that HLA-DRB1 mismatch may lead to high graft-versus-leukaemia (GvL) effect in patients transplanted in non-remission (but there is also a greater risk of GvHD).
In non-malignant disorders:
- Higher total and CD34+ cell dose is requested, and HLA match is preferable.

Cord blood units with 4/6 HLA match. HLA-A or HLA-B mismatches are better than HLA-DRB1 mismatches.
In malignant disorders:
- Nucleated cell dose:
  - at freezing >3.5 x 10^7/kg
  - after thawing >3.0 x 10^7/kg.
- CD34+ cell dose: at freezing or after thawing, approximately >1.7 x 10^5/kg
- HLA-DRB1 mismatch may lead to a high GvL effect in advanced phase of the diseases.
In non-malignant disorders:
- Nucleated cell dose:
  - at freezing, minimum cell dose 4 to 5 x 10^7/kg

- after thawing, minimum 3.5×10^7/kg.
- CD34+ cell dose: no available data, but should be higher than 2 to 2.5×10^5/kg.

CB units with 3/6 HLA match. Should be avoided, but in extremely severe cases may be considered for patients with malignant disorders; a high nucleated cell dose should be given. Not recommended for patients with non-malignant disorders.

Other considerations:
- If several cord blood units are available that fit the above criteria, the following should be taken into consideration:
  - Cord blood bank accreditation status and location
  - ABO compatibility
  - Allele HLA typing of HLA-A and -B
  - Other HLA factors such as HLA-C, high resolution HLA typing, NIMA; KIR are under study and cannot be used at this stage for donor choice.
- Double cord blood transplants can be recommended if the cell dose is insufficient with a single CBU. The total dose of both combined units should be at least 3×10^7 TNC/kg. HLA matching between the 2 units and the recipient must be as matched as possible but no firm recommendation can be given. Note that double cord transplant gives a good engraftment and survival with more GvHD and less relapse than single cord blood transplant.

4. Comparison between stem cell sources and algorithm for donor search

4.1 Bone marrow compared to PBSC
An EBMT-initiated prospective randomised trial that involved 350 patients with standard-risk leukaemia compared HLA identical sibling BM to PBSC and showed that the incidence of grades II-IV acute GvHD was significantly higher in patients who underwent PBSCT. There was a higher incidence of chronic GvHD after PBSCT (21). On the other hand, there were no significant differences in overall survival or leukaemia-free survival between the BMT and PBSCT groups at the 3-year follow-up (5).
A large retrospective International Bone Marrow Transplant Registry (IBMTR) and EBMT registry analysis involving 824 patients revealed the following data: the incidence of chronic GvHD at 1 year was significantly higher in patients after PBSCT, and treatment-related mortality rates and leukaemia-free survival rates were in favour of PBSCT in patients in advanced stages of leukaemia. A later retrospective EBMT

registry analysis of 3465 adult patients with AML and ALL again revealed a higher incidence of chronic GvHD after PBSCT. However, rates of acute GvHD, leukaemia-free survival and overall survival were similar after BMT and PBSCT (5).

In aplastic anaemia, 3 studies with HLA identical siblings or matched unrelated donors have shown that PBSC gave more GvHD and decreased survival (22, 23). Despite these results the number of PBSCT is increasing steadily. There are many possible reasons, including preference of the centres, since the logistics of organising PBSC collection are easier than organising bone marrow collection with general anesthaesia. One main reason advocated by the centres is donor safety, but a recent report on over 50,000 donations for PBSC in Europe documented a significantly higher rate of severe adverse events with PBSC collection, 10.76 per 10,000 donations for PBSC compared with 4.32 per 10,000 donations for BM. Fatalities were also higher, though not significantly, in PBSC versus BM donors (4 versus 1 fatality) (5).

4.2 HLA identical siblings versus matched unrelated transplants

To determine whether the risks of allogeneic transplantation are different when the donor is a fully matched unrelated donor based on 10/10 HLA alleles compared to an HLA-identical sibling, Woolfrey et al. performed a retrospective analysis of 1448 patients with high-risk or advanced haematologic malignancies given T-replete grafts after myeloablative conditioning. No statistically differences were found between the two groups in survival, disease-free survival and non-relapse mortality for patients with high-risk disease or those given bone marrow as a graft source. However, for patients with intermediate-risk disease receiving peripheral blood grafts, they observed higher non-relapse mortality and lower overall survival in the 10/10 MUD compared to matched sibling donors (24). A prospective French study showed no statistically significant difference between MUD and HLA matched sibling donors. The Essen group performed the same study in 101 patients who were given either a 10/10 MUD or a HLA identical sibling transplant and did not find any difference in survival. In both studies MUD transplant gave more GvHD. These studies show that use of a HLA 10/10 MUD is a good option when an HLA identical sibling donor is unavailable. A higher degree of HLA mismatches, 9 or 8/10, is often used but there are no strong data to suggest what mismatches are acceptable.

4.3 Cord blood versus unrelated bone marrow transplant

In children, with malignant diseases, two studies have compared the outcome of unrelated UCBT and BMT (25, 26). Eurocord published a study comparing the outcome of matched unrelated BMT (HLA 6 out of 6), either unmanipulated or T-depleted, with that of mismatched UCBT. Results showed that after UCBT, engraftment was delayed, GvHD was reduced similarly to T-cell depleted BMT and there was no difference in relapse or in leukaemia-free survival. Eapen et al. for the CIBMTR and the New York Cord Blood Bank (NYCBB) compared the outcomes of 503 children with acute leukaemia given an unrelated mismatched UCBT with 282 unrelated BM transplant recipients. HLA allele-mismatched BM recipients had more acute and chronic GvHD without decreasing leukaemia-free survival (LFS). Importantly, they found that even using an allele-matched BM donor, LFS was not statistically different from one or 2 HLA disparate UCBT and that an HLA-matched UCBT recipient had better outcomes compared to HLA allele-matched BM recipients. However, an increased transplant related mortality was observed in children transplanted with a low CB cell dose (<3 x 10^7/kg) and a 1 HLA disparate CB graft or in children given a 2 HLA disparate UCBT, independently of the cell dose infused. Interestingly, use of 2 HLA mismatched UCBT was associated with a lower incidence of relapse (27). The same studies were performed in adults with malignancies. Eurocord compared adults with acute leukaemia receiving either a matched unrelated bone marrow transplant (HLA 6 out of 6) or a mismatched cord blood transplant. Results showed that, despite a delay of engraftment, UCBT gave a similar leukaemia-free survival to BMT. In the same issue of the journal, CIBMTR and NYCBB showed that, in adults with malignancies, UCBT gave the same LFS survival as 1 antigen mismatched unrelated bone marrow transplant (UBMT) (25, 26). At the same time, a Japanese study showed that CBT gave better results than matched unrelated bone marrow transplants. In a meta-analysis, combining these published studies, 161 children and 316 adults undergoing UCBT, along with 316 children and 996 adults undergoing UBMT were analysed. T-cell–depleted UBMT was excluded where data were available, and only fully matched UBMT was used in the analysis. Pooled comparisons of studies of UCBT and UBMT in children found that the incidence of chronic GvHD was lower with UCBT, but the incidence of grade III–IV acute GvHD did not differ. There was no difference in 2-year overall survival in children when studies were pooled. For adults, transplantation-related mortality (TRM) and LFS were not statistically different.

Recently, Eurocord and CIBMTR performed a study comparing the outcome of unrelated HLA-matched or 1-2 antigen mismatched bone marrow (n=364) or G-CSF mobilised peripheral blood (n=728) with that of mismatched cord blood transplant (n=148) in adults with acute leukaemia. In multivariate analysis, TRM was higher after UCBT, but relapse rate and GvHD were lower, resulting in the same LFS compared to the other sources of stem cells (Figure 3) (28, 29). The results of these comparative studies and the meta-analysis (30), gathered together, showed that UCBT is feasible in adults when a cord blood unit contains a high number of cells and should be considered an option as an allogeneic stem cell source for patients lacking a HLA-matched bone marrow donor; despite increased HLA disparity, UCB

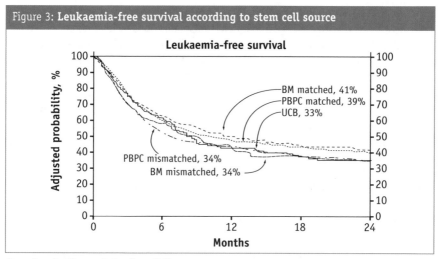

Figure 3: **Leukaemia-free survival according to stem cell source**

Reproduced with permission from (29)

from unrelated donors offers sufficiently promising results compared with matched UBMT in adults with haematological malignancies leading to the conclusion, as in children, that the donor search process for BM and UCB from unrelated donors should be started simultaneously, especially in patients with acute leukaemia, where the time factor is crucial (30, 31).

Further improvement has been obtained by the use of double cord blood transplant and of reduced intensity conditioning regimens (31).

These papers were the hallmark of the worldwide development of cord blood transplant as they clearly demonstrated that cord blood transplant could be used in adults as well as in children, and furthermore showed that unrelated mismatched cord blood transplant gave the same results as a HLA matched unrelated bone marrow transplant.

4.4 Related haploidentical transplants compared to other sources of hematopoietic stem cells

There are very few publications on the long-term results of haploidentical related transplants. Although the technology has changed over the years, large randomised studies are needed. Retrospective comparative studies show that early results are comparable to other sources of cells but long-term results are not available. Leung et al. evaluated 190 children with very high-risk leukaemia who underwent allogeneic haematopoietic cell transplantation in two sequential treatment eras to determine whether those treated with contemporary protocols had a lower risk of relapse or toxic death and whether non-HLA identical transplantations yielded poorer outcomes (32). For the recent cohorts, 5-year overall survival rates were 65% for the 37 patients with ALL and 74% for patients with AML. These rates compared favourably with those of earlier cohorts (28% and 34% respectively). The recent improvement was observed regardless of the cell source (5-yr OS for matched sibling transplants 70 versus 24%, MUD 61 versus 37% and haploidentical 88 versus 19%). This improvement was attributable to a reduction in infections, in regimen-related toxicity and in leukaemia-related death. Survival probability was dependent on leukaemia status and minimal residual disease. The authors conclude that with the improvement of results over time, bone marrow transplantation should be considered for all children with very high-risk leukaemia regardless of matched donor availability.

5. Algorithm of donor choice and conclusion (see Figure 4)

- Results of allogeneic HSCT have been markedly improving over time, due to a better expertise of the centres, better supportive care and better prevention and treatment of infections.

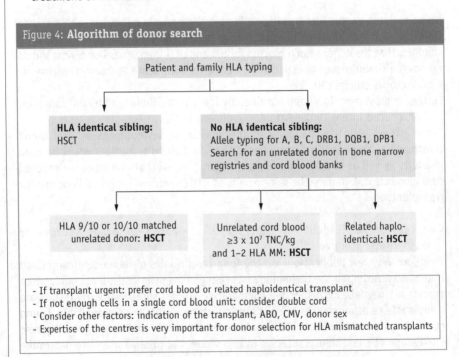

Figure 4: **Algorithm of donor search**

Patient and family HLA typing

HLA identical sibling:
HSCT

No HLA identical sibling:
Allele typing for A, B, C, DRB1, DQB1, DPB1
Search for an unrelated donor in bone marrow registries and cord blood banks

HLA 9/10 or 10/10 matched unrelated donor: **HSCT**

Unrelated cord blood ≥3 x 10^7 TNC/kg and 1–2 HLA MM: **HSCT**

Related haplo-identical: **HSCT**

- If transplant urgent: prefer cord blood or related haploidentical transplant
- If not enough cells in a single cord blood unit: consider double cord
- Consider other factors: indication of the transplant, ABO, CMV, donor sex
- Expertise of the centres is very important for donor selection for HLA mismatched transplants

- Indications have increased because of the diminution of transplant-related mortality due to reduced intensity conditioning adapted to disease status and co-morbidities.
- Choice of donor source has extended the possibility of offering HSCT to almost all patients who need a transplant. The major recent advances are due to the use of HLA mismatched transplant using either cord blood or haplo-identical family donors.
- Choice of donor source is dependent on the indication for HSCT, its urgency, the age of the patient, and the expertise and resources of the centre.
- HLA mismatched HSCT (haplo-mismatched or cord blood) should be performed in experienced centres. Centres who perform these transplants must report the outcomes to international registries in order to evaluate results.
- Transplant centres, transplant coordinators and the cell therapy laboratory should work very closely with bone marrow registries and cord blood banks in order to find the best possible donor source for each patient.

References

1. Gratwohl H, Baldomero H, Aljurf M et al. Hematopoietic stem cell transplantation. A global perspective. JAMA 2010; 303: 1617–1624.
2. Baldomero H, Gratwohl M, Gratwohl A et al. The EBMT activity survey 2009: Trends over the past 5 years. Bone Marrow Transplant 2011; 46: 485–501.
3. Halter J, Kodera Y, Ispizua AU et al. Severe events in donors after allogeneic hematopoietic donation. Haematologica 2009; 94: 94–101.
4. Shaw AU, Ball L, Beksac M et al. Donor safety: The role of the WMDA in ensuring the safety of volunteer unrelated donors: Clinical and ethical considerations. Bone Marrow Transplant 2010; 45: 832–838.
5. Korbling M, Freireich EJ. 25 years of peripheral blood stem cell transplantation. Blood 2011; 117: 6411–6416.
6. Shaw BE, Confer DL, Hwang WY et al. Concerns about the use of biosimilar granulocyte colony-stimulating factors for the mobilization of stem cells in normal donors: Position of the World Marrow Donor Association. Haematologica 2011; 96: 942–947.
7. Ballen KK, Spitzer TR. The great debate: Haploidentical or cord blood transplant. Bone Marrow Transplant 2011; 46: 323–329.
8. Barrett J, Gluckman E, Handgretinger R, Madrigal A. Point-counterpoint haploidentical family donors versus cord blood transplantation. Biol Blood Marrow Transplant 2011; 17 (Suppl 1): S89–93.
9. Tuve A, Gayoso J, Scheid C et al. Haploidentical bone marrow transplantation with post grafting cyclophosphamide multicenter experience with an alternative salvage strategy. Leukemia 2011; 25: 880–883.
10. XJ Huang, YJ Chang. Unmanipulated HLA-mismatched/haploidentical blood and marrow hematopoietic stem cell transplantation. Biol Blood Marrow Transplant 2011; 17: 197–204.

11. Leung W, Campana D, Yang J et al. High success rate of hematopoietic cell transplantation regardless of donor source in children with very-high-risk leukemia. Blood 2011; 118: 223–230.

12. Lee KH, Lee JH, Lee JH et al. Reduced intensity conditioning therapy with busulfan, fludarabine and antithymocyte globulin for HLA-haploidentical hematopoietic cell transplantation in acute leukemia and myelodysplastic syndrome. Blood 2011; 118: 2609–2617.

13. Petersdorf EW. The world Marrow Donor Association: 20 years of international collaboration for the support of unrelated donor and cord blood hematopoietic cell transplantation. Bone Marrow Transplant 2010; 45: 807–810.

14. Foeken L, Green A, Hurley CK, Marry E, Wiegand T, Oudshoorn M, on behalf of the Donor Registries Working group of the World Marrow Donor Association (WMDA). Monitoring the international use of unrelated donors for transplantation: The WMDA annual reports. Bone Marrow Transplant 2010; 45: 811–818.

15. Eapen M, Le Rademacher J, Antin JH et al. Effect of stem cell source on outcomes after adult unrelated donor transplantation in severe aplastic anemia. Blood 2011; 118: 2618–2621.

16. Gluckman E, Ruggeri A, Volt F et al. Milestones in umbilical cord blood transplantation. Br J Haematol 2011; 154: 441–447.

17. Gluckman E, Rocha V, Arcese W et al. Factors associated with outcomes of unrelated cord blood transplant: Guidelines for donor choice. Exp Hematol 2004; 32: 397–407.

18. Welte K, Foeken L, Gluckman E, Navarrete C. International exchange of cord blood units: The registry aspects. Bone Marrow Transplant 45: 825–831, 2010.

19. Barker JN, Byam C, Scaradavou A. How we search: A guide to the selection and acquisition of unrelated cord blood grafts. Blood 2011; 117: 3277–3285.

20. Barker JN, Scaradavou A, Stevens CE. Combined effect of total nucleated cell dose and HLA match on transplantation outcome in 1061 cord blood recipients with hematologic malignancies. Blood 2010; 115: 1843–1849.

21. Schrenzenmeier H, Passweg J, Marsh J et al. Worse outcome and more chronic GVHD with peripheral blood progenitor cells than bone marrow in HLA-matched sibling donor transplants for young patients with severe acquired aplastic anemia. Blood 2007; 110: 1397–1400.

22. Chu R, Brazauskas R, Kan F et al. Comparison of outcomes after transplantation of G-CSF stimulated bone marrow grafts versus bone marrow or peripheral blood grafts from HLA identical siblings donors for patients with severe aplastic anemia. Biol Blood Marrow Transplant 2011; 17: 1018–1024.

23. Bacigalupo A. Back to the OR? Blood 118: 2386.

24. Woolfrey A, Lee SJ, Gooley TA et al. HLA-allele matched unrelated donors compared to HLA matched sibling donors: Role of cell source and disease risk category. Biol Blood Marrow Transplant 2010; 16: 1362–1367.

25. Rocha V, Labopin M, Sanz G et al. Transplants of umbilical-cord blood or bone marrow from unrelated donors in adults with acute leukemia. N Engl J Med 2004; 351: 2276–2285.

26. Laughlin MJ, Eapen M, Rubinstein P et al. Outcomes after transplantation of cord blood or bone marrow from unrelated donors in adults with leukemia. N Engl J Med 2004; 351: 2265–2275.
27. Eapen M, Rubinstein P, Zhang MJ et al. Outcomes of transplantation of unrelated donor umbilical cord blood and bone marrow in children with acute leukaemia: A comparison study. Lancet 2007; 369: 1947–1954.
28. Eapen M, Rocha V, Sanz G et al. on behalf of the center for International Blood and Marrow Transplant Research, the Acute Leukemia Working Party and Eurocord (the European Group for Blood and Marrow Transplantation) and the National Cord Blood program of the New York Blood Center. Effect of graft source on unrelated donor haematopoietic stem-cell transplantation in adults with acute leukemia: A retrospective analysis. Lancet Oncol 2010; 11: 653–660.
29. Eapen M, Rocha V, Sanz G et al. Effect of graft source on unrelated donor haematopoietic stem-cell transplantation in adults with adult leukaemia: A retrospective analysis. Lancet Oncol 2010; 11: 653–660.
30. Hwang WY, Samuel M, Tan D et al. A meta analysis of unrelated donor cord blood transplantation versus unrelated donor bone marrow transplantation in adult and pediatric patients. Biol Blood Marrow Transplant 2007; 13: 444–453.
31. Brunstein CG, Fuchs EJ, Carter SL et al. Alternative donor transplantation after reduced intensity conditioning: Results of parallel phase 2 trials using partially HLA-mismatched related bone marrow or unrelated double umbilical cord blood grafts. Blood 2011; 118: 282–288.
32. Leung W, Campana D, Yang J et al. High success rate of hematopoietic cell transplantation regardless of donor source in children with very high risk leukemia. Blood 2011; 118: 223–230.

Multiple Choice Questionnaire

To find the correct answer, go to http://www.esh.org/online-training/handbook/

1. **In recent years use of peripheral blood progenitor cells has surpassed bone marrow for allogeneic haematopoietic stem cell transplantation in Europe:**
   a) True . . . . ☐
   b) False . . . . ☐

2. **Peripheral blood progenitor cell collections are associated with which of the following:**
   a) Bone pain . . . . ☐

b) Splenic rupture.. ☐
c) Haematoma... ☐
d) All of the above... ☐

3. **The following characteristics are considered when selecting a cord blood unit for transplantation:**
   a) Allele-level HLA typing at class I and II .... ☐
   b) Cell viability.. ☐
   c) Total nucleated cell dose per kilogram of patient body weight........... ☐
   d) b + c .... ☐

4. **A 35 year old gentleman with acute lymphoblastic leukemia experiences an on-therapy bone marrow relapse. He achieves a second complete remission after re-induction chemotherapy. He does not have a matched sibling and you decide the best treatment option for this gentleman is an unrelated donor transplantation. He has an adult unrelated donor who is HLA-matched at -A, -B, -C, -DRB1 and -DP1. He also has a cord blood unit with adequate total nucleated cell dose/kg and mismatched at 1-locus (5/6 HLA-matched). The waiting period to procure the adult donor graft is 3 months. Which of the donor sources would you choose for this patient?**
   a) Matched unrelated adult donor.................................... ☐
   b) Mismatched cord blood unit .... ☐

5. **Compared to bone marrow, peripheral blood stem cell transplant gives:**
   a) Better engraftment .... ☐
   b) Less GvHD .... ☐
   c) More relapse... ☐
   d) Better survival .... ☐

NOTES

✳ CHAPTER 7

Bone marrow donor registries and cord blood banks

Carlheinz Mueller, Sergio Querol

1. Introduction

In most countries where an allogeneic HSCT is a therapeutic procedure available to most patients in need, families have been so small for many decades that an HLA-identical sibling donor is available for fewer than a third of the patients. Hence the vast majority of patients have to rely on alternatives: peripheral blood stem cells (PBSC) or bone marrow (BM) from adult unrelated donors (AUDs) or frozen umbilical cord blood units (CBUs). In no other field of medicine is the fate of almost half of the patients so dependent on an efficient international collaboration. In 2010, 46% of all HSCT from AUDs involved a donor from outside the patient's country. The percentage of international unrelated HSCT has been continuously growing for many years in spite of growing national donor registries in most active countries and the presence of large evolving countries with little external interaction, both factors which decrease the percentage of international transplants.

This chapter will describe the organisational framework involved in providing unrelated stem cells and the procedures leading to obtaining a suitable graft. The complex decision tree between the three types of stem cell product and the choice between different available donors or units have been discussed in the two preceding chapters.

2. Institutions involved

Although the management of AUDs and publicly available CBUs varies between and even within countries, certain structures and functional entities are always present (see Figure 1 for a functional overview). Several, or even all, of them may exist under the roof of a single organisation, e.g. within a university or hospital, but more often are found in independent but closely collaborating institutions.

In the ideal case, a Registry is the single point of access to all AUDs and CBUs units in a region or country. It collects the relevant data from the inventories of its affiliated donor centres and cord blood banks into a single file and maintains an adequate administrative and IT infrastructure to facilitate the search process. In particular, it provides lists of suitable AUDs and/or CBUs to requesting organisations, manages the flow of information for all subsequent activities in the donor search processes and takes care of the related invoices and payments. Reflecting its central role, the registry is often also designated as the (national) hub.

A Search Unit (SU) operating within or on behalf of a Transplant Centre (TC) accesses the registry for national patients. The SU staff are in close contact with the transplant physicians responsible for the patient and the local HLA laboratory and they trigger all actions aiming at the identification of a suitable AUD or CBU. At the other end of the network, there are the providers of the stem cell sources, either the donor centres for AUDs or the cord blood banks for CBUs.

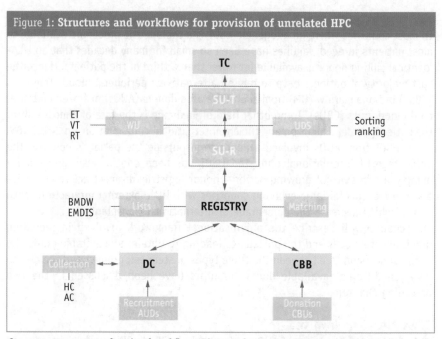

Figure 1: Structures and workflows for provision of unrelated HPC

Grey: structures; green: functional workflows. TC: transplant centre; SU-T: Search Unit interface at the Transplant Centre; SU-R: Search Unit interface at the Registry; UDS: unrelated donor search process including donor selection strategies; WU: workup usually accomplishing Extended Typing (ET), Verification Typing (VT) and Releasing Tests (RT); Registry: site of access to the donors (typically a national hub) including listing and matching algorithms; DC: donor centre for adult unrelated donors (AUDs) including affiliated collection units for bone marrow (Harvesting Centres, HC) or Mobilised Peripheral Blood (Apheresis Centres, AC); CBB: cord blood bank for cord blood units (CBUs)

The Donor Centre (DC) is responsible for recruiting new donors including generating the publicity required, obtaining the informed consent of interested volunteers and registering their personal and search relevant data (typically age and gender, CMV status, blood group, previous pregnancies). It will subsequently get back to the donors at reasonable intervals to keep them informed, motivated and contactable for the moment when they are needed. Upon the request of the SU the DC performs subsequent tests on a donor or provides a fresh blood sample to the SU's lab for further testing.

Eventually, the donation takes place in an Apheresis Centre (AC) for PBSC or in a Harvest Centre (HC) for BM. The Work-Up (WU) leading to the stem cell harvest is a fairly complex process designed to ensure a maximum of safety for both donors and patients. Therefore in particular the DC and the AC/HC have to formally define their interaction and to agree upon the delineation of their responsibilities. In many countries, all communication between the DC and the TC in the WU and transplant process has to go via the national hub, in particular for details of the harvest and transport of the product.

The Cord Blood Bank (CBB) is a multidisciplinary structure that is responsible for the recruitment and subsequent management of donors/mothers as well as the collection, processing, testing, cryopreservation, storage, listing, reservation, release, and distribution of CBUs. It is typically affiliated to a registry. To achieve these functions CBBs are usually divided into three different areas:

- Collection
- Manufacturing including processing, testing and storing
- Provision and release of the CBUs to TCs.

Finally, the cord blood bank is also responsible for evaluating clinical outcomes to ascertain that the units shipped for transplantation are safe and potent (see (1) and (2) for comprehensive reviews).

3. The search process

In the vast majority of cases, an HLA-identical sibling is regarded as the best option for an allogeneic transplant. Hence, a complete and unsuccessful donor search in the core family should always precede the search for an AUD or CBU, both called unrelated donor search (UDS) below. Moreover, the patient's HLA type must be confirmed using a second (blood) sample before UDS is initiated.

We recommend to start all donor searches not only by consulting the national registry but also Bone Marrow Donors Worldwide (BMDW) to acquire an immediate overview of the AUDs and CBUs globally available. In easier cases, this can help to quickly identify an optimal stem cell source; in more difficult cases HLA expertise and further background knowledge will be required to determine a suitable search strategy. The main questions to be discussed and decided are:

- What are the constraints with regard to duration and cost of this patient's search?
- What is a realistic target for the level of the HLA compatibility of an AUD and where should the line be drawn for accepting a mismatched donor?
- Which options exist for a single or double cord graft, taking into account the cell counts, degree of matching and the patient's weight?

The main subsequent steps in the search process are further tests to exclude donors unsuitable for the transplant or to collect other supplementary information to prioritise the donors still under consideration. These tests primarily address the HLA system and, more recently, also other genetic systems but also check markers for infectious diseases or acquired immunity. For reasons of cost and efficiency, a laboratory commissioned by the DC should perform requests of the SU whenever the chance of exclusion of the donor is high, i.e. if the patient has a rare variant many donors will need to be tested to find a suitable one and it is more efficient for testing to be done by the DC than to ask for CT samples of each and every candidate. Moreover, the number of donors requested simultaneously for further testing should take into account the chance of a favourable outcome of each test.

At the end of the donor selection process, one set of blood samples is sent to the laboratory of the SU in order to finally ensure the suitability of the donor under consideration. This process has been called confirmatory typing (CT) but the terminology has been revised recently to address its two major aspects separately: *extended typing* means refining the HLA assignments by adding more loci or typing known ones at higher resolution while *verification typing* means repeating the HLA typing to ensure the identity of the stem cell source by using a fresh sample from an AUD or an attached segment for a CBU.

4. National and international search systems

BMDW is a database with the HLA phenotypes of AUDs and more comprehensive information on CBUs from practically all registries and CBBs accessible for international transplants worldwide. BMDW is operated by the Dutch registry, Europdonor, in Leiden. In mid 2011, 66 registries from 47 countries, and 48 CBBs from 28 countries were listed on BMDW with a total number of 17.5M donors and over 0.5M CBUs. Most contributors update their data at monthly intervals. BMDW provides access to these data via a password-protected search tool on the web, providing lists of matched or acceptably mismatched AUDs or CBUs based on a patient's HLA phenotype. Access is granted to all persons/institutions involved in donor searches and access requests are to be sent to the national registry or, where no such exists, to the BMDW office in Leiden. More details can be found at *www.bmdw.org*.

First introduced in Europe, the European Marrow Donor Information System (EMDIS) is now a network connecting the computer systems of 26 registries with AUDs and CBUs on 5 continents. Typically, for every new patient requiring an international search, an EMDIS registry broadcasts the search request to all partners and receives their adequately matched AUDs and/or CBUs electronically; it can thus present to its users integrated lists based on timely information from the national and international inventories. Any subsequent activity can be triggered by no more than a mouse-click. All information pertaining to requests and results travels transparently between the partners ensuring consistent electronic patient files. Although only 40% of the registries are connected via EMDIS, over 80% of international transplant activity takes place between these partners.

As of today, BMDW and EMDIS can be regarded as complementary (3). BMDW is a pure information system easy to access and use by any TC and registry, while EMDIS provides the comprehensive automation of business processes indispensable for today's volume of activity; however EMDIS depends on an adequate national infrastructure.

5. Matching services

The primary end product of BMDW or a national computer system with or without EMDIS integration is a list of potential AUDs or CBUs for a given patient. The responsible management of the search process requires a sound understanding of the composition and internal organisation of these lists. Due to the complexity of the issue and the limited documentation of most systems in terms of matching algorithms, the experience of the users is indispensable. This is of special importance in the EMDIS network, where donors preselected in the computer system of one registry are presented by the matching services of another registry.

Typically, donor lists are shown in groups of ascending number of already identified HLA differences (see (4) for the underlying rationale), but systems vary according to which loci are considered (whether or not HLA-C and/or HLA-DQB1 are included) and to whether allelic (high resolution) differences are recognised and/or counted or not (5). Beyond the donor's identification and HLA, most lists also provide the gender and age of the donor and supplementary information like CMV status, blood group or previous donations. Some systems (like HapLogic™ or OptiMatch® developed by the US and German registries respectively) also include a statistical prognosis for the HLA identity of loci not yet typed at high resolution and use it to prioritise donors on the list (see Figure 2). This substantially helps to identify a fully matched donor or, at least, the donor with the fewest possible mismatches.

Lists of CBUs show a number of distinct features. First, they are generally grouped according to number of HLA differences for HLA-A, -B and -DRB1, where the former two are evaluated at serological or low-resolution level but for HLA-DRB1 all allelic differences are counted. Second, they provide important additional information, in particular the counts of nucleated cells (TNC) and of CD34+ cells. Either of these can be the primary sorting criterion within groups of equal HLA matching level. Ideally, an online system also provides a link to the detailed CBU report.

Figure 2: An example of a donor match list

Patient 153818	aktiv		02:DFKP	14:02:01	04:CVAF	01:02:01	05:01:01 3*02:XX
DE-YZ	1960 M AP		24:CWFP	35:BEEX	08:02	14:BCAD	05:03:01

Donor n	Identity M/P Age	Status G BG/CMV	Match 10/10 - 9/10	pA A or A*	pB B or B*	pC C or C*	pDR DR or DRB1	pDQ DQ or DQB1	DRB345	DPB1
10/10 (potential) allele matches										
DE 1	XYZ 3869184 22 M	AV	PPPAA 97 - 3	97 02:CVYA 24:ENHC	99 35:EKNR 14:BH	99 04:EKPB 08:EKPD	100 01:02:01 14:01	100 05:01 05:03		
DE 2	XYZ 758303 49 F AP	AV N 1999-07	PPPAP 73 - 21	87 2s 24s	81 65s 35s	99 4s 8s	100 01:02 14:BCAD	99 05:RV	3*02:02	
DE 3	XYZ 960604 39 M	AV	PPPPP 56 - 24	90 2s 24s	68 65s 35s	77	99 01:02 14:JFA	99	3*02:KJJ	
9/10 (potential) allele matches										
DE 4	XYZ 18529 50 F	AV	PPMPP 0 - 68	94 2s 24s	70 14s 35s	0 4s 4s	99 01:XX 14:XX	99		
DE 5	XYZ 2807994 40 M	AV	PLPPP 0 - 20	98 02:AZWD 24:XX	0 14:02 35:HNH	22	96 01:02 14:XX	98		
8/10 (potential) allele matches										
DE 6	XYZ 2745989 41 M	AV	LLPPP 0 - 0	0 02:EK 24:XX	0 14:02 35:HNH	29	96 01:02 14:XX	98		

The columns Match 10/10 and 9/10 indicate the overall probability for the respective degree of matching. The columns pA, pB, pC, pDR and pDQ indicate the probability of allele identity for the loci HLA-A, -B, -C, -DRB1 and -DQB1. Proven antigen level mismatches are shown in red, allele level mismatches in blue (screenshot from OptiMatch® and BMDnet)

6. The operation of a CBB

6.1 CB donation
Donation refers to all activities necessary to ensure the safe collection of a cellular product. This is usually divided into three phases. First, prior to labour, when an information programme should allow mothers-to-be to reach an autonomous decision on donation, based on clear and ethically sound information. This concludes in obtaining a signed consent to collect or donate or both, depending on the strategy. The second phase is during labour, when: the potential donor is evaluated by a trained health professional according to donor eligibility criteria to ensure that no risk exists for transmissible diseases. Information is directly obtained from medical charts and using a specifically driven health questionnaire to disclose risk behaviours and travel history. In general, any disease transmissible by transplantation of infectious, genetic, neoplastic or immune origin can cause donor exclusion. Eligibility criteria may vary between countries depending on local regulation. Consenting eligible donors undergo a cord blood collection that is generally performed by venepuncture of the umbilical cord vein after birth under aseptic conditions with drainage of the blood into sealed bags. There are two main collection techniques, one performed while the placenta is still *in utero* and the other performed immediately after placental delivery in a contiguous area (*ex utero* collection). Importantly, CB collection must not interfere with the management of labour and should be carried out by a dedicated collector. Once collected, units are kept in a controlled environment before transportation to the processing centre. Each CB programme must validate the

temperature range for non-frozen storage and transportation that maximises cell viability.

Finally, the last phase, post-labour, refers to donor follow-up. This is not usually mandatory unless communicating any abnormal analytical findings detected during CB production can help in the prevention or treatment of previously unknown medical conditions for either the mother, the new-born or related persons.

6.2 CB manufacturing

Cord blood tissue refers to the blood including haematopoietic progenitor cells (HPC) harvested from placental and umbilical vessels after birth. Collected products are sent to a processing centre where they are thoroughly checked before batch production of therapeutic units then called HPC, Cord Blood. Evaluation consists of inspection of both samples and documents, labelling verification and initial testing. Most banks define a minimum cellular threshold to identify which units will be processed to increase efficiency of their inventories. Various processing methods are used. Closed cord blood automated procedures increase quality by reducing the risk of product contamination and mix-up. Usually, processing methods aim to reduce volume in order to increase the number of units that can be stored in limited space. The most popular techniques extract plasma and red blood cells to concentrate nucleated cells (NC) while maintaining the original properties of the collected unit. Preparation for cryopreservation and freezing into storage requires no more than minimal manipulation. Once stored, cord blood units can be kept on inventory for many years. Inventory management should be designed to monitor the individual thermal history during the long-term storage period. Target storage temperature is < -150°C.

Products are qualified according to four main aspects: safety, identity, purity and potency. Many variables are evaluated along the process to assess cord blood unit conformity. An example of decision checkpoints are presented below:

1. Acquisition: volume, cell number and/or CD34+ cell counts and cell viability
2. Manufacturing: batch production, and cell contents (total and CD34+ cell numbers and viability tests)
3. Listing: batch production review including sterility, infectious disease markers (IDM), haemoglobin, blood group and HLA types
4. Release for transplantation: CFU, HLA verification, blood group verification, gender verification and maternal haplotype verification.

Each country has its minimal testing requirements, and other accreditation bodies have published their own recommendations. For example, Table 1 summarises the US Food and Drug Administration's guidance for industry of a minimally manipulated, unrelated, allogeneic placental/umbilical cord blood intended for haematopoietic reconstitution in patients with haematological malignancies.

Table 1: Example of requirements for CBUs intended for HSCT (US FDA)

Product characteristics	Testing	Sample (type and timing)	Results of product testing
Safety	Infectious diseases - Testing required according to national law	Maternal peripheral blood obtained within 7 days of cord blood collection - Type and timing determined according to national law	All tests negative except non-treponemal test for syphilis may be positive provided confirmatory test is negative. (*Cytomegalovirus* (CMV) results are recorded)
	Sterility - Bacterial and fungal cultures - Testing required according to national law	Cord blood* and HPC-C (pre-cryopreservation)**	Negative
	Haemoglobin electrophoresis	Cord blood*	No homozygous haemoglobinopathy
Purity and potency	Total nucleated cells (TNC)	HPC-C (pre-cryopreservation)	$\geq 5.0 \times 10^8$ TNC***/unit HPC-C
	Viable nucleated cells	HPC-C (pre-cryopreservation)	$\geq 85\%$ viable nucleated cells
	Viable CD34+ cells (flow cytometry)	HPC-C (pre-cryopreservation)	$\geq 1.25 \times 10^6$ viable CD34+ cells****/unit HPC-C
Identity	Human leukocyte antigen (HLA) typing	Cord blood	Report
	Confirmatory HLA typing	Attached segment of HPC-C	Confirms initial typing
	Blood group and Rh type	Cord blood	Report

*Cord blood: cord blood before undergoing volume reduction; **Sample may be obtained before or after addition of the cryoprotectant; ***Based on 20 kg recipient @ $\geq 2,5 \times 10^7$ nucleated cells/kg & $\geq 70\%$ post-thaw recovery = 1.7×10^7 nucleated cells/kg; ****Based on CD34+ cells $\geq 0.25\%$ of TNC prior to freezing*

6.3 CB provision

In order to make inventories available for transplantation, cord blood banks list their validated units using minimum essential data required for search procedures. Searches usually first sort potential candidates according to HLA match categories and then by cell dose. Other variables can be used to identify the best compatible donor between a few pre-selected candidates. Thus, data usually exported from the local processing databases to publicly accessible global databases are:

• HLA typing of HLA-A, –B and -DRB1 loci. For historical reasons, search databases contain units typed at different resolutions. Current standards recommend that new units are typed using molecular techniques of low resolution for class I loci and high resolution for class II loci.

- Cell dose. This is primarily evaluated by the amount of NC (including erythroblasts) contained in a CB unit. In addition, CD34+ cell count is increasingly used as an indicator of graft potency. Both parameters should be considered when analysing a product intended for transplantation.
- Qualitative data. Including cord blood bank, year of production, ABO, other HLA types, and CFU.

Once a unit is listed, cord blood banks can be contacted for different requests. These can be grouped into:

- Preliminary reports.
- Additional testing. Examples of most frequent activities related are extended typing, specific IDM to meet local regulations, and CFU post-thawing to confirm potency.
- Reservation. Allocation of a CBU for a defined patient and can include identity confirmation ideally using a segment attached to the transplant bag.
- Shipment. It is recommended not to start patient conditioning before a unit has been safely received at the transplant centre. As a CB graft is already harvested shipment can be arranged immediately, although a number of administrative and technical procedures are required before transporting the unit using a door-to-door service. Factors including export/import issues (for international deliveries) and release tests sometimes prevent the immediate use of a unit.

After shipment, the transplant centre needs to apply strict protocols of quality assurance. Temperature range during transportation, inspection for bag integrity and labelling are important aspects to review before acquiring the product. All time sample need to be maintained below temperature of -150°Celsius.

On reception, the unit needs to be transiently stored below -150°C. Finally, the way a CB should be reconstituted for infusion is still controversial; but usually CB grafts are infused after a dilution/washing step using a dextran buffer to minimise infusion toxicity. Cord blood bank tasks end when a basic clinical follow-up analysis is done. The best way to validate CB quality is to demonstrate engraftment ability and low toxicity after infusion. Therefore, every cord blood bank will require this information as part of their quality assurance plan. In this regard, Eurocord in Europe and CIBMTR in US are the main centres for retrospective studies on CB efficacy and provide important insights for future modification of standard practices.

6.4 Special issues of CBBs and CBUs
The production of cord blood grafts is expensive, thus making cord blood banking

feasible requires determination of the adequate size for an efficient inventory. According to recent publications, cord blood banks containing a few tens of thousands of thoroughly tested and diverse units may provide optimal donors for the majority of local patients. International networking is still necessary to cover the entire population of a country including minority ethnicities. Enlarging the inventory has only marginal benefits but substantially increases the cost. As the cellular threshold for a secure engraftment is now better defined, another parameter to consider when designing a cord blood bank project is the minimal cell dose acceptable for processing. For instance, to target 50 kg patient body weight and accepting 2.5×10^7 TNC per kilogram as a safe target, the cellular threshold should be at least 12.5×10^7 TNC post-processing. This decision has cost implications and affects the way collection programmes should be organised.

7. International organisations, accreditation and regulatory aspects

The World Marrow Donor Association (WMDA) is the umbrella organisation of the registries worldwide, together with a large and increasing number of independent cord blood banks. According to its mission statement *"The WMDA fosters international collaboration to facilitate the exchange of high quality hematopoietic stem cells for clinical transplantation worldwide and to promote the interests of unrelated donors"* the WMDA has published numerous guidelines and reference documents supporting registries in setting up and improving most aspects of their operation. Most importantly, the WMDA defined Standards for registries encompassing all their relevant collaborating entities and on this basis established an accreditation system; 19 registries worldwide have so far successfully been accredited. The WMDA's website *www.worldmarrow.org* gives access to all its relevant documents and provides an extensive insight into its activities.

HPC, Cord Blood is a product which is highly regulated. Many local agencies define it as a tissue or even a drug, requiring production under GMP conditions. However, most of the products are globally distributed and an important achievement has been the development of international standards for the harmonisation of this activity. Currently, the fourth edition of the NetCord-FACT International Standards for Cord Blood Collection, Banking, and Release for Administration, produced after a collaborative effort between NetCord and the Foundation for the Accreditation of Cellular Therapy (FACT), is available. NetCord is an international Foundation where leading cord blood banks collaborate to promote high quality cord blood banking and clinical use of umbilical cord blood for allogeneic stem cell transplantation, while FACT's mission is to promote quality medical and laboratory practice of cellular therapy through its peer-developed standards and voluntary inspection and accreditation program (more information in *www.netcord.org* and *www.factwebsite.org*). At present,

26 public unrelated cord blood bank programmes are accredited worldwide (*www.factwebsite.org*).

The harvest, processing and distribution of all stem cell products are subject to increasing regulation in most countries. These not only differ between the countries but also frequently between BM, PBSC and CBU within a country. Typically, the regulations for CBUs are strictest since it is a pre-produced product much like an off-the-shelf drug, whereas more lenient rules apply to the directed donation of BM and PBSC from AUDs.

The most complicated, and often legally risky, situation is the import of a foreign stem cell product for a patient. The EU Tissue Directive probably (also) aimed at harmonising the situation within Europe, but this has by no means become reality. However, in practice there is a high level of mutual trust between EU member states in this field – whatever that translates into in practice in each country. Institutions from non-EU member states issuing a stem cell product typically would have to obtain a formal license from the authorities of the importing country which, of course, is unrealistic. The only approach is to be well-informed about the pertaining regulations of your country and their practical application and to mantain good contact with the Competent Authorities at the regional and national levels. Either it is possible to agree on a practicable *modus operandi* with the authorities, or it may be necessary to operate with a degree of legal uncertainty about every case. At present there is a concern that regulatory efforts meant to safeguard the welfare of patients may seriously endanger or even harm patients in our field.

These increasing obstacles to the international exchange of stem cell products are a major concern to the WMDA. Its Regulatory Committee is actively monitoring the situation and documents current practices on the website. The WMDA Board tries to influence international decision-making processes and to foster practices of standardisation and mutual recognition, and also supports its member registries in synergistic efforts at the national level.

8. Summary/Conclusion

Allogeneic HSC transplantation is sometimes the single curative option for many haematological disorders. Access to this therapy depends on the availability of donors providing safe products. After many years of technical development and clinical improvements, it is now possible to offer HSCT to many patients in need. Integral management of AUDs and CBUs and international networking of the resources are facilitating the widespread access to this therapy worldwide.

References

1. Gluckman E, Ruggeri A, Volt F, et al. Milestones in umbilical cord blood transplantation.

Br J Haematol 2011 Jul 5. doi: 10.1111/j.1365-2141.2011.08598.x. [on line].
2. Rubinstein P. Cord blood banking for clinical transplantation. Bone Marrow Transplant 2009; 44: 635–642.
3. Mueller CR. Computer applications in the search for unrelated stem cell donors. Transpl Immunol 2002; 10: 227–240.
4. Lee SJ, Klein J, Haagenson M et al. High-resolution donor-recipient HLA matching contributes to the success of unrelated donor marrow transplantation. Blood 2007; 110: 4576–4583.
5. Bochtler W, Maiers M, Bakker JN et al. World Marrow Donor Association framework for the implementation of HLA matching programs in hematopoietic stem cell donor registries and cord blood banks. Bone Marrow Transplant 2011; 46: 338–343.

Multiple Choice Questionnaire

To find the correct answer, go to http://www.esh.org/online-training/handbook/

1. **In a search process, which of the following is correct?**
   a) The physician should start by consulting only the national registry ...... ☐
   b) Within a list of potential donors, it is not usually necessary to do further testing to identify the right donor .... ☐
   c) Transplant centres should have defined criteria for accepting a mismatched donor .... ☐
   d) In the vast majority of cases, an HLA-mismatched sibling donor is regarded as the best option for an allogeneic transplant .... ☐

2. **Regarding matching services, which sentence is *not* true?**
   a) Donor lists generated are generally grouped on ascending number of HLA differences between donor and recipient. .... ☐
   b) Lists may include statistical prognosis for HLA identity. .... ☐
   c) In CBU, either CD34 or TNC can be the primary sorting criterion .... ☐
   d) Once lists are generated, the experience of the users is no longer required. .... ☐

3. **To donate a CB unit to a public CBB, which sentence is correct?**
   a) It is not necessary to obtain signed consent. .... ☐
   b) Some diseases transmissible by stem cell transplantation can cause donor exclusion .... ☐

c) It is mandatory to perform a donor follow-up assessment before CB use .... ☐

d) CB collection must always take place after delivery of the placenta ...... ☐

4. **Related to CB manufacturing, which of the following sentences is *not* true:**
   a) Target long-term storage temperature is colder than -150°C .... ☐
   b) CB grafts are qualified based on safety, identity, purity and potency aspects .... ☐
   c) CBU release for transplantation usually require the verification of identity .... ☐
   d) A typical processing method used for reducing storage space requirement is immunomagnetic positive selection of CD34+ cells .... ☐

5. **Which of the following is *not* a functional structure within the workflow for unrelated HPC provision?**
   a) EBMT .... ☐
   b) BMDW .... ☐
   c) EMDIS .... ☐
   d) National Registry .... ☐

* CHAPTER 8

Principles of conditioning

Alois Gratwohl, Enric Carreras

1. Introduction

Conditioning plays a central part in HSCT. It is the source of the inherent dilemma in HSCT: how to get rid of the disease but without toxicity. Conditioning is a key cause of early mortality but holds out the prospect of long-term disease control or even cure. Errors in its application can have serious, even immediately fatal consequences. Quality management issues (see below) therefore have a central role in all aspects of conditioning. It is of importance to be familiar with all aspects of conditioning. The term "conditioning" in HSCT means to "condition", e.g. to prepare the patient for its transplant. Conditioning is given with three main objectives: "creation of space", immunosuppression and disease eradication (1, 2).

1.1 Creation of space

This is a somewhat controversial concept, which originated from the belief that immature progenitor cells occupy defined niches within the marrow stroma where they obtain the necessary support for proliferation and differentiation. According to this theory, existing host stem cell cells must be eradicated in order for donor stem cells to obtain access to these niches and for engraftment to occur. Experimental and clinical data do not provide a clear answer about the need to create space. There are indications that engraftment after reduced intensity conditioning (RIC) HSCT is more rapid in patients with an "empty" bone marrow compared to a "full" bone marrow.

1.2 Immunosuppression to prevent a host versus graft reaction

Immunosuppression is required to prevent rejection of the incoming donor cells by host immune cells. This is clearly not required in autologous or syngeneic HSCT. The need for immunosuppression increases with the increase of disparity in major histocompatibility antigens (HLA). The risk of rejection is increased in situations where the recipient has been "pre-sensitised" against minor histocompatibility antigens, e.g. by the administration of multiple blood products prior to HSCT. Rejection is also increased in TCD (T-cell depleted) HSCT. *Vice versa*, graft acceptance is increased by high stem cell dose and high T-cell dose.

1.3 Disease eradication

The key goal of the conditioning regimen is long-term disease control. This is the main objective for patients with malignancies, but it is also of vital importance in diseases characterised by hyperplastic marrows, e.g. thalassaemia. Partial engraftment may be sufficient in situations where only a "specific product" is required, e.g. B-cells in some immunodeficiency states or when an enzyme produced by haematopoietic cells is required, e.g. in mitochondrial neurogastrointestinal encephalopathy.

2. Historical perspective

In order to understand the diversity and multitude of today's conditioning regimens, they have to be seen in their historical context. Bone marrow transplantation was initially investigated as a tool to protect survivors of accidental high dose irradiation due to nuclear accident or atomic bomb exposure. At the same time, it was realised that total body irradiation (TBI) could be used as a tool to eliminate a leukaemic haematopoietic system without causing irreversible damage to other organs. "Condition" meant the preparation of the recipient to accept a new organ in place of the diseased and eradicated haematopoietic system. TBI proved to be sufficient for engraftment but insufficient for long-term disease control when used on its own. The addition of cyclophosphamide (Cy) to TBI and transplantation at an early stage of the disease were the main elements for successful BMT in the late seventies. At that time attempts were already being made to replace TBI with "radiomimetic" drugs or high dose "leukaemia-specific" chemotherapy, using drugs including Cy, busulfan (Bu), etoposide (VP16), cytosine arabinoside (ARA-C), carmustine (BCNU) and melphalan (MEL). The combinations Cy/TBI, Bu/Cy alone or BACT (BCNU, ARA-C, cyclophosphamide and 6TG) were the main conditioning regimens for HSCT at this time. In the 1980s, emphasis was on dose intensification and exploring alternatives to Cy in combination with TBI. New conditioning regimens were designed with the aim of reducing the risk of relapse and rejection. A number of studies defined maximum tolerable doses for single drugs in combination with TBI. Dose escalation studies suggested that up to 60 mg/kg of VP16, 110-180 mg/m^2 of MEL and 36 g/m^2 of ARA-C could be combined as individual drugs with TBI. Dose limiting toxicities were interstitial pneumonitis (IP) for TBI, stomatitis and veno-occlusive disease (VOD) for MEL/TBI and VP16/TBI, and CNS and skin toxicity for ARA-C/TBI.

Several centres evaluated the use of TBI plus more than one drug, but no consensus was reached regarding the maximum tolerated doses. None of these regimens made any significant improvements to clinical outcome. Any reduction in relapse or rejection risk was usually accompanied by an increase in TRM. OS and DFS remained unchanged or worsened. Similarly, no study with "leukaemia-specific agents" such as ARA-C or VP16, showed superiority to Cy, a drug that is not used in the conventional treatment of leukaemia. So far, no single study has shown any conditioning regimen to provide better long-term survival than Cy/TBI or Bu/Cy. In the 1990s the emphasis switched to concepts focused on reducing TRM and morbidity with improvements in QoL. Better understanding of graft versus leukaemia (GvL) effects, the recognition of the capacity of donor lymphocyte infusion (DLI) to shift the balance between donor and recipient in a predictable way and preclinical experiments which defined the minimal requirements for stable engraftment, led to the introduction of the concept of: "reduced intensity conditioning". Most of the conditioning regimens (standard, intensified or reduced) were developed as phase I/II trials and then adopted by individual institutions without formal phase III studies.

There are a few exceptions. Standard conditioning with Cy/TBI was compared with Bu/Cy in several studies in haematological malignancies. There were substantial differences in toxicities (more VOD, more permanent alopecia with Bu/Cy) but little differences in long-term survival. In ALL there is probably an advantage in the long-term with TBI containing regimens. Current strategies focus on a new concept. Until recently, most patients were given the same conditioning regimen. Today, it is believed that patients with a high risk for TRM and a low disease risk should receive a different conditioning regimen from patients with a low risk for TRM and high-risk disease. The approach should integrate conditioning, graft product and GvHD prophylaxis and treatment from the very beginning (see Table 1) (1–4).

3. RIC HSCT and the concept of "immunoablation versus myeloablation"

The concept of RIC HSCT is based on the idea of circumventing the high morbidity and mortality associated with standard conditioning in patients with advanced age or comorbidities. It evolved from preclinical studies which defined the minimal requirements for engraftment. They also made use of the potential of DLI to shift mixed chimerism to full chimerism. The goal of RIC HSCT is not tumour eradication or destruction of host haematopoiesis by cytotoxic therapy but via immune-mediated effects. The graft versus tumour potential of the approach is based on several components: initial conditioning, graft composition, prevention of post-transplant rejection and use of DLI in case of incomplete chimerism at specified time points. During recent years a large number of RIC regimens have been developed, most of them based on the use of fludarabine (Flu) and ranging from those with a minimally reduced intensity but with a clearly reduced toxicity (e.g. Flu/Bu using slightly reduced doses of iv Bu) to those where intensity is so reduced that they do not produce myelotoxicity (e.g. Flu/TBI), usually called non-myeloablative (see Table 1). RIC HSCT is an established component of transplant strategies today, especially in patients with advanced age. Despite many studies, none has shown unequivocal benefit in long-term survival compared to standard conditioning. Early organ toxicity can be reduced but impact on GvHD and infectious complications is much less and RIC HSCT is always associated with an increased risk of relapse during follow-up (see Figure 1) (5–8).

Table 1: **Conditioning regimens**

Classical regimens	Total dose (days)	Intensified regimens (allo)	Total dose (days)
Cy/TBI (allo/auto)		**Cy/VP/TBI**	
Cyclophosphamide (mg/kg)	120 (-6,-5)	Cyclophosphamide (mg/kg)	120 (-6, -5)
Total body irradiation (Gy)	12–14 (-3 to -1)	Etoposide (mg/m²)	30–60 (-4)
		Total body irradiation (Gy)	12–13.8 (-3 to -1)
Bu/Cy# (allo/auto)			
Busulfan (mg/kg)	16 (-7 to -4)	**TBI/TT/Cy**	
Cyclophosphamide (mg/kg)	120 (-3, -2)	Total body irradiation (Gy)	13.8 (-9 to -6)
		Thiotepa (mg/kg)	10 (-5, -4)
BACT (allo)		Cyclophosphamide (mg/kg)	120 (-3, -2)
BCNU (mg/m²)	200 (-6)	**Bu/Cy/MEL**	
ARA-C (mg/m²)	800 (-5 to -2)	Busulfan (mg/kg)	16 (-7 to -4)
Cyclophosphamide (mg/kg)	50 (-5 to -2)	Cyclophosphamide (mg/kg)	120 (-3, -2)
6-Thioguanine (mg/m²)	800 (-5 to -2)	Melphalan (mg/m²)	140 (-1)
BEAM (auto/allo)		**Reduced toxicity regimens***	Total dose (days)
BCNU (mg/m²)	300 (-6)	**Flu/MEL**	
Etoposide (mg/m²)	800 (-5 to -2)	Fludarabine (mg/m²)	150 (-7 to -3)
ARA-C (mg/m²)	800 (-5 to -2)	Melphalan (mg/m²)	140 (-2,-1)
Melphalan (mg/m²)	140 (-1)		
		Flu/Bu	
MEL (auto)		Fludarabine (mg/m²)	150 (-9 to -5)
Melphalan (mg/m²)	200 (-3, -2)	Busulfan (mg/kg)	8–10 (-6 to -4)
Other "standard" regimens	Total dose (days)	**Flu/Cy**	
		Fludarabine (mg/m²)	150 (-7 to -3)
TBI/VP (allo)		Cyclophosphamide (g/m²)	140 (-2,-1)
Total body irradiation (Gy)	12–13.2 (-7 to -4)		
Etoposide (mg/kg)	60 (-3)	**Flu/Bu/TT**	
		Fludarabine (mg/m²)	150 (-7 to -5)
AC/TBI (allo)		Busulfan (mg/kg)	8 (-6 to -4)
ARA-C (g/m²)	36 (-9 to -4)	Thiotepa (mg/m²)	5 (-3)
Total body irradiation (Gy)	12 (-3 to -1)	Non-myeloablative regimens	Total dose (days)
MEL/TBI (allo/auto)		**Flu/TBI**	
Melphalan (mg/m²)	110–140	Fludarabine (mg/m²)	90 (-4 to -2)
Total body irradiation (Gy)	10-14	Total body irradiation (Gy)	2 (0)
Bu/MEL (auto)		**TLI/ATG**	
Busulfan (mg/kg)	16 (-5 to -2)	Total Lymphoid Irradiation (Gy)	8 (-11 to -1)
Melphalan (mg/m²)	140 (-1)	ATG*	7 (-11 to -7)
CBV (auto)		**TBI**	
BCNU (mg/m²)	300 (-6)	Total body irradiation (Gy)	1–2 (0)
Etoposide (mg/m²)	800 (-5 to -2)		
Cyclophosphamide (g/m²)	4.8–7.2 (-5 to -2)		

Nowadays moving to Cy/iv Bu on days -7, -6 and -5 to -2, respectively; * In many cases these regimens include ATG

Figure 1: **Probability of survival, transplant-related mortality and relapse depending on the EBMT Risk Score**

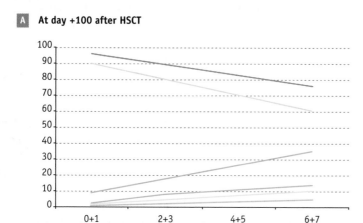

A **At day +100 after HSCT**

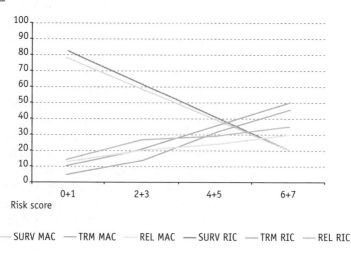

B **At 3 years after HSCT**

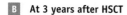

SURV MAC — TRM MAC — REL MAC — SURV RIC — TRM RIC — REL RIC

For definition of EBMT Risk Score, see Chapter 18

4. Special considerations for specific conditioning regimens

4.1 TBI

TBI requires specific knowledge and should only be applied at an experienced institution under the guidance of a specialist radiophysicist or radiation oncologist. It has the specific advantage of having access to so-called "sanctuary sites" of malignancies, e.g. CNS or gonads, where some drugs may not penetrate. TBI is most commonly delivered to the patient using a linear accelerator. Patients are placed within a single irradiation field and lie on their side or in lateral position at a specified distance from the radiation source. Irradiation is given with horizontal beams using the anterior-posterior or lateral-lateral technique. The effects of TBI depend on total dose, dose rate and fractionation. TBI is prescribed as either a single dose (1 to 8 Gy total dose); fractionated dose (10 to 14 Gy total dose in 5–6 fractions over 3 days); or "hyperfractionated" TBI (14–15 Gy total dose in 10–12 fractions over 4 days).

Dose rates differ considerably between machines and have different radiobiological effects. Lower total doses must be applied when higher dose rates are used. Fractionation reduces the incidence and severity of acute and late complications of normal tissue. As such TBI is similar to conditioning with chemotherapy. Low total doses, e.g. 6 Gy, may decrease toxicity but increase the risks of graft failure and disease recurrence. Very high doses, e.g. 15.75 Gy, may reduce the incidences of graft rejection and disease relapse, but at the expense of increased morbidity and mortality. Radiation dose is normally calculated as midline tissue dose at the level of the umbilicus, but other strategies, e.g. targeting maximum lung dose, are possible. The received radiation doses to various parts of the body are monitored by *in vivo* dosimetry using diodes and thermoluminescent detectors placed anteriorly and posteriorly on various parts of the body. In some institutions parts of the body, usually the lungs or the eyes, are protected with lead blocks during part of the application to "shield" this organ and to reduce organ specific toxicity. Other centres avoid shielding since leukaemic cells could also be protected by the shields. Dosimetry is still a difficult undertaking and measured dose is less exact than calculated delivered dose. Monitoring during TBI is essentially required to detect major technical errors, e.g. too high or too low an applied dose. Immediate side effects of TBI are nausea, vomiting and, typically, parotid swelling. Adequate preventive measures are recommended. Pilocarpine p.o. is used to reduce parotid swelling (4).

4.2 TCD and conditioning

T-cells are an essential component of the graft product including for engraftment.

Graft facilitating cells in the T-cell fraction enhance engraftment via soluble factors and by their direct effect on residual host T-cells. Simultaneously, T-cells are responsible for acute and chronic GvHD and for GvL effects. Therefore, TCD of the stem cells prior to infusion is highly effective in the prevention of acute and chronic GvHD, but at the expense of an increased risk of graft rejection and disease recurrence. The incidence of graft failure and graft rejection in TCD HLA-identical sibling HSCT is in the order of 10–20% with standard conditioning, and is higher in haploidentical, UD or RIC HSCT. Several approaches have been used to overcome the increase in graft failure associated with TCD. Some centres have intensified CT/RT by increasing dosages or adding TLI or TAI (total lymphoid/abdominal irradiation). This approach can effectively overcome graft failure but is associated with increased morbidity and mortality, resulting in similar OS rates. Because TCD is so effective at preventing GvHD, no further GvHD prevention e.g. with CsA and/or methotrexate (MTX) is given after HSCT. The re-introduction of CsA to these protocols can reduce the rate of graft failure/rejection. Other centres combine TCD with additional immunosuppressive therapy for patients prior to stem cell infusion, e.g. *in vivo* Campath-1H™, ATG or MoAb to OKT-3 for several days before HSCT. It may also be possible to overcome graft failure by increasing the SC dose as has been shown not only in murine models of transplant but also in haplo-identical family member transplants for acute leukaemia. Addition of T-cells which are depleted of alloreactive T-cells or selected NK-cells are novel approaches under current investigation (9, 10).

4.3 ATG
Anti-T-cell globulins are polyclonal antibodies of different origins (horse, rabbit, or, more rarely, goats and pigs) with a wide variety of specificities that have never been compared in controlled settings. Their primary mechanism of action is *in vivo* T-cell depletion but B-, NK-, macrophages and dendritic cells are also targeted by ATG. For that reason they have been mainly used to prevent GvHD (see Chapter 13). However, in some circumstances, ATG is included in the preparative regimen as a true conditioning agent. This is the case of transplants with a high risk of graft failure (TCD grafts, cord blood HSCT, alloimmunisation of the recipient due to multiple transfusions, RIC HSCT). In these cases ATG is used to facilitate engraftment. Despite promising results in GvHD prevention and graft facilitation its use is strongly limited by multiple side effects (anaphylaxis, cytokine release syndrome, CMV and EBV reactivation, lymphoproliferative disorders, among others) and an increased risk of relapse. Even for the rabbit preparation of ATG, the most extensively studied preparation, the "ideal" dose (highest efficacy and lowest toxicity) has not yet been defined (10, 11).

4.4 Busulfan

In the eighties, Santos et al. introduced the combination Bu/Cy into clinical practice and shortly after this regimen became the standard conditioning for centres without facilities for total body radiation. However this combination was associated with three main problems. First, due to its poor solubility Bu was only available in its oral form and this fact made it necessary to administer Bu before all other emetogenic agents. Second, the combination was hepatotoxic with a high incidence of VOD. Reduction of the Cy dose from 200 to 120 mg/kg and adjusting the oral doses of Bu according to blood levels to prevent the high inter and intra-patient variability were introduced to reduce VOD complications. Third, the high levels of Bu in the cerebrospinal fluid can produce seizures; prophylactic anticonvulsant therapy must be administrated routinely. With these precautions Bu/Cy offered results comparable, and in some series even better, than those obtained by the classical Cy/TBI (2, 3). This picture changed with the introduction of an intravenous formula. iv Bu has the following advantages: 1. is easier to administer, less emetogenic and can be given as a single daily dose; 2. has predictable pharmacokinetics; 3. causes less liver toxicity (note that 1 mg oral Bu corresponds to 0.8 mg iv Bu). In addition, theoretical and pharmacological data indicate that Bu triggers liver toxicity of subsequent Cy. Bu reduces hepatic glutathione, so that toxic metabolites of Cy can no longer be eliminated. They induce sinusoidal damage, the initial event of VOD. Cy induced emesis is no longer a contraindication for Bu when given iv, hence these drugs can today be administered in the reverse order. Animal studies and several initial clinical series have confirmed this hypothesis showing an almost complete absence of VOD when using Cy/iv Bu (12).

4.5 Paediatric transplants

There are two main differences between adult and paediatric patients in relation to conditioning. Children in general tolerate side effects better than older patients and higher total doses may be applied. In contrast, conditioning affects growth and endocrine development. Retarded growth and failed or retarded puberty are the main late sequelae in paediatric HSCT patients. There is no general consensus between the various paediatric groups about the optimal conditioning regimen. Nevertheless, a general outline of the strategies used in children can be given. Since many reports comparing TBI containing conditioning regimens with those containing only CT show similar outcomes, TBI should be avoided in small children, whenever possible. It should probably never be given to children below 2 years of age. TBI (2 doses per day) in combination with Cy and/or VP16 is commonly used in children (>2 years of age) undergoing HSCT for ALL. These children have usually already received all the drugs useful in this disease and TBI is thought to have an additional antileukaemic effect in ALL (13).

5. Disease specific aspects (see also Chapters 19 and 20)

5.1 Inborn errors of the lymphohaematopoietic system

In patients with profound deficiencies of the lymphoid immune system, such as SCID, the capacity for graft rejection is extremely low or absent. Preparative regimens are therefore unnecessary but HSCT results in an unusual form of lympho-haematopoietic chimerism. Donor cell engraftment after HLA-identical sibling HSCT is usually restricted to the lymphocytes, whilst the myeloid system remains of host cell origin. The same approach in TCD HLA-mismatched HSCT has led to more variable results. Here, complete or partial graft failure, in particular failure of B-cell reconstitution, has been observed. This experience has resulted in the use of CT-based preparative regimens in patients transplanted for SCID from HLA-mismatched donors. The regimen most frequently employed is that of Bu 2 mg/kg/day for 4 d + Cy 50 mg/kg/day for 4 d. In the presence of serious clinical conditions, e.g. pulmonary infections prior to the transplant, the use of chemotherapy may greatly increase the morbidity and mortality of the procedure. In these cases, HSCT may be performed without conditioning, as even partial immunological reconstitution may be of therapeutic benefit to the child. In less severe variants of lymphoid deficiencies and in all other inborn errors, conditioning is required for myeloablation and to prevent graft rejection and disease recurrence. Some young patients come to transplant with a number of complications related to their underlying disease, in particular poorly controlled chronic infections. The use of non-CT based conditioning protocols which allow stable engraftment remains a long-term goal (14).

5.2 Severe aplastic anaemia

The marrow is empty in patients with SAA and the sole aim of the conditioning protocol is to provide immunosuppression. Cy 50 mg/kg/d for 4 successive days is an appropriate conditioning regimen. It is very immunosuppressive and its use involves few serious long-term side-effects. Rejection remains a concern, especially in patients sensitised to their donors via blood products. The addition of ATG has reduced risk of rejection in one pilot study but prospective randomised and retrospective multicentre analyses have failed to confirm its value in non-sensitised recipients. Still, it is the most frequently used approach at the present time. The optimal conditioning regimen for patients with SAA receiving alternative donor transplants still needs defining. Several recent studies suggest that the addition of Flu and low dose TBI (2 Gy) to the conditioning might permit to reduce the dose of Cy improving the results and reducing the toxicity (15). All long-term follow-up studies have shown a higher incidence of late malignancies in SAA patients given TBI or TAI during conditioning.

5.3 Fanconi's anaemia

Fanconi's anaemia is a genetic disorder associated with diverse congenital abnormalities, progressive BM failure and increased risk of leukaemia and other cancers. HSCT is an effective treatment. The underlying molecular defects are heterogeneous but all result in defective DNA repair mechanisms.

These patients are therefore extremely susceptible to the effects of CT/RT, in particular to irradiation and alkylating agents. Conditioning regimens must be reduced in intensity. Most regimens contain Cy 5–10 mg/kg/d for 4 days. Some centres add low dose TBI or TAI (400–450 cGy) and/or ATG to overcome graft rejection. However, there is concern that the addition of TBI may increase the incidence of secondary malignancies in a group of patients already susceptible to further malignant disease. More recent approaches investigate the use of Bu or the addition of Flu.

5.4 Lymphoma and myeloma

The conditioning regimens for high dose therapy in both have been based on custom and practice rather than proof or confirmation by randomised trials.

Auto-HSCT is the type of transplant most commonly performed in both diseases as it can cure many patients with aggressive lymphoma or significantly prolong the duration of the response in those with myeloma. BEAM has been the most commonly used regimen both for NHL and HD. The standard BEAM uses a total dose of VP of 800 mg/m^2/d for 4 days. Several groups have attempted to change the individual components. None has proved superior and there is no evidence that any other regimen has more anti-tumour effect than BEAM. For myeloma patients MEL 200 mg/m^2 given over 1-2 days is the standard regimen. No other regimen has shown better results. In some patients with myeloma who are not candidates for an allo-HSCT a double auto-HSCT has been used with controversial results.

Allo-HSCT: This option should be considered in patients with NHL or HD relapsing, or with a high-risk of relapse. The same applies to younger people with high-risk myeloma. Standard allo-HSCT was used in the nineties in preference to auto-HSCT but was abandoned, as results were unsatisfactory. Today, the usual practice in these cases is to perform a tandem HSCT (auto followed by allo-RIC) in a planned manner or at progression of the disease. However, no study has ever confirmed in any disease that this separation of cytoreduction and allogeneic effect is indeed superior to direct, full-conditioning allo-HSCT. The best RIC regimen and interval between procedures are not known but the most frequently applied are Flu/MEL, Flu/Bu and Flu/TBI with an interval between HSCTs ranging between 3 and 6 months. The possible role of new agents, as proteasome inhibitors, in the conditioning of patients with myeloma is unknown at the present time (14, 16, 17).

5.5 Solid tumours

Dose intensification was the underlying rationale for the introduction of auto-HSCT as an investigational tool for treatment of solid tumours. Initial results appeared promising and there was huge interest in the mid-nineties. Conditioning regimens were developed with "tumour specific" drugs in mind and a multitude of regimens appeared.

None has proved to be superior to any other and HSCT in solid tumours with very few exceptions is still considered investigational. Conditioning regimens should follow those specified in clinical protocols (14). They are discussed in Chapters 19.11 and 20.10. Allo-HSCT has been investigated in more recent years as a tool for promoting graft vs tumour effects. Hence, primarily RIC regimens are chosen with the aim of establishing donor type engraftment. Any RIC regimen can be used without a need for tumour specific therapy. RIC HSCT for solid tumours is still to be considered investigational (18).

6. Conditioning induced organ damage

The desirable effects of conditioning regimens are offset by their highly predictable toxicities, which are responsible for considerable morbidity and mortality (see Table 2). These involve the GI, renal, hepatic, pulmonary and cardiac systems and include cardiac toxicity (Cy >1.5 $g/m^2/d$; BCNU), pulmonary toxicity (TBI >8 Gy), mucositis, hepatic toxicity, bladder toxicity, renal toxicity and neurological toxicity (3). Prevention and treatment of early and late complications are discussed in detail in Chapters 11 and 15.

7. Quality management issues

Application of high dose therapy in the context of HSCT is a complex and challenging therapy. It is prone to errors and all possible strategies should be undertaken to minimise such risks. This includes specifically the following points, as indicated in the JACIE standards and as outlined in Chapter 3. Each institution administering high dose CT in the context of HSCT must establish a quality management system for administration of this therapy. Such a system must be established in close cooperation with the institutional pharmacy and the nursing team. Conditioning has to be based on pre-printed orders. Regular check points at different levels and immediately prior to administration have to safeguard that the right patient is given the specified drugs at the correct dose and appropriate timing.

All check points include the "4 eyes" principle (at least two people must witness or approve a certain activity). Similar considerations apply to the administration of TBI (19).

	RI	TRM	LFS	OS
Disease factors				
Stage: increasing stage	↑	↑	↓	↓
Interval: Dx-HSCT >12 months*	↑	↑	↓	↓
Dx-1st CR long**	↑	↑	↓	↓
1st CR-HSCT short**	↑	↑	↓	↓
Patient-related factors		↑		
Age (higher)	?	↑	↓	↓
Sex (male)	—	↑	↓	↓
Race	?	?	?	?
Viral status (CMV positivity)	—	↑	↓	↓
Donor-related factors				
Histocompatibility (vs HLA-id sibling)				
Identical twin	↑	↓	↓	↑
Unrelated	↓	?	?	?
Mismatched	↓	↑	↓	↓
Sex (female D for male R)	↓	↑	↓	↓early/↑late
Viral status (CMV positivity)	?	↑	↓	↓
Peri-transplant factors				
Conditioning (intensified)	↓	↑	—	—
(reduced)	↑	↓	↓	?
GvHD prevention (intensified)	↑	↓	—	—
(reduced)	↓	↑	—	—
Cell content (CD34) high	↓	↓	↑	↑
low	—	↑	↓	↓
Stem cell source: BM vs PB	↑	↑	?	?
Post-transplant factors				
Acute GvHD (increasing grade)	↓	↑	↓	↓
Chronic GvHD (none vs any)	↓	↑	↓	↓

D: donor; R: recipient; Dx: diagnostic; 1st CR: first complete remission. *does not apply to patients receiving HSCT in first CR; **applies only to patients receiving HSCT in first CR. Please note that the worse outcome for patients with a short interval from first CR to HSCT does not imply that transplant should be delayed. The lower relapse risk for patients with a long delay is primarily due to the fact that some patients in long-term CR1 may already be cured before HSCT

References

1. Thomas ED. A history of allogeneic hematopoietic cell transplantation. In: Thomas' Hematopoietic Cell Transplantation, 4th Edition (Appelbaum FR, Forman SJ, Negrin RS, Blume KG Eds.), Wiley-Blackwell Publishing Chichester, West Sussex, UK, 2009, pp 3–7.
2. Santos GW, Tutschka PJ, Brookmeyer R. Marrow transplantation for acute non-lymphocytic leukemia after treatment with busulfan and cyclophosphamide. N Engl J Med 1983; 309: 1347–1353.

3. Bensinger WI. High-dose preparatory regimens. In: Thomas' Hematopoietic Cell Transplantation, 4th Edition (Appelbaum FR, Forman SJ, Negrin RS, Blume KG Eds.), Wiley-Blackwell Publishing Chichester, West Sussex, UK, 2009, pp 316–332.
4. Young JYC, Schultheiss T. Radiotherapeutic principles of hematopoietic cell transplantation. In: Thomas' Hematopoietic Cell Transplantation, 4th Edition, Appelbaum FR, Forman SJ, Negrin RS, Blume KG Eds., Wiley-Blackwell Publishing Chichester, West Sussex, UK, 2009, pp 333–350.
5. Slavin S, Nagler A, Naparstek E et al. Non-myeloablative stem cell transplantation and cell therapy as an alternative to conventional bone marrow transplantation with lethal cytoreduction for the treatment of malignant and non-malignant hematologic diseases. Blood 1998; 3: 756–763.
6. Giralt S, Estey E, Albitar M et al. Engraftment of allogeneic hematopoietic progenitor cells with purine analog-containing chemotherapy: Harnessing graft-versus-leukemia without myeloablative therapy. Blood 1997; 89: 4531–4536.
7. Blaise D, Vey N, Faucher C, Mohty M. Current status of reduced-intensity-conditioning allogeneic stem cell transplantation for acute myeloid leukemia. Haematologica 2007; 92: 533–541.
8. Bacigalupo A, Ballen K, Rizzo D et al. Defining the intensity of conditioning regimens: Working definitions. Biol Blood Marrow Transplant 2009; 15: 1628–1633.
9. Ho VT, Soiffer RJ. The history and future of T-cell depletion as graft-versus-host disease prophylaxis for allogeneic hematopoietic stem cell transplantation. Blood 2001; 98: 3192–3204.
10. Soiffer RJ, Lerademacher J, Ho V et al. Impact of immune modulation with anti–T-cell antibodies on the outcome of reduced-intensity allogeneic hematopoietic stem cell transplantation for hematologic malignancies. Blood 2011; 117: 6963–6970.
11. Mohty M, Gaugler B. Advances in umbilical cord transplantation: The role of thymoglobulin/ATG in cord blood transplantation. Best Pract Res Clin Haematol 2010; 23: 275–282.
12. Cantoni N, Gerull S, Heim D et al. Order of application and liver toxicity in patients given BU and CY containing conditioning regimens for allogeneic hematopoietic SCT. Bone Marrow Transplant 2011; 46: 344–349.
13. Satwani P, Cooper N, Rao K et al. Reduced intensity conditioning and allogeneic stem cell transplantation in childhood malignant and nonmalignant diseases. Bone Marrow Transplant 2008; 41: 173–182.
14. Ljungman P, Bregni M, Brune M et al. Allogeneic and autologous transplantation for haematological diseases, solid tumours and immune disorders: Current practice in Europe 2009. Bone Marrow Transplant 2010; 45: 219–234.
15. Bacigalupo A, Socié G, Lanino E et al. Severe Aplastic Anemia Working Party of the European Group for Blood and Marrow Transplantation. Fludarabine, cyclophosphamide, antithymocyte globulin, with or without low dose total body irradiation, for alternative donor transplants, in acquired severe aplastic anemia: A retrospective study from the EBMT-SAA working party. Haematologica 2010; 95: 976–982.
16. Cavo M, Rajkumar S, Palumbo V et al. International Myeloma Working Group consensus

approach to the treatment of multiple myeloma patients who are candidates for autologous stem cell transplantation Blood 2011; 117: 6063–6073.

17. Gratwohl A. Allogeneic hematopoietic stem-cell transplantation for myeloma: It's time for the appropriate studies. J Clin Oncol 2011; 29: e483.

18. Secondino S, Carrabba MG, Pedrazzoli P et al.; European Group for Blood and Marrow Transplantation Solid Tumors Working Party. Reduced intensity stem cell transplantation for advanced soft tissue sarcomas in adults: A retrospective analysis of the European Group for Blood and Marrow Transplantation. Haematologica 2007; 92: 418–420.

19. Gratwohl A, Brand R, Niederwieser D et al. Introduction of a quality management system and outcome after hematopoietic stem-cell transplantation. J Clin Oncol 2011; 29: 1980–1986.

Multiple Choice Questionnaire

To find the correct answer, go to http://www.esh.org/online-training/handbook/

1. **Total body irradiation (TBI) is frequently used for conditioning in HSCT. Its biological effects depend primarily on:**
   a) Radiation source . . . . ☐
   b) Total radiation dose applied . . . . ☐
   c) Combination of dose rate and fractions of doses . . . . ☐
   d) Combination of total dose, dose rate and fractions of doses . . . . ☐

---

2. **The type of conditioning regimen is more important in autologous than in allogeneic HSCT, because:**
   a) Graft versus tumour reaction is the only element in allogeneic HSCT for tumour control . . . . ☐
   b) Dose intensification of tumour specific therapy is the key element of autologous HSCT . . . . ☐
   c) There is no specific chemotherapy in allogeneic HSCT . . . . ☐
   d) Monoclonal antibodies, such as CD20+ antibodies can only be integrated in the conditioning in autologous HSCT . . . . ☐

---

3. **Which of the following statements about reduced intensity conditioning (RIC) is correct?**
   a) RIC has a specific advantage in patients with advanced malignancies . . . ☐

b) RIC has a specific advantage in patients with non-malignant conditions where no graft-versus-disease effect is required .... ☐
c) RIC has a specific advantage in CMV positive patients with CMV negative donors .... ☐
d) Peripheral blood as a stem cell source is associated with less rejection than bone marrow in patients with RIC .... ☐

4. **There is an inherent dilemma in allogeneic HSCT: increasing conditioning decreases risk of rejection and risk of relapse at the expense of increased toxicity; *vice versa*, decreased conditioning decreases direct regimen related toxicity at the expense of increased risk of rejection and relapse. Which of the following statements about this dilemma is true?**
a) Different regimens should be employed for patients with high-risk disease and low transplant risk compared to patients with low-risk disease but high transplant risk .... ☐
b) T-cell depletion can abolish this dilemma .... ☐
c) The statement does not hold true for unrelated cord blood transplants .. ☐
d) The statement is not correct for non-malignant disorders .... ☐

5. **Which one of the following can reduce the toxicity of busulfan?**
a) To use intravenous busulfan .... ☐
b) To adapt the doses of busulfan to the blood levels .... ☐
c) To administrate busulfan after cyclophosphamide .... ☐
d) All of the above .... ☐

* CHAPTER 9

Transfusion support in patients undergoing HSCT

Rachel Pawson, Derwood Pamphilon

1. Introduction

Haematopoietic stem cell transplant (HSCT) patients may require intensive blood component support. Complications of transfusions include transmission of viral and bacterial infections, transfusion-associated (TA)-GvHD and transfusion-related acute lung injury. Alloimmunisation (AI) to red cell antigens may cause difficulties in selecting compatible blood whilst AI to human leucocyte antigens (HLA) expressed on platelets may cause subsequent platelet transfusion refractoriness. It is essential to define robust transfusion policies and procedures and these should be regularly audited. This chapter reviews blood component transfusion in the setting of HSCT and describes policies for selection and testing of high quality blood components, blood component specification and appropriate use, the prevention of platelet transfusion refractoriness, TA-GvHD and *Cytomegalovirus* (CMV) transmission, the use of granulocyte transfusions and the management of ABO-mismatched HSCT with specific reference to the impact of reduced intensity conditioning (RIC).

2. Selection and testing of blood components in Europe in the era of regulation and quality

The European Union (EU) Directive 2002/98/EC sets standards for the collection, testing, processing, storage and distribution of human blood and blood components (1). It requires that Blood Establishments should be licensed and this is of importance for both Blood Centres in EU countries that undertake these activities as well as hospitals that collect and issue components such as granulocytes for transfusion. The most important aspects of the Directive are:

- The fate of each unit of all blood components should be recorded and this record kept for 30 years. i.e. vein-to-vein traceability
- Robust quality systems should be in place
- The processing of blood and blood components should be undertaken by licensed blood establishments (see above)
- Training should be provided for hospital transfusion laboratory staff
- Haemovigilance systems should be established to include the reporting of adverse events.

Establishments are licensed by the Competent Authorities in EU Member States following inspection by a regulatory body – in the UK this is the Medicines and Healthcare Products Regulatory Authority (MHRA) – and reports of compliance must be submitted.

2.1 Microbiological testing

Concerns about overall product quality and transfusion transmitted infection (TTI) has driven the implementation of quality initiatives and regulation. The EU Directive

(1) requires that all blood donations and components for clinical use have mandatory testing for HBsAg, anti-HIV 1 and 2, anti-HCV, HCV NAT, anti-HTLV I/II and syphilis antibodies. Further additional discretionary testing may be undertaken to increase the safety of transfusion for particular donors or recipients e.g. CMV serology to provide a supply of CMV seronegative components. In addition, there are also strict donor selection criteria to increase the safety of the blood supply. In the UK, universal leucodepletion (LD) has been in place since 1999 to reduce the risk of transfusion-transmitted variant CJD and is widely used in Austria, France, Germany and the Netherlands. An alternative is to use pathogen reduction (PR) to reduce transfusion-transmitted infections and in recent years, several approaches to PR have been developed including solvent-detergent treatment, methylene blue and visible light, psoralen S-59 and UVA light and riboflavin treatment. Examples of the latter two technologies are CE-marked and in use for treatment of platelets in Belgium, France and Italy. These strategies are attractive since the inactivation of nucleic acid would, in addition, eliminate the likelihood of other complications such as alloimmunisation to HLA and TA-GvHD.

2.2 Blood grouping and antibody testing

The ABO and Rhesus D type of all donated blood is determined by standard techniques. All donations are tested to exclude the presence of immune IgG antibodies that are reactive with common blood groups and which occur after an immunising stimulus such as pregnancy or transfusion. Selected units of red cells are more extensively phenotyped (Kell, Duffy, Kidd, MNSs antigens) to be used for patients with red cell alloantibodies.

3. General principles of transfusion support

The appropriate use of blood components according to pre-defined policies helps to minimise complications, many of which are not specific to HSCT patients. Transplant centres should have policies based on national and international guidelines and consensus documents describing the thresholds and doses to be used for transfusion; they should also conduct regular audits to ensure that blood components are used appropriately.

3.1 Red cell support

3.1.1 Red cell concentrates (RCC)
These may be:
• Suspended in additive solutions, usually a combination of saline, adenine,

glucose and mannitol (SAG-M): haematocrit 0.5–0.7, volume 220–340 mL.
- Derived from whole blood from which a proportion of the plasma has been removed - plasma reduced blood (PRB): haematocrit 0.5–0.6, volume 200–450 mL. A haematocrit of >0.7 is used for intrauterine transfusions.
- Unmodified whole blood: volume 420–560 mL.

The last term is misleading since platelets and labile coagulation factors deteriorate rapidly in stored blood. The storage period for red cells is 35–49 days and for whole blood is 28–35 days at 4 ± 2°C. RCC in additive solutions are the product of choice. Specifications above are taken from Guidelines for UK Blood Transfusion Services and the EU Guide to the Preparation, Use and Quality Assurance of Blood Components (2).

3.1.2 Red cell transfusion policy

- Red cells should be matched for ABO and Rhesus D type.
- Extended patient phenotyping eg for Kell, Duffy, Kidd, MNSs antigens is advisable in patients having long-term transfusion support eg patients with sickle cell disease, thalassaemia, severe aplastic anaemia and myelodysplastic syndromes. This allows selection of red cell units matched for some significant antigens e.g. Rhesus and Kell and aids antibody identification if it occurs.
- Red cells should be cross-matched against the patients serum by standard techniques prior to transfusion.
- Thresholds should be defined for haemoglobin and haematocrit below which red cell transfusions are always given although the evidence on which to base these is sparse. Suggested arbitrary cut off points are Hb <8.0 g/dL and haematocrit <25% unless there is significant cardiac impairment or symptoms of anaemia.
- In adults 1 unit of red cells raises the Hb by 1.0 g/dL whereas in children the volume of blood to be transfused is derived from the formula:
Volume = Increase in Hb (g/dL) required x 4 x weight (kg)

3.2 Platelet support

3.2.1 Platelet concentrates (PC)

These can be produced in three ways:
- By centrifuging units of whole blood in a "top-top" pack format to obtain platelet rich plasma (PRP), which is then further concentrated. PRP-PCs may be transfused individually or pooled in multiples - usually 6. The average content is >55 x 10^9 per whole blood donation (so 6 times this for a pool of 6).
- By centrifuging units of whole blood in a "bottom & top" (BAT) pack format to separate the buffy coat (BC), pooling 4 BCs (usually between 4 and 6) and recentrifuging to separate PRP which is then expressed into a secondary storage

container. The average content of platelets: 3×10^{11}; WBC $<1 \times 10^6$.

- By collecting PCs directly on a cell separator with an inherently low WBC content as a result of the process. The average content of platelets: 3×10^{11}; WBC $<1 \times 10^6$.

The storage period is 5 days at $22 \pm 2°C$ although this may be extended to 7 days if either pathogen activation or bacterial screening is used.

3.2.2 Platelet transfusion policy

Historically prophylactic platelet transfusions have been used to prevent severe haemorrhage. Clinical Practice Guidelines from North America and Europe - reviewed in reference (3) - recommend a platelet transfusion threshold of $<10 \times 10^9/L$ for prophylaxis and the higher threshold of $20 \times 10^9/L$ for patients who have mucosal bleeding or a temperature $>38°C$. These recommendations are based on evidence from randomised controlled trials showing that the lower threshold is not detrimental in terms of bleeding, red cell and platelet transfusion requirements and overall outcome (4). However, given improvements in both the quality of platelet components and other aspects of supportive care, debate has centred on whether prophylactic platelet transfusion is necessary at all and an important clinical trial, the Trial of Prophylactic Platelets Study (TOPPS) is currently recruiting patients in the UK and Australia aiming to answer this question. Specific advice is as follows:

- PCs should be ABO and Rh compatible wherever possible since ABO incompatibility may reduce the expected count increment (CI) by 10–30%.
- Group O PCs should be tested for high titre anti-A, B and if positive should only be transfused to group O recipients to avoid haemolysis caused by passive administration of antibody.
- If Rh D positive platelets are given to an Rh D negative woman of child-bearing potential it is recommended that 250 IU polyclonal anti-Rh (D) immunoglobulin should be given. This dose would cover up to 5 adult therapeutic doses of platelets given over 6 weeks and should be given subcutaneously in thrombocytopenic patients. Since the chance of Rh immunisation is probably <5% anti-D may be omitted and the patient's serum screened at intervals or prior to a red cell transfusion.

The established guidelines for platelet transfusion are:

- A threshold of $10 \times 10^9/L$ for prophylactic platelet transfusion.
- A higher threshold of $20 \times 10^9/L$ in patients with fever, sepsis, splenomegaly and other well established causes of increased platelet consumption.
- A threshold of $>50 \times 10^9/L$ if an invasive procedure is planned, e.g. central line insertion.

PCs are contraindicated in patients with thrombotic thrombocytopenic purpura (TTP). In adults the usual dose of platelets is 3×10^{11} (adult therapeutic dose - ATD) in a volume of 200–300 mL; in children 15–30 kg transfuse 0.5 ATD (volume 100–150 mL); in children <15 kg a proportionately smaller volume is given.

- Rate of transfusion:
  - Adults 1 ATD is given usually in <60 minutes
  - Children e.g. 2–5 mL/kg/hr
- Outcome - monitor by:
  - Looking for cessation of bleeding
  - Measuring the platelet count the following day. A persistent value $<20 \times 10^9/L$ suggests refractoriness
- If the patient is refractory to transfusion of PCs, consider clinical causes. If none are present, samples should be taken to test for HLA antibodies
- HLA-matched platelets collected by apheresis of HLA-typed donors should be used in patients with HLA alloimmunisation
- If the platelet count remains $<10 \times 10^9/L$ and/or bleeding persists then:
  - Check for non-immune causes of refractoriness
  - Look for platelet-specific antibodies - this is a rare cause of refractoriness in HSCT patients
  - Consider using cross-matched platelets: HLA-typed or random units of platelets are cross-matched against the patients serum usually by an immunofluorescent technique and unreactive units selected if possible
  - If the platelet count remains $<10 \times 10^9/L$ following transfusion of HLA matched PCs and the patient is not bleeding then withhold platelet transfusion
  - If refractoriness is due to non-immune causes, particularly if there is significant clinical bleeding then either give 2 or 3 ATD or give 1 ATD twice or three times daily.

3.3 Fresh frozen plasma and cryoprecipitate

3.3.1 Products

Fresh frozen plasma (FFP) is made by centrifuging whole blood and freezing separated plasma within 24 hours of collection. The volume is 200–340 mL and factor VIII level should be >70 IU/mL (usually in >75% units).

Cryoprecipitate is made by controlled thawing of FFP at 4°C and centrifugation after which cryoproteins are separated and resuspended in approximately 20–30 mL plasma. This is then refrozen. The fibrinogen and factor VIII levels should be >140 mg/dL and >70 IU/mL respectively (usually in >75% units). FFP and cryoprecipitate have a storage period of 24–36 months at < -25°C.

3.3.2 Transfusion policy
- FFP transfusion is indicated after HSCT in the following circumstances:
  - Liver disease causing significant defects of coagulation factors
  - Severe DIC
  - As replacement fluid in TTP where plasma exchange is undertaken.
- FFP transfusion may be indicated after HSCT where:
  - Large volume blood transfusion, e.g. after haemorrhage, has caused a dilutional coagulopathy
  - The volume transfused is 10–15 mL/kg.
- Cryoprecipitate transfusion is indicated in severe DIC with bleeding and fibrinogen <100 mg/dL.
- Outcome - monitor the clinical response and prothrombin time (PT) and activated partial thromboplastin time (APTT). The ratios compared to control should correct to <1.5. In DIC the fibrinogen should be >100 mg/dL.

3.4 Granulocyte transfusion

3.4.1 Products
Granulocytes for transfusion can be prepared in three ways: by apheresis of unstimulated donors, by apheresis after stimulation of donors with G-CSF and/or dexamethasone and by pooling of buffy coats from whole blood donations with or without an optimisation step. Donors are stimulated with G-CSF and dexamethasone 12–24 hours prior to apheresis to increase the circulating number of granulocytes. Granulocyte yields of 36–84 x 10^9 can be obtained by this method, compared to 5.4 x 10^9 in unstimulated donors (5). Pooled buffy coats can give yields of up to 10 x 10^9 granulocytes from 10 donations (5).

3.4.2 Transfusion policy
HSCT patients are at high risk of neutropenic sepsis due to the duration and depth of neutropenia. Granulocyte transfusions (GT) are given as secondary prophylaxis to patients with a history of severe fungal or (rarely) bacterial infection prior to HSCT or as therapy in those in whom such infection develops post-transplant and who are unresponsive to appropriate antimicrobial therapy. Not all blood services permit the administration of G-CSF and steroids to voluntary unrelated donors due to the small but potential risks to donors, in particular the possible risk of developing haematological malignancies (6). A recent report of 10 year follow up of unrelated volunteer granulocyte donors suggested that stimulation with G-CSF and dexamethasone is not associated with significant differences in the occurrence of malignancies, coronary artery disease, and thrombosis (7). The authors concluded

that, although the number of granulocyte donors studied is small and continued surveillance of healthy individuals after G-CSF is prudent, the data suggest that G-CSF plus dexamethasone stimulation appears to be safe.

There is still no conclusive evidence of the clinical efficacy of GT either in the treatment of neutropenic sepsis or as prophylaxis for high risk patients. A recent Cochrane review concluded that there is a possibility that prophylactic GT at a dose of $\geq 10 \times 10^9$ may reduce the risk of mortality from infection but overall mortality was not affected. The majority of the studies included were performed many years ago and both supportive care and the yields of granulocytes have improved since then (8). The review found it difficult to recommend prophylactic GT outside the setting of clinical trials.

Similarly, the evidence for GT in the treatment of neutropenic sepsis does not provide conclusive evidence of efficacy in reducing mortality and improving outcome from infection. Many studies have reported a beneficial effect with use of GT but further clinical randomised trials are required (9).

4. ABO incompatibility and selection of appropriate blood components

15–25% of HLA matched sibling allografts are ABO mismatched and the figure is higher in unrelated allografts. In the peri- and post-transplant period changing blood groups and persistence of recipient alloagglutinins provide challenges to ensure compatible blood components are provided. Types of ABO incompatibility are defined as:

- Major
  - alloagglutinins anti-A, -B or -AB reactive to donor red cells present in recipient plasma e.g. recipient Group O, donor Group A
- Minor
  - alloagglutinins anti-A, -B or -AB reactive to recipient red cells present in donor plasma e.g. recipient Group A, donor Group O
- Bidirectional
  - presence of reactive alloagglutinins in both recipient and donor plasma e.g. recipient Group B, donor Group A.

4.1 Problems encountered in ABO mismatched HSCT

4.1.1 Acute haemolysis when the graft is given
In major ABO incompatibility there is the potential for an immediate haemolytic reaction to occur during transfusion of stem cells. Modification during apheresis collection or processing of stem cells to reduce red cell contamination significantly

reduces this. It is recommended practice that red cell contamination should be reduced to less than 20 mL where the host anti-donor ABH alloagglutinin titre is 1 in 32 or greater. In minor ABO incompatibility where alloagglutinin titres are 1 in 256 or greater, plasma should be removed from bone marrow products (10).

4.1.2 Pure red cell aplasia, delayed erythropoietic recovery and increased transfusion requirements

RIC schedules spare more B-cells and plasma cells than myeloablative regimes such that recipient anti-donor alloagglutinins can persist for a long time post-transplant. Evidence suggests that this might increase the occurrence of pure red cell aplasia (PRCA) and delayed erythropoietic recovery and may increase transfusion requirements in the ABO-mismatched setting, reviewed in reference (3).

In one study early establishment of myeloid donor chimerism in the absence of PRCA led the authors to postulate that the type of conditioning, specifically the use of alemtuzumab, and degree of B-cell suppression achieved could be important. Mijovic et al. reported no difference in erythroid recovery, disappearance of recipient isohaemagglutinins, emergence of donor red cells or incidence of PRCA between RIC and recipients, reinforcing the view that alemtuzumab played a critical role in dampening immune reactions in the host and donor (3). A retrospective analysis of 153 patients undergoing major/bidirectional ABO incompatible HSCT with two different regimes, either (i) pre-transplant reduction of anti-donor isoagglutinin titre and post-transplant transfusion of donor type red cells or (ii) removal of RBC from the graft followed by post transplant recipient type red cells, concluded that PRCA and delayed red cell engraftment depended on the pre-transplant anti-donor isoagglutinin titres and could be prevented by pre-transplant removal of anti-donor isoagglutinins (11).

4.1.3 Passenger lymphocyte syndrome

Delayed haemolytic reactions can occur in minor ABO mismatch because of a secondary (amnestic) response, termed the passenger lymphocyte syndrome, mediated via memory B-cells in the graft that are re-stimulated by recipient ABO antigens. This phenomenon is rarely seen in T-cell depleted grafts or when CD34 positive selection is used in stem cell processing. It develops 7–14 days post-transplant with anaemia and jaundice as the principal clinical features (10).

4.1.4 Overall outcome of transplant

ABO mismatching might not only impact red cell engraftment and haemolysis, but also overall survival (OS), disease-free survival (DFS) and the occurrence of GvHD and other complications; available reports, some from large studies, disagree on this. Seebach et al. reported equivalent outcomes for OS, treatment-related mortality (TRM) and incidence of GvHD in a series of 3,103 patients where 995 were ABO mismatched (451 minor, 430 major and 114 bidirectional (12)). However, a report from the Japan Marrow Donor Program in 5,549 recipients found reduced OS (ABO identical 63%; major mismatch 56.9%; minor mismatch 57.1%) at 1 year, increased TRM, delayed trilineage engraftment and increased severe GvHD (13). These differences are not explained at present. A recent meta-analysis of 6 published studies and 1 unpublished study found no overall difference in OS between recipients of ABO matched or mismatched grafts and no differences with regard to outcome from related donor allografts. In unrelated donor transplants there was a marginally reduced OS in patients who received bidirectionally or minor mismatched transplants, particularly those with acute leukaemia, patients transplanted after 1998 and in Asian transplant centres (14).

4.2 Blood groups used for transfusion support in ABO mismatched HSCT
Pre-transplant: blood component support should be with recipient type blood components.
Post-transplant: selection of the appropriate group is more complicated (see Figure 1). The requirements for platelet and FFP support are also shown. The following groups should be given post-transplant until engraftment when ABO antibodies to the donor ABO group are undetectable and the direct antiglobulin test is negative:
Major ABO incompatibility: red cells of group O or recipient's own ABO group should be given. Plasma and platelets should be of donor-type blood group.
Minor ABO incompatibility: red cells of donor ABO group should be given. Plasma and platelets should be of recipient-type blood group.
Bidirectional ABO incompatibility: give group O red cells, group AB plasma and platelets of recipient-type blood group.

5. Leucodepletion and alloimmunisation
Transfused leucocytes may provoke AI to HLA class 1 antigens. This can be manifest clinically as febrile non-haemolytic transfusion reactions, although these may also be caused by antibodies to neutrophils, platelets, plasma proteins and by cytokines such as interleukin (IL)-1, IL-6, IL-8 and tumour necrosis factor (TNF)-α which accumulate in stored blood components, especially platelet concentrates (15). HLA sensitisation may result in accelerated destruction of HLA-incompatible platelets and platelet transfusion refractoriness. Donor dendritic cells in red cell and platelet transfusions are responsible for sensitisation to HLA and studies show that removal of leucocytes to less than 5×10^6 per blood component prevents primary HLA AI

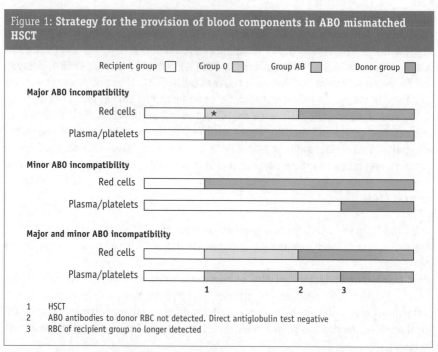

Figure 1: **Strategy for the provision of blood components in ABO mismatched HSCT**

1 HSCT
2 ABO antibodies to donor RBC not detected. Direct antiglobulin test negative
3 RBC of recipient group no longer detected

Or recipient-type red cells. Modified from Practical Transfusion Medicine with permission (Figure 27.3, page 138). Practical Transfusion Medicine (Third Edition) Murphy MF, Pamphilon D, Wiley-Blackwell Publishers 2009; 138

in >97% of patients with haematological malignancies (16). The use of leucodepleted blood components also reduces secondary AI and refractoriness (17). More than 50% of refractoriness results from non-immune causes such as fever, splenomegaly, disseminated intravascular coagulation and concurrent amphotericin therapy (16). HLA AI is associated with the development of red cell alloantibodies in patients with sickle cell disease, an increased chance of graft failure after unrelated or haploidentical HSCT and delayed neutrophil recovery after umbilical cord blood transplantation (3). HLA sensitisation can be reduced by filtration of whole blood or individual components which should be done in Blood Centres and hospital blood banks. Data from studies where leucocytes were filtered from blood components at the bedside show that this may be ineffective in preventing or reducing FNHTR, AI and refractoriness (18). Photo- or photochemical inactivation of blood components also reduces AI but are not yet widely use for this indication (17).

• If the patient is refractory to transfusion of PCs, consider clinical causes. If none

are present, samples should be taken to test for HLA antibodies.
- HLA-matched platelets collected by apheresis of HLA-typed donors should be used in refractory patients with HLA alloimmunisation.
- If there are no increments in the platelet count and/or bleeding persists then:
  - Check for non-immune causes of refractoriness
  - Look for platelet-specific antibodies - this is a rare cause of refractoriness in HSCT patients
  - If there is no increment following transfusion of HLA matched PCs and the patient is not bleeding then withhold platelet transfusion
  - If refractoriness is due to non-immune causes, particularly if there is significant clinical bleeding, then either give 2 or 3 ATD or give 1 ATD twice or three times daily.

6. Prevention of CMV transmission

CMV reactivation and disease is a major cause of morbidity and mortality in HSCT patients. Transmission of CMV through blood products has been shown to be an important cause of primary CMV infection in the HSCT population. In immunocompetent individuals the virus remains latent in leucocytes and if transfused into immunocompromised patients can cause significant infection. It is important that measures are taken to reduce transmission of CMV through blood components. Current technologies include:
- *Provision of CMV seronegative blood components*. In certain areas the prevalence of CMV seropositivity is high in the donor population making provision of CMV seronegative components difficult. Maintaining a CMV seronegative blood component inventory is also expensive. Studies have shown that using CMV seronegative blood products in CMV seronegative patients who have received CMV seronegative stem cells reduces the risk of primary infection to 0–7% (19–21). In CMV seropositive patients or those that have received CMV seropositive stem cells CMV infection is mostly due to reactivation from previous exposure such that the use of seronegative components has little impact (19).
  The use of CMV DNA testing is under consideration or use in some countries. However, variation in the sensitivity and specificity of PCR assays has been associated with widely varying estimates of the frequency of detection of CMV DNA in blood donations (22). The recent introduction of an international reference standard for CMV viral load measurement will facilitate assessment of the usefulness of this methodology.
- *Leucodepleted (LD) blood components*. The American Association of Blood Banks (AABB) suggests that levels of less than 5×10^6 leucocytes per blood component

may significantly reduce transfusion transmitted (TT)-CMV. Some studies have suggested that LD is as effective as CMV seronegative components (19, 21) but there is no conclusive evidence as to what level of LD is required to prevent TT-CMV. The authors of a meta-analysis concluded that CMV seronegative blood components are more effective than LD in preventing TT-CMV. However, only 3 controlled studies in HSCT patients were identified, only one of which was randomised and another used bedside filtration which is thought to be less efficient at removing CMV than pre-storage LD (21). It has been suggested that CMV seronegative components can be abandoned if pre-storage LD is used but this remains controversial. A survey of practice in 183 institutions in USA reports wide variability in the use of LD versus CMV seronegative products (23). A European Survey on provision of CMV safe components performed in 2010 found 5 of 15 responding countries do not perform CMV serology testing at all but rely on LD. Of the 10 countries who did screen for CMV, 8 provided CMV negative units for bone marrow transplant patients where both the donor and recipient are CMV seronegative but 2 did not (S. MacLennan, personal communication). One of the largest bone marrow transplant centres in the USA abandoned the use of CMV seronegative components for its transplant patients in 2010 and no increase in post-transplant CMV infection has been seen (T. Gernsheimer, personal communication). In the UK, the Department of Health has called for a review of the provision of CMV-safe blood components, the results of which are awaited. In summary, both LD and the use of CMV seronegative products are effective in the prevention of TT-CMV but neither provide complete protection. Centres should establish their own policies and monitor outcome.

7. Transfusion associated graft-versus-host disease
Viable donor lymphocytes in blood components can proliferate in the recipient and cause TA-GvHD which is fatal in >90% of cases. The clinical symptoms are fever, rash, diarrhoea, liver dysfunction and pancytopenia. Diagnosis may be confirmed by skin, gut or liver biopsy or evidence of persistence of third party (transfusion donor) lymphocytes in recipient tissues (24). Short tandem repeat analysis on peripheral blood or biopsies from affected and non-affected skin areas in patients showing persistent donor cells can be diagnostic (24). Although this complication has also been reported in non-immunocompromised patients due to haplotype sharing, HSCT patients are at high risk, including recipients of autologous HSCT. Gamma- or X-irradiation of cellular blood components inhibits lymphocyte proliferation. In the UK the current recommended dose is that a minimum of 25 Gy is given to all parts of the blood component pack. The American Association

of Blood Banks (AABB) recommend a dose of 25 Gy to the central area of the component with no portion receiving less than 15 Gy (25). The blood components that require irradiation are summarised in Table 1. The need for irradiated blood products depends on the tempo of immune reconstitution, but serial measurements of this are impractical in the context of determining the requirement for irradiated blood components. The current European Group for Blood and Marrow Transplantation (EBMT) Guideline (2008) is:

- Autologous HSCT: 3 months, 6 months if TBI used
- Allogeneic HSCT: from time of initiation of chemoradiotherapy until immunosuppression stopped or lymphocytes >1 x 10^9
- It is also recommended that stem cell donors receive irradiated blood components from 7 days prior to harvest
- At present leucodepletion is not considered sufficient to prevent TA-GvHD in immunocompromised individuals (26).

In the UK, no cases of TA-GvHD have been reported to SHOT (Serious Hazards of Transfusion) the UK national haemovigilance scheme for 8 years. Two cases of TA-GvHD following transfusion of leucodepleted components have been reported to SHOT, one in 1998–1999 before the introduction of universal leucodepletion (in 1999) and the other in 2000–2001. In the last 7 years, 596 cases have been reported where irradiated blood components were indicated but the patients were inadvertently transfused with non-irradiated components; none of them developed TA-GvHD (26). However, the report emphasises that the absence of new cases is a testament to the successful prevention of TA-GvHD and that it would be imprudent to interpret it as a sign that there is no longer a risk of TA-GvHD (27).

Table 1: **Blood components that require irradiation**

Blood components requiring irradiation to prevent TA-GvHD

- Whole blood
- Red cells
- Platelets (pooled and apheresis)
- Granulocytes

Blood components that do not require irradiation

- Fresh frozen plasma
- Cryoprecipitate
- Fractionated plasma products
- Albumin
- Intravenous immunoglobulin
- Deglycerolised red cells

Acknowledgements
The authors are grateful to Carol Griffin for her invaluable assistance in preparing the manuscript.

References

1. European Union Directive 2002/98/EC http://eurlex.europa.eu/LexUriServ/site/en/oj/ 2003/l_033/l_03320030208en00300040.pdf
2. European Directorate for Quality of Medicines and Healthcare, Strasbourg. EU Guide to Preparation, Use and Quality Assurance of Blood Components 2010.
3. Radia R, Pamphilon D. Transfusion strategies in patients undergoing stem-cell transplantation. Expert Rev Hematol 2011; 4: 213–220.
4. Rebulla P, Finazzi G, Marangoni F et al. The threshold for prophylactic platelet transfusions in adults with acute myeloid leukaemia. N Engl J Med 1997; 337: 1870–1875.
5. Standard Advisory Committee on Blood Components, Stanworth S, Cardigan R, Massey E. Position Statement: Granulocyte Therapy. Joint UKBTS/ NIBSC Professional Advisory Committee, 2008.
6. Pamphilon D, Nacheva E, Navarrete C et al. The use of granulocyte-colony-stimulating factor in volunteer unrelated hemopoietic stem cell donors. Transfusion 2008; 48: 1495–1501.
7. Quillen K, Byrne P, Yau YY, Leitman SF. Ten year follow-up of unrelated volunteer granulocyte donors who have received multiple cycles of granulocyte colony-stimulating factor and dexamethasone. Transfusion 2009; 49: 513–518.
8. Massey E, Paulus U, Doree C, Stanworth S. Granulocyte transfusions for preventing infections in patients with neutropenia or neutrophil dysfunction. Cochrane Database Syst Rev, CD005341 2009.
9. Robinson SP, Marks DI. Mini Review: Granulocyte transfusions in the G-CSF era. Where do we stand? Bone Marrow Transplant 2004; 34: 834–846.
10. Rowley SD, Donato ML, Bhattacharyya P. Red blood cell-incompatible allogeneic hematopoietic progenitor cell transplantation. Bone Marrow Transplant 2011; 46: 116–1185.
11. Stussi G, Halter J, Bucheli E et al. Prevention of pure red cell aplasia after major or bi-directional ABO blood group incompatible hematopoietic stem cell transplantation by pre-transplant reduction of host anti-donor isoagglutinins. Haematologica 2009; 94: 239–248.
12. Seebach JD, Stussi G, Passweg JR et al. ABO blood group barrier in allogeneic bone marrow transplantation revisited. Biol Blood Marrow Transplant 2005; 11: 1006–1013.
13. Kimura F, Sato K, Kobayashi S et al. Impact of ABO-blood group incompatibility on the outcome of recipients of bone marrow transplants from unrelated donors in the Japan Marrow Donor Program. Haematologica 2008; 93: 1686–1693.
14. Kanda J, Ichinohe T, Matsuo K et al. Impact of ABO mismatching on the outcomes of allogeneic related and unrelated blood and marrow stem cell transplantations for hematologic malignancies: IPD-based meta-analysis of cohort studies. Transfusion 2009; 49: 624–635.

15. Yazer MH, Podlosky L, Clarke G, Nahirniak SM. The effect of prestorage WB reduction on the rates of febrile nonhemolytic transfusion reactions to platelet concentrates and RBC. Transfusion 2004; 44: 10–15.
16. Slichter SJ. Platelet refractoriness and alloimmunization. Leukemia 1998; 1 (Suppl 1): S51–53.
17. Leukocyte reduction and ultraviolet B irradiation of platelets to prevent alloimmunization and refractoriness to platelet transfusions. The Trial to Reduce Alloimmunization to Platelets Study Group. N Engl J Med 1997; 337: 1861–1869.
18. Williamson LM, Wimperis JZ, Williamson P et al. Bedside filtration of blood products in the prevention of HLA alloimmunisation - a prospective randomised study. Alloimmunisation Study Group. Blood 1994; 83: 3028–3035.
19. Bowden RA, Sayers M, Fluornoy N et al. Cytomegalovirus immune globulin and seronegative blood products to prevent primary cytomegalovirus infection after marrow transplantation. N Engl J Med 1986; 314: 1006–1010.
20. Nichols WG, Price TH, Gooley T et al. Transfusion-transmitted cytomegalovirus infection after receipt of leuko-reduced blood products. Blood 2003; 10: 4195–4200.
21. Vamvakas EC. Is white blood cell reduction equivalent to antibody screening in preventing transmission of cytomegalovirus by transfusion? A review of the literature and meta-analysis. Transfus Med Rev 2005; 19: 181–199.
22. Roback JD, Drew WL, Laycock ME et al. CMV DNA is rarely detected in healthy blood donors using validated PCR assays. Transfusion 2003; 43: 302–305.
23. Smith D, Lu Q, Yuan S et al. Survey of current practice for prevention of transfusion-transmitted cytomegalovirus in the United States: Leucoreduction vs. cytomegalovirus seronegative. Vox Sang 2010; 98: 29–36.
24. Shaz BH, Hillyer CD. Transfusion-associated graft-versus-host disease and microchimerism. In: Practical Transfusion Medicine (Third Edition). Murphy MF, Pamphilon D (Ed.), Wiley-Blackwell Publishers 2009; 107–116.
25. Standards for Blood Banks and Transfusion Services, 26th edition. American Association of Blood Banks, 2009.
26. Williamson LM, Stainsby D, Jones H et al. The impact of universal leukodepletion of the blood supply on hemovigilance reports of posttransfusion purpura and transfusion-associated graft-versus-host disease. Transfusion 2007; 47: 1455–1467.
27. Steering Group. Serious Hazards of Transfusion: SHOT Annual Report 2009.

Multiple Choice Questionnaire

To find the correct answer, go to http://www.esh.org/online-training/handbook/

1. The EU Directive for Blood and Blood Components (2002/98/EC) requires that hospitals collecting therapeutic granulocytes by apheresis:

a) Keep a record of the fate of each unit for 10 years............... ☐
b) Are licensed by the national competent authority............... ☐
c) Have the option to report adverse events............... ☐
d) Should test all blood components for anti-hepatitis B core antibodies... ☐

2. **The strategy with proven efficacy in the prevention of transfusion-associated graft-versus-host disease in BMT patients is:**
   a) Leucodepletion by filtration .... ☐
   b) Photoinactivation with a psoralen and ultraviolet light .... ☐
   c) X- or gamma-irradiation .... ☐
   d) HLA matching of blood components .... ☐

3. **Platelet concentrates:**
   a) May be stored for up to 10 days if they are tested for bacterial contamination .... ☐
   b) New trial data suggests that prophylactic transfusions are unnecessary............... ☐
   c) The accepted threshold for platelet transfusion in stable thrombocytopenic patients is 20 x 10^9/L............... ☐
   d) The accepted threshold for platelet transfusion in febrile (T >38°C) thrombocytopenic patients is 20 x 10^9/L .... ☐

4. **Refractoriness to platelet transfusion is best managed by:**
   a) HLA typing all patients pre-transplant and transfusing HLA matched platelets to prevent it occurring .... ☐
   b) Transfusing 2–3 therapeutic doses of random platelet concentrates each day if there is clinical bleeding .... ☐
   c) Transfusing crossmatched random platelet concentrates each day if there is clinical bleeding .... ☐
   d) Excluding non-immune causes and transfusing HLA-matched platelet concentrates .... ☐

5. **A group O Rh(D) positive patient with AML is about to receive reduced intensity conditioning and a bone marrow allograft from her**

HLA-identical sister who is A Rh(D) positive. The patient's anti-A titre is 1:128. It is the case that:
a) The graft can be infused unmanipulated with attention to hydration and urinary output .... ☐
b) Passenger lymphocyte syndrome is a likely complication .... ☐
c) Post-transplant red cell transfusions should be group O Rh(D) positive .. ☐
d) The decline in recipient anti-donor alloagglutinin titre would the same as if the patient received myeloablative conditioning .... ☐

6. **A patient with aplastic anaemia and suspected fungal infection remains pyrexial after transplant from an unrelated donor and appropriate anti-microbial therapy. Granulocyte transfusions:**
a) Will give the best results if obtained from pooled buffy coats .... ☐
b) Do not require irradiation .... ☐
c) A Cochrane review recommended the use of prophylactic granulocytes in this situation .... ☐
d) Should be obtained from healthy volunteers who have received G-CSF priming .... ☐

* CHAPTER 10

Supportive care

Tamás Masszi, Arno Mank

1. Introduction

Supportive care comprises all treatments given to prevent, control, or relieve complications and side effects in the HSCT process. Supportive care in HSCT is essential in optimising the outcome of the treatment. This chapter will focus on protective issues including protective isolation and hygiene aspects, nutritional support including low bacterial diet, the use of central venous devices and their consequences and complications, the use of haematopoietic growth factors, intervention pre- and post-transplant to prevent and treat oral mucositis, and anti-emesis strategies.

2. Protective issues

Patients with haematologic malignancies treated with HSCT are at great risk of developing infective complications because of marked immunosuppression and prolonged pancytopenia, together with mucosal injury. In addition to antimicrobial prophylaxis, there are other important strategies to prevent infections, together building up a network of infection control measures. Key points of these are: protective environment, protective clothing and equipment, hand hygiene, low microbial diet, vaccination and exclusion policy and monitoring infectious complications.

2.1 Protective environment (isolation) and cleaning

A variety of practices exist regarding the use of isolation for immunocompromised patients; however, the effectiveness of protective isolation has not been established. Numerous studies have assessed the effect of laminar airflow or HEPA filtration with conflicting results. Most of these studies tested several interventions simultaneously (e.g., chemoprophylaxis, protective clothing, and sterile food), making it difficult to determine whether independent effects of individual interventions were present. However, it has been shown that there is some protective effect of laminar airflow and HEPA filtration against infections, particularly aspergillosis, especially during hospital building programmes (1). Patient transport to diagnostic facilities or other wards should be avoided if possible or at least time spent outside the protective environment should be minimised. In addition it is important to improve hygiene measures such as daily cleaning and changing of bed linen. Fresh or potted flowers/plants should be banned from the patient's area.

2.2 Personal and hand hygiene, protective clothing and equipment

Because a large proportion of infections in patients with neutropenia is associated with the patient's own microbial flora, the patient's personal hygiene is of outstanding importance. Hand washing and hand disinfection of nursing and other personnel is also important and has been proven by multiple, well-designed studies to be one of the most effective ways to prevent the transmission of infection. There have also been studies of the benefit of antiseptic baths, but the evidence for an association between antiseptic bathing and reduced risk of infection is contradictory. Although several studies with gowns or other protective clothing have not been shown to reduce the risk of infections it seems to be prudent to discourage visitors from wearing coats or other outerwear in the patient's room.

2.3 Basics of hand hygiene
- This is important for patients as well as staff. All patients should regularly wash their hands with soap and water or use an antiseptic hand rub.
- Personnel should wash hands with soap and water between each patient contact, if hands are visibly dirty or contaminated. The same procedure should be followed if *C. difficile* is present. In all other cases alcohol-based hand rubs alone can be used.
- Hands may remain colonised with microorganisms after hand washing if hands are not dried properly.

2.4 Low bacterial diet
It has been argued that a diet containing food with low levels of bacteria can possibly help to reduce the number and/or severity of infections in cancer patients. However, there is no clear evidence that the use of a low bacterial diet (LBD) actually decreases the number of infections.

It is clear from numerous surveys of current practice that the majority of hospitals place neutropenic patients on a restricted diet. The range and level of restrictions regarding indications for starting and stopping LBD and the specific dietary products allowed showed large variations and contradictions (2). Moreover, compliance with restricted diets is inconsistent. In a randomised clinical trial of 153 patients a low bacterial diet did not prevent major infection or death (3). Other studies on smaller patient populations also failed to find significant difference in the amount of infections with a low bacterial diet compared to a normal diet. In spite of the current routine practice of applying LBD in most transplant wards, the true scientific proof for food restrictions remains lacking.

2.5 Vaccination and exclusion policy
It is advisable that health care workers and visitors in contact with transplant patients should be vaccinated for influenza, especially during the flu season. Personnel should also possess protective titers for *Varicella-zoster virus* (VZV). Individuals showing

signs and symptoms of a respiratory, gastrointestinal or muco-cutaneous infection should be excluded from work or should not be allowed to visit the patient.

2.6 Monitoring infection rate and antimicrobial resistance
Every centre should have a policy for monitoring the incidence of infections. At the same time trends of antimicrobial resistance must carefully be followed. The incidence of invasive fungal infections must be monitored, and a twofold increase within a six month period should prompt examination of possible environmental and logistic factors.

3. Nutritional and metabolic support
Nutritional and metabolic support prevent loss of lean body mass, fluid and electrolyte imbalance, increase patient comfort and improve survival for patients who are unable to eat or absorb nutrients for a prolonged period of time. The goal is to enable the patient to recover the ability to take in and absorb food orally as quickly as possible following transplantation.

3.1 Caloric and metabolic alterations
Most HSCT patients develop significant mucositis and have difficulties in maintaining adequate oral nutrition. Decreased oral intake caused by nausea, vomiting and diarrhoea, decreased nutrient absorption and loss of nutrients from the gut result in a negative nitrogen balance. This is further complicated by the catabolic effects on skeletal muscle exerted by the underlying disease, the conditioning regimen and subsequently by transplant complications such as GvHD and sepsis.

3.2 Nutritional support
Impaired nutritional status before transplantation is a negative prognostic factor for outcome after HSCT and better nourished patients have a shorter time to engraftment. Irrespective of nutritional status, however, parenteral nutritional support is commonly administered prophylactically after HSCT until patients are able to maintain an adequate oral nutritional intake, usually following bone marrow recovery. Although hypothetically enteral nutrition is possible, total parenteral nutrition (TPN) is largely favoured in HSCT patients because nausea, vomiting and oro-oesophageal mucositis prevent the insertion and subsequent tolerability of nasogastric tubes. Moreover, virtually all patients undergoing HSCT have a central venous catheter in situ through which TPN can be easily administered. Finally, parenteral nutrition probably allows better modulation of fluid, electrolyte, and nutrient administration which can be of critical importance when complications such as GvHD or VOD arise.

3.3 Total parenteral nutrition

The routine use of TPN during transplantation is based on a study that randomly assigned 137 previously well nourished patients undergoing BMT to either prophylactic TPN or intravenous maintenance fluids (dextrose, electrolytes, minerals, trace elements and vitamins). Treatment started during conditioning, and continued for 4 weeks following transplantation. Compared to the control arm, patients receiving TPN had significantly better overall and disease-free survival, and a longer time to relapse. Notably, 61% of control patients eventually required TPN because of a decline in their nutritional status (4). In contrast, other studies have not provided strong support for the routine use of TPN in patients with HSCT. However, the care of recipients of HSCT has changed significantly over the last twenty years, e.g. hospital stays are shorter due to the increasing use of peripheral blood stem cell transplantation and the use of recombinant haematopoietic growth factors, and a number of questions remain unanswered regarding nutritional support. For instance in a prospective randomised trial, 57 patients undergoing BMT received either prophylactic TPN or an enteral feeding programme. TPN was associated with significantly more days of diuretic use, more frequent hyperglycaemia and more catheter-related complications. Although the patient cohort was small this study suggests that the role of TPN in patients undergoing HSCT deserves further investigation (5). In a double blind study, 258 patients were randomly assigned to receive either TPN or hydration in an outpatient setting. Patients who received TPN had a delay in the resumption of 85% of their caloric requirement (16 versus 10 days), suggesting that the administration of TPN may suppress normal appetite (6). Another study attempted to define subgroups of patients who were likely to require TPN, using the following three criteria to define the need for TPN: severe malnutrition at admission, a prolonged (at least 7–10 days) period of minimal oral intake and clinical weight loss exceeding 10% during treatment. TPN was found to be necessary in only 55% of patients undergoing HSCT, with a range of 37% for autologous recipients to 92% for those receiving an HLA mismatched allograft (7).

According to the European Society for Clinical Nutrition and Metabolism (ESPEN) guideline (2009), parenteral nutrition (PN) in HSCT patients should be reserved for those with severe mucositis, ileus, or intractable vomiting. PN should start either when oral feeding falls below 60–70% of requirements for three days or may be started on the day following stem cell infusion if the patient is malnourished and it should be generally maintained for 15–20 days (8).

3.4 Caloric, protein and other necessities

Energy requirements in HSCT patients may exceed 130–150% of the estimated basal energy expenditure. Protein needs are also elevated. The recommended amino acid dose in TPN is 1.5–2 g/kg/day. A balanced caloric intake with both fat and carbohydrate is recommended. Long chain triglycerides (LCT), containing saturated, fatty acid moieties of 20-24 carbons or a mixture of long chain and medium chain triglycerides (MCT, 6-12 carbons) should provide 30% of caloric intake. MCT seem to be advantageous in TPN over LCT because they are more water soluble, more rapidly cleared from plasma, have protein sparing effects and do not accumulate in the liver or adipose tissue. Clinical studies have suggested that mixtures of MCT and LCT are advantageous in patients with respiratory illnesses, hepatic dysfunction, and sepsis with multi-system organ failure compared to LCT alone. Electrolytes, minerals, vitamins and trace elements (chromium, zinc, copper, manganese, selenium) are added to the TPN according to the recommended daily amount.

Glutamine supplementation of TPN has been addressed recently as glutamine is an important precursor for nucleotide synthesis and thus can be a source for rapidly dividing cells, such as gastrointestinal epithelial cells. Although several studies have evaluated the effect of enteral or parenteral administration of glutamine on gastrointestinal toxicity, none have shown a clear preventative or curative effect on intestinal mucositis. On the other hand, prospective studies have suggested positive effects of glutamine administration after HSCT on nitrogen balance, infectious complications and length of hospital stay (9). Preliminary data support the concept that parenteral glutamine may preserve hepatic function in HSCT recipients by maintaining hepatic glutathione concentrations which in turn protects hepatocytes from the oxidant stress of the conditioning regimen. Glutamine supplementation may also have a role in preventing and possibly treating VOD. A meta-analysis of 29 studies confirmed some beneficial effects of adding glutamine to parenteral nutrition in HSCT recipients (10).

3.5 Evaluation of nutritional status and monitoring nutritional support
Nitrogen balance is considered the most accurate way of assessing nutritional status in HSCT recipients as it is the direct expression of the imbalance existing between protein breakdown and synthesis. From studies published of TPN in HSCT some kind of consensus can be derived concerning nutritional status/support monitoring parameters. Daily monitoring of weight (primarily to judge hydration status) is essential, together with electrolytes, BUN, creatinine, and glucose. Liver function tests, serum albumin, transferrin, triglyceride and nitrogen balance are also helpful (Table 1).

3.6 Timing of nutritional support
The current practice of the timing of TPN is heterogeneous. In the study of Weisdorf (which became the scientific basis of routine administration of TPN in HSCT

Table 1: **Monitoring of nutritional support during the in-patient stay**		
Daily	**Two times a week**	**Once a week**
- weight (fluid balance)	- liver function tests	- nitrogen balance
- blood glucose	- serum calcium	- serum transferrin
- serum electrolytes	- serum magnesium	- serum albumin
- BUN	- serum phosphorus	- serum triglyceride
- serum creatinine		- serum zinc
- calorie and protein intake		

patients), parenteral nutrition was started before the conditioning regimen and continued to day 28 following HSCT. However, in many centres TPN is started only when severe mucositis develops. Others initiate TPN on day 1 post-transplant and continue for 2–3 weeks according to the intensity and duration of mucositis. TPN is usually not administered routinely to recipients of autologous transplantation unless prolonged mucositis occurs.

3.7 Complications of TPN
Complications essentially can be divided into two types: those related to the central venous catheter, and metabolic complications.

3.7.1 Metabolic complications
The most remarkable metabolic complications are hepatic enzyme elevations. The initial manifestation is usually an elevation of transaminases 1–2 weeks after the start of TPN. Increases in serum bilirubin and alkaline phosphatase generally occur 1 or 2 weeks later. These changes often resolve spontaneously without long-term consequences especially if the period of administration of TPN is short (not longer than 3 months). However elevated liver enzymes have multiple causes in HSCT patients and the differential diagnosis may be difficult. Drug toxicity, infections, GvHD, VOD, or recurrence of the original malignancy should also be considered (Table 2). If all

Table 2: **Common causes of elevated liver enzymes in the post-transplant period**
• Side effects of drugs (methotrexate, cyclosporin-A)
• Infections (bacterial, fungal, viral)
• Veno-occlusive disease of the liver
• Graft versus host disease
• Relapse of malignancy
• Parenteral nutrition

these possible causes are excluded various other measures can be initiated e.g. shortening the period of infusion of TPN from 24 hours to 12–20 hours, introducing some oral feeding, decreasing the non-protein caloric intake and commencing treatment with ursodeoxycholic acid (Table 3).

Table 3: **Treatment approach to elevated liver enzymes during TPN**
• Search for causes other than TPN (see Table 2)
• Shorten TPN cycle to 12-20 from 24 hours/day
• Reduce the non-protein caloric intake by 10-15% of the total daily calories
• Initiate some oral intake if possible
• Treat with ursodeoxycholic acid
• Utilise oral metronidazole to decrease enteral endotoxin formation

3.8 Diet in graft versus host disease of the gut

Patients suffering from intestinal graft versus host disease may benefit from glutamine-supplemented PN. The optimal dose of glutamine is not established but studies have suggested around 0.6 g/kg/day.

The oral diet should be adjusted to the severity of GvHD in general: avoid fat, fibre and lactose.

A 4-step schedule is recommended:

Step 1 - bowel rest; glutamine-supplemented PN

Step 2 - liquid oral diet

Step 3 - solid food; lactose-free, low fibre, fat reduced

Step 4 - slowly increase the amount of solid foods. Lactose-containing products are often the last to be tolerated (11).

3.9 Conclusions

Nutritional support is an integral part of the supportive care of patients receiving HSCT and the main tool remains TPN. It seems to be prudent to administer TPN to patients undergoing HSCT if they have severe mucositis or gastrointestinal manifestations of GvHD, when a long period of insufficient oral intake is anticipated. The most common complications of TPN are central venous catheter related.

4. Central venous devices

Health-care institutions purchase millions of intravascular catheters each year. Central venous catheters (CVC) are the devices most frequently used for vascular access in HSCT. Although CVC are indispensable in HSCT, they also represent a significant source of complications including catheter-related bloodstream infections, complications of insertion, venous thromboembolism, mechanical obstruction, dislodgment and leakage. The most important of these complications are bloodstream infections with an estimated incidence of 5/1000 patient days and a mortality rate between 3–25%.

4.1 Catheter related blood stream infection
Catheter related blood stream infection (CRBSI), is defined as bacteraemia or fungaemia in a patient with an intravascular catheter with more than one positive blood culture obtained from a peripheral vein, clinical manifestation of infections (i.e. fever, chills, and/or hypotension) and no apparent source of the blood stream infection other than the catheter. The incidence of CRBSI varies considerably by type of catheter, frequency of catheter manipulations, and disease-related factors. The incidence of CRBSI remains high despite of the use of aseptic techniques. In a prospective study of 111 HSCT recipients, representing 143 Hickman catheter placements, 44% of patients had positive blood cultures. Most of these (40/63) were coagulase-negative *Staphylococci* suggesting a primary line infection rather than a secondary contamination from a blood-borne source. Other frequently involved microorganisms are *Staphyloccus aureus*, Gram-negative bacteria and *Candida species*.

The clinical diagnosis of CRBSI is difficult as there are no specific clinical signs. The fever itself is a sensitive, but non-specific sign, while exit site reactions are specific but not sensitive. In the absence of other foci a positive blood culture is suspicious, and resolution of fever following removal of the catheter makes the diagnosis even more probable, although not proven.

Full proof diagnosis of CRBSI is possible only after removal and culture of the catheter:
- Roll plate technique used by the microbiology laboratory (semiquantitative, >5 CFU)
- Flush or ultrasound technique used by the microbiology laboratory (quantitative, >10^2 CFU)
- Same isolate from blood and catheter tip.

If the catheter is not removed, the diagnosis of CRBSI is established if:
- Same isolate with simultaneous blood cultures from peripheral vein and from catheter blood, with a ratio higher than 3:1 CFU ratio between CVC and peripheral sample
- Same isolate from both lumens with a ratio higher than 3:1 CFU between the two lumens
- Using an automated blood culture system the differential time to positivity of CVC culture versus peripheral blood culture positivity being greater then 2 hours is highly predictive for CRBSI.

There are four main possible mechanisms for developing a CVC related infection:

- Migration of skin organisms at the insertion site into the cutaneous catheter tract with colonisation of the catheter tip
- Contamination of the catheter hub leading to intraluminal colonisation
- Occasionally, catheters may be haematogenously seeded from another focus of infection and rarely
- Infusate contamination.

The most important recommendations concerning the prevention of CVC related blood stream infections are listed in Table 4, based on the guidelines developed in the USA by a working group led by the Infectious Disease Society (12).

5. Haematopoietic growth factors

5.1 G-CSF

Prolonged neutropenia and subsequent infections are the most frequent causes of morbidity and mortality following HSCT. The administration of G-CSF post-transplantation results in a clear clinical benefit by shortening time to engraftment and hence reducing complications associated with neutropenia. However, the optimal way of administration is still debated.

5.1.1 Autologous transplantation

G-CSF has been shown to shorten the time to neutrophil engraftment in several randomised phase III trials. The reduction ranged from 2–9 days. This proved to be independent of the number of CD34+ cells infused. In spite of the common concern that G-CSF administration may delay platelet engraftment, in most of the studies this was not the case. Although most studies did not find significant difference in days of febrile neutropenia, half of the studies demonstrated a reduction of the length of hospitalisation. Several studies aimed to find the optimal time to start G-CSF following autologous PBSCT, assuming that progenitors responsive to G-CSF are not immediately present after PBSCT, so that early post-transplant G-CSF administration might be unnecessary. When comparing the time to neutrophil engraftment between early (from day 0 to day +4) initiation of administration to delayed (from day +5 to day +7) there were no significant differences. Neither were there any differences in days of febrile neutropenia, time to platelet engraftment or in the length of hospital stay. Therefore, delayed starting of G-CSF administration following autologous PBSCT is proved to be equally effective. A few randomised studies compared the safety and efficacy of pegfilgrastim and filgrastim in the auto PBSCT setting. No differences were found in terms of time to neutrophil and platelet engraftment, or in the length of hospitalisation, showing that pegfilgrastim may be an acceptable alternative.

Table 4: **Recommendations for prevention of CVC related blood stream infections**	
Education	Health-care worker education and training for the insertion and maintenance of CVCs is essential. Moreover, periodic assessment of their knowledge of and adherence to guidelines is strongly recommended. Trained personnel for the insertion and maintenance of CVCs should be designated.
Catheters and materials	An important pathogenetic determinant is the material from which the device is made. *In vitro* studies demonstrate that CVCs made of polyethylene or polyvinyl chloride are less resistant to adhesion of micro-organisms than are CVCs made of teflon, silicone or polyurethane. The number of ports must be kept to the minimum required for the patient's management. Cuffed and tunnelled CVCs should be employed if their use is to be prolonged (e.g. allogeneic transplant).
Site of catheter insertion	In adults, a subclavian site is preferred as lower extremity sites are associated with a higher risk of infection (and deep venous thrombosis). Subclavian sites also reduce the risk of infection compared to jugular sites.
Maximal sterile barrier precautions during insertion	Full aseptic techniques should be used at the time of insertion. 2% aqueous chlorhexidine gluconate (preferably), tincture of iodine, or 70% alcohol can be used to prepare the skin before CVC insertion. Organic solvents (e.g. acetone and ether) should not be applied.
Catheter and catheter site care	One port should be designated exclusively for hyperalimentation if a multilumen catheter is used. The routine use of prophylactic intranasal or systemic antibiotics before insertion or during the use of the CVC and antibiotic lock solutions are not recommended. The catheter site can be covered by sterile gauze or a sterile, transparent semi-permeable dressing and the dressings should be replaced whenever they become damp or loosened. Gauze dressings should be replaced at least every two days and transparent dressings every 7 days. The catheter sites must be monitored visually or by palpation regularly and if patients have tenderness at the insertion site and/or fever without obvious source, the dressing should be removed for thorough examination.
Replacement of catheter	Catheters that are no longer essential should be removed promptly. However routine replacement of CVCs to prevent catheter related infections is not advised. CVCs must not be removed on the basis of fever alone. Clinical judgement is required to assess the appropriateness of catheter removal if infection is evidenced elsewhere or if a non-infectious cause of fever is suspected.
Administration set replacement	• Following administration of blood, blood products immediately • Following total parenteral nutrition – after 24 hours • Other fluid sets – after a maximum of 72 hours

5.1.2 Allogeneic transplantation

Several studies have addressed the efficacy of using G-CSF to reduce the post-transplant neutropenic period in allogeneic bone marrow or peripheral blood stem cell transplantation. In the PBSCT setting all studies demonstrated an improvement of 1–4 days in neutrophil engraftment compared to the control arm. Neither platelet engraftment, nor the number of days with febrile neutropenia differed. The median time period of hospitalisation following transplantation was also similar. Similar results were reported in retrospective observations of patients receiving bone marrow as the source of stem cells. The only different observation concerned the incidence of GvHD. While there was no significant difference in the PBSCT setting, a significant increase in acute GvHD was detected in patients with post transplant G-CSF in two retrospective studies with bone marrow transplantation. However, a meta-analysis including 1198 allo-transplanted patients (with 88% bone marrow graft) did not find an increased incidence of GvHD associated with G-CSF use, so no clear conclusion can be drawn whether the use of G-CSF following allogeneic transplantation has any effect on GvHD incidence (13).

5.2 Erythropoietin
Erythropoietin (EPO) has been used with the aim to accelerate the recovery of red blood cells following stem cell transplantation. This idea was based on the observation that EPO levels after transplantation were lower than calculated for the degree of anaemia. However studies not show any major benefits. In allogeneic transplantation some studies showed a reduction in the median time to transfusion independence, but transfusion requirements were not different. However, in subsets at high risk for transfusion EPO reduced transfusion needs. There may be some benefit in the reduced intensity transplant setting where EPO responsive erythroid precursors may persist following conditioning, but prospective studies are lacking. Because of the modest and mixed results of the studies, most centres do not use EPO in the early post-transplant setting. A few randomised trials have addressed the efficacy of EPO following autologous transplantation. None found a significant reduction of transfusion requirements. The lack of benefit is particularly evident with peripheral blood stem cell transplantation (14).

5.3 Conclusion
Evidence exists in favour of the use of G-CSF in some transplantation settings. Besides stem cell mobilisation, G-CSF accelerates engraftment following autologous bone marrow and peripheral blood stem cell transplantation, thus decreasing hospital stay and overall costs. In allogeneic transplantation the administration of G-CSF is acceptable following PBSCT, but because of a potential risk of GvHD its use is not recommended following allogeneic bone marrow transplantation unless future controlled studies generate more favourable results.

6. Oral mucositis

Oral mucositis (OM) occurs in most patients treated with high-dose therapy and stem cell transplantation. It has been associated with an increased need for total parenteral nutrition and opioid analgesics, prolonged hospitalisation, and increased risk of infection.

Despite the benefits of TPN, mucositis *per se* remains an important clinical problem. It is characterised by mucosal damage ranging from mild inflammation to extensive ulceration, which may affect the oral cavity and other parts of the alimentary tract. Typically, oral mucositis peaks between day 6 and 12, and resolution coincides with engraftment. Mucositis is associated with an increased risk of systemic infection resulting from bacteraemia associated with the breakdown of mucosal barriers. Mucositis-associated pain and infection cause significant morbidity and mortality. Both the severity and the duration of oral mucositis are decreased in reduced-intensity conditioning (RIC) regimens compared to myeloablative HSCT, although considerable differences may exist between different RIC protocols.

6.1. Interventions for the prevention of mucositis

Management of oral mucositis requires a multidisciplinary approach. Basic oral care consists of a pre-transplant oral/dental examination aimed at decreasing the oral infectious and inflammatory burden. It also minimises the need for invasive dental procedures in the immune reconstitution phase. Routine mouth care typically consists of daily assessments by trained nurses using standardised tools to evaluate oral mucositis, pain and other oral complaints. Bland rinses (e.g. water, saline, sodium bicarbonate) are used routinely to remove debris and keep the oral tissues moist. Patients should use a soft toothbrush or dental plaque accumulation should be prevented chemically using chlorhexidine-digluconate solutions (0.05 or 0.12%).

6.2 Intervention for the treatment of mucositis

6.2.1 Pain management

Many patients require narcotics and the length of time of intravenous narcotic need is one of the best indicators of the severity of mucositis. Morphine is recommended as the opioid of choice.

Topical agents are available with or without analgesics including diphenhydramine, corticosteroids, antacids, sodium hyaluronate gel, and mucoadhesive protectants. Unfortunately, the evidence supporting benefit for any of these interventions is absent or weak. One single centre study reported a beneficial effect of a supersaturated calcium phosphate oral rinse solution on the duration and severity of mucositis and pain (15). Amifostine is a phosphorylated aminothiol, which has a protective effect on normal tissues against radiation and alkylating agent toxicity. It has been reported to reduce mucositis associated with high-dose melphalan in one prospective study and several retrospective studies. There is increasing evidence for the use cryotherapy (e.g. ice cubes) to prevent oral mucositis in conditioning protocols containing high dose melphalan, and some studies indicate a positive effect when used in other conditioning regimens (16, 17).

A biological approach aimed to prevent mucositis is the use of recombinant keratinocyte growth factor (KGF, palifermin, Kepivance®). The efficacy of prophylactic intravenous palifermin was demonstrated in a double blind multicentre trial of 212 patients undergoing autologous HSCT for haematological malignancies. Significantly fewer patients receiving palifermin had grade 3 or 4 mucositis (63 vs 98% with placebo) and the duration of mucositis was shorter (median 6 vs 9 days) (18). These benefits were associated with significantly less use of opioid analgesics and less frequent requirement for TPN support. On the basis of this study palifermin was approved in Europe for the prevention of oral mucositis associated with autologous HSCT.

6.3 Other oral complications

6.3.1 Infection
Oral mucosal infections may be associated with a wide variety of other microorganisms including anaerobic bacteria, fungi and viruses. Dental infections, particularly chronic periodontitis, may also give rise to infectious complications. However, periodontitis can be easily overlooked particularly during neutropenia when local signs of infection are reduced. Chronic GvHD and its treatment increase the risk for oral infections. In oral GvHD, systemic therapies may be combined with local immunosuppressive agents, or local measures alone. Patients with oral cGvHD should be seen regularly by a dental professional as caries is very common (19).

6.3.2 Bleeding
In addition, gingivitis and periodontitis may contribute to bleeding risk during profound thrombocytopenia.

6.3.3 Dry mouth
Reduced saliva production increases risk of dental caries, oral mucosal injury and infections, and affects taste. Palliation includes sugarless gum or sweets, frequent water sipping, non-alcoholic mouthwashes and lip balm or systemic sialogogues (pilocarpine hydrochloride). Because of increased mucosal sensitivity, spices, alcohols, and flavouring agents (especially mint flavours in toothpaste and oral care products) should be avoided. There are also difficulties with chewing and swallowing.

6.4. Conclusion

Oral care should be performed before, during and after HSCT. Several approaches have been tried for the prophylaxis or therapy of mucositis. Although progress has been made, the problem has not yet been solved. A number of new agents promise clinical benefit, either single or in combination therapy.

7. Prevention and treatment of chemotherapy induced nausea and vomiting

7.1 Introduction, classification

The objective of antiemetic treatment is the perfect prevention of nausea and vomiting during the course of the transplant.

For the classification of chemotherapy induced vomiting and the emetic potential of cytotoxic therapy see Table 5 and Table 6.

The high dose chemo/radiotherapy used in standard conditioning regimens (see

Table 5: **Classification of CT induced emesis**		
Acute emesis	**Delayed emesis**	**Anticipatory emesis**
Occurs during the first 24 h following CT	Occurs later than 24 h	Conditioned response of patients who developed significant nausea and vomiting during previous CT

Table 6: **Emetogenic potential of intravenous antineoplastic agents**	
Probability of vomiting*	**Agent**
High (>90%)	Cisplatin Cyclophosphamide $\geq$1500 mg/m² Carmustine
Moderate (30–90%)	Cytarabine >1 mg/m² Ifosfamide Cyclophosphamide <1500 mg/m²
Low (10–30%)	Mitoxantrone Etoposide Methotrexate
Minimal (<10%)	Busulfan Fludarabine

*in the absence of antiemetic prophylaxis

Chapter 8) has high emetic potential. In addition, there are several other factors that may further increase the risk of vomiting (consecutive day administration, prior cytotoxic treatment, and other medication, e.g. opiate analgesics).

7.2. Prophylaxis and treatment
The main principles of emesis control are:
- Nausea and vomiting are far easier to prevent than to treat
- Antiemetic therapy should be adjusted for the drug with the highest emetic risk
- The risk for emesis following highly emetogenic chemotherapy lasts approximately 4 days
- Patients must be protected throughout the full period of risk
- Oral and IV formulations have equivalent efficacy.

There are few randomised trials specifically studying the issue of nausea/vomiting in the transplant setting. The neurokinin-1 receptor antagonist aprepitant represents a new class of antiemetic drugs. When used in combination with serotonin antagonists and corticosteroids, aprepitant appears to provide better protection against both acute and delayed emesis in very highly emetic chemotherapy. There is a general consensus that a combination of a serotonin receptor antagonist (ondansetron, granisetron, tropisetron, palonosetron or dolasetron) plus aprepitant and dexamethasone should be the standard prophylaxis during conditioning. Recently, a water soluble form of aprepitant (fosaprepitant) has been approved and can be administered as parenteral alternative to oral aprepitant. In case of failure of the prophylaxis the addition of further dexamethasone (max 20 mg/day) and/or a benzodiazepine (e.g. lorazepam max 4 mg iv) may help to counter increased patient anxiety and possible anticipatory emesis. An alternative is to switch to a different serotonin antagonist, since there is an incomplete cross-resistance between agents (Table 7 and Table 8) (20).

Table 7: **Prevention of conditioning induced nausea/vomiting**	
Drug (start before conditioning)	**Administration**
Aprepitant	125 mg PO on day 1 and 80 mg on days 2-3
Dexamethasone	12 mg PO or iv on days 1- until end of conditioning +2 days
5HT3 antagonist (setron)	PO or iv
+ Proton pump inhibitor	All days
+/- Lorazepam or clonazepam (0.5–2 mg)	All days

Table 8: **Treatment of breakthrough emesis**
General principle: give an additional agent from a different drug class
- Metoclopramide 10–40 mg PO or iv every 4–6 h - Lorazepam or clonazepam 0.5–2 mg every 4–6 h - Promethazine 12.5–25 mg PO or iv or iv every 4 h - Haloperidol 1–2 mg PO or iv every 4–6 h - Change 5H3 antagonist
Exclude other causes:
- GvHD - *Candida/herpes* esophagitis - other drugs (imipenem) - bowel obstruction - uraemia, etc.

7.3 Conclusion

The conditioning regimens used in HSCT are known to have a high emetogenic risk. A com-bination of a serotonin antagonist (setron) plus a neurokinin-1 antagonist (aprepitant) together with dexamethasone is considered to be the standard prophylaxis.

References

1. Nihtinen A, Anttila VJ, Richardson M et al. The utility of intensified environmental surveillance for pathogenic moulds in a stem cell transplantation ward during construction work to monitor the efficacy of HEPA filtration. Bone Marrow Transplant 2007; 40: 457 –460.
2. Mank AP, Davies M, for the EBMT-NG. Examining low bacterial dietary practice: A european survey on low bacterial food. Eur J Oncol Nurs 2008; 12: 342–348.
3. Gardner A, Mattiuzzi G, Faderl S et al. Randomized comparison of cooked and noncooked diets in patients undergoing remission induction therapy for acute myeloid leukemia. J Clin Oncol 2008; 26: 5684–5688.
4. Weisdorf SA, Lysne J, Wind D et al. Prophylactic total parenteral nutrition on long-term outcome of bone marrow transplantation. Transplantation 1987; 48833–838.
5. Szeluga DJ, Stuart RK, Brookmeyer R et al. Nutritional support of bone marrow transplant recipients: A prospective, randomized clinical trial comparing total parenteral nutrition to an enteral feeding program. Cancer Res 1987; 47: 3309–3316.
6. Charuhas PM, Fosberg KL, Breummer B et al. A double blind randomized trial comparing outpatient parenteral nutrition with intravenous hydration: Effect on resumption of oral intake after marrow transplantation. J Parenter Enteral Nutr 1997; 21: 157–161.
7. Iestra JA, Fibbe WE, Zwinderman AH et al. Parenteral nutrition following intensive cytotoxic therapy: An exploratory study on the need for parenteral nutrition after various treatment approaches for haematological malignancies. Bone Marrow Transplant 1999; 23: 933–939.
8. Bozzetti F, Arends J, Lundholm K et al. ESPEN Guidelines on parenteral nutrition: Non-

surgical oncology. Clin Nutrition 2009; 28: 445–454.

9. Ziegler TR, Young LS, Benfell K et al. Clinical and metabolic efficacy of glutamine supplemented parenteral nutrition after bone marrow transplantation. A randomized, double-blind, controlled study. Ann Intern Med 1992; 116: 821–828.

10. Murray SM, Pindoria S. Nutrition support for bone marrow transplant patients. Cochrane Database Syst Rev 2009; Jan 21: CD002920.

11. Imataki O, Nakatani S, Hasegawa T et al. Nutritional support for patients suffering from intestinal graft-versus-host disease after allogenic hematopoietic stem cell transplantation. Am J Hematol 2006; 81: 747–752.

12. O'Grady NP, Alexander M, Burns LA et al. Guidelines for the prevention of intravascular catheter-related infections. Clin Inf Dis 2011; 52: e162–193.

13. Trivedi M, Martinez S, Corringham S et al. Optimal use of G-CSF administration after hematopoietic SCT. Bone Marrow Transpl 2009; 43: 895–908.

14. Ivanov V, Faucher C, Mohty M et al. Early administration of recombinant erythropoietin improves haemoglobin recovery after reduced intensity conditioned allogeneic stem cell transplantation. Bone Marrow Transplant 2005; 36: 901–906.

15. Papas AS, Clark RE, Martuscelli G et al. A prospective, randomized clinical trial for the prevention of mucositis in patients undergoing hematopoietic stem cell transplantation. Bone Marrow Transplant 2003; 31: 705-12.

16. Clarkson JE, Worthington HV, Furness S et al. Interventions for treating oral mucositis for patients with cancer receiving treatment. Cochrane Database Syst Rev 2011 Apr 13: CD000978.

17. Worthington HV, Clarkson JE, Bryan G et al. Interventions for preventing oral mucositis for patients with cancer receiving treatment. Cochrane Database Syst Rev 2010 Dec 8: CD000978.

18. Spielberger R, Stiff P, Bensinger W et al. Palifermin for oral mucositis after intensive therapy for hematologic cancers. N Engl J Med 2004; 351: 2590–2598.

19. Couriel D, Carpenter PA, Cutler C et al. Ancillary therapy and supportive care of chronic graft-versus-host disease: National Institutes of Health consensus development project on criteria for clinical trials in chronic graft-versus-host disease: V. Ancillary Therapy and Supportive Care Working Group Report. Biol Blood Marrow Transplant 2006; 12: 375–396.

20. Roila F, Herrstedt J, Aapro M et al. Guideline update for MASCC and ESMO in the prevention of chemotherapy- and radiotherapy-induced nausea and vomiting: Results of the Perugia consensus conference. Ann Oncol 2010; 21(Suppl 5): 232–243.

Multiple Choice Questionnaire

To find the correct answer, go to http://www.esh.org/online-training/handbook/

1. Which of the following is the most accurate for assessing nutritional status in HSCT recipients?

a) Serum cholesterol ☐
b) Serum glucose ☐
c) Nitrogen balance ☐
d) Anthropometric measurements ☐

2. **What is the most common complication of TPN?**
   a) Elevated liver enzymes ☐
   b) Hypertriglyceridaemia ☐
   c) Elevated serum creatinine ☐
   d) Catheter-related complications ☐

3. **What is the most important handling regarding protective environment for all transplant patients?**
   a) No visitors ☐
   b) Use alcohol hand rub ☐
   c) Use of gowns and other protective clothing ☐
   d) Antiseptic bathing ☐

4. **Which of the following is *not* considered a standard indication for the use of G-SF?**
   a) Stem cell mobilisation ☐
   b) To accelerate engraftment following allo-HSCT ☐
   c) To accelerate engraftment following auto-HSCT ☐
   d) Treatment of secondary neutropenia following transplant due to drug toxicity ☐

5. **Which statement is true concerning oral mucositis?**
   a) Oral mucositis a significant cause of morbidity and mortality after HSCT ☐
   b) A pre-transplant oral/dental evaluation prior to HSCT is only necessary in patients with oral complaints ☐
   c) Tooth brushing should be discontinued during pancytopenia ☐
   d) Oral GvHD is a contraindication to preventative dental care ☐

NOTES

* CHAPTER 11

Early complications after HSCT

Enric Carreras

1. Introduction

The high doses of RT and/or CT included in conditioning regimens (see Chapter 8) affect all organs and tissues of the recipient, producing several early and late secondary effects of variable intensity. The most common early effects such as nausea, vomiting, mucositis and pain are discussed in Chapter 10, and late effects are covered in Chapter 15. Here we summarise some other early complications that, albeit infrequent, are an important cause of morbidity and mortality.

2. Haemorrhagic cystitis

Haemorrhagic cystitis (HC) can be a serious complication of HSCT and causes significant morbidity, prolongation of hospitalisation, and, occasionally, death. Various additional complications have been described in patients with HC: obstructive uropathy, hydronephrosis, tubulointerstitial nephritis, acute renal failure and bladder perforation.

2.1. Clinical features

Haematuria, symptomatic or asymptomatic, is graded as follows: grade I, microscopic; grade II, macroscopic; grade III, with clots; and grade IV, requiring instrumentation for clot evacuation or leading to urinary retention or requiring surgical intervention (1).

2.2 Pathogenesis

Early bleeding (up to 72 hrs after CT agents) occurs almost exclusively when using conditioning therapies including Cy, whose metabolite acrolein produces direct toxicity to the urothelium. The risk of developing HC after Cy is dose dependent. Occasionally, other agents such as ifosfamide, Bu (especially if associated with Cy), VP16 or TBI have been implicated.

Episodes of HC occurring late (usually more than 2 weeks after HSCT) are classically attributed to BK polyomavirus infection (and exceptionally to infections with other polyomaviruses, adenovirus or CMV). However, the role of BK viraemia and viruria on the development of HC is not clear, as many patients with BK infection do not develop HC. This fact, and the higher incidence of late-onset HC in allo-HSCT from alternative donors and in patients with advanced age, GvHD and thrombocytopenia, suggests that the pathogenesis of HC may be multifactorial. Several - but not all - authors have observed a similar incidence of late-onset HC in patients receiving RIC and in those undergoing MAC-HSCT (1, 2).

2.3 Incidence

HC secondary to Cy is seen in 5–25% of cases, depending on the preventive measures adopted. Late HC was reported in a recent series as occurring in 7% of patients with RIC vs 17% of those undergoing MAC-HSCT and up to 58% in patients receiving MAC-HSCT from haplo or cord blood HSCT who had positive BK viruria (2).

2.4 Prophylaxis

Continuous irrigation of the bladder has been abandoned because it produces more haematuria and urinary tract infections than does Mesna. Although most centres use Mesna as a prophylaxis for Cy-based regimens, several randomised studies have shown that this drug does not offer additional benefits if hydration and diuresis are adequate. The recommended daily dose for hydration is 3 L/m^2. If used, the daily dose of Mesna should be 1.0–1.5 × the daily dose of Cy, administered iv using one of the following schedules:

a. As a continuous infusion in 1 L of 0.9% saline over 12–24 hrs, beginning 4 h prior to the 1st dose of Cy;

b. As bolus injections of 20% of the daily dose of Cy administered as a bolus ½–1 hr before Cy and the remaining daily dose divided into bolus injections q 2–3 hrs;

c. By combining continuous infusion with intermittent bolus injections.

Whichever regimen is used, the presence of acrolein in the bladder 24 hrs after Cy makes it advisable to prolong mesna administration for 24 hrs after the last Cy dose.

2.5 Treatment

Treatment should be based on a three-step approach as follows:

a. Forced hydration plus intensive platelet support. The use of procoagulant agents such as aminocaproic acid is contraindicated as they favour clot formation in the bladder.

b. Continuous bladder irrigation (via transurethral or suprapubic cystotomy) with saline. Some success has been reported with bladder instillation of formalin, alum, silver nitrate, sodium hyaluronate, prostaglandin E2, GM-CSF or fibrin glue as well as with the administration of palifermin, hyperbaric oxygen, oestrogens, or recombinant FVIIa. Similarly, systemic or intravesical cidofovir, ciprofloxacin (reduces BK replication) or ribavirin have been reported as effective for cases of HC attributable to BK or adenovirus.

c. If the above measures do not alleviate HC, other salvage approaches can be considered: selective embolisation of bladder arteries (one of the simplest and most effective measures in the hands of an expert angioradiologist); catheterisation of both ureters to rest the bladder; hypogastric bond (which can produce sexual impotence) or, as a last resort, cystectomy.

3. Early complications of endothelial origin

There are a number of complications where injury to the vascular endothelium seems to be the most important initial event. These have imprecise diagnostic criteria and overlapping clinical features and are observed within the first 30–60 days after HSCT. The best-defined syndromes resulting from this endothelial injury are: 1. veno-occlusive disease of the liver; 2. capillary leakage syndrome; 3. engraftment syndrome; 4. diffuse alveolar haemorrhage; and 5. HSCT-associated thrombotic microangiopathy (3). This endothelial injury seems also to have a relevant role in the pathogenesis of GvHD (see Chapter 13). Figure 1 shows their common pathogenesis.

Figure 1: **Common pathogenesis of early complication of vascular origin after HSCT**

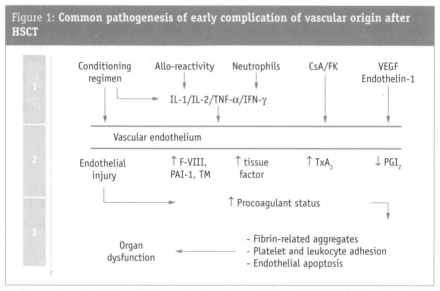

VEGF: vascular endothelial growth factor; Tx: thromboxane; PG: prostaglandin; TM: thrombomodulin; PAI-1: plasminogen activator inhibitor type 1

3.1 Hepatic veno-occlusive disease

3.1.1 Definition

Hepatic veno-occlusive disease (VOD) is the term used to designate the symptoms and signs that appear early after HSCT as a consequence of conditioning regimen-related hepatic toxicity. This syndrome is characterised by jaundice, fluid retention and tender hepatomegaly appearing in the first 35–40 days after HSCT (4–7).

3.1.2 Pathogenesis

The hepatic metabolism of certain drugs (e.g. Cy) by the cytochrome P450 enzymatic system produces several toxic metabolites (e.g. acrolein). These toxic metabolites are converted into stable (non-toxic) metabolites by the glutathione (GSH) enzymatic system and eliminated. When this process occurs in patients with a reduced GSH activity caused by previous liver disease or by the action of agents such as Bu, BCNU or TBI, which consume GSH, toxic metabolites are not metabolised. Toxic metabolites are predominantly located in area 3 of the hepatic acinus (around the centrilobular veins) because this area is rich in P450 and poor in glutathione. Consequently, damage to hepatocytes and sinusoidal endothelium occurs predominantly in this zone. The remaining factors listed in Figure 1 can also contribute to endothelial injury.

Experimental models show that the first events after endothelial injury caused by toxic metabolites are loss of *fenestrae* in sinusoidal endothelial cells (SEC), formation of gaps within and between SEC and rounding up or swelling of SEC. Consequently, red blood cells penetrate into the space of Disse and dissect off the sinusoidal lining cells, which embolise downstream and block the sinusoids, reducing the hepatic venous outflow and producing post-sinusoidal hypertension. Based on all these observations, some authors have proposed the term of sinusoidal obstruction syndrome for this complication (8).

3.1.3 Clinical features

Classical VOD. Several days after conditioning (from days −1 to +21) there is the presence of jaundice (in almost 100% of cases), hepatomegaly and/or right upper quadrant pain and weight gain (not attributable to an excessive fluid administration) together with oedema and ascites (4).

Late VOD. This shows the same clinical manifestations as classical VOD but develops late after HSCT (one-third of cases occur after patient discharge). It is mainly observed after conditioning including the use of one of several alkylating agents (e.g. busulfan, melphalan or thiotepa). One-third of cases show a biphasic course with an initial and transitory peak followed by a definitive late phase (9).

VOD with multi-organ failure. This shows the previously described clinical manifestations plus thrombocytopenia (refractoriness to platelet transfusions); pleural effusion, pulmonary infiltrates, progressive renal, cardiac and pulmonary failure, confusion, encephalopathy, and coma (6, 7).

3.1.4 Incidence

This has ranged from 3% to 54% in the largest series. This variability is a consequence of the presence or absence of the well-known risk factors for this complication (see below). In the only prospective multi-centre study published, the incidence of VOD was 8% in cases of allo-HSCT and 3% in cases of auto-HSCT (5). In a large single-centre study, the cumulative incidences of VOD in cases of allo-HSCT in the last decade were 14% and 8% using Seattle or Baltimore criteria, respectively. The incidence in patients undergoing RIC-HSCT seems to be less than 2% (7).

3.1.5 Risk factors
See Table 1 (4, 6, 7, 9).

Table 1: **Risk factors for VOD**	
Risk	**Lower risk < Higher risk**
Transplant type	Syngeneic or autologous < allogeneic
Donor type	Sibling < another relative < unrelated
HLA compatibility	HLA match < any mismatch
Stem cell origin	Peripheral blood < bone marrow
T-cell depletion	With TCD < without TCD
Diagnosis	Non-malignant disease < malignant disease
Status of the disease	Remission < relapse
Conditioning	
- Intensity	Cy alone < Cy + TBI < BVC [a]
- TBI	Fractionated TBI < single dose TBI
	Less than 12 Gy < more than 12 Gy
	Low dose rate < high dose rate
- Busulfan	iv Bu < adjusted oral Bu < non adjusted oral Bu
- Timing	Interval Cy – TBI 36 hours < 12 hours
Age/Sex	Younger < older/men < women
Karnofsky index	100–90 < lower than 90
ASAT/ALAT before HSCT	Normal < high
Transplant number	First < second
Previous hepatic irradiation	No < yes
Previous Mylotarg	No < yes [b]
Status of the liver	Normal < fibrosis < cirrhosis or infiltration
CMV serological status	Negative < positive
Fever in conditioning	Absent < present
Hepatotoxic drugs	Progestogens, ketoconazole, CsA, methotrexate, amphotericin B, vancomycin, acyclovir, iv Ig [c]
Genetic predisposition	GSTM1 positive < GSTM1 null genotype [d]

The most important risk factors are indicated in bold type. (a) BVC (BCNU, VP, Cy). (b) VOD incidence up to 64% (Wadleigh et al. Blood 2003). (c) Higher incidence of VOD with high-dose iv Ig (Cordonier et al. Ann Intern Med 2003). (d) Srivastava et al. Blood 2004

As for any syndrome, the diagnosis of VOD must be established clinically. All teams employing HSCT use one of the following two sets of clinical criteria (4, 6, 7).

Seattle criteria. In the first 20 days after HSCT, the presence of two or more of the following: bilirubin >2 mg/dL (>34 mmol/L); hepatomegaly or pain in the right upper quadrant; weight gain (>2% basal weight).

Baltimore criteria. In the first 21 days after HSCT, the presence of bilirubin at >2 mg/dL (>34 mmol/L) plus two or more of the following: painful hepatomegaly, ascites or weight gain (>5% basal weight).

In both diagnostic criteria, other possible causes of these clinical features should be excluded before accepting a diagnosis of VOD (see differential diagnosis). Additionally, it is necessary to remember that some cases of VOD can appear late after HSCT. Other studies that can complement the diagnosis are as follows.

Haemodynamic studies of the liver. These are carried out through the jugular or femoral veins (10). Despite its usefulness, this procedure is only indicated to confirm the diagnosis of VOD if it is required to decide on a therapeutic approach, as it can be potentially hazardous for the patient. An hepatic venous gradient pressure (HVGP) of ≥10 mmHg in a patient without a previous liver disease allows a precise differential diagnosis with a high degree of specificity. However, a normal HVGP does not exclude this syndromic diagnosis.

Liver biopsy. The thrombocytopenia usually present in this phase after HSCT precludes a transparietal liver biopsy. Consequently, hepatic tissue can only be obtained by means of a transvenous biopsy in the course of a haemodynamic study. In addition to the classical histological changes seen with VOD (concentric non-thrombotic narrowing of the lumen of small intrahepatic veins), other less specific abnormalities can be observed (e.g. eccentric narrowing of the venular lumen; phlebosclerosis; sinusoidal fibrosis or hepatocyte necrosis). Because of the patchy nature of VOD, a normal biopsy does not exclude this syndromic diagnosis.

Ultrasonography. A variety of abnormalities can be observed, such as gallbladder wall thickening, ascites, hepatomegaly and attenuated or reversed portal flow, but they are all non-specific.

Biological studies. Although the serum of patients with VOD shows an increase in levels of plasminogen activator inhibitor (PAI)-1 (marker with the highest specificity and sensitivity for VOD), vWF, thrombomodulin, E-selectin, sICAM, aminopropeptides of type III collagen and hyaluronic acid, they are all of little utility in daily clinical practice (4).

3.1.7 Differential diagnosis

To accept a diagnosis of VOD, all of the following possible causes of similar clinical features should be excluded as far as possible.

Infections. These include *Cholangitis lenta* (sepsis of the liver), fungal infections and viral hepatitis.

Immune dysfunction. This can lead to hepatic GvHD or autoimmune hepatitis.

Drug toxicity. This can arise from CsA, azoles, MTX, progestogens, trimethoprim-sulfamethoxazole and TPN, among others.

Reduction of venous outflow. This can lead to increased volume, constrictive pericarditis, congestive heart failure, fluid overload or renal failure.

Other causes. These include pancreatic ascites, chylous ascites or infiltration of the liver.

3.1.8 VOD prophylaxis
See Table 2 (4, 11).

Table 2: **VOD prophylaxis**
To avoid risk factors
• When possible, delay HSCT if an acute hepatitis exists; adjust Bu dose or use iv Bu; use first Cy than Bu; fractionate TBI; avoid hepatotoxic drugs, etc.
• In high risk patients, consider RIC allo-HSCT (incidence of VOD <2%) (7)
Pharmacological
• Sodium heparin: 100 U/kg/day by continuous infusion. Despite two randomised studies showing a beneficial effect others have suggested that it is ineffective and dangerous.
• Prostaglandin E1: 0.3 µg/kg/h by continuous infusion. Evaluated in several clinical trials usually combined with heparin. When administered alone no beneficial effect was observed.
• Ursodeoxycholic acid: 600–900 mg/day *per os*. Four randomised trials and 2 historically controlled studies have shown a reduction in VOD and TRM.
• Low molecular weight heparin: enoxaparin 40 mg/day or fraxiparin 5000 U/day s.c. Relatively safe, may have some effect; a randomised study is needed.
• Defibrotide. Only one randomised study in children showing a clear reduction in the incidence of VOD and GvHD (11).

3.1.9 VOD treatment
See Table 3 (4, 6, 12).

3.1.10 VOD evolution
See Table 4 (4, 6, 7, 12).

3.2 Capillary leak syndrome (CLS)

3.2.1 Pathogenesis
Injury to the capillary endothelium (probably caused by cytokines and VEGF)

Table 3: VOD treatment

First line therapy	
Symptomatic [a]	• Restriction of salt and water intake ± diuretics • Maintain intravascular volume and renal perfusion by means of albumin, plasma expanders and transfusions (haematocrit >30%)
Specific	• DF: 6.25 mg/kg iv in 2 h infusion q 6 h x 14 d → 50-55% CR in severe VOD with MOF and 47-60% of survival at day +100 with no secondary effects (15) • Other agents [b, c]
Other measures	
Symptomatic [a]	• Analgesia • Paracentesis/thoracocentesis • Haemodialysis/haemofiltration • Mechanical ventilation
Specific	• TIPS (transvenous intrahepatic portosystemic shunt) [d] • Surgical shunt • Liver transplantation

DF: defibrotide; MOF: multiorgan failure. (a) Symptomatic treatment should be established first, reserving specifies measures for most severe cases. (b) rt-PA (recombinant tissue plasminogen activator) (0.05 mg/kg/h in 4 h (max. 10 mg/d) during 2-4 d) usually combined with sodium heparin (20 U/kg as a bolus (max. 1000 U) followed by 150 U/kg/day by continuous infusion for 10 days) was frequently used before defibrotide became available. Although rt-PA is effective in some cases, its use is contraindicated in patients with multiorgan failure, haemorrhage or severe hypertension. (c) Occasional successes have been reported with antithrombin III, prostaglandin, corticosteroids, glutamine/vitamin E, N-acetylcysteine, and human recombinant soluble thrombomodulin but the reported series are small precluding any recommendation. (d) Although portal hypertension and ascites improve, long term efficacy and survival are extremely poor.

produces a loss of intravascular fluids to the interstitial space, which leads to the clinical manifestations of CLS (13).

3.2.2 Incidence
The absence of well-established clinical criteria for the diagnosis of CLS precludes an adequate estimation of its incidence. Additionally, the differential diagnosis from VOD, engraftment syndrome (ES) or DAH can be very difficult.

3.2.3 Clinical features
This is characterised by the development in the first 15 days after HSCT of weight

Table 4: **VOD evolution**		
	Classification [a]	**Frequency** [b]
CR at day +100 without treatment	Mild VOD	8–23%
CR at day +100 with treatment	Moderate VOD	48–64%
Non-CR before death [c] or day +100	Severe VOD	23–28%
Mortality attributable to VOD by day +100 in classical series (4) [d]	1–3% of all HSCT 18–28% of all VOD 75–95% of severe VOD	
Cumulative incidence of dying from VOD by day +100 in HSCT performed since 1997 (7) [e]	2% of all HSCT 14% of all VOD 50% of severe VOD	
Mortality of severe VOD with MOF (7)	without DF: 78%	with DF: 25%

CR: complete remission; DF: defibrotide; MOF: multi-organ failure; (a) Classification described by Seattle group to evaluate VOD retrospectively. (b) Values observed in the two largest series. (c) In many cases VOD is not the direct cause of death but contributes to it. (d) Data from pre-defibrotide era. (e) Using Baltimore clinical criteria

gain (>3% within 24 hrs) and generalised oedematous syndromes (e.g. ascites, pleural effusion or pericarditis) that characteristically do not respond to furosemide treatment. Other features occasionally observed are tachycardia, hypotension, renal insufficiency of pre-renal origin and hypoalbuminaemia (13, 14).

3.2.4 Differential diagnosis
From ES: its earlier development, the absence of skin rash and the poor response to corticosteroids. From VOD: the absence of jaundice and painful hepatomegaly and the poor response to furosemide. From DAH: generalised oedema.

3.2.5 Risk factors
The use of G-CSG, GM-CSF or K-CSF; high cumulative doses of CT in the pre-HSCT phase; unrelated or HLA-mismatched donor grafts.

3.2.6 Treatment
Withdraw any growth factors. Despite being used systematically, corticosteroids offer poor responses. iv Ig and bevacizumab (anti-VEGF) have been used successfully in some cases (14).

3.2.7 Evolution
There is a high mortality rate if CLS progresses to multi-organ failure.

3.3 Engraftment syndrome

This syndrome has received other names in the literature: capillary leak syndrome at engraftment; auto-aggression syndrome; peri-engraftment respiratory distress syndrome (PERDS); and aseptic shock syndrome (15-17).

3.3.1 Pathogenesis

This involves a massive release of pro-inflammatory cytokines (e.g. IL-2, TNF-α, IFN-γ and IL-6), M-GSF, EPO, products of degranulation and oxidative metabolism of neutrophils and systemic endothelial damage.

3.3.2 Incidence

ES is almost exclusively diagnosed after auto-HSCT. In this setting, the incidence ranges from 5% to 25% (13% in the largest series). It is rarely seen after conventional allo-HSCT, but is occasionally described after RIC allo-HSCT and CB-HSCT (18).

3.3.3 Clinical features and diagnostic criteria

The clinical manifestations and the Spitzer and Maiolino diagnostic criteria are listed in Table 5 (13, 16). A recent study showed that the Maiolino criteria - when correctly applied - are the best tool to establish an early diagnosis, despite being less specific than the Spitzer criteria. A sudden and significant increase in the level of C-reactive protein can help to establish the diagnosis (17).

Table 5: Clinical criteria for diagnosis of ES	
Major clinical criteria	**Minor clinical criteria**
Non-infectious fever[1] Skin rash[2] Pulmonary oedema[3], hypoxaemia	Weight gain[4] Hepatic or renal dysfunction[5] Transient encephalopathy[6]
Spitzer criteria (15)	**Maiolino criteria** (16)
3 major criteria, or 2 major and 1 minor criteria, within 96 h of engraftment	Non-infectious fever[1] + skin rash, or pulmonary infiltrates, or diarrhoea[7], from 24 h before or at any time after the first appearance of neutrophils[8]

[1]New fever (>38°C) without clinical or microbiological documentation or response to antimicrobial treatment. [2]Maculo-papular exanthema involving >25% body surface area. [3]Documented by X-ray or CT without signs of infection, cardiac failure or pulmonary embolism. [4]Higher than 2.5% of basal. [5]Bilirubin $\geq$ 2 mg/dL (34 μmol/L) or ASAT/ALAT $\geq$ 2 times or creatinine $\geq$ 2 times normal. [6]If unexplainable by other causes. [7]At least two episodes of liquid stools/day without microbiological documentation of infection. [8]The original sentence "24 h before or after" is confusing and has generated incorrect interpretations in some papers

3.3.4 Risk factors

Most cases of ES were described following the introduction of growth factors and PBSCT. Nowadays, ES is mainly observed in patients who have not received intensive chemotherapy before undergoing auto-HSCT or in those receiving less intensive conditioning, as occurs in cases of breast cancer, amyloidosis, myeloma, POEMS or autoimmune diseases (17).

3.3.5. Treatment

Methyl-PDN 1 mg/kg q 12 hrs (for 3 days) with progressive tapering off over 1 week. Because of the difficulty of excluding an infectious origin of the fever, this treatment should not be started until it has been confirmed that the fever does not respond to empirical antibiotic therapy and that cultures are negative.

3.3.6 Evolution

There is complete resolution in 1–5 days in >80% of the cases if steroids are introduced early. In some cases the symptoms reappear after stopping steroid therapy.

3.4 Diffuse alveolar haemorrhage (DAH)

The systematic use of bronchoscopy and bronchoalveolar lavage (BAL) to study these patients has permitted the recognition of DAH as a major entity after HSCT and allowed it to be differentiated from idiopathic pneumonia syndrome (IPS) (19, 20).

3.4.1 Pathogenesis

DAH seems to originate from the disruption of the alveolar–capillary basement membrane by conditioning, immune-mediated events and the return of neutrophils with marrow recovery. The pathological observations on small arteries are very similar to those observed in veins affected by VOD (20).

3.4.2 Incidence

The reported incidence ranges from 1% to 21% in cases of auto-HSCT and from 2% to 17% in cases of allo-HSCT.

3.4.3 Clinical features

The median times to onset in patients undergoing allo- and auto-HSCT are 19 and 12 days, but episodes after the first month are not uncommon. The main manifestations are as follows:
- Shortness of breath and non-productive coughing with or without fever; haemoptysis is rare.

- Hypoxaemia that can require oxygen therapy.
- Chest X-ray or CT findings with focal or diffuse interstitial or alveolar infiltrates located in the middle and inferior lung fields.

3.4.4 Diagnosis
This is based on BAL findings becoming progressively bloodier but not attributable to infection (absence of pathogens in BAL), on thrombocytopenia, fluid overload or heart failure. Successive aliquots of 20 mL, in at least three segmentary bronchi, become progressively more blood stained (indicating blood in the alveoli). The presence of hemosiderin-laden macrophages is usual but their mere presence is insufficient to diagnose DAH and their absence does not exclude the diagnosis as they can take 72 hrs to appear in the BAL.

3.4.5 Differential diagnosis
The differential diagnosis from IPS is very difficult. IPS usually appears after engraftment, predominantly in patients undergoing allo-HSCT. It does not respond to corticosteroids and progresses to fibrosis and respiratory failure in 85% of cases (only 15% in those with DAH). The differential diagnosis from PERDS (a form of ES) is almost impossible clinically but 2/3 of patients with PERDS do not show a progressively bloodier BAL.

3.4.6 Risk factors
DAH is not related to low platelet counts. Factors that favour this complication are older age, previous thoracic radiation, TBI and myeloablative conditioning.

3.4.7 Treatment
After some small retrospective series, high-dose methyl-PDN (250–500 mg q 6 hrs, 4–5 days and tapering over 2–4 weeks) was considered the treatment of choice. However, many other authors have failed to observe any benefit of corticosteroids on the poor outcome associated with DAH (19). No other measures have proved to be effective.

3.4.8 Evolution
The overall mortality rate ranges from 60% to 100% (80–100% if patients require mechanical ventilation). With steroid therapy, many patients do not develop respiratory failure (85%) but most of them die from multi-organ dysfunction syndrome or sepsis. Recent reports using non-invasive ventilation, lung-protective strategies and early diagnosis and treatment show that at the present the mortality

rate is around 50%. The prognosis is clearly better in patients with DAH appearing early after HSCT and in those receiving auto-HSCT (>70% of survivors) than those observed later or in an allo-HSCT setting (<25%) (19).

3.5 HSCT-associated thrombotic microangiopathy (TMA)

3.5.1 Pathogenesis
Conditioning regimens and other less well-known triggering factors produce a generalised endothelial dysfunction causing microangiopathic haemolytic anaemia and platelet consumption, resulting in thrombosis and fibrin deposition in the microcirculation. Unlike that seen in patients with classical TTP, ADAMTS13 activity in patients with TMA rarely decreases to below 10% of normal (21, 22).

3.5.2 Incidence
This is less than 4% in cases of auto-HSCT but up to 15% in cases of allo-HSCT (7% in an EBMT survey). There is a similar incidence after RIC and MAC-HSCT (22).

3.5.3 Clinical features
TMA usually develops around day +60, but early (day +4) and late (2 years) episodes have been described. It is characterised as follows.
a. Microangiopathic haemolytic anaemia (MHA), defined as anaemia with >2–4% schistocytes, together with raised LDH and other markers of haemolysis.
b. Thrombocytopenia or increased requirement for platelet transfusions.
c. Renal dysfunction and/or neurological abnormalities such as cortical blindness, seizures and typical images in CT scans of the CNS.
In addition to these classical findings, experts insist on the relevance and high frequency of elevated blood pressure, diarrhoea secondary to intestinal TMA and proteinuria, as well as in the possible absence of renal and neurological symptoms (22).

3.5.4 Diagnosis
Table 6 shows the most used frequently clinical criteria, including a recently described category of "possible" TMA (23–25).

3.5.5 Risk factors
A higher incidence has been observed in patients receiving TBI, calcineurin inhibitors (CNI), sirolimus, unrelated or HLA-mismatched donor grafts, or developing GvHD or aspergillus, CMV or adenovirus infections. The intensity of conditioning does not seem to play a role in the development of TMA.

Table 6: **Diagnostic criteria for HSCT-associated TMA**

Blood & Marrow Transplant Clinical Trials Network consensus (23)
1) RBC fragmentation and 2 schistocytes per high-power field on PB smear
2) Concurrent increased serum LDH
3) Concurrent renal [a] and/or neurologic dysfunction w/o other explanations
4) Negative direct and indirect Coombs test

International Working Group of the EBMT (24)
1) Increased percentage (>4%) of schistocytes in peripheral blood
2) Thrombocytopenia <50 x 10^9/L or a ≥50% decrease in platelet count
3) Sudden and persistent increase in LDH
4) Decrease in Hb concentration or increase in RBC transfusion requirement
5) Decrease in serum haptoglobin concentration

Probable TMA (25)
1) Increased percentage (>4%) of schistocytes in peripheral blood
2) Concurrent increased serum LDH
3) Thrombocytopenia <50 x 10^9/L or a ≥50% decrease in platelet count
4) Negative direct and indirect Coombs test
5) Decrease in serum haptoglobin concentration
6) Absence of coagulopathy

[a] *Doubling of serum creatinine or 50% decrease in creatinine clearance from baseline pre-HSCT*

3.5.6 Clinical forms

Two main forms of TMA can be observed, as follows.

CNI-associated TMA is defined as MHA with or without (probable TMA) nephrotoxicity (or neurotoxicity). Classically, TMA develops early after HSCT. It is associated with the use of CNI and is usually reversible after stopping their administration. The relevance of recognising cases of probable TMA is that patients have an excellent prognosis.

TMA not associated with CNI toxicity presents with two clinical forms: a. TMA mimicking a haemolytic uraemic syndrome, primarily affecting the kidney and often causing oliguric or anuric renal failure with hypertension, MHA and thrombocytopenia; and b. fulminating multifactorial TMA, i.e. early after HSCT, characterised by renal failure, CNS disturbances, hypertension, MHA and thrombocytopenia, and associated with GvHD, viral or fungal infections. Most cases have a fatal evolution because the patients do not respond to treatment.

3.5.7 Prevention

The only reasonable measure is to keep close observation (2–3 times per week) of the CNI, LDH and creatinine levels. If any of these markers increase, peripheral blood smears, haptoglobin levels and Coombs tests (direct and indirect antiglobulin tests) should be evaluated.

3.5.8 Treatment
The most effective measure is to stop CNI immediately (no dose reduction) by changing GvHD prophylaxis/treatment to another drug (corticosteroids, mycophenolate). Plasma exchange usually offers a poor response (median 35%; range 20–80%) probably because TMA is not associated with an absence or severe reduction of plasma ADAMTS13 activity and has a high associated mortality (80%). Some authors have reported successful results with defibrotide, rituximab, daclizumab and basiliximab therapies.

4. Idiopathic pneumonia syndrome (IPS)

4.1 Pathogenesis
IPS is the consequence of non-infectious lung injury after HSCT caused by the toxic effects of conditioning, immunological cell-mediated injury, inflammatory cytokines, flora-derived LPS and - probably - occult pulmonary infections (26, 27).

4.2 Incidence
Thanks to improvements in diagnostic methods, the incidence of IPS has fallen from more than 20% in earlier series of allo-HSCT to less than 10% at the present (around 8% and 2% after conventional and allo-RIC, respectively) (26). It is uncommon in the setting of auto-HSCT. Similarly, the median time of onset after allo-HSCT has moved from day +40–50 to day +18–21.

4.3 Clinical features
IPS is characterised by the development around day +20 of fever and non-productive cough, tachypnoea and hypoxaemia, and diffuse alveolar or interstitial infiltrates on X-rays or CT scans.

4.4 Diagnosis
Today, this diagnosis is accepted when there is evidence of:
a. Widespread alveolar injury (clinical, radiological and/or functional); and
b. Absence of active lower respiratory tract infection (all cultures and tests in BAL or lung biopsies are negative); and
c. Absence of cardiac dysfunction, acute renal failure or iatrogenic fluid overload.

4.5 Clinical spectrum of IPS

Sometimes, additional studies allow the distinction of other entities among patients fulfilling IPS criteria. Categorised by the presumed site of the primary lung injury, the following are routinely included under the classification of IPS (26).

a. Pulmonary parenchyma: acute interstitial pneumonitis, acute respiratory distress syndrome or delayed pulmonary toxicity syndrome.
b. Airway endothelium: bronchiolitis obliterans syndrome or cryptogenic organising pneumonia (formerly bronchiolitis obliterans organising pneumonia) (see Chapter 15).
c. Vascular endothelium: PERDS (a form of ES), CLS, or DAH.

4.6 Risk factors

These include the intensity of conditioning, use of TBI, allo-HSCT, older recipient age, acute leukaemia or MDS and the presence of GvHD.

4.7 Treatment

Supportive care measures (including non-invasive and invasive mechanical ventilation and haemofiltration), broad-spectrum antimicrobial agents and corticosteroids. Low or high doses of methyl-PDN seem to have limited efficacy (except in DAH forms of IPS). Preclinical and translational studies indicate that neutralisation of TNF-α might be a useful strategy. Etanercept given s.c. at the dose of 0.4 mg/kg twice weekly for a maximum of eight doses in combination with systemic corticosteroids seems to be well tolerated and efficacious in two-thirds of patients and to improve survival (28).

4.8 Evolution

Up to 60–80% of patients with IPS (95% if requiring mechanical ventilation) will die from progressive impairment of respiratory function.

References

1. Hingorani S. Kidney and bladder complications of hematopoietic cell transplantation. In: Thomas' Hematopoietic Cell Transplantation, 4th Edition (Appelbaum FR, Forman SJ, Negrin RS Blume KG Eds.), Wiley-Blackwell Publishing Chichester, West Sussex, UK, 2009, pp 1473–1486.
2. Silva Lde P, Patah PA, Saliba RM et al. Hemorrhagic cystitis after allogeneic hematopoietic stem cell transplants is the complex result of BK virus infection, preparative regimen intensity and donor type. Haematologica 2010; 95: 1183–1190.
3. Carreras E, Diaz-Ricart M. The role of the endothelium in the short-term complications of hematopoietic SCT. Bone Marrow Transplant 2011 Apr 4. [Epub ahead of print.]

4. Carreras E. Veno-occlusive disease of the liver after hemopoietic cell transplantation. Eur J Haematol 2000; 64: 281–291.
5. Carreras E, Bertz H, Arcese W et al. Incidence and outcome of hepatic veno-occlusive disease after blood or marrow transplantation: A prospective cohort study of the European Group for Blood and Marrow Transplantation. Blood 1998; 92: 3599–3604.
6. Coppell JA, Richardson PG, Soiffer R et al. Hepatic veno-occlusive disease following stem cell transplantation: Incidence, clinical course, and outcome. Biol Blood Marrow Transplant 2010; 16: 157–168.
7. Carreras E, Díaz-Beyá M, Rosiñol L et al. The incidence of veno-occlusive disease following allogeneic hematopoietic cell transplantation has diminished and the outcome improved over the last decade. Bone Marrow Transplant 2011 Jun 24. [Epub ahead of print].
8. DeLeve LD, Shulman HM, McDonald GB. Toxic injury to hepatic sinusoids: Sinusoidal obstruction syndrome (veno-occlusive disease). Semin Liver Dis 2002; 22: 27–42.
9. Carreras E, Rosiñol L, Terol MJ et al. Veno-occlusive disease of the liver after high-dose cytoreductive therapy with busulfan and melphalan for autologous blood stem cell transplantation in multiple myeloma patients. Biol Blood Marrow Transplant 2007; 13: 1448–1454.
10. Carreras E, Grañena A, Navasa M et al. Transjugular liver biopsy in BMT. Bone Marrow Transplant 1993; 11: 21–26.
11. Corbaciogly S, Cesaro S, Fareci M et al. Defibrotide prevents hepatic VOD and reduces significantly VOD–associated complications in children at high risk: Final results of a prospective phase II/III multicentre study. Bone Marrow Transplant 2010; 45 (Suppl 2): S1.
12. Ho VT, Revta C, Richardson PG. Hepatic veno-occlusive disease after hematopoietic stem cell transplantation: Update on defibrotide and other current investigational therapies. Bone Marrow Transplant 2008; 41: 229–237.
13. Nürnberger W, Willers R, Burdach S, Göbel U. Risk factors for capillary leakage syndrome after bone marrow transplantation. Ann Hematol 1997; 74: 221–224.
14. Yabe H, Yabe M, Koike T et al. Rapid improvement of life-threatening capillary leak syndrome after stem cell transplantation by bevacizumab. Blood 2010; 115: 2723–2724.
15. Spitzer TR. Engraftment syndrome following hematopoietic stem cell transplantation. Bone Marrow Transplant 2001; 27: 893–898.
16. Maiolino A, Biasoli I, Lima J et al. Engraftment syndrome following autologous hematopoietic stem cell transplantation: Definition of diagnostic criteria. Bone Marrow Transplant 2003; 31: 393–397.
17. Carreras E, Fernández-Avilés F, Silva L et al. Engraftment syndrome alter auto-SCT: Analysis of diagnostic criteria and risk factors in a large series from a single center. Bone Marrow Transplant 2010; 45: 1417–1422.
18. Gorak E, Geller N, Srinivasan R et al. Engraftment syndrome after nonmyeloablative allogeneic hematopoietic stem cell transplantation: Incidence and effects on survival. Biol Blood Marrow Transplant 2005; 11: 542–550.
19. Afessa B, Tefferi A, Litzow MR et al. Diffuse alveolar hemorrhage in hematopoietic stem cell transplant recipients. Am J Respir Crit Care Med 2002; 166: 641–645.

20. Majhail NS, Parks K, Defor TE, Weisdorf DJ. Diffuse alveolar hemorrhage and infection-associated alveolar hemorrhage following hematopoietic stem cell transplantation: Related and high-risk clinical syndromes. Biol Blood Marrow Transplant 2006; 12: 1038–1046.
21. Batts ED, Lazarus HM. Diagnosis and treatment of transplantation-associated thrombotic microangiopathy: Real progress or are we still waiting? Bone Marrow Transplant 2007; 40: 709–719.
22. Laskin BL, Goebel J, Davies SM, Jodele S. Small vessels, big trouble in the kidneys and beyond: Hematopoietic stem cell transplant associated-thrombotic microangiopathy. Blood 2011; 118: 1452–1456.
23. Ho VT, Cutler C, Carter S et al. Blood and marrow transplant clinical trials network toxicity committee consensus summary: Thrombotic microangiopathy after hematopoietic stem cell transplantation. Biol Blood Marrow Transplant 2005; 11: 571–575.
24. Ruutu T, Barosi G, Benjamin RJ et al.; European Group for Blood and Marrow Transplantation; European LeukemiaNet. Diagnostic criteria for hematopoietic stem cell transplant-associated microangiopathy: Results of a consensus process by an International Working Group. Haematologica 2007; 92: 95–100.
25. Cho BS, Yahng SA, Lee SE et al. Validation of recently proposed consensus criteria for thrombotic microangiopathy after allogeneic hematopoietic stem-cell transplantation. Transplantation 2010; 90: 918–926.
26. Panoskaltsis-Mortari A, Griese M, Madtes DK et al.; American Thoracic Society Committee on Idiopathic Pneumonia Syndrome. An official American Thoracic Society research statement: Noninfectious lung injury after hematopoietic stem cell transplantation: Idiopathic pneumonia syndrome. Am J Respir Crit Care Med 2011; 183: 1262–1279.
27. Yanik GA, Ho VT, Levine JE et al. The impact of soluble tumor necrosis factor receptor etanercept on the treatment of idiopathic pneumonia syndrome after allogeneic hematopoietic stem cell transplantation. Blood 2008; 112: 3073–3081.
28. Fukuda T, Hackman RC, Guthrie KA et al. Risks and outcomes of idiopathic pneumonia syndrome after nonmyeloablative and conventional conditioning regimens for allogeneic hematopoietic stem cell transplantation. Blood 2003; 102: 2777–2785.

Multiple Choice Questionnaire

To find the correct answer, go to http://www.esh.org/online-training/handbook/

1. Late onset haemorrhagic cystitis usually is produced by:
a) The direct action of cyclophosphamide on the bladder ☐
b) A polyomavirus infection ☐
c) A bacterial infection of the urinary tract ☐
d) The neutropenia ☐

2. **Which of the following complications could *not* be attributed to an endothelial dysfunction?**
   a) Engraftment syndrome ☐
   b) Veno-occlusive disease of the liver ☐
   c) Haemorrhagic cystitis ☐
   d) Thrombotic microangiopathy ☐

3. **Which of the following is not a clinical manifestation of VOD?**
   a) Weight gain ☐
   b) Ascites ☐
   c) Platelet refractoriness ☐
   d) Diarrhoea ☐

4. **All but one of the following are classical manifestations of engraftment syndrome**
   a) Skin rash ☐
   b) Back pain ☐
   c) Fever ☐
   d) Hypoxaemia ☐

5. **Which is the main cause of thrombotic microangiopathy after HSCT?**
   a) Bacterial infection ☐
   b) Graft allo-reaction ☐
   c) Cyclosporin toxicity ☐
   d) Renal failure ☐

* CHAPTER 12

Infections after HSCT

Montserrat Rovira, Josep Mensa, Enric Carreras

1. Introduction

Infections remain a main cause of morbidity and mortality in patients undergoing HSCT. In recent years, improvement in supportive care measures, better understanding of the mechanism of immunosuppression, the introduction of reduced intensity conditioning (RIC) regimens and new anti-infectious agents and prophylactic strategies have decreased infectious morbidity and mortality; however, there is still room for improvement (1).

The principal risk factors for infections after HSCT are the status of the haematological disease at HSCT, the co-morbidities of the patient, the degree of neutropenia, the disruption of anatomical barriers (mucositis and indwelling catheters), depressed T- and B-cell function and immunosuppressive therapy. The reconstitution of immune status after HSCT depends on the type of transplantation (autologous or allogeneic), the source of progenitor cells (bone marrow, peripheral blood or cord blood), the conditioning regimen (myeloablative, RIC, or non-myeloablative), the degree of histocompatibility between the donor and the recipient (sibling, unrelated or mismatch), the type of GvHD prophylaxis (calcineurin or mTOR inhibitors, mono- or polyclonal antibodies or T-cell depletion) and the presence and grade of GvHD and its treatment. Depending on these factors, the patient can be immunodeficient for months or years after HSCT (see Chapter 14). There is a clear relationship between the type of immunodeficiency after HSCT and the incidence of certain infections. According to this, three different periods can be distinguished, with a predominance of specific pathogens in each phase (Figure 1) (2).

2. Chronology of infections after HSCT

2.1 Early or neutropenic phase (days 0 to +30)

This first period spans from conditioning up to engraftment. During this period, all risk factors for infections are present. Although neutropenia and disruption of anatomical barriers (mucosal damage and vascular devices) are the most relevant risk factors in this phase, cellular and humoral immunodeficiency and, in patients receiving TBI, functional asplenia are also present. The principal pathogens observed in this phase are Gram-positive and -negative bacteria, *Candida* spp. and the *Herpes simplex virus* (HSV) and the most frequent type of infections are bacteraemia/sepsis, pneumonia, oropharingitis, sinusitis, proctitis and cellulitis. The types of infectious complication in this period are the same after autologous and allogeneic HSCT. However, after autologous HSCT, the risk of bacterial infections and their mortality rate are lower due to the usually less intensive mucositis and the shorter neutropenia. In the autologous setting, the infection risk almost completely disappears after neutrophil recovery.

Figure 1: Chronology of predominant infections after HSCT

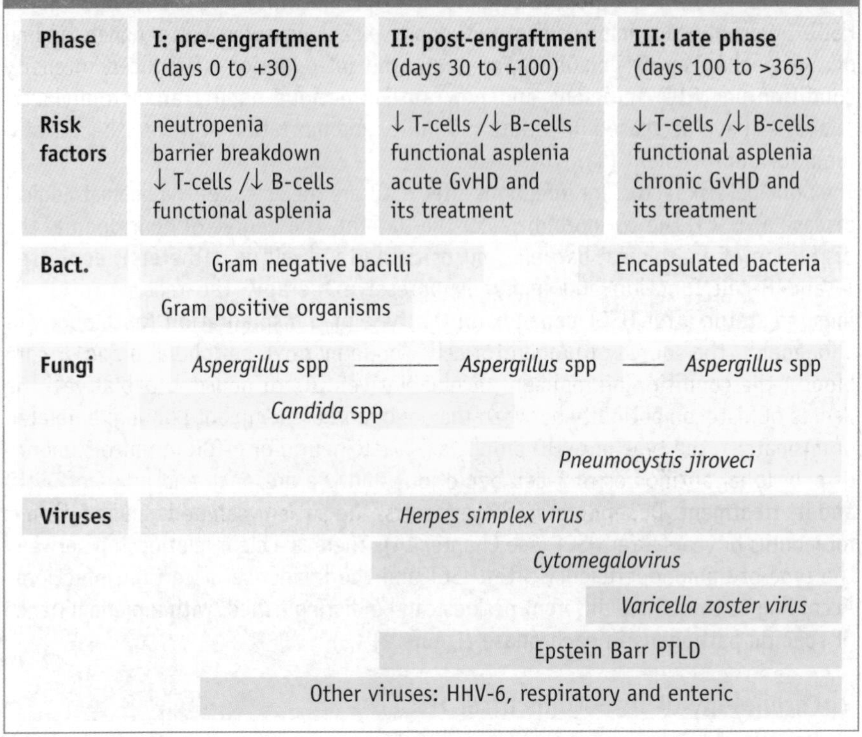

Phase	I: pre-engraftment (days 0 to +30)	II: post-engraftment (days 30 to +100)	III: late phase (days 100 to >365)
Risk factors	neutropenia barrier breakdown ↓ T-cells /↓ B-cells functional asplenia	↓ T-cells /↓ B-cells functional asplenia acute GvHD and its treatment	↓ T-cells /↓ B-cells functional asplenia chronic GvHD and its treatment
Bact.	Gram negative bacilli Gram positive organisms		Encapsulated bacteria
Fungi	*Aspergillus* spp ——— *Aspergillus* spp —— *Aspergillus* spp *Candida* spp		
			Pneumocystis jiroveci
Viruses	*Herpes simplex virus*		
		Cytomegalovirus	
			Varicella zoster virus
		Epstein Barr PTLD	
	Other viruses: HHV-6, respiratory and enteric		

Adapted from (2). PTLD: post-transplant lymphoproliferative disorder

2.2 Intermediate phase (days +30 to +100)

The second phase starts at marrow engraftment. At this time, neutropenia and mucositis have disappeared but central lines, immunodeficiency and functional asplenia, which may be worsened and maintained by GvHD and its treatment, persist. This favours the development of viral and fungal infections. *Cytomegalovirus* (CMV), adenovirus, BK polyomavirus, respiratory viruses, *Pneumocystis jiroveci* (Pj), *Candida* spp., *Aspergillus* spp. and other moulds are responsible for infections in this phase.

For decades, CMV disease was the principal infectious complication in this phase; however, with the introduction of good surveillance techniques that allow anticipated diagnosis and pre-emptive treatment, the mortality due to CMV has decreased notably (see below) (3). Currently, invasive aspergillosis (IA) is observed in 5–15% of allogeneic HSCT recipients, 60% of whom will die because of this infection despite the efficacy of the new antifungal agents (4).

2.3 Late post-transplantation phase (days > +100)

Infections occurring during this period are associated with the presence and severity of chronic GvHD, which prevents the normal recovery of cellular and humoral immunity. In addition, functional asplenia persists in patients with GvHD and in those receiving TBI. For this reason, in this phase, infections are generally secondary to encapsulated bacteria (*Streptococcus pneumoniae* and *Haemophilus influenzae*), *Aspergillus* spp. and other moulds, *Pj* and *Varicella zoster virus* (VZV).

In this late phase, a clear relationship exists between the degree of recovery of cellular immunity and infectious complications. Thus, the number of CD4+ cells correlates with certain infections/reactivations (Figure 2). Clear examples of this are the reactivation of *Toxoplasma gondii* in sero-positive patients and the *Pj* pneumonia observed when TMP-SMZ prophylaxis is stopped before CD4+ recovery (2).

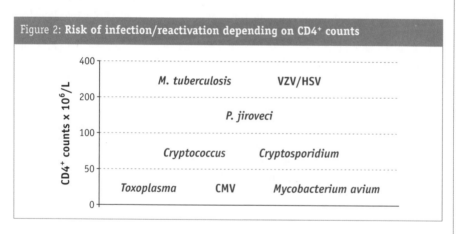

Figure 2: **Risk of infection/reactivation depending on CD4+ counts**

2.4 Some considerations about this chronology

The chronology of infections mentioned previously was described in patients receiving a myeloablative HSCT, but some differences can be observed in recipients of autologous HSCT or RIC-HSCT. Thus, in the autologous setting, as mentioned previously, bacterial infections are less frequent and severe and the other infections mentioned are exceptional. However, patients receiving immunosuppressive agents (steroids, purine analogues or monoclonal antibodies such as rituximab or alemtuzumab) or with severe hypogammaglobulinaemia prior to the auto-HSCT are at risk of developing infections similar to those observed in the allogeneic setting. In the past decade, RIC-HSCT has been used increasingly worldwide (see Chapter 8). Infections related to neutropenia and mucositis are less frequent with this modality of HSCT than after conventional HSCT. However, viral and fungal infections occurring in the intermediate and late period are comparable because the incidence and severity of GvHD is similar to that observed in myeloablative HSCT. Additionally, RIC-HSCT is usually applied to older patients, who have worse general condition and co-morbidities; for all these reasons, the infection-related mortality has not decreased in this setting (5).

3. Bacterial infections

3.1 Early phase after HSCT (neutropenic phase)
The main sources of bacterial infections in neutropenic patients are the normal endogenous flora in the gastrointestinal tract, which is responsible for infections by Gram-negative bacteria, and the exogenous acquisition of organisms from vascular devices, which is the main cause of infections by Gram-positive microorganisms. Analysis of catheter-related infections is beyond the scope of this chapter; for those interested, guidelines for the diagnosis and management of intravascular catheter-related infection have been published recently (see reference 6).

Interestingly, only 30–35% of febrile episodes in neutropenic patients can be documented microbiologically; in the remaining cases, the cause of the fever cannot be demonstrated. In the 1990s, Gram-positive bacteria were the pathogens isolated most frequently in cultures; in contrast, since the beginning of the current century, Gram-negative bacteria are re-emerging. Because most of these bacterial infections occur while the patient is treated in hospital, they can have a nosocomial origin; consequently, the epidemiology and protective measures used in the centre acquire special relevance.

3.1.1 Prophylaxis
Anti-bacterial prophylaxis has been general practice in this phase of HSCT. It is based on the elimination of endogenous gastrointestinal flora and on the prevention of the acquisition of exogenous organisms. The most important measures are hand-washing, oral hygiene, low-bacterial diets and gastrointestinal decontamination (GID) using oral antibiotics. Hand-washing is the only environmental measure with proven efficacy (level of recommendation AI) and should be used systematically in all cases. In this phase, the use of masks is indicated for all visitors and health care personnel in close contact with the patient, or if they present symptoms of upper

respiratory tract infection and contact with the patients cannot be avoided. The effectiveness of other protective measures (gowns, caps and leggings) has not been proven in this context (7).

The value of a low-bacterial diet has been questioned recently by the results of a randomised trial that compared cooked versus non-cooked food. In that study, cooked food was not associated with any survival advantages (8). Nevertheless, low-bacterial diets continues to be a general and reasonable practice in HSCT units.

GID has changed with the years. Up to the 1980s, this prophylaxis was achieved using non-absorbable antibiotics (i.e., gentamicin, vancomicin and nystatin (GVN)) that produced a complete GID; however, because of poor compliance and high cost, it has been generally abandoned. After the introduction by Van der Vaaij of the concept of "resistance to colonisation" (the presence of anaerobic bacteria in the intestine prevents the proliferation and, consequently, hampers the risk of aerobic bacteria translocation), co-trimoxazole (TMP-SMZ) and quinolones were used to destroy intestinal aerobic flora selectively. Because of the haematopoietic toxicity of TMP-SMZ, quinolones have been adopted systematically in HSCT since the 1980s. Many randomised studies and meta-analyses have been published on this topic (9) and the European Conference on Infections in Leukaemia (ECIL) guidelines recommend prophylaxis with fluoroquinolones during all the neutropenic phase for patients with acute leukaemia or for recipients of HSCT, with a strength of recommendation and level of evidence of AI (10).

3.1.2 Diagnosis

In the diagnostic work-up for any immunocompromised patient with fever the following aspects must be analysed systematically:

a. Epidemiological exposures (epidemic outbreaks and contact with children or other patients) and the status of the patient's microbiological flora (knowledge of previous antibiotics and infections); the possibility of reactivations (history of travelling, positive serologies, past tuberculosis, endemic mycoses, etc.)

b. The predominant type of immunosuppression (neutropenia, mucositis, type of immunodeficiency, function of the spleen, etc.) and

c. The preventive measures used (prophylactic agents, type of isolation and vaccines received).

This information must be completed by obtaining samples from blood, urine, stools and other possible foci of infection for cultures, PCR studies, antigen detection, biochemical analyses (basic and C-reactive protein), blood gases, and imaging techniques (chest-X ray, CT, MRI and ultrasound). As catheter-associated infections are a leading cause of blood-stream infections in this phase, the observation of a differential growing time greater than 2 hours between cultures obtained simultaneously from catheter and from peripheral blood using automated blood culture systems can be very useful for establishing a correct diagnosis without removing the line (6).

3.1.3 Treatment

In a neutropenic patient with fever, antibiotic treatment should be started immediately, based on an empirical approach and adapted to the flora usually observed in each centre, to the expected flora of the patient and to his/her clinical situation (11). The patient's flora changes during the time course of treatment and it is not the same after receiving antibiotics for several days or when treated in an ICU as it was during the first febrile episode in the neutropenic phase. Similarly, the approach must be completely different if the patient has an evident focus of infection (e.g., pneumonia, meningitis, abscess or cellulitis) - a situation in which the bacterial burden is high - rather than if a simple bacteraemia or a catheter infection with a low bacterial burden are present. This is why a standard febrile neutropenic patient without a focus of infection can be treated with monotherapy using a beta-lactam antibiotic active against Gram-positive and Gram-negative agents (including *Pseudomonas aeruginosa*), such as piperacillin/tazobactam, carbapenem or cefepime. However, in centres with a high incidence Gram-negative pathogens producing extended-spectrum beta-lactamases, the initial treatment must include a carbapenem (imi-, mero-, or doripenem). In this phase, neither an aminoglucoside nor a glycopeptide are recommended (as they exhibit more toxicity than survival benefit). Similarly, in the case of a persistent fever with negative cultures and absence of focal signs, the addition of a glycopeptide is not recommended (as Gram-positive agents are usually detected in blood cultures and have a low mortality rate). A neutropenic patient with a catheter infection, a severe mucositis or colonisation by MRSA is a completely different scenario; in these cases, a glycopeptide (or one of the new agents as doripenem or linezolid) should be added to the beta-lactam antibiotic (10).

If an infectious focus (e.g., pneumonia, typhlitis or cellulitis) exists, or if the patient has received antibiotics recently, or is colonised with resistant Gram-negative agents, an aminoglucoside must be added to the initial treatment. In the case of neutropenic patients presenting sepsis, shock or worsening after the first days of treatment, a treatment with a beta-lactam antibiotic, aminoglucoside and glycopeptide (or doripenem) should be started promptly (11).

In all cases, it is important to note that fever can persist up to 5–7 days after starting the antibiotic treatment. In this situation, if the patient is in a good clinical condition, there is no need to change the initial treatment. The reduction in the levels of C-reactive protein and/or procalcitonin can help to confirm that the infection is resolving.

3.2 Late infections

Bacterial infections occurring in this period are generally secondary to encapsulated bacteria (*Streptococcus pneumoniae, Haemophilus influenzae* and *Neisseriae meningitidis*) and are favoured by chronic GvHD and its treatment, functional asplenia, hypogammaglobulinaemia and the absence of specific antibodies. Patients receiving total body irradiation (TBI) also have a higher risk of pneumococcal sepsis (12).

3.2.1 Prophylaxis

Measures against encapsulated bacteria are well established: vaccination 6–12 months after HSCT (or when chronic GvHD is controlled) (see Table 1), administration of penicillin (or a macrolide) while under immunosuppressive treatment and immunoglobulin replacement (if severe hypogammaglobulinaemia and repeated infections are observed).

When evaluating an HSCT patient with fever in this late phase, it is necessary to remember that other "rare" bacterial infections produced by *Mycobacterium, Nocardia, Listeria* and *Legionella* are observed occasionally in these patients (2).

Table 1: **Vaccinations recommended after autologous and allogeneic HSCT**

Vaccine	Recommended after HSCT	Time to vaccine	Doses
Pneumococcal (conjugated)*	Yes (BI)	3–6 months	3*
Tetanus	Yes (BII)	6–12 months	3
Diphtheria	Yes (BII)	6–12 months	3
Pertussis (acellular)	Yes (CIII)	6–12 months	3
Haemophilus (conjugated)	Yes (BII)	6–12 months	3
Meningococcal (conjugate)	National recommendations (BII)	6–12 months	1
Polio (inactivated)	Yes (BII)	6–12 months	3
Hepatitis B (recombinant)	National recommendations (BII)	6–12 months	3
Influenza (inactivated)	Yearly (AII)	4–6 months	1–2
Measles	Yes (BII)	24 months	1–2
Mumps	Yes (CIII)	24 months	1–2
Rubella	Yes (BIII)	24 months	1–2

*Adapted from (2) and (13). *Followed by 2 doses of polysaccharide vaccine at 12 and 24 m (14)*

4. Fungal infections

4.1 Pathogenesis and epidemiology

As mentioned previously, fungal infections also follow a chronological pattern after HSCT (see Figure 1). In the first period, with neutropenia as the main risk factor, infections due to Candida spp. are the most common. The most relevant fungal infections occur in the intermediate/late phase and are favoured by the presence of GvHD and its treatment. Approximately 5–15% of HSCT patients develop invasive aspergillosis (IA) and 60% of them will die because of this, rendering it the main cause of infectious mortality after HSCT (15). Yeasts (with *Candida* as a representative) are acquired by translocation from intestinal mucosa or through the catheters. In contrast, *Aspergillus* spp. and other moulds are usually acquired by inhalation of spores (conidia) present in the air, causing rhinosinusitis or pneumonias. Rarely, they can be acquired through the skin, causing onychomycoses or mucosal infections. In normal conditions, the *Aspergillus* agents reaching the lung via inhalation are phagocytosed by pulmonary macrophages. If these macrophages are non-functional because of cellular immunosuppression or the use of steroids, *Aspergillus* can grow by germination, producing hyphae. Neutrophils are capable of stopping this growth; however, if neutropenia exists, *Aspergillus* continues to grow and, because of its angioinvasive capacity, can disseminate and occlude small vessels, producing avascular spaces.

4.2 Prophylaxis

Because mould infections are acquired mainly by inhalation, protective environment measures can be extremely relevant. The use of isolation rooms equipped with HEPA filters (filters that retain 99.97% of air particles with more than 0.3 μm, including bacteria, fungi and even viruses adherent to dust) permit the reduction of the risk of mould acquisition. Several studies have demonstrated their usefulness in reducing *Aspergillus* in the air and the incidence of IA. Unfortunately, these isolation measures are only applicable when patients are hospitalised, and the risk of infection by moulds lasts for several months after HSCT, when patients are no longer hospitalised (see Figure 1). Only one registry study has shown a survival benefit of HEPA/LAF rooms for patients receiving an allogeneic HSCT for leukaemia (16); however, many other authors have questioned their efficacy (7) or have reported large series of HSCT performed without protective environmental measures with a low incidence of IA (17). The low incidence of conidia in the air of centres situated in geographical areas with a high latitude, frequent rain and cold climate may be an explanation for these differing observations. Despite their theoretical effectiveness, there is limited experience with the use of portable HEPA filters and FFP3 masks. Regarding pharmacological antifungal prophylaxis, fluconazole has been the gold standard for many years as a consequence of some initial studies showing a survival advantage for auto- and allo-HSCT recipients receiving this prophylaxis. Fluconazole is excellent for most *Candida* spp. and for *Cryptococcus*, but is ineffective against *C. glabrata* and *krusei*, *Aspergillus* and other moulds. Further studies demonstrated that itraconazole may be a good alternative to fluconazole, but its low tolerance and its toxicity hamper its use. Micafungin has an efficacy that is similar to that of fluconazole. Prophylaxis with voriconazole did not yield better survival than that using fluconazole or itraconazole, but decreased the incidence of *Aspergillus* infections (18). Finally, prophylaxis with posaconazole offered a better survival compared with standard azoles in HSCT patients with GvHD (19). Consequently, the ECIL-3 guidelines strongly recommend posaconazole (AI) or voriconazole (for patients who already have a provisional AI) prophylaxis for HSCT patients with GvHD (Table 2) (4). Recently, a randomised, placebo-controlled trial has shown the effectiveness of aerosolised liposomal amphotericin B for prophylaxis of invasive pulmonary aspergillosis in neutropenic and HSCT patients (20).

Prophylaxis against *Pneumocystis jiroveci* is a mandatory practice in autologous and allogeneic HSCT, from the beginning of the procedure until CD4+ T-cell counts are above 200–400 x 10^6/L. The best prophylactic regimen is oral TMP-SMX 2–3 days/week (if administered 3 days/week, the prophylaxis is also effective against *Toxoplasma*). If this drug cannot be administered, aerosolised pentamidine (using a previous bronchodilator and administrating half of the dose in the Trendelenburg position), dapsone or atovaquone are good alternatives.

Table 2: ECIL-3 primary antifungal prophylaxis in HSCT recipients. Quality and evidence of recommendations

Antifungal drug	Initial neutropenic phase	With severe GvHD
Fluconazole (400 mg/d oral)	AI	CI
Itraconazole (400 mg/d oral*)	BI	BI
Voriconazole (400 mg/d oral)	AI (provisional)	AI (provisional)
Posaconazole	No data	
Echinocandins (iv)	--	Insufficient data
Micafungin (50 mg/d iv)	CI	--
Polyenes (iv)	CI	CI
Aerosolised L-AmB + fluco oral	BII	Insufficient data

*L-AmB: liposomal amphotericin B; *200 mg iv followed by oral solution*

4.3 Diagnosis

The diagnosis of fungal infections is based on histopathology, imaging techniques and microbiology. Histopathology remains the gold standard for diagnosis because it is the proof that there is a fungal infection in a tissue; however, although a description of the fungi can be made, the diagnosis of the species relies on the microbiology.

Microbiology is the hall-mark in the diagnosis of fungal infections. There are several techniques. Direct examination of sputum, BAL and skin samples with different staining often allows diagnosis on the same day. Although they require a few days, cultures (with specific media for moulds and yeasts) lead to the identification of the species of the fungi. The development of serological methods has been the most important advance in this field. Among them, the detection of *Aspergillus* galactomannan (GM) antigen and beta-D-glucan are the most relevant. GM detection has become a standard technique in the follow-up of patients at risk of IA. With a cut-off value of 0.5, it permits the detection of IA some days before the classical clinical/radiological manifestations appear (21). The sensitivity of GM decreases under prophylaxis against moulds. Possible false-positive results are another caveat of this test, especially after the ingestion of some foods or when receiving certain antibiotics, such as piperacillin/tazobactam.

Regarding imaging techniques, conventional radiology has many limitations. Although an abnormal chest X-ray is sufficient to suspect the diagnosis, an unremarkable X-ray must be followed by a CT scan. The observation of the so-called halo and crescent signs is compatible with the diagnosis of IA and, recently, the reverse halo sign has also been described as suggestive of zygomycosis. The halo sign appears early in the development of the infection and, after 3 days, most images in CT scans become less specific. This observation stress the relevance of a prompt CT scan to evaluate these patients because the probability of survival improves notably if the treatment is started when the halo sign is observed (22). Biopsy guided by CT scan is a complementary intervention that can allow the diagnosis.

The stratification for investigational purposes of invasive fungal infections as proven, probable and possible using clinical, histopathological, imaging and microbiological data has been a relevant step in this field (see Figure 3) (23).

4.4 Treatment

In recent years, there has been an increasing interest in antifungal treatment because of the introduction of new agents and the development of different therapeutic approaches using confusing terminologies. Empirical antifungal treatment can be defined as antifungal treatment administered to a patient with fever after 5–7 days of anti-bacterial therapy with negative clinical, microbiological and radiological

Figure 3: Main criteria for proven, probable and possible invasive fungal infection

Proven IFI	Probable IF	Possible IFI
Histological or culture evidence (in sterile material)	Host factors (neutropenia, immunosuppressants) **+** **Mycological criteria** (direct - cytology, culture of non sterile material - or indirect tests - GM or βDG) **+** Clinical criteria (+CT/MRI, FBS, retinal)	Host factors **+** **Clinical criteria**

GM: galactomannan; βDG: beta-D-glucan; FBS: fibrobronchoscopy. Retinal: retinal images suggestive of IFI. For complete description of host, clinical and microbiological criteria see reference (22)

results. This strategy was established 30 years ago based on two small studies and became a standard in haematological practice. The main criticism of this approach is that about 70–80% of the patients treated empirically do not have a fungal infection. Several randomised studies were designed to compare the different new agents when used for empirical treatment; all they yielded similar results (see Table 3).

Table 3: Double-blind clinical trials on empirical antifungal therapy

Author, year	Drugs compared	Outcome baseline IFI	Breaktrough IFI	Nephro-toxicity
White, 1998	ABCD* vs AmB-d	NS	NS	* Less
Walsh, 1999	Lipo-AmB* vs AmB-d	NS	* Less	* Less
Wingard, 2000	ABCD* vs Lipo-AmB	NS	NS	* More
Walsh, 2002	Vori* vs Lipo-AmB	NS	* Less	NS
Walsh, 2004	Caspo* vs Lipo-AmB	* Better	NS	* Less

ABCD: amphotericin B colloidal dispersion; Lipo-AmB: liposomal amphotericin B; AmB-d: amphotericin B deoxycholate; Vori: voriconazole; Caspo: caspofungin; NS: no significant difference

If using this empirical approach, ECIL-3 guidelines recommend the use of caspofungin or liposomal amphotericin B (degree of recommendation AI) (4).

However, because of the improvement of diagnostic techniques, the same ECIL guidelines suggest the transition to an early or anticipated antifungal treatment. The aim of this approach is to start antifungal treatment when the patient is at risk of invasive fungal infection and there is a positive antigen test (GM or beta-D-glucan) or a CT scan that is compatible with a fungal infection (24). Therapeutic strategies based on this approach are clearly effective and markedly reduce the cost of the treatment. Unfortunately, this strategy can only by applied in centres able to perform GM determinations twice a week and a CT scan promptly when requested. Directed antifungal treatment is used to treat patients with a proven diagnosis of fungal infection. Despite the fact that *Candida albicans, tropicalis* and *parapsilosis* are sensitive to all antifungals, the guidelines on candidaemia treatment in HSCT recipients recommend the initiation of treatment using a broad spectrum antifungal agent, followed by adjustment of the agent when the *Candida* species is identified (4). In patients with invasive candidiasis with criteria of severe sepsis, presence of metastasis or focal infection, colonisation by *C. krusei* or under prophylaxis with fluconazole, the recommendation is to start treatment using a candin, voriconazole or amphotericin B, whereas fluconazole is the drug of choice in the remaining situations. Catheter removal is recommended whenever possible in haematological patients with candidaemia or with *C. parapsilosis*.

Voriconazole is recommended as the first-line treatment for IA and offers a response rate of ~50% (25). For salvage treatment, the global response to the different antifungals is ~40% (Table 4). Although antifungal combinations are not recommended routinely for IA treatment, this approach should be considered in patients with severe sepsis, respiratory failure or CNS involvement; however, at present no randomised study has been performed to support this policy. It is important to remember that, during the first days of treatment of IA, the image of the pulmonary lesion can grow; this represents the normal kinetics of the infection and does not correlate with a poor outcome. The reduction in GM levels confirms a good response to treatment.

5. Viral infections

Viral infections after HSCT also follow a specific chronology (see Figure 1). Limitations of space in this chapter preclude the analysis of all the viruses that can affect HSCT recipients. We summarise the more relevant in the allogeneic setting (CMV, EBV and HHV-6); BK polyomavirus is covered in chapter 11 and the remainder can be consulted in the references attached (2, 3, 27).

Table 4: First line pharmacological treatment of invasive aspergillosis after HSCT. Quality and evidence of recommendation for different working groups

Antifungal agent	IDSA	ECIL-3	SEIMC
Voriconazole (6 mg/kg/d iv)	AI	AI	AI
L-AmB (3 mg/kg/d iv)	AI	BI	AI
ABLC (5 mg/kg/d iv)		BII	No data
Caspofungin (50 mg/d iv)		CII	CII
Micafungin (100 mg/d iv)			No data
Itraconazole (200 mg/d iv)		CIII	DIII
Posaconazole		No data	No data
Combination of antifungals	BII	DIII	CIII

Adapted from (26). IDSA: Infectious Diseases Society of America; ECIL: European Conference on Infections in Leukemia; SEIMC: Sociedad Española de Enfermedades Infecciosas y Microbiología Clínica; L-AmB: lipsosomal amphotericin; ABLC: amphotericin B lipid complex

5.1 Cytomegalovirus

Around 40–80% of people (depending on the country) are infected by CMV (herpes virus type 5) in childhood. After infection (positive IgM serology), CMV becomes latent for life (positive IgG serology). Under certain circumstances, as in immunosuppression following HSCT, latent CMV can reactivate.

5.1.1 Diagnosis

CMV infection/reactivation can be detected using several techniques (mainly CMV antigenaemia and PCR using blood samples). A positive result indicates an active CMV infection/reactivation. The diagnosis of CMV disease can be established when this infection/reactivation is accompanied by clinical manifestations. There are well-defined criteria for the diagnosis of CMV disease in each of the organs which are commonly affected, e.g., lung, gastrointestinal tract, brain, and eye (28).

5.1.2 Management

For decades, CMV disease was the most important cause of infectious morbidity and mortality after HSCT. The development of good reliable techniques for the diagnosis of CMV infection (antigenaemia and PCR) allows the treatment of the infection/reactivation before the development of CMV disease (pre-emptive or anticipated treatment) (29).

It is very important to prevent infection in patients with a negative CMV IgG serology before HSCT. For this purpose, transfusions using filtered products or from seronegative donors are mandatory. These patients have to be trained to avoid sharing cups, glasses and eating tools, to use condoms if not monogamous and to perform regular hand-washing. When possible, a CMV seronegative donor should be chosen because the outcome of HSCT is improved in these cases.

In a patient with a positive CMV IgG serology, there are two possible strategies:

a. Primary prophylaxis: administration of universal prophylaxis using high-dose acyclovir or ganciclovir to all seropositive patients. This is an effective but toxic and non-cost-effective approach that usually is reserved for populations with a very high risk of CMV disease (i.e. cord blood HSCT);

b. Pre-emptive approach: treatment of the infection detected by antigenaemia or PCR before the development of CMV disease using either ganciclovir or foscarnet. This approach is preferred by most teams, but requires the monitoring of CMV twice a week during the period at risk (at least until day +100).

It is important to note that, although the mortality due to CMV has decreased using this strategy, an increase of late CMV disease, which has the same mortality as early disease, has been observed. The median time of appearance of these late cases is around day +180, and patients with low numbers of CD4+ T-cells and with chronic GvHD are at higher risk. The selection of sero-positive donors for sero-positive patients is preferred.

5.1.3 Treatment

Although CMV management has improved the outcome of HSCT, the mortality of CMV disease remains high. Thus, the mortality of CMV pneumonia, which to date has been the most frequent clinical presentation of CMV infection, can increase up to 50–70%. Currently, gastrointestinal CMV disease seems to be more frequent than its pulmonary forms among patients receiving RIC-HSCT. First-line treatment depends on the organ affected:

a. CMV pneumonia: ganciclovir (or foscarnet if a pancytopenia exists) associated with high dose of intravenous immunoglobulin (500 mg/kg every 48 h; seven to 10 doses, followed by a weekly maintenance dose for 2–4 weeks);

b. Other forms of CMV disease: either ganciclovir or foscarnet, without immunoglobulin.

The oral presentation of ganciclovir (valganciclovir) is used extensively but should be used with caution. As a fixed dose is recommended, the monitoring of peripheral counts and renal function is mandatory, especially in patients with low body weight, because of its excellent bioavailability. Second-line treatment is based on cidofovir or the combination of ganciclovir with foscarnet.

5.2 Epstein-Barr virus

Another herpes virus, Epstein-Barr virus (EBV), is associated with post-HSCT lymphoproliferative disease (EBV-PTLD), which is a life-threatening complication. The following risk factors increase the risk of PTLD: unrelated and/or mismatched HSCT; use of T-cell depletion, ATG or OKT3; EBV serology mismatch between the donor and the recipient (increased risk for sero-negative patients with a sero-positive donor); primary EBV infection and splenectomy. Monitoring of EBV reactivation using quantitative PCR (at least once a week for 3 months) is recommended for this high-risk population to allow pre-emptive treatment if a rise in viral load is observed. The ECIL-2 recommendations for pre-emptive treatment are: rituximab (375 mg/m², one or two doses), reduction of immunosuppression, when possible, and donor EBV-specific cytotoxic T-lymphocytes, if available. Antiviral drugs are not recommended. In cases of established EBV-PTLD, the same measures must be applied; if there is no response, donor lymphocyte infusions or chemotherapy are additional options (24).

5.3 Human herpes virus 6

Human herpes virus 6 (HHV-6) in the setting of allogeneic HSCT reactivates in 50–70% of patients (typically earlier than CMV) and has distinctive clinical manifestations that can help its diagnosis: encephalitis, with characteristic limbic- and hippocampus-derived symptoms, can be confirmed using MRI studies, EEG changes and demonstration of the presence of HHV-6 DNA in the CNS; marrow suppression is observed as a delayed engraftment or graft failure together with positive HHV-6 PCR in blood; and skin rash, which is predominant in cheeks and resembles an acute GvHD, is also characteristic. Any of these symptoms/signs is suspicious of HHV-6 reactivation. Treatment consists of either foscarnet or ganciclovir (30).

References

1. Gratwohl A, Brand R, Frassoni F et al. Cause of death after allogeneic haematopoietic stem cell transplantation (HSCT) in early leukaemias: An EBMT analysis of lethal infectious complications and changes over calendar time. Bone Marrow Transplant 2005; 36: 757–769.
2. Tomblyn M, Chiller T, Einsele H et al. Guidelines for preventing infectious complications among hematopoietic cell transplantation recipients: A global perspective. Biol Blood Marrow Transplant 2009; 15: 1143–1238.
3. Ljungman P, de la Cámara R, Cordonnier C et al. European Conference on Infections in Leukemia. Management of CMV, HHV-6, HHV-7 and Kaposi-sarcoma herpesvirus (HHV-8) infections in patients with hematological malignancies and after SCT. Bone Marrow Transplant 2008; 42: 227–240.
4. Maertens J, Marchetti O, Herbrecht R et al. Third European Conference on Infections in Leukemia. European guidelines for antifungal management in leukemia and hematopoietic

stem cell transplant recipients: Summary of the ECIL 3-2009 update. Bone Marrow Transplant 2011; 46: 709–718.

5. Scott BL, Sandmaier BM, Storer B et al. Myeloablative vs nonmyeloablative allogeneic transplantation for patients with myelodysplastic syndrome or acute myelogenous leukemia with multilineage dysplasia: A retrospective analysis. Leukemia 2006; 20: 128–135.

6. Mermel LA, Allon M, Bouza E et al. Clinical practice guidelines for the diagnosis and management of intravascular catheter-related infection: 2009 Update by the Infectious Diseases Society of America. Clin Infect Dis 2009; 49: 1–45.

7. Hayes-Lattin B, Leis JF, Maziarz RT. Isolation in the allogeneic transplant environment: How protective is it? Bone Marrow Transplant 2005; 36: 373–381.

8. Gardner A, Mattiuzzi G, Faderl S et al. Randomized comparison of cooked and noncooked diets in patients undergoing remission induction therapy for acute myeloid leukemia. J Clin Oncol 2008; 26: 5684–5688.

9. Imran H, Tleyjeh IM, Arndt CA et al. Fluoroquinolone prophylaxis in patients with neutropenia: a meta-analysis of randomized placebo-controlled trials. Eur J Clin Microbiol Infect Dis 2008; 27: 53–63.

10. Guidelines from the first European Conference on Infections in Leukaemia: ECIL1. Cordonier C, Calandra T, Meunier F (Eds.). Eur J Cancer Supplements 2007; 5: 1–59.

11. Freifeld AG, Bow EJ, Sepkowitz KA et al. Clinical practice guideline for the use of antimicrobial agents in neutropenic patients with cancer: 2010 update by the infectious diseases society of america. Clin Infect Dis 2011; 52: e56–93.

12. Kulkarni S, Powles R, Treleaven J et al. Chronic graft versus host disease is associated with long-term risk for pneumococcal infections in recipients of bone marrow transplants. Blood 2000; 95: 3683–3686.

13. De la Cámara R, Mensa J, Carreras E et al. Antifungal prophylaxis in oncohematologic patients: Literature review and recommendations. Med Clin (Barc) 2010; 134: 222–233.

14. Cordonnier C, Labopin M, Chesnel V et al. Randomized study of early versus late immunization with pneumococcal conjugate vaccine after allogeneic stem cell transplantation. Clin Infect Dis 2009; 48: 1392–1401.

15. Kontoyiannis DP, Marr KA, Park BJ et al. Prospective surveillance for invasive fungal infections in hematopoietic stem cell transplant recipients, 2001-2006: Overview of the Transplant-Associated Infection Surveillance Network (TRANSNET) Database. Clin Infect Dis 2010; 50: 1091–1100.

16. Passweg JR, Rowlings PA, Atkinson KA et al. Influence of protective isolation on outcome of allogeneic bone marrow transplantation for leukemia. Bone Marrow Transplant 1998; 21: 1231–1238.

17. McDiarmid S, Hutton B, Atkins H et al. Performing allogeneic and autologous hematopoietic SCT in the outpatient setting: Effects on infectious complications and early transplant outcomes. Bone Marrow Transplant 2010; 45: 1220–1226.

18. Wingard JR, Carter SL, Walsh TJ et al. Randomized, double-blind trial of fluconazole versus voriconazole for prevention of invasive fungal infection after allogeneic hematopoietic cell transplantation. Blood 2010; 116: 5111–5118.

19. Ullmann AJ, Lipton JH, Vesole DH et al. Posaconazole or fluconazole for prophylaxis in

severe graft-versus-host disease. N Engl J Med 2007; 356: 335–347.

20. Rijnders BJ, Cornelissen JJ, Slobbe L et al. Aerosolized liposomal amphotericin B for the prevention of invasive pulmonary aspergillosis during prolonged neutropenia: A randomized, placebo-controlled trial. Clin Infect Dis 2008; 46: 1401–1408.

21. Maertens J, Van Eldere J, Verhaegen J et al. Use of circulating galactomannan screening for early diagnosis of invasive aspergillosis in allogeneic stem cell transplant recipients. J Infect Dis 2002; 186: 1297–1306.

22. Greene RE, Schlamm HT, Oestmann JW et al. Imaging findings in acute invasive pulmonary aspergillosis: Clinical significance of the halo sign. Clin Infect Dis 2007; 44: 373–379.

23. De Pauw B, Walsh TJ, Donnelly JP et al. Revised definitions of invasive fungal disease from the European Organization for Research and Treatment of Cancer/Invasive Fungal Infections Cooperative Group and the National Institute of Allergy and Infectious Diseases Mycoses Study Group (EORTC/MSG) Consensus Group. Clin Infect Dis 2008; 46: 1813–1821.

24. Maertens J, Theunissen K, Verhoef G et al. Galactomannan and computed tomography-based preemptive antifungal therapy in neutropenic patients at high risk for invasive fungal infection: A prospective feasibility study. Clin Infect Dis. 2005; 41: 1242–1250.

25. Herbrecht R, Denning DW, Patterson TF et al. Voriconazole versus amphotericin B for primary therapy of invasive aspergillosis. N Engl J Med 2002; 347: 408–415.

26. Fortún J, Carratalá J, Gavaldá J et al. Guidelines for the treatment of invasive fungal disease by Aspergillus spp. and other fungi issued by the Spanish Society of Infectious Diseases and Clinical Microbiology (SEIMC). 2011 Update. Enferm Infecc Microbiol Clin 2011; 29: 435–454.

27. Styczynski J, Reusser P, Einsele H et al. Management of HSV, VZV and EBV infections in patients with hematological malignancies and after SCT: Guidelines from the Second European Conference on Infections in Leukemia. Bone Marrow Transplant 2009; 43: 757–770.

28. Ljungman P, Griffiths P, Paya C. Definitions of cytomegalovirus infection and disease in transplant recipients. Clin Infect Dis 2002; 34: 1094–1097.

29. Boeckh M, Ljungman P. How we treat cytomegalovirus in hematopoietic cell transplant recipients. Blood 2009; 113: 5711–5719.

30. Zerr DM, Corey L, Kim HW et al. Clinical outcomes of human herpes virus 6 reactivation after hematopoietic stem cell transplantation. Clin Infect Dis 2005; 40: 932–940.

Multiple Choice Questionnaire

To find the correct answer, go to http://www.esh.org/online-training/handbook/

1. **Regarding the chronology of infections after HSCT, which of the following is not a risk factor in the early or neutropenic phase?**
   a) Neutropenia . . . . □
   b) Disruption of anatomical barriers . . . . □

c) Cellular and humoral immunodeficiency ☐
d) Chronic GvHD ☐

2. **In the late post-transplantation phase, which of the following agents is not a frequent cause of infection?**
    a) *Candida* ☐
    b) *Varicella zoster virus* ☐
    c) *Aspergillus* ☐
    d) *Haemophilus influenzae* ☐

3. **Which of the following statements is false?**
    a) The main sources of bacterial infections in neutropenic patients are the normal endogenous flora in the gastrointestinal tract ☐
    b) Vascular devices are not associated with infections by Gram-positive microorganisms ☐
    c) Only 30–35% of febrile episodes in neutropenic patients can be documented ☐
    d) Most of the bacterial infections can have a nosocomial origin ☐

4. **In a neutropenic patient with fever, which of the following statements is false?**
    a) Treatment should be started immediately ☐
    b) Treatment should be adapted to the flora of each hospital ☐
    c) It is not important to start antibiotics immediately, wait until the results of cultures ☐
    d) A neutropenic patient without an infectious focus can be treated with monotherapy ☐

5. **In a case of invasive aspergillosis, which of the following antifungal agents is not effective?**
    a) Fluconazole ☐
    b) Voriconazole ☐
    c) Candins ☐
    d) Amphotericin B ☐

NOTES

* CHAPTER 13

Graft-versus-host disease

Jane Apperley, Tamás Masszi

1. Introduction

Graft-versus-host disease (GvHD) was first recognised in murine models of HSCT, when in the absence of knowledge of the HLA-system, it was termed "secondary" or "runt" disease on the basis of anorexia, reduced weight, diarrhoea, ruffled fur and eventual death. Billingham established the criteria for the occurrence of secondary disease in the 1960s, i.e.:
- The administration of a graft containing immunocompetent cells
- Immunological disparity between host and donor
- The administration of the graft to an immunosuppressed host.

In the human setting we traditionally recognise two forms of GvHD, acute (aGvHD) and chronic (cGvHD). The original distinction of acute from chronic GvHD, namely the occurrence before or after day 100 post stem cell infusion, has become blurred recently due to the development of an aGvHD-like illness beyond day 100 after reduced-intensity conditioning (RIC) regimens and/or after donor lymphocyte infusions (usually given after day 100). Nevertheless the underlying combination of symptoms and signs affecting the skin, liver and gastrointestinal tract form a classical clinical syndrome enabling the diagnosis and a helpful guide to the appropriate terminology is provided in Table 1.

Table 1: **Distinguishing acute and chronic graft-versus-host disease**			
Category	**Time of symptoms**	**Acute GvHD features**	**Chronic GvHD features**
Acute GvHD			
Classic acute	≤100 days	Yes	No
Persistent, recurrent or late-onset acute	>100 days	Yes	No
Chronic GvHD			
Classic chronic	No time limit	No	Yes
Overlap syndrome	No time limit	Yes	Yes

2. Acute graft-versus-host disease

2.1 Definition

aGvHD remains, directly or indirectly, the major cause of short-term (day 100) mortality after allogeneic HSCT. The pathology of aGvHD has been attributed to a three phase process comprising initial tissue damage from the conditioning regimen which in turn leads to activation of host antigen-presenting cells and activation and proliferation of donor T-cells (afferent phase) and finally to the release of inflammatory cytokines such as interleukin-1 and tissue necrosis factor (TNF)-α that eventually produce tissue necrosis (efferent phase). The action of this pathogenetic process in the induction of aGvHD is modulated in part by the presence of cells capable of inhibiting immune responses, most notably T-regulatory cells (T-regs).

2.2 Risk factors
As aGvHD is a result of an alloimmune effect the major risk for occurrence is the presence of HLA disparity, and increasing degrees of HLA-mismatching increase the probability of more severe disease. Other important and consistent risk factors include older patient age, the use of female donors for male recipients, prior alloimmunisation of the donor and the nature of GvHD prophylaxis. A number of publications have variously reported risk factors such as increasing donor age, increasing intensity of the preparative regimen, the use of peripheral blood stem cells as opposed to bone marrow, and recipient seropositivity for cytomegalovirus. A recent study of 2941 recipients of allogeneic HSCT in Seattle confirmed the importance of the degree of HLA-mismatching, the use of unrelated donors and the administration of total body irradiation in predicting the occurrence of moderate to severe aGvHD. In contrast they found that increasing donor age, cytokine-mobilised stem cells and the use of female donors for male recipients did not impact on the likelihood of aGvHD but were associated with the occurrence of cGvHD (1).

More recently we have begun to appreciate the importance of non-HLA genetic factors in the development of GvHD. Examples include polymorphisms in the genes encoding cytokines such as the tumour necrosis factors, the interleukins (IL-1, IL-6 and IL-10), interferon (IFN)-γ and transforming growth factor (TGF)-β and the expression of the killer cell immunoglobulin-like receptors (KIR) (discussed more extensively in Chapter 5). Interestingly one of the common features of the organs involved in aGvHD is that they are all exposed to microbial pathogens through the intestinal mucosa, epidermis and portal circulation and early murine studies confirmed a reduction in the severity and incidence of GvHD in animals that received antibiotic prophylaxis to "decontaminate" the gastrointestinal tract or those kept in germ-free environments. This has led to the speculation that potential differences within individuals in the interactions of antigens derived from infective organisms and pathogen recognition receptors (PRR) might protect or predispose to the occurrence of GvHD. To date the most extensively studied of these receptors is NOD2 (CARD15) which detects muramyl dipeptide (MDP), a by-product of peptidoglycan, which is itself a cell wall component of most bacteria. Single nucleotide polymorphisms (SNPs) in NOD2 are present in approximately 15% of the population and several investigators have studied their potential association with the occurrence of GvHD. Results are so far conflicting and further work is required to determine their real significance (reviewed in Penack et al. (2)).

2.3 Diagnosis and scoring

aGvHD is manifested by one or more of the following features: an erythematous skin reaction, cholestatic liver disease and gastrointestinal dysfunction. The variety of presentations in each organ is provided in more detail in Table 2; the syndrome ranges from a mild self-limiting condition to a serious and potentially fatal disorder. Because of the complexity of care of an allogeneic transplant recipient it is often very difficult to distinguish the characteristic features of aGvHD from those of other complications such as veno-occlusive disease, drug toxicity and infection, and consequently to determine the appropriate choice of treatment. For this reason it is essential to establish the diagnosis by biopsy of one or more affected organs and confirmation of the characteristic histopathological features (Table 3). The targets of the immune response in aGvHD are the epithelial cells including basal and suprabasal cells of the epidermis, the intestinal epithelium and the biliary duct epithelium, and the characteristic feature is identical, i.e. the presence of infiltrating immune cells close to apoptotic cells known as "satellite cell necrosis".

The first classification of aGvHD was developed by Glucksberg et al. in 1974. Each organ was staged from 0 to 4 (Table 4) and the resultant stages were combined to provide an overall grade (Table 5) (3). In 1994 Przepiorka et al. described the outcome of a Consensus Workshop to develop an improved scoring system that retained most of the characteristics of Glucksberg but dropped the use of the clinical performance score and included upper intestinal symptoms within the definition of aGvHD (4). Subsequently the IBMTR prospectively evaluated a "severity index" against the

Table 2: **Clinical manifestations of acute graft-versus-host disease**	
Organ	**Clinical manifestations**
Skin	Erythematous maculopapular rash, often initially involving the palms and soles May progress to involve entire body surface May be pruritic and/or painful In severe cases, bullae may form leading to desquamation
Liver	Cholestasis with or without frank jaundice Cholestatic enzymes comparatively more deranged than transaminases
Gastrointestinal tract	Anorexia, nausea and vomiting Diarrhoea, typically green and watery In severe cases diarrhoea contains fresh blood and mucosa and is accompanied by abdominal pain and on occasions followed by paralytic ileus

Table 3: Histopathological features of acute graft-versus-host disease

Organ	Histopathological features
Skin	The diagnostic feature is a lichenoid infiltration of the upper dermis and lower epidermis with vacuolation, degeneration and individual cell necrosis of the cells of the basal layer of the epidermis Grade 1: vacuolation of epidermal basal cells Grade 2: presence of individually necrotic keratinocytes Grade 3: confluent areas of keratinocyte necrosis forming bullae Grade 4: sloughing of the epidermis
Liver	The most consistent histological feature is small bile duct damage, which is usually seen in association with cholestasis and is rare in other complications of HSCT. The biliary epithelial cells have enlarged hyperchromatic nuclei or small pyknotic nuclei and vacuolated cytoplasm Periportal and midzone hepatocellular necrosis and minimal lymphocytic infiltrates in the portal tract Although there is a histological grading for liver histology but it has no proven prognostic value
Gastrointestinal tract	"Exploding crypts" within which are necrosis of individual epithelial cells at the periphery of the crypt leaving fragments of nuclear and cytoplasmic debris Grade 1: individual cell necrosis Grade 2: loss of individual crypts Grade 3: loss of two or more adjacent crypts with ulceration Grade 4: denudation of epithelium

Table 4: Staging of acute graft-versus-host disease

Stage	Skin based on maculopapular rash	Liver based on serum bilirubin	Gastrointestinal tract based on quantity of diarrhoea
+	<25% of body surface	34–50 µmol/L	>500 <1000 mL
++	25–50% of body surface	51–102 µmol/L	>1000 <1500 mL
+++	Generalised erythroderma	103–255 µmol/L	>1500 mL
++++	Generalised erythroderma with bullae and desquamation	>255 µmol/L	Severe abdominal pain with or without ileus

Table 5: **Overall grading of acute graft-versus-host disease**	
Grade	**Organ and stage of involvement**
I	Skin + to ++
II	Skin + to +++ Gastrointestinal tract and/or liver + Mild decrease in clinical performance
III	Skin ++ to +++ Gastrointestinal tract and/or liver ++ to +++ Marked decrease in clinical performance
IV	Skin ++ to ++++ Gastrointestinal tract and/or liver ++ to ++++ Extreme decrease in clinical performance

Glucksberg criteria but were unable to identify any particular advantage for the new system (5). In fact the Glucksberg score was a better predictor of survival and remains in regular use.

2.4 Epidemiology
Moderate to severe aGvHD occurs in approximately 40% of all recipients of allogeneic HSCT, but the precise incidence varies considerably depending predominantly on the nature of the donor and the method of GvHD prophylaxis. Without effective prophylaxis it is an almost inevitable complication of unrelated matched donor and mismatched family grafts.

2.5 Prevention
Grade III-IV aGvHD has an extremely poor prognosis despite therapeutic intervention and consequently considerable efforts are made to try and prevent its occurrence (Table 6). The rationale of prophylaxis was originally directed towards prolonged immunosuppression of donor T-cell function through the peri- and post-transplant administration of immunosuppressive agents. Early studies identified the superiority of a combination of the calcineurin inhibitor, cyclosporin, with methotrexate over methotrexate alone. In practice this combination remains the most frequently used method of prophylaxis although some investigators have replaced cyclosporin with tacrolimus since large two phase III randomised studies reported a reduction in the incidence of grade II-IV aGvHD at 32% in recipients of sibling transplants and 56% in those who received unrelated donor grafts in patients who received tacrolimus plus methotrexate compared to 44% (sibling) and 74% (unrelated) in

Table 6: Agents used in the prevention of acute graft-versus-host disease

Agent	Mechanism of action	Dose
Cyclosporin	Calcineurin inhibition i.e. blockade of T-cell activation	3 mg/kg iv
Tacrolimus	Calcineurin inhibition i.e. blockade of T-cell activation	0.02 mg/kg iv
Methotrexate	Antimetabolite	15 mg/m^2 day +1, 10 mg/m^2 day +3, 6 and 11
Methylprednisolone	Receptor mediated lympholysis and other unidentified actions	0.5–1.0 mg/kg
Mycophenolate mofetil	Inhibition of DNA synthesis, lymphocyte apoptosis	1.5–3 g/day
Sirolimus	Macrolide antibiotic; blockade of T-and B-cell activations	12 mg day -3 then 4 mg/day
Antithymocyte globulin	Rabbit or equine polyclonal antibodies recognising T-cells	2.5 mg/kg/day x 4
Monoclonal antibodies eg. alemtuzumab (anti-CD52)	Humanised monoclonal antibodies recognising T-cells	10 mg/kg/day, usually for 5 days
Cyclophosphamide	Cytotoxic agent inducing death of proliferating cells	50 mg/kg/day on days +3 and +4

those who were randomised to cyclosporin and methotrexate. However there was no difference in survival that could be attributed to the nature of the GvHD prevention (6, 7). Recently investigators have also reported the efficacy of newer agents such as mycophenolate mofetil (MMF) and sirolimus, and the combination of tacrolimus and sirolimus is currently being compared with that of tacrolimus and methotrexate in a phase III randomised study.

An alternative approach to GvHD prophylaxis is to consider removal of donor T-cells either *ex vivo* prior to infusion or *in vivo* before and/or after infusion using polyclonal (anti-thymocyte globulin, ATG) or monoclonal antibodies. A similar effect can also be achieved by positive selection of CD34+ stem cells. These techniques, collectively known as T-cell depletion, are extremely efficient in preventing acute and chronic GvHD and were in widespread use in the 1980s and 1990s. Unfortunately they were rapidly identified as contributing to an increased risk of infection and disease relapse, and subsequently became confined to situations in which the risk of GvHD is particularly high, e.g. recipients of mismatched and haploidentical transplants where the risk of death from GvHD outweighs the risk of later disease recurrence. In particular ATG contributes substantially to the risk of developing EBV-related post-transplant lymphoproliferative disease (PTLD) necessitating regular molecular monitoring and prophylaxis or pre-emptive treatment with rituximab.

Other studies have explored alternative methods of acute GvHD prophylaxis including the infusion of an expanded population of T-regulatory cells at the time of stem cell infusion, the use of extracorporeal photophoresis and most recently the administration of high dose cyclophosphamide, particularly in the context of haploidentical transplantation (reviewed in Perez et al. (8)).

2.6 Treatment

Grade I aGvHD, by definition affecting only the skin, can often be effectively treated with topical steroids alone. More advanced grades require systemic therapy and the mainstay of treatment remains high dose methylprednisolone, usually at a dose of 2 mg/kg/day, continued for 7–14 days and followed by a gradual reduction in dose. The chance of response decreases with increasing grade of GvHD but in general approximately 40–50% of patients will demonstrate a response. Reductions in steroid doses are often followed by an exacerbation of symptoms that can sometimes be settled by simply increasing the dose and reducing more slowly on the second occasion. Achieving a balance between the level of immunosuppression required to control aGvHD and retaining a degree of immunocompetence against microbial infection is challenging, and viral and fungal infections are frequent complications of prolonged steroid therapy. Anti-infective prophylaxis should be considered for all such patients. The Blood and Marrow Transplant Clinical Trials Network (BMT-CTN) recently completed a randomised phase II study of four agents, etanercept, MMF, denileukin diftitox, or pentostatin, each in combination with methylprednisolone 2 mg/kg/day. The complete remission rates at day 28 after initiation of therapy were 26, 60, 53 and 38% respectively (9). The interpretation of the study was complicated by the fact that many eligible patients had received MMF as GvHD prophylaxis and therefore could not be randomised to the arm containing MMF. Patients randomised to any of the other three arms contained a significant proportion that had previously failed MMF, raising the possibility that the results would be biased in favour of MMF. Nevertheless the combination of steroids and MMF has been taken forward to a phase III study against steroids alone.

Failure to respond to standard steroid doses (defined as progression within 3 days of starting treatment or an incomplete response by 14 days) or refractory recurrence after initial dose reduction will necessitate second line treatment. In this context many agents have been tried alone or in combination with corticosteroid. None have shown convincing long-term efficacy. The most frequent choice of second line therapy involves one or more monoclonal antibodies recognising T-cells, or ATG. Monoclonal antibodies include alemtuzumab for the pan T-cell marker, CD52, daclizumab, for the alpha sub-unit of the IL-2 receptor expressed on activated T-cells and now no longer available in Europe and infliximab and etanercept for TNF-α. These agents often result in short-term control but durable effects are relatively infrequent and the outcome of refractory aGvHD is dismal with approximately 80% mortality. Newer approaches currently under evaluation include immunotoxin-based agents such as denileukin difitox. Responses have been reported with extracorporeal photopheresis but this is a difficult treatment to deliver at regular intervals (at least twice a week) to individuals who are seriously unwell.

In 2006, Ringden et al. reported the successful use of mesenchymal stromal cells (MSC) in a small group of patients with refractory severe aGvHD (10) and later this group described a response rate of 40% in a larger group of patients (11), MSC exert immunosuppressive effects in a non-HLA restricted manner and like T-regs offer interesting and novel strategies for the management of this potentially fatal complication.

3. Chronic graft-versus-host disease

3.1 Definition and pathology

cGvHD is an immunoregulatory disorder occurring after allogeneic HSCT and shares features of autoimmunity and immunodeficiency. Features of cGVHD resemble other autoimmune diseases such as Sjögren syndrome, scleroderma, primary biliary cirrhosis and immuncytopenias. Similarly to aGVHD, cGVHD is also thought to be induced by the immune cells of the donor but the pathophysiology is even less well understood. Although autoreactive T-lymphocytes are considered to play the key role, recent data revealed the importance of B-cells (12). cGVHD is the main cause of late non-relapse mortality and morbidity after allogeneic HSCT. Mortality is primarily caused by infections either due to the immunodeficiency of cGVHD or its treatment.

3.2 Risk factors

The major risk factors for the development of cGVHD are prior acute GvHD, higher degree of HLA mismatch, older patient age, previous splenectomy, CMV seropositivity, female donor to male recipient and mobilised peripheral blood stem cell graft (Table 7) (1, 13).

3.3 Diagnosis and scoring

The diagnosis of cGvHD is based on its clinical manifestations. The signs and symptoms of cGvHD may occur in any organ but the most frequently affected

Table 7: **Major risk factors for the development of chronic graft-versus-host disease**	
Given factors	**Variable factors**
Older age of recipient	Higher degree of HLA mismatch
CMV seropositivity of recipient	Older age of donor
Previous splenectomy	CMV seropositivity of donor
Prior acute GvHD	Female donor to male recipient
	Mobilised blood stem cell graft

organs/sites are the skin, nails, mouth, eyes, female genitalia, gastrointestinal tract, liver, lungs, muscles, fascia and joints. The disease may be mono-symptomatic, but can also be widespread and leading to debilitating consequences such as end stage lung disease or joint contractures. Since the NIH consensus development project on cGvHD in 2005 new diagnostic and staging criteria has been established (14). The consensus group defined diagnostic signs (any one of these signs itself establishes the diagnosis of cGvHD without further investigation), distinctive signs (should be confirmed by pertinent biopsy or other relevant test, e.g. Schirmer), other features of cGvHD which are not specific, and common signs that occur both in acute and chronic GvHD (Table 8). There is no time limit for setting the diagnosis of cGvHD in contrast to the previous definition when cGvHD could be diagnosed exclusively only after 100 days following the transplant (Table 1).

Until the NIH proposal cGvHD grading was based on a retrospective study of 20 patients (15). This divided cGvHD into limited (only localised skin involvement and/or hepatic dysfunction) and extensive disease. This classification was very easy to use in the daily routine, but was insufficiently robust and reproducible to allow for appropriate comparisons between clinical studies. The NIH global scoring system includes two components. First each organ system (skin, mouth eyes, GI tract, liver, lungs, joints and fascia and female genital tract) receives a score from 0 to 3 precisely described according to the severity of the effected organ. Second, the number of affected sites/organs is calculated and these together establish three categories (mild, moderate and severe) according to the score generated.

Mild cGvHD reflects the involvement of no more than 1 or 2 organs/sites (except for lung) with a maximum score of 1.

Moderate cGvHD involves at least 1 organ/site with a score of 2 or three or more organs/sites with a score of 1 (or lung score 8).

Severe cGvHD is diagnosed when a score of 3 is given to any organ (or score of 2 to lungs) (Table 9).

Table 8: Signs and symptoms of chronic graft-versus-host disease

Organ/Site	Diagnostic	Distinctive	Other features*	Common (both acute and chronic)
Skin	Poikiloderma Lichen planus-like features Sclerotic features	Depigmentation	Sweat impairment Hypopigmentation Hyperpigmentation	Erythema Maculopapular rash Pruritus
Nails		Dystrophy Longitudinal ridging splitting, or brittle features		
Scalp/hair		Alopecia	Premature gray hair	
Mouth	Lichen planus type features	Xerostomia		Mucositis
Eyes		Dry eyes Keratoconjunctivitis sicca	Photophobia Blepharitis	
Genitalia	Lichen planus type features	Erosions, fissures, ulcers		
Gastrointestinal tract	Esophageal web Stricture or stenosis of the esophagus		Exocrine pancreatic insufficiency	Nausea Vomiting Anorexia, weight loss
Liver				Bilirubin or alkaline phosphatase, ALT or AST >2 x upper limit of normal
Lung	Bronchiolitis obliterans			Bronchiolitis obliterans organising pneumonia (BOOP)
Muscles, fascia, joints	Fasciitis, joint stiffness secondary to sclerosis	Myositis Polymyositis	Oedema Muscle cramps Arthralgia, arthritis	
Haematopoietic and immune			Thrombocytopenia Eosinophilia Lymphopenia Hypo- or hyper-gammaglobulinemia Autoantibodies	
Other			Peripheral neuropathy Myasthenia gravis Ascites, pericardial or pleural effusion	

Can be considered the part of cGvHD symptomatology if the diagnosis is confirmed

Table 9: **NIH consensus for global grading of chronic graft-versus-host disease**			
Number of organs/sites	**Mild**	**Moderate**	**Severe**
1 site	Score 1	Score 2	Score 3
2 sites	Score 1	Score 2	Score 3
3 or more sites		Score 1	Score 3
Lung involvement		Score 1	Score 2

Besides the NIH Global Scoring Akpek et al. established a very simply applicable and useful cGvHD grading in 2001 for assessing prognosis. With the help of the following three risk factors (progressive onset of cGvHD, platelet count lower then 100,000 and more than 50% of body surface involvement of the skin) patients are divided into low risk (no risk factor) intermediate risk (1 or 2 risk factors) and high risk (3 risk factors) categories with significantly different probabilities of long term survival (over 80%, approximately 50%, and less than 20%) respectively (16). Recently, a much more detailed risk score has been proposed by the CIBMTR following a review of 5343 patients with cGvHD. Ten variables (age, prior acute GvHD, time from transplant to cGvHD, donor type, disease status at transplant, GvHD prophylaxis, gender mismatch, serum bilirubin, Karnofsky score and platelet count) were identified resulting in 6 risk groups with significantly different non-relapse mortality and overall survival. This may be a useful tool to precisely identify different risk category patients at the diagnosis of cGvHD and making appropriate decisions regarding further therapy and possible enrolment in clinical trials (17).

3.4 Epidemiology

cGvHD occurs in 40% of HLA identical sibling unmanipulated SCT, more than 50% of HLA- non-identical related SCT and in 70% of matched unrelated SCT. A study from Seattle showed that the higher the degree of HLA disparity, the earlier the onset of symptoms, with a median of 201 days in HLA identical siblings, and 133 days in matched unrelated donors transplanted with bone marrow and after standard conditioning (18). The most frequently involved sites of the clinical manifestations of 324 pts were the mouth (89%), skin (81%), gastrointestinal tract (48%), liver (47%), eyes (47%). The disease started with a quiescent onset (followed acute GvHD with a remission period) in 60%, with a progressive onset (cGvHD transformed from acute) in 13%, and with *de novo* onset (no prior acute GvHD) in 27% of the cases. Symptoms usually start no later than 3 years following transplant.

3.5 Treatment

Limited disease necessitates only local treatment, and this avoids further immunosuppression which might result in infectious complications and the other side effects of long term steroids. In the case of extensive disease systemic treatment is necessary and patience and appropriate evaluation of response is very important. Most patients require immunosuppressive treatment for up to 1 year, with more than half of them still on therapy after 2 years.

3.5.1 First line treatment
Standard first line systemic treatment is orally administered prednisolone 1 mg/kg and cyclosporin (CsA) 10 mg/kg with the dose of CSA adjusted to plasma levels. The corticosteroid component is the main part of the therapy while the addition of CsA had the advantage of less avascular necrosis in a prospective randomised study (19, 20). Attempts to add a third immune-suppressive drug (azathioprine, thalidomide or mycophenolate mofetil) to the standard initial treatment did not improve results and should be avoided (21, 22). Because of the significant morbiditiy caused by long-term steroid treatment the dose of prednisolone should be tapered according to response. In practice this usually starts 2 weeks after evidence of improvement of clinical manifestations. The tapering should be very slow with a typical approach starting with 0.25 mg/kg reduction on alternating days reaching no steroid on every second days by 2 months. Then after a 4 months interval an even slower taper may be initiated reaching steroid-free status by the end of the first year but still on CSA treatment (23).

Steroid-refractory cGvHD is defined as progression on prednisolone at 1 mg/kg/day for 2 weeks or stable disease on >0.5 mg/kg/day prednisolone for 4–8 weeks or an inability to taper prednisolone below 0.5 mg/kg/day.

3.5.2 Second line treatment
There is no standard salvage treatment of cGvHD. A large number of options have been tested in rather small phase II clinical trials with different enrolment and response criteria making their comparative evaluation difficult. Possibilities include mycofenolate mofetil, tacrolimus, rapamycin, rituximab, thalidomide, extracorporeal photopheresis, pulsed high dose steroids (10 mg/kg/day for 4 days), total lymphoid irradiation (1 Gy), alemtuzumab, pentostatin, revlimid, anti-IL-2 receptor Ab, anti-TNF receptor Ab, and recently tyrosine kinase (PDGFR, TGF-β) inhibitors such as imatinib, nilotinib, or dasatinib (Table 10) (24).

3.5.3 Ancillary treatment
As the primary cause of death of patients with cGvHD is infection, antimicrobial prophylaxis is of outstanding importance. Prevention from encapsulated bacteria, *Pneumocystis pneumonia*, CMV, *Varicella zoster*, and fungal infections should be

Table 10: Treatment of steroid-refractory chronic graft-versus-host disease

Agent	Side effects	Comments
High dose steroids	Osteoporosis, avascular necrosis, diabetes	Important but need to spare steroids because of side effect profile
Extracorporeal photopheresis (ECP)	Venous access required	Spares steroids, excellent safety profile
Sirolimus	Hyperlipidemia, rash, renal dysfunction, infections, thrombotic macroangiopathy (TMA)	Increased risk for TMA in combination with calcineurin inhibitors, lower efficacy in thrombocytopenia, requires frequent monitoring
Tacrolimus	Renal toxicity, hypertension	Spares steroids, should be avoided in renal impairment
Mycophenolate mofetil (MMF)	Nausea Diarrhoea Neutropenia	Increased risk of viral reactivation, spares steroids, GI toxicity may mimic GvHD clinically and histologically
Pentostatin	Cytopenias, infectious risk	Best results in children, caution in presence of impaired marrow function, long-term immunosuppression
MTX	Cytopenias	Best response in mucocutaneous cGvHD, spares steroids
Imatinib	Fluid retention	Best results in sclerotic skin lesions, potentially effective in mild and moderate bronchiolitis obliterans
Thalidomide	Neurotoxicity, sedation, constipation	May be used in concomitant relapse of multiple myeloma
Azathioprine	Cytopenias, infectious risk	Increased risk for oral malignancies
Retinoids	Skin toxicity, hyperlipidemia	Effective in sclerotic skin lesions
Anti-CD20	Infectious risk	Effective in autoantibody-mediated manifestations and cutaneous and musculoskeletal cGvHD
Anti-CD52	Infectious risk	Last choice

considered and adjusted to the actual immunosupressive status. Systemic therapy always should be accompanied with appropriate local treatment of the affected organs and sites accordingly (Table 11) (25).

Table 11: Ancillary therapy of chronic graft-versus-host disease

Organ system	Prevention/Treatment
Skin and appendages	Avoidance of sun exposure, topical emollients, steroids, antipruritic agents, topical antimicrobials
Mouth and oral cavity	Topical steroids and analgesics, tacrolimus ointment, cyclosporin/tacrolimus rinses, salivary stimulants (sugar-free gum)
Eyes	Artificial tears, ocular ointments, topical steroids, cyclosporin eye-drops, topical antimicrobials, punctal occlusion
Vulva and vagina	Avoid chemical irritants (eg. soap), clean genital area with warm water. Water-based lubricants, topical estrogens, tacrolimus ointment
GI tract and liver	Dietary modifications, enzyme supplementation for malabsorption, gastroesophageal reflux management, esophageal dilatation, ursodeoxycholic acid
Lungs	Inhaled steroids, bronchodilators, supplementary oxygen, pulmonary rehabilitation, lung transplantation in appropriate candidates
Haematopoietic	Haematopoietic growth factors, immunoglobulin for immune cytopenias
Musculoskeletal	Physical therapy, bisphosphonates for osteopenia and osteoporosis

4. Conclusion

Acute GvHD is a common complication of allo-HSCT and is a leading cause of early morbidity and mortality. First-line therapy is single agent methylprednisolone which is effective in 40–50% of cases. Second line treatment for steroid refractory disease is largely unsatisfactory and therefore major efforts are exerted to prevent the occurrence of aGvHD. The most effective method of prophylaxis is T-cell depletion but in good risk transplants is accompanied by an unacceptable level of infection and relapse of the original disease. The most frequently used regimen for aGvHD prevention remains methotrexate and a calcineurin inhibitor. Manipulation of cellular sub-populations with immunosuppressive properties are promising new strategies for both prevention and treatment.

Chronic GvHD is a common (30 to 70%) complication after allo-HSCT and is a leading cause of late morbidity and mortality. The standard treatment is steroid and a calcineurin inhibitor. Prolonged steroid use is required with fewer than 50% of patients discontinuing immunosuppression by 2 years. There is no standard salvage therapy for cGvHD. cGvHD and its treatment are associated with severe complications including infections, osteoporosis, hypertension, hyperglycemia, hyperlipidemia and renal insufficiency. Infections are the leading cause of death and antimicrobial prophylaxis is necessary. Careful management of complications require multidisciplinary treatment.

References

1. Flowers MED, Inamoto Y, Carpenter PA et al. Comparative analysis of risk factors for acute graft-versus-host disease and for chronic graft-versus-host disease according to National Institutes of Health consensus criteria. Blood 2011; 117: 3214-3219.
2. Penack O, Holler E, van den Brink MRM. Graft-versus-host disease: Regulation by microbe-associated molecules and innate immune receptors. Blood 2010; 115: 1865-1872.
3. Glucksberg H, Storb R, Fefer A et al. Clinical manifestations of graft-versus-host disease in human recipients of marrow from HL-A-matched sibling donors. Transplantation 1974; 18: 295-304.
4. Przepiorka D, Weisdorf D, Martin P et al. Consensus Conference on Acute GvHD Grading. Bone Marrow Transplant 1995; 15: 825-828.
5. Rowlings PA, Przepiorka D, Klein JP et al. IBMTR Severity Index for grading acute graft-versus-host disease: Retrospective comparison with Glucksberg grade. Br J Haematol 1997; 97: 855-864.
6. Nash RA, Antin JH, Karanes C et al. Phase 3 study comparing methotrexate and tacrolimus with methotrexate and cyclosporine for prophylaxis of acute graft-versus-host disease after marrow transplantation from unrelated donors. Blood 2000; 96: 2062-2068.
7. Ratanatharathorn V, Nash RA, Przepiorka D et al. Phase III study comparing methotrexate and tacrolimus (prograf, FK506) with methotrexate and cyclosporine for graft-versus-host disease prophylaxis after HLA-identical sibling bone marrow transplantation. Blood 1998; 92: 2303-2314.
8. Perez L, Anasetti C, Pidala J. Have we improved in preventing and treating acute graft-versus-host disease? Curr Opin Hematol 2011; 18: 408-413.
9. Alousi AM, Weisdorf DJ, Logan BR et al. Etanercept, mycophenolate, denileukin, or pentostatin plus corticosteroids for acute graft-versus-host disease: A randomized phase 2 trial from the Blood and Marrow Transplant Clinical Trials Network. Blood 2009; 114: 511-517.
10. Ringden O, Uzunel M, Rasmusson I et al. Mesenchymal stem cells for treatment of therapy-resistant graft-versus-host disease. Transplantation 2006; 81: 1390-1397.
11. LeBlanc K, Frassoni F, Ball L et al. Mesenchymal stem cells for treatment of steroid-resistant, severe, acute graft-versus-host disease: A phase II study. Lancet 2008; 371: 1579-1586.
12. Shimabukuro-Vornhagen A, Hallek MJ, Storb RF, Bergwelt-Baildon MS. The role of B cells in the pathogenesis of graft-versus-host disease. Blood 2009; 114: 4919-4927.
13. Carlens S, Ringden O, Remberger M et al. Risk factors for chronic graft-versus-host disease after bone marrow transplantation: A retrospective single centre analysis. Bone Marrow Transplant 1998; 22: 755-761.
14. Filipovich AH, Weisdorf D, Pavletic S et al. National Institutes of Health consensus development project on criteria for clinical trials in chronic graft-versus-host disease: I. Diagnosis and staging working group report. Biol Blood Marrow Transplant 2005; 11: 945-956.
15. Shulman HM, Sullivan KM, Weiden PL et al. Chronic graft versus host syndrome in man - A long-term clinicopathologic study of 20 Seattle patients. Am J Med 1980; 69: 204-217.

16. Akpek G, Zahurak ML, Piantadosi S et al. Development of a prognostic model for grading chronic graft-versus-host disease. Blood 2001; 97: 1219–1226.

17. Arora M, Klein JP, Weisdorf DJ et al. Chronic GVHD risk score: A Center for International Blood and Marrow Transplant Research analysis. Blood 2011; 117: 6714–6720.

18. Sullivan KM, Agura E, Anasetti C et al. Chronic graft-versus-host disease and other late complications of bone-marrow transplantation. Semin Hematol 1991; 28: 250–259.

19. Sullivan KM, Witherspoon RP, Storb R et al. Alternating-day cyclosporine and prednisone for treatment of high-risk chronic graft-v-host disease. Blood 1988; 72: 555–561.

20. Koc S, Leisenring W, Flowers MED et al. Therapy for chronic graft-versus-host disease: A randomized trial comparing cyclosporine plus prednisone versus prednisone alone. Blood 2002; 100: 48–51.

21. Arora M, Wagner JE, Davies SM et al. Randomized clinical trial of thalidomide, cyclosporine, and prednisone versus cyclosporine and prednisone as initial therapy for chronic graft-versus-host disease. Biol Blood Marrow Transplant 2001; 7: 265–273.

22. Martin PJ, Storer BE, Rowley SD et al. Evaluation of mycophenolate mofetil for initial treatment of chronic graft-versus-host disease. Blood 2009; 113: 5074–5082.

23. Flowers MED, Lee SE, Vogelsang AG. An update on how to treat chronic GVHD. Blood 2003; 102: 2312.

24. Wolff D, Schleuning M, von Harsdorf S et al. Consensus Conference on clinical practice in chronic GVHD: Second-line treatment of chronic graft-versus-host disease. Biol Blood Marrow Transplant 2011; 17: 1–17.

25. Couriel D, Carpenter PA, Cutler C et al. Ancillary therapy and supportive care of chronic graft-versus-host disease: National Institutes of Health Consensus Development Project on Criteria for Clinical Trials in Chronic Graft-versus-Host Disease: V. Ancillary Therapy and Supportive Care Working Group report. Biol Blood Marrow Transplant 2006; 12: 375–396.

Multiple Choice Questionnaire

To find the correct answer, go to http://www.esh.org/online-training/handbook/

1. **Which of the following statements is *untrue*?**
   a) The incidence and severity of GvHD increases with increasing HLA disparity .... ☐
   b) One of the prerequisites for the occurrence of GvHD is lack of immunocompetence in the patient .... ☐
   c) GvHD can only be diagnosed within the first 100 days of transplant ..... ☐
   d) Epithelial tissue damage is modulated through cytokines .... ☐

2. **Which of the following is *not* a feature of acute GvHD?**

a) Nausea..☐
b) Raised alkaline phosphatase..☐
c) Lichen planus ....☐
d) Bullae...☐

3. **Which of the following has *not* been reported as a risk factor for acute GvHD?**
   a) Older patient age ....☐
   b) The use of fludarabine in the conditioning regimen....................☐
   c) CMV seropositivity..☐
   d) Gender disparity between donor and recipient..........................☐

4. **Which of the following statements is *untrue*?**
   a) Keratoconjunctivitis sicca is a feature of chronic GvHD...............☐
   b) The most frequent cause of mortality in patients with chronic GvHD
      is infection ....☐
   c) Prior splenectomy is associated with an increased risk of chronic GvHD .☐
   d) The organ demonstrating the best response to imatinib is the mucosa...☐

5. **Which of the following features has *not* been used in a scoring system for chronic GvHD?**
   a) Thrombocytopenia...☐
   b) Number of organs involved ....☐
   c) Time from transplant to occurrence of acute GvHD......................☐
   d) Extent of skin involvement ....☐

* CHAPTER 14

Immune reconstitution after allogeneic HSCT

Antoine Toubert

1. Introduction

Allogeneic haematopoietic stem cell transplantation (allo-HSCT) is widely used in the treatment of haematological malignancies as a form of immunotherapy acting through a graft-versus-leukemia (GvL) reaction. This curative allogeneic response can be associated with severe drawbacks, such as frequent and severe graft-versus-host disease (GvHD). Another main concern is the profound and long-lasting immunodeficiency which follows this procedure, especially now with the development of innovative strategies such as umbilical cord blood transplantation (CBT) or transplants from haplo-identical family donors (haplo-HSCT). In the long-term follow-up of these patients, severe post-transplant infections, relapse or secondary malignancies may be directly related to persistent immune defects (1).

Reconstitution of the different lymphocyte populations (B, T, NK, NKT) and antigen presenting cells of myeloid origin (monocytes, macrophages and dendritic cells) should be considered not only quantitatively but especially qualitatively, in terms of functional subsets. Immune deficiency leading to an increased susceptibility to infections lasts for more than a year. The post-transplant period is subdivided in different phases in relation to the occurrence of infections (see Chapters 11, 12). Although infections that occur in the first month mostly result from a deficiency in both granulocytes and mononuclear cells (MNC), later post-engraftment infections are due to a deficiency in MNC subsets, primarily CD4 T-cells and B-cells. T-cell reconstitution has been extensively studied because of the central role of T-cells in mediating both GvHD, evidenced by the reduced incidence of this complication following T-cell depletion (TCD), and a GvL effect as shown by DLI (see Chapters 16, 17). In the recent years there has been renewed interest in the role of NK-cells, especially in the context of haplo-HSCT, and in B-cell reconstitution.

2. General considerations

New approaches have been developed during recent years to minimise the likelihood of graft failure, conditioning toxicity, GvHD, and infections (2). The addition of T-cell–depleting agents (e.g. antithymocyte globulin, ATG, or alemtuzumab [Campath®]) to conditioning regimens has been associated with a reduced incidence of GvHD and diminished risk of graft rejection but may delay immune reconstitution (IR). Non-myeloablative preparative regimens that use cytotoxic drugs or low-dose total body irradiation (TBI) in conditioning regimens have been associated with reduced non-relapse mortality and have provided new options for HSCT among the elderly and in patients with substantial co-morbidities. Although the degree of myelosuppression is milder following non-myeloablative regimens, the depth and extent of lymphodepletion tends to be similar, with prolonged periods of immune incompetence observed in recipients of both myeloablative and non-myeloablative regimens. This is because engraftment of allogeneic haematopoietic progenitor cells requires significant recipient immunosuppression to prevent graft rejection, even in the context of full HLA matching. With some regimens, virtually complete eradication of recipient lymphocytes is accomplished by the preparative regimen itself. However, with other regimens depletion of recipient lymphocytes occurs more gradually via the use of donor leucocyte infusions following transplant. In both cases, the vast majority of HSCT recipients experience near-total lymphocyte depletion, and thus must undergo lymphoid reconstitution via mature lymphocytes and lymphoid progenitors contained in the graft.

Many factors relating to the donor and/or the recipient can affect IR (Table 1). Reconstitution of the major lymphocyte subsets (T, B, NK) will be discussed separately for clarity, but IR has to be considered as a whole, each population being included in a global functional network with effector and regulatory properties. Finally, this re-view does not claim to be exhaustive. In particular, it will only indirectly cover the reconstitution of antigen-presenting cells of myeloid origin (monocytes, macro-phages, dendritic cells) and of "non-classical" lymphocyte populations (γδ T-cells, NKT-cells) where more knowledge is still needed about their roles in the physiology of the immune system.

Table 1: **Main factors affecting immune reconstitution (IR)**	
Host factors	Age, sex, conditioning regimen (myeloablative or not, use of lymphocyte-depleting antibodies such as ATG or Campath®). Initial pathology
Genetic differences	Degree of genetic differences between donor and recipient including HLA, minor histocompatibility Ag and genes associated with immune responses to microorganisms (see Chapter 5)
Source of HSC	Source of HSC: CB, BM, PBSC, haplo-identical HSCT. Transplant manipulation: TCD, double and multiple CBT, adoptive therapy with antigen-specific lines or clones (EBV, CMV)
Post-HSCT events	aGvHD and cGvHD, relapse and infectious complications (EBV or CMV viruses, fungal infections, toxoplasmosis). Effects of biotherapies (such as CD20-specific monoclonal antibodies)

3. T-cell reconstitution

3.1 Naive and memory T-cells
Memory T-cells are the first to expand after HSCT (Figure 1); they may be either of donor origin in the case of a non-TCD graft or, in the case of a TCD graft, originate

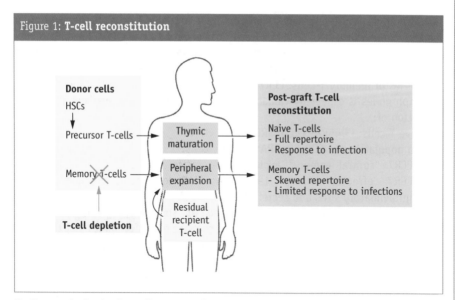

Figure 1: **T-cell reconstitution**

T-cell reconstitution involves a first wave, a thymic-independent pathway giving rise to memory T-cells and, in a longer and more sustainable way, a thymic-dependent pathway giving rise to naive T-cells (or recent thymic emigrants) with a broad repertoire and reactivity. The respective importance of these two pathways will depend on the graft (T-cell depletion, source) and the recipient (age, residual T-cells)

from host T-cells that have survived the conditioning regimen. They respond quickly to previously encountered pathogens, are easier to trigger, faster to respond and enter tissues more readily than naive T-cells. They are frequently directed towards periodically reactivated herpes viruses, CMV or EBV, which they keep under control. They constitute the majority of oligoclonal T-cell expansions found in healthy adults, especially in the CD8+ population.

In the long term, immune responses need the reconstitution of a naive T-cell repertoire able to respond to a broad range of pathogens encountered by the host and to tumour antigens. Reconstitution of this compartment is an ongoing process which requires a functional thymus for the recovery of a complete T-cell ontogeny. The thymus itself may be a target of the alloreactive immune attack with possible consequences on thymic selection, escape of self-reactive T-cell clones and perpetuation of GvHD, as will be discussed later.

3.2 The evaluation of naive and memory T-cell populations
The current immunological tests assess naive and memory lymphocyte populations:

CD45RO for memory T-cells and CD45RA or CD62L for naive T-cells are the most usual markers. However, memory CD45RO+ T-cells may revert to a naive CD45RA+ phenotype, especially in case of persistent infection with herpes viruses. Therefore, other markers should be added to definitely assess naive T-cells and the different categories of memory T-cells. CCR7, a molecule involved in the homing of T-cells to lymph nodes is especially valuable. A combination of these markers allows the definition of:

- Naive T-cells: CD45RA[high] CD45RO- CCR7+ CD28+
- Two populations of CD8+CD45RA- memory cells:
  - CCR7+ "central memory", expressing L-selectin (CD62L)
  - CCR7- "effector memory", L-selectin-, IL-2 dependent, which migrate to inflammatory sites and secrete IFN-γ.

Various approaches known as "immunoscope" or "spectratyping" may be used to evaluate T-cell diversity. They are based on the size diversity analysis of the CDR3 β-chain region as an index of the diversity of the whole $\alpha\beta$ T-cell population. Overall, early after HSCT (within 6 months post-transplant) many abnormalities of the T-cell repertoire are demonstrable, but these are difficult to correlate with the clinical status of the patient. Conversely, later after the graft (after 1 yr at least) and ongoing for at least 2 to 3 yrs post-transplant, it is possible to correlate repertoire dis-turbance with the occurrence of GvHD, severe infectious complications or relapse. T-cell repertoire reconstitution is delayed in case of TCD or in CD34+ purified grafts and is improved where there is full donor haematopoiesis. Techniques of TCR β-chain sequencing have clearly separated T-cell clones mediating GvHD and GvL and could be used in the future to monitor GvHD-causing clones in HSCT recipients.

3.3 The thymus is a critical organ in T-cell immune reconstitution after allo-HSCT

As we stated above, a *bona fide* T-cell reconstitution is dependent on the recapitula-tion of T-cell ontogeny from progenitors of donor origin in the recipient thymus. Lymphocyte leaving the thymus or "recent thymic emigrants" (RTE) can now be ev-aluated directly *ex vivo* by measuring the episomal DNA excision circles of the TCR δ locus deleted during recombination of the α locus present in the vast majority (>70%) of functional $\alpha\beta$ T-cells. This is the signal-joint T-cell receptor rearrangement excision DNA circles or "sjTREC" assay which is a totally non-invasive technique requiring only a small amount of blood and suitable for cohort follow-up (Figure 2). Excision circles are episomal DNA which are not replicated during cell division. sjTREC values reflect thymic output and should be calculated as copy numbers/CD3+ T-cell counts and as absolute numbers of sjTREC/mL of peripheral blood, which are directly proportional to the number of RTE. Thymic function based on sjTREC

Figure 2: *Ex-vivo* thymic function analysis

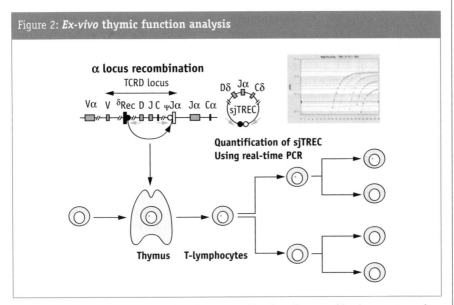

sjTREC are produced during TCR α-chain locus recombination. The recombination events produce episomal DNA fragments carried out of the thymus with recent T-cell emigrants when they exit the organ. They can be quantified by real-time PCR reaction directly from a blood sample

values in the recipient before allo-HSCT has been associated with a better clinical outcome (3).

The sjTREC assay as *ex vivo* markers of thymic function has been used in allo-HSCT monitoring by different groups showing that sjTREC levels are low until 3–6 months after allo-BMT. Low sjTREC values are associated with increasing patient age and T-cell depletion but also mainly with GvHD, leukaemia relapse or opportunistic infections (4, 5). As shown by different groups in different myeloablative and non-myeloablative conditioning, patients affected with chronic GvHD (cGVHD) have a very low and usually undectable thymic function. High sjTREC levels and a broad T-cell repertoire have been associated with an efficient immune reconstitution after CB transplantation in the long term (6). Interestingly, the level of recovery of thymopoiesis has been directly linked to CMV clearance and survival after double CBT (7). Experimental models in mice showed that the thymus is very sensitive to an allogeneic attack, notably through IFN-γ induced apoptosis of thymic epithelial cells (TEC) (8). We recently defined further some mechanisms of thymic impairement during acute GvHD (aGvHD) in an intrafamilial HLA-genoidentical HSCT setting in adults (5).

Acute GvHD delays the thymic dependent T lymphocyte recovery.
Although total T-cell number recovery was not significantly affected by the occurrence of aGvHD, the reconstitution of the CD4+ CD45RA+ CD62L+ naive compartment and the level of RTE assessed by sjTREC were significantly lower in patients with aGvHD at 6 and 12 months after graft.

Acute GvHD effect on thymic function is reversible in younger adult patients.
Age-related thymic involution begins with the increase in sex steroid levels seen at puberty. Therefore age could synergise with aGvHD to delay immune reconstitution after allo-HSCT in adults. Indeed, we observed that patients older than 25 years had the lowest sjTREC levels before transplantation and showed also a minimal recovery in presence or absence of aGvHD up to 1 year after graft. Recovery of sjTREC level was much more efficient in younger patients. aGvHD had a significant impact on thymic output at month 6 after HSCT but thereafter thymic function recovered, reaching pretransplant values at one year after graft. Therefore we concluded that in younger patients (<25 years of age), the thymic impact of an episode of aGvHD may be fully reversible. Conversely, cGvHD had a persistent effect on thymic function independently of the recipient's age.

3.4 How is the Ag-specific immune response reconstituted after allo-HSCT?
Naive T-cell reconstitution is a key issue for the long-term recovery of immune responses but memory T-cells are also needed for an efficient and timely response towards pathogens. Therefore, especially in some graft settings (TCD, CBT, HLA mismatch UD), adoptive immunotherapy can be used in an attempt to compensate for the lack of Ag-specific immunocompetent T-cells (2). In order to do this, it is necessary to evaluate patients at risk and to be able to monitor Ag-specific immune responses towards pathogens. Herpes viruses (CMV, EBV) are of primary importance in HSCT because reactivation of EBV can result in potentially fatal EBV-associated lymphoproliferative disease and because of the frequency of late CMV reactivation in the host even under pre-emptive therapy. It is possible:
- To monitor EBV and CMV-specific cytotoxic responses by Elispot functional assays or intracellular cytokine staining which are easier to perform than the conventional ^{51}Cr release cytotoxic assay in a routine laboratory.
- To use the tetramer technology to stain directly *ex vivo* CD8+ T-cells reactive with peptide/HLA complexes and to characterise these cells in terms of phenotype and function. This is a very sensitive method which can stain 1/5000 CD8+ T-cells (or $1/5 \times 10^4$ PBMC). It may also be used to isolate Ag-specific T-cells by cell sorting and to expand them *in vitro* (9). Although becoming more easily available, these techniques have not yet defined a consensus cut-off value which can predict future reactivations in the recipient.

4. NK-cell reconstitution

4.1 The haplo-HSCT KIR/ligand mismatch concept

NK-cells are lymphocytes that act early in the immune response against infection and tumour-transformed cells. Based on phenotyping (CD16 and CD56), they are the first lymphocyte subpopulation to be reconstituted in all graft settings, usually within 3 months.

The genetic organisation and function of NK receptors, either inhibitory or activating, has been unravelled in the past few years. NK-cell receptors are encoded by two structurally distinct families of molecules: the killer immunoglobulin-like receptors (KIR) and the lectin-like CD94:NKG2 heterodimers. Every NK-cell expresses at least one inhibitory receptor specific for autologous HLA class I, thereby ensuring self-tolerance. As KIR and HLA segregate independently and as unrelated individuals almost always have different KIR genotypes, we predict that approximately 25% of transplants between HLA-identical siblings involve KIR identity and approximately 75% KIR disparity. For transplantation with an HLA matched unrelated donor, the frequency of KIR incompatibility approaches 100%. In allo-HSCT, a GvL effect has been assigned to NK-cells of donor origin after a haplo-HSCT TCD transplant (10). Pertinently, the acute myeloid leukaemia relapse rate was dramatically lowered when an HLA ligand for an inhibitory KIR was present in the donor and absent in the recipient.

4.2 Reconstitution of NK-cell subsets and NK "education" or "licensing"

Different NK subsets are now more precisely defined and especially the CD56^{bright}CD16- and CD56^{dim}CD16+, respectively prone to cytokine production or cytotoxicity. The rapid recovery of NK-cells post-transplant is due to an expansion of CD56^{bright}CD16- (11). At the level of KIR and lectin-like NK receptors, expression level and function showed that CD94:NKG2A may be expressed earlier than KIR and that most patients reconstitute a donor-type NK repertoire depending on their KIR genotype.

Finally, the concept of NK-cell "education" or "licensing" has more recently emerged, which should be taken into account in the haplo-HSCT context. In mice and humans, some NK-cells did not express any inhibitory receptor for self HLA but nonetheless had impaired responsiveness. The emerging concept is that signals dependent on self-specific inhibitory receptors are required for the acquisition and/or maintenance of NK-cell responsiveness, in a process called "licensing" or "education". Data on NK-cell education after allogeneic HSCT are still scarce, controversial, and concern only KIR-ligand-matched HSCT at rather early time points. Yu et al. (12) showed results interpreted as breaking of NK-cell tolerance to self during the first 100 days after HSCT followed by a progressive functional education. Notwithstanding, Björklund et al. (13) showed that NKG2A-negative NK-cells expressing KIRs for non-self HLA ligands remain self-tolerant during the first 6 months after HLA-identical sibling HSCT. Haas et al. assessed long-term NK-cell education after KIR-ligand-matched or mismatched allo-HSCT and found that the NK-cell-education process is fully effective after HSCT and is dependent on donor ligands, since a donor-like education pattern ensued and persisted for at least 3 years post-HSCT (14). This means that NK-cells specific to a ligand present in the donor but absent in the recipient should remain responsive even long after transplant, and may therefore exert a long-term GvL effect.

5. B-cell reconstitution

This aspect of IR is gaining more interest now, in the light of advances in the knowledge of B-cell ontogeny and the availability of surface markers suitable to follow B-cell subsets in mice and humans. The major area of interest is cGvHD, which is clinically close in some aspects to autoimmunity (scleroderma or systemic lupus) and where autoantibodies or B-cell monoclonal expansions are frequently found.

5.1 Quantification of serum total IgG, IgM and IgA and of IgG subclasses

After a decline in the first several months after HSCT, levels of specific antibodies to protein Ag frequently encountered after transplantation (e.g. CMV) return to pre-transplantation levels within the first year. In contrast, antibodies to protein Ag that are unlikely to be encountered after HSCT (e.g. tetanus, measles, polio) continue to decline. This supports the recommendation of post-HSCT vaccination. Antibody levels in the first year are affected primarily by pre-HSCT antibody levels in the recipient. A persistent defect in IgA, especially in patients with cGvHD, explains mucosal infections of the respiratory and digestive tracts. IgG2 and IgG4 subclasses are also deficient in the case of GvHD, accounting for the increased susceptibility to infections, primarily those due to encapsulated bacteria (e.g. *Streptococcus pneumoniae* or *Haemophilus influenzae*). PBSC recipients do not have higher antibody levels than BM recipients.

5.2 Vaccinations

Vaccinations with inactivated or conjugated vaccines (see Chapter 12) should be initiated when CD4 and B-lymphocyte counts are sufficient (>200/μL) to expect efficacy, usually from 6 months post-transplant onwards.

5.3 B-lymphocyte phenotyping and physiopathology of cGvHD

Classical surface markers include B-lineage markers (CD19, CD20, CD21) and activation or differentiation markers (CD5, CD27). CD19+ B-cells normalise by one year after transplant. B-cell regeneration may be associated with transient appearance of monoclonal B-cell expansions. Low total B-cell counts are associated with high infection rates and cGvHD (15). Surface phenotypic markers may help to define functional B-cell subsets: CD27 is considered a marker of memory B-cells, CD21^{low}CD10^{high} belong to the so-called "transitional" B-cell compartment. This is actually a heterogeneous population, some transitional B-cells expressing the B-cell activation factor (BAFF) receptor. Based on several recent publications (16), the emerging picture of B-cell abnormalities in cGvHD is the following: increased BAFF serum level and delay in naïve B-cells with a relatively increase in BAFF/B-cells ratio. This would favour the emergence of autoreactive B-cells. Interestingly, naïve B-cell recovery and a decrease in BAFF/B-cell ratio has been associated with clinical response after rituximab therapy (16). The role played by "immature" or "transitional" B-cells in cGvHD will still need further assessment based on phenotypic and molecular analysis.

6. From monitoring to immune intervention

The combination of these innovative approaches (comprehensive phenotyping, TREC for thymic function, Elispot, tetramer staining) should enable more precise immune monitoring of patients at risk of relapse or persistent severe infectious complications. The objective would to be able to tailor individual follow-up according to guidelines (1) in a so-called "personalised medicine" approach.

The tetramer approach has direct benefits for the identification of patients with impaired CD8+ specific cytotoxic responses who may be eligible for cellular adoptive immunotherapy against CMV or for CD20-specific MoAb treatment (rituximab) to prevent post-HSCT lymphoproliferative disorder during EBV reactivation. The transfer of virus-specific CTL is possible with tetramer-sorted CTL without culture (9).

Based on experimental models, other attempts could be pursued to improve immune reconstitution and graft outcome:

- Improve thymic function recovery, by growth factors such as KGF, Flt3l or androgen blockade, or in vitro expansion of early thymic progenitors (17).
- Genetic modification of T lymphocytes, with a TK suicide gene to control GvHD (18).
- Haploidentical NK immunotherapy based on the KIR/ligand mismatch concept (10).
- Immune modulation through alternative stem cell sources such as mesenchymal stem cells or "regulatory" dendritic cells (see Chapter 23).
- Manipulation of immune system homeostasis to facilitate the emergence of regulatory CD4+CD25^{high} T-cells (or T_{reg}) which have been shown in animal models to control GvHD without impairing GvL (19). In humans, T_{regs} could be

expanded *in vitro* and keep their functional properties. Pilot studies in haplo-HSCT have been recently reported with encouraging results (20).
Key Points relating to immune reconstitution are shown below.

Key Points

Immune reconstitution is not only a matter of numbers: T, B and NK-lymphocytes have to be evaluated at the level of functional subsets

T-cell reconstitution involves 2 different pathways:
- Thymic independent: cytokine driven (IL-7, IL-15) expansion of CD4 and CD8 memory T-cells, mostly with herpes virus reactivity (CMV, EBV) reactivity
- Thymic dependent: generation of recent T-cell emigrants, naive T-cells with a broad repertoire and reactivity. Long process (>1 year) dependent on recipient age and HSCT outcome (GvHD)

NK-cells: rapid reconstitution (<6 months) with expansion of the NK CD56[bright] subset endowed with cytokine production

B-cells: slow process (6 months-1 year), affected by GvHD. B-cell defects may be linked to late mucosal infection

Acknowledgements
This work was supported by research grants from the Cancéropôle Ile-de-France, AP-HP grant "Recherche Clinique Translationnelle 2010", EC programs EURO-BANK, EUROCORD and FP6 ALLOSTEM (#503319).

References

1. Mackall C, Fry T, Gress R et al. Background to hematopoietic cell transplantation, including post transplant immune recovery. Bone Marrow Transplant 2009; 44: 457–462.
2. Seggewiss R, Einsele H. Immune reconstitution after allogeneic transplantation and expanding options for immunomodulation: An update. Blood 2010; 13: 3861–3868.
3. Clave E, Rocha V, Talvensaari K et al. Prognostic value of pretransplantation host thymic function in HLA-identical sibling hematopoietic stem cell transplantation. Blood 2005; 105: 2608–2613.
4. Weinberg K, Blazar BR, Wagner JE et al. Factors affecting thymic function after allogeneic hematopoietic stem cell transplantation. Blood 2001; 97: 1458–1466.
5. Clave E, Busson M, Douay C et al. Acute graft-versus-host disease transiently impairs thymic output in young patients after allogeneic hematopoietic stem cell transplantation. Blood 2009; 113: 6477–6484.

6. Talvensaari K, Clave E, Douay C et al. A broad T-cell repertoire diversity and an efficient thymic function indicate a favorable long-term immune reconstitution after cord blood stem cell transplantation. Blood 2002; 99: 1458–1464.
7. Brown JA, Stevenson K, Kim HT et al. Clearance of CMV viremia and survival after double umbilical cord blood transplantation in adults depends on reconstitution of thymopoiesis. Blood 2010; 115: 4111–4119.
8. Hauri-Hohl MM, Keller MP, Gill J et al. Donor T-cell alloreactivity against host thymic epithelium limits T-cell development after bone marrow transplantation. Blood 2007; 109: 4080–4088.
9. Cobbold M, Khan N, Pourgheysari B et al. Adoptive transfer of cytomegalovirus-specific CTL to stem cell transplant patients after selection by HLA-peptide tetramers. J Exp Med 2005; 202: 379–386.
10. Ruggeri L, Capanni M, Urbani E et al. Effectiveness of donor natural killer cell alloreactivity in mismatched hematopoietic transplants. Science 2002; 295: 2097–2100.
11. Dulphy N, Haas P, Busson M et al. An unusual CD56^{bright}CD16^{low} NK cell sub-set dominates the early posttransplant period following HLA-matched hematopoietic stem cell transplantation. J Immunol 2008; 181: 2227–2237.
12. Yu J, Venstrom JM, Liu XR et al. Breaking tolerance to self, circulating natural killer cells expressing inhibitory KIR for non-self HLA exhibit effector function fol-lowing T-cell depleted allogeneic hematopoietic cell transplantation. Blood 2009; 113: 3875–3884.
13. Björklund AT, Schaffer M, Fauriat C et al. NK cells expressing inhibitory KIR for non-self ligands remain tolerant in HLA-matched sibling stem cell transplantation. Blood 2010; 116: 3853–3864.
14. Haas P, Loiseau P, Tamouza R et al. NK-cell education is shaped by donor HLA genotype after unrelated allogeneic hematopoietic stem-cell transplantation. Blood 2011; 173: 1021–1029.
15. Corre E, Carmagnat M, Busson M et al. Long-term immune deficiency after allogeneic stem cell transplantation: B cell deficiency is associated with late infec-tions. Haematologica 2010; 95: 1025–1029.
16. Sarantopoulos S, Stevenson KT, Kim HT et al. Recovery of B-cell homeostasis after rituximab in chronic graft versus host disease (cGVHD). Blood 2011; 117: 2265–2274.
17. Zakrzewski JL, Kochman AA, Lu SX et al. Adoptive transfer of T-cell precursors enhances T-cell reconstitution after allogeneic hematopoietic stem cell trans-plantation. Nature Med 2006; 12: 1039–1047.
18. Bondanza A, Valtolina V, Magnani Z et al. Suicide gene therapy of graft-versus-host disease induced by central memory human T lymphocytes. Blood 2006; 107: 1828–1836.
19. Edinger M, Hoffmann P, Ermann J et al. CD4+ CD25+ regulatory T cells pre-serve graft-versus-tumor activity while inhibiting graft-versus-host disease after bone marrow transplantation. Nature Med 2003; 9: 1144–1150.
20. Di Ianni M, Falzetti F, Carotti A et al. Tregs prevent GVHD and promote immune reconstitution in HLA-haploidentical transplantation. Blood 2011; 117: 3921–3928.

Multiple Choice Questionnaire

To find the correct answer, go to http://www.esh.org/online-training/handbook/

1. **After allo-HSCT the earliest lymphocyte population to recover is:**
   a) NK-lymphocytes. ☐
   b) T CD4+ naïve T-cells. ☐
   c) T CD8+ memory T-cells ☐
   d) All recover at the same time. ☐

2. **Among the following lymphocyte phenotypic markers, which is the most precise to define memory T-cells:**
   a) CD45 RA+ ☐
   b) CD45RO+ CCR7⁻ ☐
   c) CD45RA+ CCR7+ ☐
   d) CD16+ CD56+ ☐

3. **Which is the main factor directly affecting thymic recovery after allo-HSCT?**
   a) Sex mismatch ☐
   b) CMV infection ☐
   c) HLA mismatch ☐
   d) GvHD ☐

4. **After allogeneic HSCT, the risk of EBV-induced proliferative disease (PTLD) is especially increased in which one of the following situations:**
   a) T-cell depletion ☐
   b) Genoidentical sibling donor ☐
   c) Sex-mismatch between donor and recipient ☐
   d) Aplastic anaemia as primary disease ☐

5. **Among the following lymphocyte phenotypic marker(s), which is the most precise to define naïve T-cells:**
   a) CD45RA+ ☐

b) CD45RO+ CCR7⁻ .... ☐
c) CD45RA+ CCR7+ .... ☐
d) CD16+ CD56+ .... ☐

* **CHAPTER 15**

Late effects in patients treated with HSCT

André Tichelli, Gérard Socié
on behalf of the Late Effects Working Party of the EBMT,
with the contribution from Alicia Rovó, Jakob Passweg,
Carl Philippe Schwarze, Maria Teresa Van Lint, Mutlu Arat

1. Introduction

With increasing number of transplants performed yearly, and improvement in outcome, long-term survivorship of patients treated with HSCT has become increasingly important. The main aim of the HSCT is still to cure the primary disease. However, long-term survivors expect to return to normal health, with adequate physical and psychological functioning and social integration in the family and at work, as well as subjective well-being. Despite improvement in the results of HSCT, the proportion of patients surviving two years after HSCT is decreased when compared to a matched general population, and after allogeneic HSCT death rate remains higher than expected even more than 20 years after transplantation. This higher death rate is necessarily associated with increased morbidity.

2. General aspects of long-term survivorship

The likelihood of long-term survivorship depends on the patient's characteristics (age, gender, comorbidity before HSCT), the primary disease, its risk category and remission status before transplantation, the conditioning regimen (MAC, RIC, use of TBI), the cell source (bone marrow, mobilised peripheral stem cells, umbilical stem cells), as well as the onset of GvHD and the drugs used for its treatment in patients receiving allogeneic HSCT (1, 2).

The pattern of late effects after HSCT may change over time. One reason is the change in practice regarding the conditioning regimen and the transplant procedure. While TBI was universally used for more than two decades, today non-irradiation protocols and RIC conditioning regimens have become established. Therefore, cataract, which was an almost universal late complication after HSCT, has been decreasing in frequency over the last decade. On the other hand, the increasing age of the patients receiving allogeneic HSCT, as well as more frequent use of an alternative donor, has led to an increased incidence of late effects related to chronic GvHD and its treatment. Accordingly, the incidence of late avascular necrosis of the bone and chronic kidney disease may increase. Although TBI may no longer form part of standard condition regimens, the knowledge of its late consequences is mandatory, because patients who received TBI many years ago remain at risk of radiation-related late effects. Indeed, some radiation-related late effects, such as non-squamous solid tumours or cardiovascular complications are very late effects appearing more than 10 or even 20 years after HSCT, and will therefore continue increasing during the next decades.

Late effects may be the direct consequences of the transplantation procedure and its conditioning regimen. Typical examples are cataract formation, infertility or secondary malignancies. It has also become apparent that there may be secondary late effects, occurring as the consequence of a primary late effect or its treatment. Osteoporosis and dental caries are such secondary late effects, while post-transplant osteoporosis is in part the consequence of gonadal failure occurring after TBI and may also result from steroid treatment of chronic GvHD. Likewise, dental caries occur in patients with decreased salivary flow, due to conditioning with TBI and/or chronic GvHD. Cardiovascular events after HSCT have emerged as very late effects, and can be considered as tertiary late effects, due to the increased incidence of cardiovascular risk factors appearing after HSCT (secondary late effects), which are in turn the consequence of primary late effects, such as gonadal insufficiency, insulin resistance and/or growth hormone deficiency after HSCT.

Late effects are defined as those that occur after the first three months post-transplant and provoke health restriction during long-term survivorship. They are usually divided into non-malignant and malignant late effects. In fact, any organ and any tissue can be the target of a late effect. The chapter will focus on practical screening and management issues of non-malignant and malignant late effects (3, 4). Each of the main late effects will be discussed systematically in four parts: 1. scientific background and risk factors, 2. clinical presentation and diagnosis, 3. prevention, 4. treatment.

3. Late ocular effects

There are two main non-malignant late effects, cataracts and kerato-conjunctivitis.

3.1 Scientific background and risk factors

Cataracts are closely related to TBI and to a lesser extent to the use of steroids. With single dose irradiation of ≥10 Gy the probability of cataract is up to 80% or more. Fractionation of the dose and lower dose rate greatly reduced the risk of cataract to 30% at 3 years. With a conditioning regimen of cyclophosphamide alone or busulfan and cyclophosphamide the risk is about 20% at 5 years.

Kerato-conjuctivitis sicca syndrome is part of a global sicca syndrome affecting ocular, oral, anal and genital mucosa. These manifestations are closely related to chronic GvHD, which may lead in its most extensive form to a Sjögren-like syndrome. The cumulative incidence of late-onset kerato-conjunctivitis sicca syndrome is 20% by fifteen years after HSCT. It reaches nearly 40% in patient with chronic GvHD, but is less than 10% in those without GvHD.

3.2 Clinical presentation and diagnosis

Cataracts usually develop gradually, and are painless. Symptoms include decrease in vision, particularly in bright or low light, as well as decreased contrast, and altered colour appreciation. The diagnosis is made by slit lamp examination.

The ocular manifestations of kerato-conjuctivitis sicca syndrome include reduced tear flow, dryness and irritation of the eyes, sterile conjunctivitis, corneal epithelial defects, and corneal ulceration. The diagnosis can be confirmed by Schirmer's test.

3.3 Prevention

The risk of cataracts can be greatly reduced by the use of a non-radiation conditioning regimen, or by fractionation of the TBI, as well as by reduced use of steroids.

General hygiene measures help to prevent superinfection in kerato-conjunctivitis sicca syndrome.

3.4 Treatment

The only treatment for cataract is to surgically remove the opacified lens from the eye to restore transparency of the visual axis. Today, cataract surgery is a low risk procedure and improves visual acuity in 95% of eyes that have no other pathology. The treatment of isolated kerato-conjunctivitis of the eye is based on the management of chronic GvHD with regular use of topical lubricants. Virus or bacterial infections have to be treated promptly and adequately. If the ocular manifestation is part of an extensive chronic GvHD, systemic treatment must be instituted.

4. Skin and appendages

Non-malignant late effects may involve skin, nails, and hair.

4.1. Scientific background and risk factors

Sustained involvement of the skin, including mucosal and skin appendages (nails and hair) is common after allogeneic HSCT and is most often related to chronic GvHD. Persistent cutaneous lesions play a central role in late morbidity and quality of life in long-term survivors. Cutaneous GvHD can develop spontaneously, or can be triggered by events such as UV irradiation, physical trauma, or infections.

4.2 Clinical presentation and diagnosis

Dryness of the skin is a frequent early manifestation of chronic GvHD. Chronic cutaneous GvHD may present as lichenoid or sclerodermoid GvHD. In the lichenoid form, the skin is usually intact and presents as dry skin, pruritus, rash, dyspigmentation, or a lichen planus-like eruption. Chronic sclerodermoid GvHD can lead to more disabling skin complications with ulcerated areas, which are prone to superinfections, and sclerotic changes of the subcutaneous tissues. In advanced cases sclerosis provokes functional impairment with severe joint contractures. Nail dystrophy, longitudinal ridging, nail splitting or nail loss are distinctive signs of chronic GvHD. Scalp alopecia, loss of body hair, and premature greying are all characteristics of chronic GvHD, but these findings are not diagnostic. The diagnosis of cutaneous chronic GvHD is usually based on clinical examination. Histological examination may support the diagnosis.

4.3 Prevention
Patients should be encouraged to reduce direct UV skin exposure. Photoprotection including protective clothing and high-potency sun-screen should be used and direct-exposure to sunlight should be avoided.

4.4 Treatment
Limited lichenoid GvHD lesions may respond to topical corticosteroids and calcineurin inhibitors as well as to phototherapy. Systemic immunosuppressive treatment is necessary in case of more advanced disease. In addition to the immunosuppressive treatment, early physiotherapy with stretching becomes essential, in order to prevent contractures and to improve range of motion.

5. Oral and dental complications
There are a number of non-malignant late effects of the oral cavity, including dental complications.

5.1 Scientific background and risk factors
Late oral complications are strongly associated with chronic GvHD and conditioning with TBI. They are characterised by mucosal atrophy, erythema, lichenoid-hyperkeratinoid lesions, salivary gland dysfunction, taste disorders, and dental complications. Late sclerotic changes may result in decreased oral opening. Saliva plays a major role in maintaining oral health. Abnormal salivary composition and reduced salivary flow can be the consequence of TBI and/or chronic GvHD. In long-term survivors, salivary gland dysfunction is associated with an increased risk of rampant dental decay. Poor oral hygiene associated with oral discomfort is an additional contributing factor.

5.2 Clinical presentation and diagnosis
The symptoms most often reported are pain, sensitivity to normally tolerated items, and xerostomia. Secondary oral infections, such as candidiasis, herpes simplex and cytomegalovirus can complicate and exacerbate oral lesions. Painful

mucosal ulcers hinder normal food ingestion. Rampant dental decay may occur in patients with sicca syndrome, poor dental hygiene and large-scale consumption of sugar-containing food or drinks.

5.3 Prevention
Maintaining oral and dental health is critical. Basic oral care include brushing of teeth with a soft toothbrush twice a day, the use of fluoride-containing toothpaste, daily flossing between teeth and under any bridges, the use of remineralising solutions, and avoidance of regular sugar-containing beverages.

5.4 Treatment
Topical corticosteroids such as budesonide mouthwash may be used as adjunctive therapy for oral GvHD. Systemic treatment of chronic GvHD is usually required. Regular dental review is important.

6. Thyroid dysfunction
Endocrine dysfunction is a frequent non-malignant late effect on the thyroid gland (5).

6.1 Scientific background and risk factors
Thyroid dysfunction is frequent, appearing within the first 2 to 3 years after HSCT. TBI plays a key role, and the risk of thyroid dysfunction depends on the dose and type of irradiation. The risk is 5–6 time higher when single dose instead of fractionated TBI is applied. The incidence after conditioning with busulfan and cyclophosphamide is 11%. The median time to diagnosis of hypothyroidism is about 4 years after HSCT.

6.2 Clinical presentation and diagnosis
Asymptomatic compensated hypothyroidism with increased TSH and normal fT4 levels is the most common form of thyroid dysfunction. In some patients these will normalise spontaneously. Overt hypothyroidism is variable and depends on the risk factors to which the patient has been exposed. Autoimmune diseases such as Hashimoto's thyroiditis and Graves' disease due to adoptive transfer or chronic GvHD have been reported. Yearly screening of TSH is indicated in patients at risk for thyroid dysfunction (previous radiation therapy of the neck, TBI), or if relevant symptoms develop.

6.3 Prevention
The use of a non-TBI conditioning regimen is the only preventive measure.

6.4 Treatment

Patients with overt hypothyroidism should receive hormonal substitution. Periodic adjustment of the dose, based on thyroid assessment, should be done with the help of an endocrinologist. Treatment of asymptomatic hypothyroidism remains controversial, but should be considered if TSH levels remain high or increase.

7. Fertility and gonadal dysfunction

Non-malignant late effects due to gonadal damage include endocrine dysfunction and infertility (6, 7).

7.1 Scientific background and risk factors

Gonadal damage after HSCT is dependent on the age of the patient, the dose and schedule of TBI, and the use of chemotherapy. Ovaries are more vulnerable than testes. In female patients, infertility and hyper gonadotropic hypogonadism is almost universal after TBI, with elevated serum FSH and LH. Fractionation of TBI has a sparing effect on the ovaries. Busulfan is one of the most gonadotoxic chemotherapeutic agents. In contrast, conditioning with cyclophosphamide alone is associated with a high probability of recovery of gonadal function and fertility. The age at transplantation is of major significance: the younger the age, the better the chances for gonadal recovery.

In male recipients, endocrine dysfunction of the testis is less pronounced. Testosterone levels are usually normal, since the Leydig cells are more resistant to chemotherapy and irradiation than the Sertoli cells. Usually serum FSH levels are increased, but with normal LH levels. The absence of spermatozoa is a common long-term sequel in male patients receiving chemotherapy and irradiation prior to HSCT. Azoospermia is less frequent in patients conditioned with busulfan and cyclophosphamide (50%) and is uncommon in patients treated with cyclophosphamide alone (10%). Even when conditioned with standard dose TBI, male recipients surviving more than 10 years, younger than 25 years at HSCT, and without chronic GvHD have a reasonable likelihood of spermatogenesis.

7.2 Clinical presentation and diagnosis

In young adult women gonadal dysfunction leads to a premature menopausal state after HSCT with menopausal symptoms. Untreated gonadal failure can in long-term survivors lead to secondary late complications, such as osteoporosis and metabolic syndrome. Male HSCT recipients are usually asymptomatic. Symptoms suggestive of hypogonadism are erectile dysfunction, low libido and bone loss. Females in whom hormonal substitution is discontinued should be assessed regularly for FSH and LH.

7.3 Prevention

The impact of treatment on fertility and symptoms due to gonadal failure must be discussed with patients before HSCT and repeatedly throughout the treatment period after HSCT. In young women healthcare providers should provide menopause-related symptoms and management of menopausal issues. Consideration should be given to sperm or embryo preservation before HSCT. Paradoxically, the potential recovery of spermatogenesis should also alert staff about the need for counseling regarding birth control during post-transplantation follow-up.

7.4 Treatment

The main reason to treat hypogonadism after transplantation is the prevention of osteoporosis and prevention of symptoms in pre-menopausal-aged women. Up to 90% of adult female patients require sex-hormone replacement therapy after HSCT. This replacement therapy can be interrupted every 1-2 years to evaluate spontaneous recovery. Sex-hormone replacement will not be necessary in most of the male patients, despite reduced or absent spermatogenesis.

8. Noninfectious respiratory tract complications

Non-malignant late effects of the lung (8) include obstructive and restrictive problems.

8.1 Scientific background and risk factors

Late-onset non-infectious pulmonary complications involving both the airway and lung parenchyma are frequent after HSCT, appearing usually between 3 months and 2 years post-transplant; however, functional consequences may persist for years. The most common delayed pulmonary complications include bronchiolitis obliterans (BO), cryptogenic organising pneumonia (COP), and idiopathic pneumonia syndrome (IPS). BO is a severe obstructive pulmonary manifestation characterised by a nonspecific inflammatory injury affecting primarily the small airways. In advanced stages, due to the progressive peri-bronchiolar fibrosis, restrictive functional changes also develop. BO is considered as the main pulmonary manifestation of chronic GvHD. COP is a clinico-pathological syndrome involving bronchioles, alveolar ducts, and alveoli and presents as a restrictive respiratory complication. COP appears mainly between 1 and 12 months post transplant, with an incidence of <2%. There is a strong association between COP and GvHD. IPS usually occurs within 120 days after transplantation and is associated with TBI, GvHD, and older age at HSCT. Patients conditioned with busulfan and cyclophosphamide have lower rates of IPS. Delayed-onset IPS occurring years after HSCT has been reported.

8.2 Clinical presentation and diagnosis

The clinical presentation of BO is usually insidious with dry cough, progressive dyspnea, and wheezing. In pulmonary function tests, a decline of >20% in FEV1 from the pre-transplant value, or <80% of the predicted FEV1 should alert transplant physicians. High resolution CT of the chest with inspiratory and expiratory phase images shows a characteristic mosaic pattern. The clinical presentation of COP is usually acute, with dry cough, dyspnea and fever. The chest X-ray presents peripheral patchy consolidation, ground glass attenuation and nodular opacities. Pulmonary function tests show a restrictive pattern. Bronchoalveolar lavage is recommended to rule out infection. The definitive diagnosis is based on histopathology. Regular pulmonary function tests should be performed regularly after allogeneic HSCT. If a decrease of the function tests is observed, further evaluation is warranted. IPS presents with pulmonary function tests showing a restrictive pattern. High resolution computed tomography shows a diffuse pulmonary parenchymal disease.

8.3 Prevention

Avoidance of smoking tobacco should be recommended for all patients.

8.4 Treatment

For the treatment of BO and COP corticosteroids should be started without delay. Other treatment for chronic GvHD may be required. Prophylaxis for VZV and PCP should be continued. Bacterial and fungal infections have to be treated appropriately. There is no specific treatment for IPS.

9. Late cardiac complications

Non-malignant late effects of the heart may lead to heart failure (9, 10).

9.1 Scientific background and risk factors

Experiences of cancer survivorship in the non-transplant setting may anticipate the magnitude of risk in patients treated with HSCT. In long-term survivors with Hodgkin's lymphoma, the risk of cardiac failure is 3 to 5 times increased compared to an age-matched general population. Pre-transplant anthracycline exposure and the presence of post-transplant comorbidities are the main risk factors for late cardiac failure after HSCT. Conditioning-related chemotherapy does not contribute significantly to late cardiac complications.

9.2 Clinical presentation and diagnosis

Dyspnea on exertion is the most common presenting symptom, followed by fatigue, orthopnea and weight gain. Routine cardiac surveillance and screening may be of limited value. However, patients at risk, and those with symptoms should be monitored clinically. ECG should be performed and extended cardiac investigation including echocardiogram should be discussed with a cardiologist.

9.3 Prevention
Cardiac disease occurs 10 years or later after treatment. This means that these effects are slow to develop, and may be partially prevented with the control of other cardiovascular risk factors, including arterial hypertension. Endocarditis prophylaxis in patients with valvular anomaly is recommended.

9.4 Treatment
Heart failure should be managed as for non-transplant patients.

10. Late vascular complications
Non-malignant vascular late effects include cerebrovascular and cardiovascular disease (11, 12).

10.1 Scientific background and risk factors
The cumulative incidence of an arterial event, such as cerebrovascular, coronary artery or peripheral arterial disease is 22% at 25 years after allogeneic HSCT. It is higher after allogeneic than after autologous HSCT, supporting the hypothesis that the alloreactive transplant is involved in the atherosclerotic process. The established cardiovascular risk factors appearing after HSCT (hypertension, dyslipidemia, diabetes, smoking, physical inactivity) are the main risk for a premature late cardiovascular complication post-transplant.

10.2 Clinical presentation and diagnosis
The clinic manifestations of late cardiovascular complications after HSCT are similar to those observed in a general population. However, the events may occur at an earlier age that expected. Cerebrovascular disease may present as transient ischaemic attack, stroke or symptoms related to lacunar infarcts of the brain. Clinical manifestations of coronary artery disease are angina pectoris, myocardial infarction, and symptoms due to chronic coronary heart disease. Patients with peripheral arterial disease can present with claudication, rest pains, acute ischemia or gangrene. Silent myocardial infarction is not uncommon, due to the possible damage of the autonomous nervous system.

10.3 Prevention
Control of cardiovascular risk factors is the main focus of preventive measures, and

starts with education and counseling for a heart-healthy lifestyle. Patients should be encouraged to undertake regular physical activity, stop smoking tobacco, avoid passive smoking and maintain a healthy body weight. Proper management of cardiovascular risk factors should be started early during follow-up, and not be postponed until the patient is off immunosuppression.

10.4 Treatment
Cardiovascular symptoms should undergo appropriate investigation and early treatment as for non-transplanted patients.

11. The metabolic syndrome in long-term survivors
Non-malignant late effects occurring in long-term survivors after HSCT include hypertension, dyslipidemia, and diabetes (13). As previously discussed, these predispose to vascular complications.

11.1 Scientific background and risk factors
Dyslipidaemia, hypertension, and diabetes occurring after HSCT and also physical inactivity and ongoing smoking are related to the increased risk of cardiovascular disease in long-term survivors. Two or more cardiovascular risk factors are associated with a more than 5-fold increase of late cardiovascular complications. Retrospective studies have reported a prevalence of diabetes mellitus to be between 7 and 13% after allogeneic HSCT. The prevalence of dyslipidaemia is even higher, ranging between 9 and 39%. The reason for the high prevalence after allogeneic HSCT is not yet well understood. It could be the consequence of prolonged and intensified immunosuppressive treatment, post-transplant, endocrine dysfunction or leptin resistance. However, the use of immunosuppressive treatment cannot explain alone the increase of these risk factors after allogeneic HSCT, since it is observed even in patients off immunosuppressive treatment.

11.2 Clinical presentation and diagnosis
Patients with abnormal cardiovascular risk factors are usually asymptomatic until a late cardiovascular complication occurs. Therefore, regular screening for cardiovascular risk factors should be included for all patients. Checking blood pressure at every clinic visit and measuring of fasting blood sugar and lipid profile at the yearly assessment are recommended. Efficacy of the treatment for a cardiovascular risk factor should be monitored adequately. Cardiovascular risk factors and particularly dyslipidaemia are undiagnosed and undertreated in long-term survivors. Treatment for cardiovascular risk factors should not be postponed until discontinuation of immunosuppressive treatment.

THE EBMT HANDBOOK 2012 EDITION

11.3 Prevention
Counseling for a heart-healthy life style (stop smoking; regular exercise; maintaining healthy weight; dietary counseling) to prevent cardiovascular risk factors has become an essential part of the long-term management. Patients should be encouraged to reduce modifiable risk factors such as obesity, to perform aerobic exercise, and to eat a well-balanced diet.

11.4 Treatment
Management should focus on controlling dysplipidaemia, diabetes and hypertension. Proper management of risk cardiovascular factors reduces the risk of a cardiovascular event and improves survival in a non-HSCT population, and will probably reduce morbidity and mortality in long-term survivors after HSCT. For the management of dyslipidaemia, ATP III guidelines (Adult treatment Panel III from the National Cholesterol Education Program, NCEP) should be applied. Patients with increased LDL-cholesterol and risk for cardiovascular disease should be treated with statins. Patients with elevated triglycerides should be treated appropriately.

12. Chronic kidney disease
A number of factors may lead to progressive loss of renal function and ultimately to end-stage renal disease (14).

12.1 Scientific background and risk factors
Chronic kidney disease is defined as a sustained decrease in glomerular filtration rate (GFR) below 60 mL/min/1.73 m^2. Among 1190 long-term adult patients who underwent HSCT and survived for ≥1 year, the estimated cumulative incidence of chronic kidney disease was 4.4% at 5 years, and 5.7% at 10 years after HSCT. Older age at transplantation, exposure to calcineurin inhibitors for GvHD prophylaxis or treatment, a diagnosis of multiple myeloma, and nephrotoxic drugs used before HSCT, during conditioning and in the early phase post-transplant are the main risk factors. In a large cohort study of 1635 patients treated with HSCT, a strong association was observed between acute and chronic GvHD and renal dysfunction. However, it is not possible to distinguish whether GvHD itself or its treatment is the major factor responsible for chronic kidney disease. Severe kidney disease, with GFR below 30 mL/min/1.73 m^2, has been reported in 3% of patients; and half of these have end-stage disease needing chronic dialysis. Nephrotic syndrome is a rare complication after allogeneic HSCT. It has been described in patients after discontinuation of cyclosporin and is thought to be a renal complication of chronic GvHD.

12.2 Clinical presentation and diagnosis

Most patients are asymptomatic, and chronic kidney disease remains unnoticed if renal function is not checked regularly. Blood pressure should be checked regularly and hypertension investigated immediately. Renal function should be evaluated at least once yearly after HSCT. Screening assessment should include blood urea nitrogen, creatinine, calculation of GFR, and urine protein analysis. Renal biopsy should be considered if there is persistent renal dysfunction of uncertain cause.

12.3 Prevention

The use of nephrotoxic drugs should be minimised in patients at risk for chronic kidney disease.

12.4 Treatment

Arterial hypertension should be managed aggressively. Angiotensin converting enzyme inhibitors and angiotensin receptor blockers are the treatment of choice for hypertension and chronic kidney disease. In end-stage chronic kidney disease dialysis may become indicated. Rare cases of successful of kidney transplantation after HSCT have been reported.

13. Liver complications and iron overload

Non-malignant late effects of the liver include viral hepatitis and chronic GvHD, and consequences of iron overload after HSCT (15, 16).

13.1 Scientific background and risk factors

The most common causes of late hepatic dysfunction after HSCT are chronic GvHD, iron overload, and viral infections. Several causes of liver disease may coexist in the same patient. Hepatitis B (HBV) and hepatitis C (HCV) infection may be asymptomatic or progress to fulminant hepatitis, chronic active hepatitis or cirrhosis. Before systematic HCV screening by PCR was introduced in1990 the prevalence of hepatitis C infection was high. Today the risk of acquiring HBV or HBV infection from blood transfusion is greatly reduced. However, reactivation of HBV has been reported. Patient with HBV usually exhibit mild to moderate liver disease, and progression to cirrhosis is rare. The long-term outcome of HCV infected patients after HSCT is worse. Patients surviving more than 10 years after HSCT are at higher risk of chronic hepatitis, and earlier development of cirrhosis as compared to HCV infected patients without HSCT. Liver disease is seen in 90% of patients with chronic GvHD.

Iron overload due to multiple transfusions and increased iron absorption is common in long-term survivors. Iron overload may be associated with liver toxicity and organ dysfunction. Elevated ferritin before transplant is related with increased transplant related mortality and GvHD, and iron overload increases the risk of infections, veno-occlusive disease and hepatic dysfunction.

13.2 Clinical presentation and diagnosis
Chronic HCV hepatitis is often asymptomatic during the first decade post-HSCT, with fluctuating transaminase levels. However, patients surviving more than 10 years after HSCT may present clinical manifestation of liver cirrhosis, and are at risk for hepatocellular carcinoma. Liver GvHD typically presents as cholestasis, with increased bilirubin or alkaline phosphatase, but it may also present as acute hepatitis and rarely progress to biliary cirrhosis. In all long-term survivors, liver function tests (total bilirubin, alkaline phosphatase, transaminases) should be performed at least once a year. For patients with known hepatitis B or C, monitoring of HbsAG and viral load by PCR is advised. Because of the unspecific presentation of chronic liver disease after HSCT, liver biopsy is often required. Iron overload can be assessed by measuring serum ferritin, and if indicated by liver biopsy. MRI is a very sensitive, non invasive method to assess iron overload.

13.3 Prevention
The use of hepatotoxic drugs should be limited in patients at risk for chronic liver disease. Abuse of alcoholic beverages should be avoided.

13.4 Treatment
Patients with chronic HCV infection should be carefully monitored because of the risk of an accelerated progression to cirrhosis. Data on HCV treatment after HSCT are scarce, but patients may benefit from combination therapy with ribavarin and pegylated interferon. New HCV-specific protease inhibitors have been recently developed; no data are available yet in HSCT survivors but caution on their use is advised given their haematological toxicities. Despite a clear correlation between iron overload and persistent hepatic dysfunction, the clinical consequences of therapeutic iron depletion in transplant recipients have not been extensively evaluated. Nevertheless, it is reasonable to treat patients with persistent high ferritin, over 2500 ng/L, or more than 7 mg/g dry weight liver iron for iron overload. Patients without anaemia can undergo therapeutic phlebotomy (450–500 mL every 6 to 8 weeks). Iron chelation with desferroxamine or desferasirox should be initiated for the other patients.

14. Late complications of bone
Non-malignant late effects after HSCT include avascular necrosis (AVN) of the bone and osteoporosis (17, 18).

14.1 Scientific background and risk factors

The incidence of AVN varies from 4 to over 10%. The mean time from transplant to AVN is 18 months. The main risk factors for AVN are the use of steroids (total dose and duration), and TBI, mainly with receipt of single doses of 10 Gy or higher or >12 Gy in fractionated doses. In a recent series involving more than 1300 patients at the City of Hope Hospital, the cumulative incidence of AVN at 10 years was 4% after autologous HSCT, 6% after allogeneic sibling donor HSCT, and 15% after unrelated donor HSCT. For allogeneic transplant recipients, male sex, primary diagnosis of Hodgkin's lymphoma or multiple myeloma, presence of chronic GvHD and exposure to CSA, FK506, prednisone and MMF rendered patients at increased risk.

Osteopenia and osteoporosis are both characterised by a reduced bone mass and increased susceptibility to bone fracture. HSCT can induce bone loss via the toxic effects of TBI, chemotherapy, and hypogonadism. The cumulative dose and number of days of glucocorticoid therapy and the number of days of cyclosporin or tacrolimus therapy showed significant associations with loss of bone density. Non-traumatic fractures occurred in 10% of patients. Nearly 50% of the patients have low bone density, a third have osteopenia and roughly 10% have osteoporosis, 12–18 months post-transplant.

14.2 Clinical presentation and diagnosis

Pain is usually the first sign of AVN of the bone. Early diagnosis can rarely be made using standard radiography and MRI is the investigation of choice. The hip is affected in over 80% of cases, with bilateral involvement in 60% cases. Other locations include the knee, wrist and ankle.

Osteoporosis remains often asymptomatic until the moment a fracture of the bone occurs. Non-traumatic fractures may occur in 10% of the patients. The degree of reduction in bone mass can be quantified on dual photon densitometry.

14.3 Prevention

The best preventive measure for AVN of the bone is to reduce the dose and duration of steroid treatment. The application of a non-TBI conditioning regimen is an additional preventive measure.

Patients should be advised to take regular exercise. Preventive measures for osteoporosis must include sex-hormone replacement in patients with gonadal failure. Additionally, decrease of bone loss and therefore prevention of osteoporosis can be obtained by reducing the duration and dosage of steroid therapy. Elemental calcium intake as well as vitamin D should be initiated particularly in patients on chronic steroid treatment.

14.4 Treatment

Symptomatic relief of pain and measures to decrease the pressure on the affected joints are of value, but most adult patients with advanced damage will require surgery. The probability of total hip replacement following a diagnosis of AVN is approximately 80% at 5 years. While the short-term results of joint surgery are excellent in the majority (>85%) of cases, long term follow-up of the protheses is needed in young patients who have a long life expectancy.

Treatment with bisphosphonate should be initiated in patients with proved osteopenia and osteoporosis. The duration of the treatment in long-term survivors after HSCT remains unclear. However, before starting treatment, dental assessment should be performed and treatment given if indicated, because of the risk of osteonecrosis of the jaw.

15. Late haematological malignancies after HSCT

Late malignant complications may occur in long-term survivors, including haematological malignancies (19).

15.1 Scientific background and risk factors

Three type of late haematological malignancies may be observed in long-term survivors: late relapse of the primary disease, therapy-related MDS/AML (t-MDS/AML) after autologous HSCT, and donor-type leukaemia after allogeneic HSCT. Relapse of a haematological malignancy usually occurs during the first two years after HSCT. The risk is higher after autologous than allogeneic HSCT and depends on the type of leukaemia, the risk profile and the state of the disease before HSCT. However, late relapse can be observed at any time after HSCT, with a decreasing probability with longer follow-up. In a cohort of 1475 long-term survivors, 241 deaths were observed after 2 years 29% of which were attributed to relapse of the primary malignant disease. Of the 70 deaths due to relapse, 67% occurred between the second and fifth year of follow-up, 27% in the next 5 years, and only 6% after 10 years from HSCT.

Lymphoma patients treated with autologous HSCT are particularly at risk for t-MDS/AML. The cumulative incidence of t-MDS/AML at 10 years has been reported to be between 6.8 and 36%. The higher risk of t-MDS/AML, when compared to other indications such as breast cancer, multiple myeloma or germ cell tumors has largely been attributed to the extent of pre-transplant treatment. The use of alkylating agents and a higher number of chemotherapy courses before HSCT as well as prior radiotherapy contribute substantially to secondary MDS/AML in transplant recipients. In up-front transplantation relatively low rates of secondary t-MDS/AML have been observed. However the use of TBI as conditioning was associated with an increased risk of t-MDS/AML.

Donor-type leukaemia refers to leukaemia of donor cell origin after allogeneic HSCT. Although described more than 2 decades ago, most of the first reports probably involved relapse of the original leukaemia because the "donor" origin of the leukaemia was based on classical cytogenetics of leukaemic cells in a transplant setting with donor/recipient sex-mismatch, in which the origin of the leukaemia cells was demonstrated by sex chromosome typing. However we now know that loss of the Y chromosome and duplication of the X chromosome can occur in leukaemic cells. Thus nowadays only molecular proof of the donor origin can be accepted, most often using PCR of VNTRs. Using these stringent criteria malignancies of donor cell origin, although rare, do exist. A further complexity was recently demonstrated by a study from the Seattle group showing that malignancies could also be transmitted through the graft either at a premalignant stage or as a minimal clone undetectable before transplantation.

15.2 Clinical presentation and diagnosis

Relapse or a secondary leukaemia may present as asymptomatic peripheral blood changes or in contrast with the full clinical manifestation of a leukaemia. The presence of macrocytosis, abnormal dysplastic neutrophils, immature haematopoietic cells, cytopenia or blasts in peripheral blood should raise suspicion. In case of unexplained blood changes a full bone marrow investigation is indicated. Regular bone marrow aspiration to detect early relapse is not useful in patients with a long-term survivorship of more than 2 years after HSCT. The monitoring of a molecular marker present at primary diagnosis may be useful. However, in AML negativity for a marker in peripheral blood does not exclude early relapse in the bone marrow, while the re-appearance of a marker should arouse attention and initiate further investigations.

15.3 Prevention

There are few measures to prevent relapse, secondary MDS/AML or the appearance of donor-type leukaemia. In allogeneic HSCT immunosuppressive treatment should be tapered and stopped as soon as possible. Preemptive DLI infusions and the use of post-transplant maintenance treatment in high risk patients is currently under investigation. However its efficacy has still to be proven.

15.4 Treatment

The management of late haematological malignancies after HSCT depends on the time of appearance, the type of leukaemia, the extent of the disease and the comorbidity of the patient. Possibilities include stopping immunosuppressive treatment for patients still on immunosuppressive drugs, adoptive immunotherapy, re-transplant or experimental treatment.

16. Secondary solid tumors after HSCT
Late malignant complications in long-term survivors also include solid tumours (20, 21).

16.1 Scientific background and risk factors
Long-term survivors of HSCT have an increased risk of developing new solid cancers, with the risk rising from 2 to 6% at 10 years after transplantation. Several factors contribute to this increase, including TBI, primary disease, male sex, and pre-transplantation therapy. Chronic GvHD and immunosuppressive therapy have also been shown to contribute to excess risk, particularly for squamous cell carcinomas of the buccal cavity and the skin.

The largest studies today include a multi-institutional cohort of 28,874 allogeneic transplant recipients with 189 solid malignancies. Overall, patients developed new solid cancers at twice the rate expected based on general population rates, with the risk increasing over time; the risk reached 3-fold among patients followed for 15 years or more after transplantation. New findings showed that the risk of developing a non-squamous cell carcinoma following conditioning radiation was highly dependent on age at exposure. Among patients irradiated at ages under 30 years, the relative risk of non-squamous cell carcinoma was 9 times that of non-irradiated patients, while the comparable risk for older patients was 1.1. Chronic GvHD disease and male sex were the main determinants for risk of squamous cell carcinoma.

The probability of solid tumour type might be under-estimated, since some of them tend to develop very late after transplantation. Among 3,337 female 5-year survivors who underwent an allogeneic transplantation at the Fred Hutchinson Cancer Research Center or at one of 82 centres reporting to the EBMT, 52 females developed breast cancer at a median of 12.5 years following HSCT (standardised incidence = 2.2). Twenty-five-year cumulative incidence was 11.0%, and was higher among survivors who received TBI (17%) than those who did not receive TBI (3%). In multivariate analysis, increased risk was associated with longer time since transplantation, use of TBI, and younger age at transplantation. The hazard ratio for death associated with breast cancer was 2.5. Extrapolating from the existing data, it is likely the risk of solid cancers will continue to increase during the next decades.

16.2 Clinical presentation and diagnosis
Early detection of a secondary solid cancers is essential. At that time patients are usually asymptomatic. Regular self-examination and systematic yearly assessment allow early detection of secondary cancers of the skin, the oral cavity, gynaecological organs and the thyroid gland. Young female patients who received local irradiation

or TBI should have regular mammography from the age of 30 years or from 8 years post-transplant. Patients with head and neck irradiation should be regularly screened for thyroid gland abnormalities. In case of abnormal nodules, fine needle aspiration is recommended. Women, particularly those with chronic GvHD, should have a yearly gynaecological examination including a cervical smear. Patients with oral chronic GvHD should be regularly examined for secondary squamous oral cancers.

16.3 Prevention
Prevention is based on early detection of solid cancer. Therefore, patients should be counseled about the risk of late secondary cancers and shown how to perform self examination of the skin, the oral cavity and the breasts. Furthermore, patients should be advised not to expose themselves to active or passive tobacco smoking, and to avoid direct exposure of the skin to UV irradiation.

16.4 Treatment
Appropriate cancer management should be discussed with the specialised team.

References
1. Socié G, Salooja N, Cohen A et al. Nonmalignant late effects after allogeneic stem cell transplantation. Blood 2003; 101: 3373–3385.
2. Tichelli A, Rovo A, Passweg J et al. Late complications after hematopoietic stem cell transplantation. Expert Rev Hematol 2009; 2: 583–601.
3. Rizzo JD, Wingard JR, Tichelli A et al. Recommended screening and preventive practices for long-term survivors after hematopoietic cell transplantation: Joint recommendations of the European Group for Blood and Marrow Transplantation, Center for International Blood and Marrow Transplant Research, and the American Society for Blood and Marrow Transplantation (EBMT/CIBMTR/ASBMT). Bone Marrow Transplant 2006; 37: 249–261.
4. Savani BN, Griffith ML, Jagasia S, Lee SJ. How I treat late effects in adults after allogeneic stem cell transplantation. Blood 2011; 117: 3002–3009.
5. Sanders JE, Hoffmeister PA, Woolfrey AE et al. Thyroid function following hematopoietic cell transplantation in children: 30 years' experience. Blood 2009; 113: 306–308.
6. Rovo A, Tichelli A, Passweg JR et al. Spermatogenesis in long-term survivors after allogeneic hematopoietic stem cell transplantation is associated with age, time interval since transplantation, and apparently absence of chronic GvHD. Blood 2006; 108: 1100–1105.
7. Salooja N, Szydlo RM, Socié G et al. Pregnancy outcomes after peripheral blood or bone marrow transplantation: A retrospective survey. Lancet 2001; 358: 271–276.
8. Yoshihara S, Yanik G, Cooke KR, Mineishi S. Bronchiolitis obliterans syndrome (BOS), bronchiolitis obliterans organizing pneumonia (BOOP), and other late-onset noninfectious pulmonary complications following allogeneic hematopoietic stem cell transplantation. Biol Blood Marrow Transplant 2007; 13: 749–759.

9. Armenian SH, Bhatia S. Cardiovascular disease after hematopoietic cell transplantation - lessons learned. Haematologica 2008; 93: 1132–1136.
10. Tichelli A, Bhatia S, Socié G. Cardiac and cardiovascular consequences after haematopoietic stem cell transplantation. Br J Haematol 2008; 142: 11–26.
11. Tichelli A, Bucher C, Rovo A et al. Premature cardiovascular disease after allogeneic hematopoietic stem-cell transplantation. Blood 2007; 110: 3463–3471.
12. Tichelli A, Passweg J, Wojcik D et al. Late cardiovascular events after allogeneic hematopoietic stem cell transplantation: A retrospective multicenter study of the Late Effects Working Party of the European Group for Blood and Marrow Transplantation. Haematologica 2008; 93: 1203–1210.
13. Annaloro C, Usardi P, Airaghi L et al. Prevalence of metabolic syndrome in long-term survivors of hematopoietic stem cell transplantation. Bone Marrow Transplant 2008; 41: 797–804.
14. Choi M, Sun CL, Kurian S et al. Incidence and predictors of delayed chronic kidney disease in long-term survivors of hematopoietic cell transplantation. Cancer 2008; 113: 1580–1587.
15. Majhail NS, Lazarus HM, Burns LJ. Iron overload in hematopoietic cell transplantation. Bone Marrow Transplant 2008; 41: 997–1003.
16. Peffault de LR, Levy V, Asselah T et al. Long-term outcome of hepatitis C infection after bone marrow transplantation. Blood 2004; 103: 1618–1624.
17. Campbell S, Sun CL, Kurian S. Predictors of avascular necrosis of bone in long-term survivors of hematopoietic cell transplantation. Cancer 2009; 115: 4127–4135.
18. Petropoulou AD, Porcher R, Herr AL et al. Prospective assessment of bone turnover and clinical bone diseases after allogeneic hematopoietic stem-cell transplantation. Transplantation 2010; 89: 1354–1361.
19. Sala-Torra O, Hanna C, Loken MR et al. Evidence of donor-derived hematologic malignancies after hematopoietic stem cell transplantation. Biol Blood Marrow Transplant 2006; 12: 511–517.
20. Rizzo JD, Curtis RE, Socié G et al. Solid cancers after allogeneic hematopoietic cell transplantation. Blood 2009; 113: 1175–1183.
21. Socié G, Curtis RE, Deeg HJ et al. New malignant diseases after allogeneic marrow transplantation for childhood acute leukemia. J Clin Oncol 2000; 18: 348–357.

Multiple Choice Questionnaire

To find the correct answer, go to http://www.esh.org/online-training/handbook/

1. The pattern may of late effects after HSCT changes over time, because
a) Conditioning regimens are changing . . . . ☐
b) Fewer patients with CML are treated since the availability of
   tyrosine kinase inhibitors . . . . ☐

c) TBI is increasingly used . . . . □
d) The proportion of female donors is changing . . . . □

2. **TBI is the main risk factor for**
   a) Late cardiac complications after HSCT . . . . □
   b) Aseptic necrosis of bone . . . . □
   c) Secondary cancer of the oral cavity . . . . □
   d) Gonadal dysfunction in females . . . . □

3. **GvHD is the main risk factor for**
   a) Cataract formation . . . . □
   b) Bronchilitis obliterans syndrome (BOS) . . . . □
   c) Secondary breast cancer . . . . □
   d) Thyroid dysfunction . . . . □

4. **Which one of the following statements is not correct:**
   a) Dental decay after HSCT may occur in patients with sicca syndrome, poor dental hygiene and large-scale consumption of sugar-containing drinks . . . . □
   b) Male patients surviving more than 10 years, younger than 25 years at HSCT, and apparently without chronic GvHD have a reasonable likelihood of spermatogenesis after HSCT . . . . □
   c) There exists a strong correlation between chronic kidney disease after HSCT and the use of prolonged corticosteroid therapy at increased doses for chronic GvHD . . . . □
   d) It is reasonable to treat patients with persistent high ferritin, over 2500 ng/L, or more than 7 mg/g dry weight liver iron for iron overload . . . . □

5. **One of the following post-transplant managements is not advisable in respect of late effects**
   a) Female patients conditioned with TBI should have regular mammography from the age of 30 years or from 8 years post-transplant . . . . □

b) All long-term survivors after HSCT should receive regularly bisphosphonates as a prevention of post-transplant osteoporosis .... ☐

c) To prevent therapy-related vascular late effects, patients should be encouraged to undertake regular physical activity, stop smoking tobacco, avoid passive smoking and maintain a healthy body weight .... ☐

d) For the treatment of cryptogenic organising pneumonia (COP) corticosteroids should be started without delay .... ☐

* CHAPTER 16

Molecular monitoring after HSCT

---

* 16.1

Molecular monitoring of minimal residual disease

Jean-Michel Cayuela

1. Introduction

A large number of studies have shown that detection of morphologically occult leukaemic cells, i.e. minimal residual disease (MRD), significantly correlates with clinical outcome in many haematological malignancies. For example, in childhood acute lymphoblastic leukaemia (ALL) the International Berlin-Frankfurt-Muenster group (I-BFM) reported a 10-year event free survival of 93% for patients who were MRD negative on both day 33 and 78 compared to 16% for those with MRD levels of 0.1% or higher (1). Therefore, in an increasing number of categories of haematological malignancies, including childhood and adult ALL, acute promyelocytic leukaemia (APL), acute myeloid leukaemia (AML) with inv(16)(p13.1q22) or t(16;16)(p13.1;q22), AML with NPM1 mutation and chronic myeloid leukaemia (CML), MRD information is critical for clinical decision-making. Based on these data MRD detection is now becoming routinely implemented in several treatment protocols and is increasingly used for guiding therapy. For example, for CML patients treated with tyrosine kinase inhibitors (TKI) it is now widely accepted that achieving major molecular response (MMR) is associated with favourable progression-free survival and it has been proposed that treatment should be reviewed in patients who faile to achieve a MMR by 18 months (2).

Quantitative MRD data appear to be crucial for the appropriate evaluation of treatment response. They can be obtained by three main techniques: flow cytometric immunophenotyping using leukaemia-associated aberrant immunophenotypes, PCR techniques using tumour-specific DNA targets (e.g. immunoglobulin (Ig) and T-cell receptor (TCR) gene rearrangements), and reverse transcriptase (RT) PCR techniques using tumour-specific RNA targets (e.g. fusion gene transcripts). In this review we will focus on PCR-based techniques which are generally based on real-time quantitative PCR (RQ-PCR).

2. RQ-PCR analysis

In contrast to classical end-point PCR, RQ-PCR allows accurate quantification of DNA target sequences during the exponential phase of the PCR amplification process. Moreover, quantitative data can be obtained directly without any post-PCR processing, due to real-time detection of fluorescent signals during each PCR cycle. Classically, fluorescent signals are produced by sequence specific oligonucleotide probes conjugated with a reporter fluorochrome and positioned within the target sequence. The cycle threshold (CT) (sometimes referred to as crossing point) i.e. the PCR cycle at which the fluorescence exceeds the threshold line is directly proportional to the amount of target sequence present in the sample. Using serial dilutions of titrated samples (e.g. tumour samples from diagnosis or titrated commercially available DNA samples), a standard curve can be drawn. The amount of target sequence present in a sample can be calculated by plotting CT values on the standard curve. Numerous RQ-PCR platforms are currently available, but until proven otherwise, it appears that RQ-PCR techniques give comparable results with different instruments (3).

3. MRD-PCR targets

Leukaemia-cell associated molecular features amplifiable by PCR and allowing quantification of MRD belong to 4 main categories: rearrangements of Ig and TCR genes; fusion regions of other rearranged genes or of fusion-gene transcripts; over-expressed genes; and mutated alleles or transcripts of genes (Table 1).

In lymphoid malignancies, rearrangements of Ig and TCR genes are universal targets. They are produced during early B- and T-cell differentiation by somatic recombination of germline variable (V), diversity (D), and joining (J) segments of the Ig and TCR

Table 1: **Technical approaches, applicability and sensitivity of main MRD-PCR targets available in different type of haematological malignancies**

Haematological malignancies	MRD-PCR targets	Technical approaches	Nucleic acid	Applicability	Sensitivity
Precursor B-ALL	Ig/TCR gene rearrangements	Patient specific RQ-PCR	DNA	Children: 95% Adults: 90%	10^{-4}–10^{-5}
	TEL-AML1	RT-RQ-PCR	RNA	Children: 20–25% Adults: <5%	10^{-5}–10^{-6}
	BCR-ABL1	RT-RQ-PCR	RNA	Children: <5% Adults: 20–25%	10^{-5}–10^{-6}
T-ALL	Ig/TCR gene rearrangements	Patient specific RQ-PCR	DNA	Children: >95% Adults: 90%	10^{-4}–10^{-5}
	Tald1	RQ-PCR	DNA	10–15%	10^{-4}–10^{-5}
APL	PML-RARA	RT-RQ-PCR	RNA	>95%	10^{-3}–10^{-4}
AML	AML1-ETO	RT-RQ-PCR	RNA	10–12%	10^{-5}–10^{-6}
	CBFb-MYH11	RT-RQ-PCR	RNA	8–10%	10^{-4}–10^{-5}
	WT-1	RT-RQ-PCR	RNA	70–80%	10^{-2}–10^{-3}
	NPM1 mutated	ASO-RQ-PCR ASO-RT-RQ-PCR	DNA RNA	Children: 8–10% Adults: 30–35%	10^{-4}–10^{-5}

THE EBMT HANDBOOK 2012 EDITION

genes, and due to extensive combinatorial diversity and deletion of germline nucleotides by trimming the ends of the rearranging gene segments as well as random insertion of nucleotides between the joined gene segments, the junctional regions of these rearrangements can be considered as DNA-fingerprints of the malignant cells. Identification of Ig and TCR rearrangements present in each patient at diagnosis is performed by PCR and fluorescent gene scanning. Each rearrangement is then sequenced by direct sequencing of PCR products. The sequence information allows the design of junctional region-specific oligonucleotides or allele-specific oligonucleotides (ASO) that are used in specific RQ-PCR assays. Virtually all Ig and TCR gene rearrangements can be analysed relatively easily with a restricted number of oligonucleotide primers. It is of note that these rearrangements, especially in ALL, are prone to clonal evolution, because of a certain degree of oligoclonality at diagnosis or because of ongoing or secondary Ig/TCR gene rearrangements. Moreover if Ig genes are used, one should be aware of somatic hypermutations that can affect the binding sites of the primers used, especially in post-germinal centre-derived lymphoid malignancies.

Other rearranged genes can be used as tumour-specific MRD-PCR targets. This is only feasible when the breakpoints are tightly clustered among patients. This is the case for the BCL2-JH and BCL1-JH rearrangements which are detectable in two-third of the patients with follicular lymphoma and one-third of the patients with mantle cell lymphoma, respectively (4, 5). This is also feasible for the sub-microscopic TAL1 deletions present in up to 15% of T-ALL.

Chromosome aberrations resulting in fusion-gene transcripts that are similar between patients despite distinct breakpoints at the DNA level are widely present in at least some haematological malignancies. After reverse transcription into cDNA these fusion-gene transcripts can be used as targets for MRD-PCR analysis using primers that are located on each side of the breakpoint fusion region. This is the case for the BCR-ABL1 fusion transcripts that are observed in CML and in some adult ALL, but also for PML-RARA in APL or CBFB-MYH11 and AML1-ETO in core-binding-factor (CBF) AML. These MRD-PCR targets are deemed very stable during the evolution of the disease (6, 7).

The Wilm's tumour gene WT-1 is over-expressed in most patients with AML and its over-expression can therefore be considered as a specific feature of the leukaemia cells. However it should be noted that WT-1 is expressed at low level by normal bone marrow cells and, to a lesser extent, by peripheral blood leukocytes. This nonspecific background noise must be taken into account for interpretation of RQ-PCR data (8).

Mutations in the nucleophosmin (NPM1) gene represent some of the most common gene mutations in AML, especially in AML with normal cytogenetics. In up to 95%

of the patients, only 3 different mutations are found. Therefore the NPM1 mutated allele or its transcripts represents an attractive target for MRD monitoring in AML (9).

4. Control genes and expression of data

To obtain quantitative MRD-PCR data, it is crucial that control genes are included in the analysis to correct for the quantity and the quality of the nucleic acid. When DNA MRD-PCR targets are used, one should select a control gene located on a chromosome that is not frequently gained or lost in the studied type of malignancy. The albumin (ALB) gene located on chromosome 4 is often used. MRD data are then normalised according to the ALB copy number and expressed as the percentage of remaining leukaemia cells in the follow-up sample. When an RNA MRD-PCR target is used, ABL appears to be the most appropriate gene, since its expression is stable and comparable between bone marrow and peripheral blood as well as between normal and leukaemia samples. MRD data are expressed as the normalised copy numbers of the MRD-PCR target-transcripts (4, 6, 10).

5. Advantages and disadvantages of MRD-PCR targets

In lymphoid malignancies, Ig/TCR gene rearrangements are frequently used MRD-PCR targets since they are (i) widely applicable; (ii) developed in a network of highly standardised laboratories and (iii), at least in ALL, they are a well-established stratification tool in various treatment protocols. However, the identification of Ig/TCR rearrangements at diagnosis and the design of patient specific oligonucleotides for the subsequent MRD quantification during follow-up is time consuming and requires insight in the immunobiology of Ig/TCR gene rearrangements. Moreover one must keep in mind that these rearrangements can be lost during the course of the disease (i.e. risk of false negative result) and that non-specific background may greatly hamper sensitive detection (i.e. risk of false positive result). Fusion gene-transcripts (i) can be easily identified at diagnosis with a limited set of primers; (ii) are very stable MRD-targets, as they are related to oncogenesis; and (iii) there is no (or very low) background in normal cells. But they are not widely applicable and there is an increased risk of contamination of the samples since they are not patient-specific. Over-expression of WT-1 is very easy to diagnose. But expression of WT-1 is not tumour-specific and there is a background of expression in normal cells that precludes MRD quantification in bone marrow samples. Unlike WT-1, mutated NPM1 transcripts are tumour-specific, but a certain degree of non-specificity in the ASO-PCR system may produce non-specific results that must not be over-interpreted (3).

6. Blood versus bone marrow

With the exception of chronic phase CML and T-ALL, MRD levels are usually higher in bone-marrow samples than in blood. However, this does not mean that peripheral blood MRD assays are clinically useless.

For instance, they could help identifying some aggressive leukaemia subtypes associated with high risk of recurrence, occurrences of extra-medullary relapses or on the contrary, help monitoring patients once bone marrow samples have become MRD negative (11). Moreover for some MRD-PCR targets, like WT-1, blood samples are more suitable than bone marrow for MRD assessments, because of a lower background noise (8).

7. Examples of the clinical value of quantitative MRD in the context of allogeneic haematopoietic stem cell transplantation

In childhood ALL, it has been reported that MRD level prior to allogeneic HSCT is a powerful predictor of post-transplant outcome. It is therefore important to reduce as much as possible the MRD burden before proceeding to a bone marrow transplant. However, in the same study, the authors reported a minority of children with a high burden of MRD prior to allogeneic HSCT who enter a long lasting remission.

They speculated that graft-versus-leukaemia might play a role for these children and that a transplant protocol favouring development of significant graft-versus-host disease could be an alternative approach (12).

Ph-positive ALL is a subgroup of ALL with a poor prognosis and, at least in adults, HSCT in first CR is considered to be one of the best treatment options. However, detection of BCR-ABL transcripts after HSCT is associated with a high risk of subsequent relapse.

Recent data suggest that, for these patients, early administration of imatinib triggered by molecular evidence of leukaemia recurrence is associated with prolonged disease free survival (DFS) and that treatment outcomes can be anticipated on the basis of BCR-ABL transcripts levels determined during the first months of imatinib initiation (13, 14). It has also been suggested that the extent of MRD reduction before allogeneic HSCT may allow the identification of patients at high risk of relapse (15). Of course, it is of utmost importance that only reliable MRD results are used for any therapeutic decisions. It means that those results are produced by accredited laboratories involved in standardisation programs and regularly participating in external quality evaluation programs.

Key points are summarised below.

Key points

Quantitative assessment of MRD is a major prognostic factor for outcome in leukaemia patients

Ig/TCR gene rearrangements are the most prevalent MRD-PCR targets in ALL

BCR-ABL1 fusion transcripts are suitable MRD-PCR targets in CML and in Ph+ ALL

NPM1 mutations and over-expression of WT-1 are the most prevalent MRD-PCR targets in AML

In the context of HSCT, MRD status prior to, and after transplantation is critical for outcome

References

1. Conter V, Bartram CR, Valsecchi MG et al. Molecular response to treatment redefines all prognostic factors in children and adolescents with B-cell precursor acute lymphoblastic leukemia: Results in 3184 patients of the AIEOP-BFM ALL 2000 study. Blood 2010; 115: 3206–3214.
2. Baccarani M, Cortes J, Pane F et al. Chronic Myeloid Leukemia: An update of concepts and management recommendations of European Leukemia Net. J Clin Oncol 2009; 27: 6041–6051.
3. van der Velden VH, Hochhaus A, Cazzaniga G et al. Detection of minimal residual disease in hematologic malignancies by real-time quantitative PCR: Principles, approaches, and laboratory aspects. Leukemia 2003; 17: 1013–1034.
4. van der Velden VH, Cazzaniga G, Schrauder A et al. Analysis of minimal residual disease by Ig/TCR gene rearrangements: Guidelines for interpretation of real-time quantitative PCR data. Leukemia 2007; 21: 604–611.
5. van Dongen JJ, Langerak AW, Bruggemann M et al. Design and standardization of PCR primers and protocols for detection of clonal immunoglobulin and T-cell receptor gene recombinations in suspect lymphoproliferations: Report of the BIOMED-2 Concerted Action BMH4-CT98-3936. Leukemia 2003; 17: 2257–2317.
6. Gabert J, Beillard E, van der Velden VH et al. Standardization and quality control studies of 'real-time' quantitative reverse transcriptase polymerase chain reaction of fusion gene transcripts for residual disease detection in leukemia - a Europe Against Cancer program. Leukemia 2003; 17: 2318–2357.
7. van Dongen JJ, Macintyre EA, Gabert JA et al. Standardized RT-PCR analysis of fusion gene transcripts from chromosome aberrations in acute leukemia for detection of minimal residual disease. Report of the BIOMED-1 Concerted Action: Investigation of minimal residual disease in acute leukemia. Leukemia 1999; 13: 1901–1928.
8. Cilloni D, Renneville A, Hermitte F et al. Real-time quantitative polymerase chain

reaction detection of minimal residual disease by standardized WT1 assay to enhance risk stratification in acute myeloid leukemia: A European LeukemiaNet study. J Clin Oncol 2009; 27: 5195–5201.

9. Kronke J, Schlenk RF, Jensen KO et al. Monitoring of minimal residual disease in NPM1-mutated acute myeloid leukemia: A study from the German-Austrian acute myeloid leukemia study group. J Clin Oncol; 29: 2709–2716.

10. Beillard E, Pallisgaard N, van der Velden VH et al. Evaluation of candidate control genes for diagnosis and residual disease detection in leukemic patients using "real-time" quantitative reverse-transcriptase polymerase chain reaction (RQ-PCR) - a Europe against cancer program. Leukemia 2003; 17: 2474–2486.

11. Coustan-Smith E, Sancho J, Hancock ML et al. Use of peripheral blood instead of bone marrow to monitor residual disease in children with acute lymphoblastic leukemia. Blood 2002; 100: 2399–2402.

12. Bader P, Hancock J, Kreyenberg H et al. Minimal residual disease (MRD) status prior to allogeneic stem cell transplantation is a powerful predictor for post-transplant outcome in children with ALL. Leukemia 2002; 16: 1668–1672.

13. Spinelli O, Peruta B, Tosi M et al. Clearance of minimal residual disease after allogeneic stem cell transplantation and the prediction of the clinical outcome of adult patients with high-risk acute lymphoblastic leukemia. Haematologica 2007; 92: 612–618.

14. Wassmann B, Pfeifer H, Stadler M et al. Early molecular response to posttransplantation imatinib determines outcome in MRD+ Philadelphia-positive acute lymphoblastic leukemia (Ph+ ALL). Blood 2005; 106: 458–463.

15. Lee S, Kim YJ, Chung NG et al. The extent of minimal residual disease reduction after the first 4-week imatinib therapy determines outcome of allogeneic stem cell transplantation in adults with Philadelphia chromosome-positive acute lymphoblastic leukemia. Cancer 2009; 115: 561–570.

Multiple Choice Questionnaire

To find the correct answer, go to http://www.esh.org/online-training/handbook/

1. **Minimal residual disease is defined by:**
   a) The amount of undifferentiated cells remaining in bone marrow after initiation of therapy .... ☐
   b) The amount of leukaemic cells remaining in patients who do not reach complete remission .... ☐
   c) The amount of morphologically occult leukaemic cells remaining after initiation of therapy .... ☐
   d) The amount of leukaemic cells detected in bone marrow at relapse ...... ☐

2. **In ALL, the most prevalent MRD-PCR targets are:**
   a) BCR-ABL1 fusion transcripts .... ☐
   b) Ig and TCR gene rearrangements .... ☐
   c) WT-1 overexpression .... ☐
   d) NPM1 mutations .... ☐

3. **In ALL, Ig and TCR gene rarrangements are:**
   a) MRD-PCR targets related to oncogenesis .... ☐
   b) Can easily be identified at diagnosis with a limited set of primers ...... ☐
   c) Very stable MRD-PCR targets .... ☐
   d) Well-established stratification tools in various treatment protocols ..... ☐

NOTES

✳ CHAPTER 16

Molecular monitoring after HSCT

✳ 16.2
Chimerism

Thomas Lion

1. Introduction

Monitoring of the ratio of donor- and recipient-derived cells (chimerism) has become an indispensable diagnostic tool in the surveillance of allogeneic hematopoietic stem cell transplant (allo-HSCT) recipients. The increasing employment of reduced intensity conditioning (RIC) regimens and cord blood transplants, which require very careful surveillance of the graft, has further reinforced the clinical importance of chimerism testing. Analysis of chimerism during the post-transplant period permits the assessment of immunological interactions between donor and recipient, providing potentially important information for pre-emptive therapeutic interventions. In addition to enabling the assessment of successful engraftment, analysis of chimerism can provide an early indication of the risk of graft rejection (1–3), and in patients with malignant haematologic disorders, a timely alert of impending relapse (4–6).

2. Technical aspects

Current methodological approaches to chimerism analysis are rather diverse. In the sex-mismatched transplant setting, fluorescence *in situ* hybridization (FISH) analysis of the X and Y chromosomes in interphase nuclei is regarded as a highly accurate technique for quantitative investigation of chimerism. Technical approaches that can be employed regardless of donor-recipient gender are commonly based on molecular methods including primarily the polymerase chain reaction (PCR). Techniques based on PCR amplification of polymorphic DNA sequences facilitating unequivocal distinction and quantitative assessment of recipient- and donor-derived cells have been the preferred approach to chimerism testing at most centres. Despite the introduction of single nucleotide polymorphism (SNP) and insertion/deletion (Indel) polymorphism analysis by real-time PCR for the investigation of chimerism several years ago, DNA microsatellites [also referred to as short tandem repeats (STRs)] have remained the most commonly used source of polymorphic markers for quantitative assessment of donor/recipient haemopoiesis after allo-HCST. Amplification of STR markers by PCR coupled with fluorescence detection of the donor/recipient alleles using capillary electrophoresis has been a widely used approach to the monitoring of haematopoietic chimerism (7). The main advantages of automated fluorescence-based detection of STR markers over the use of conventional gel electrophoresis include greater precision and easier performance of quantitative analysis, reduced manual handling of PCR products, and higher sensitivity.

2.1 Criteria for the selection of suitable STR markers for chimerism analysis

The accuracy and reliability of quantitative chimerism analysis in post-transplant samples are greatly affected by factors such as the homozygosity/heterozygosity of STR alleles, shared alleles between donor and recipient, and the positional relationship between alleles. The EuroChimerism (EUC) consortium, an international working party (see below), has therefore established criteria facilitating selection of eligible STR markers for chimerism testing. The EUC group has developed a common descriptive nomenclature for allelic configurations termed the RSD (Recipient-Shared-Donor) code with the aim to facilitate rapid identification of STR markers displaying optimal allele constellations for accurate and reproducible chimerism analysis (8).

2.2 Multiplex versus singleplex PCR assays for chimerism analysis

Multiplex PCR assays are commonly used for initial recipient/donor genotyping to select one or more informative STR markers for the subsequent monitoring of chimerism. Moreover, investigation of post-transplant peripheral blood samples with multiple STR markers may improve the reproducibility and accuracy of quantitative chimerism analysis. The accuracy of quantitative chimerism assays can be increased by testing each sample with more than one marker and calculating mean values (9). Some investigators therefore perform clinical testing of chimerism with commercial multiplex kits facilitating co-amplification of several microsatellite markers in a single PCR reaction (9). However, the indicated advantages may be counterbalanced by the higher cost of consumables and the lower sensitivity resulting from the high number of different fragments co-amplified. Most diagnostic centres therefore rely on the use of singleplex PCR reactions for sensitive assessment and quantitative monitoring of chimerism.

2.3 Chimerism testing within total leukocytes versus analysis of specific cell lineages

PCR-based chimerism assays analysing highly polymorphic STR markers mostly permit the detection of residual autologous cells with a sensitivity limit in the range of 1%. When investigating chimerism in total leukocyte preparations from PB, this level of sensitivity may not be sufficient to allow early assessment of impending complications. It is possible to overcome this problem by investigating chimerism in specific leukocyte subsets of interest isolated by flow-sorting or by immunomagnetic bead separation. Since residual recipient-derived cells can be detected within the individual leukocyte fractions with similar sensitivity, it is possible to identify and monitor minor autologous populations that would escape detection in total PB leukocyte samples. The overall sensitivity of chimerism assays achievable by investigating specifically enriched leukocyte subsets is in a range of 0.1–0.01% (4)

i.e. one to two logs higher than analysis of total leukocyte preparations. Investigation of individual leukocyte fractions therefore not only provides more specific information, but also permits the assessment of impending complications at a significantly higher sensitivity, thus providing a basis for earlier treatment decisions.

2.4 Heterogeneity of current methods and approaches to harmonisation

The methods for STR-PCR analysis of chimerism performed in most diagnostic laboratories are based on various in-house assays. The heterogeneity of technical approaches and the diversity of STR markers used render the comparison of results generated at different centres difficult. Attempts have therefore been made to introduce a commercially available platform for chimerism testing (*http://www.bio-type.de*) or to exploit existing commercial microsatellite kits designed for forensic purposes which, however, are not optimally suited for chimerism testing (8). To address the urgent need for a standardised technology specifically adapted to the requirements of quantitative chimerism analysis, twelve leading centres from ten European countries have established the EuroChimerism consortium to perform a collaborative study supported by the European Commission within the 5th Framework Program. The paramount goal of the consortium was to establish a standardised approach to quantitative chimerism testing, with the aim to facilitate harmonisation of chimerism diagnostics between European centres, and to provide a basis for appropriate quality control. Following extensive analysis of a large set of microsatellite (STR) loci, the EuroChimerism (EUC) marker panel was established. The panel comprises 13 STR markers selected to optimally meet the specific requirements of quantitative chimerism analysis. Based on highly stringent selection criteria (8), the EUC panel provides multiple informative markers in any transplant setting. The EuroChimerism assay provides standardised STR-PCR tests permitting detection of donor- or recipient-derived cells with a sensitivity limit of 0.8–1.6%. Moreover, the assay facilitates accurate and reproducible quantification of donor and recipient haematopoietic cells (*Lion et al., submitted*). Based on the collaboration of the EUC consortium with an industrial partner (Miltenyi Biotech, Germany) a multiplex PCR kit for the identification of informative STR markers (ChimerXplain™) and a singleplex PCR kit specifically adapted for quantitative chimerism analysis (ChimerXact™) will soon be commercially available, and may serve as a tool for the harmonisation of post-transplant monitoring between diagnostic laboratories. Implementation of the kits in the clinical monitoring of chimerism could help eliminate the problems of heterogeneity in the currently used technical approaches, and could greatly improve the comparability of data and the exchange of information between centres.

3. Detection of imminent leukaemia relapse post-transplant by chimerism analysis

In most instances, surveillance of residual or reappearing leukaemic cells after allo-HSCT is performed by leukaemia- or clone-specific markers. In instances in which specific markers are not available, the exploitation of chimerism testing may be instrumental for the assessment of impending relapse. Investigation of chimerism in total leukocyte fractions from PB was shown to reveal reappearance of autologous cells (mixed chimerism) before the diagnosis of relapse (6), thus providing a basis for timely initiation of appropriate treatment. In a number of instances, however, chimerism testing within total leukocytes may not show any changes indicative of impending relapse (4). Based on its greater sensitivity, investigation of specific leukocyte subsets derived from PB or bone marrow (BM) has a greater potential of revealing informative changes in patients who later experience haematological relapse. Patients with imminent leukaemia relapse can reveal persistence or reappearance of autologous allelic patterns within cell subsets expected to harbour leukaemic cells, if present. These cell populations can be specifically enriched for chimerism testing by targeting the original immunophenotype of the leukaemic clone. The stem cell marker CD34 is commonly expressed by leukaemic cells in combination with lineage-specific markers. For example, tumour cells in B-cell precursor acute lymphocytic leukaemia typically display co-expression of CD34 and CD19. Cell populations expressing these markers can therefore be specifically targeted for the assessment of residual disease by monitoring the presence and the kinetics of recipient chimerism. In some instances, however, the only observation made before haematological relapse is lineage-specific chimerism kinetics suggestive of graft rejection (4). This observation may be attributable to the loss of the graft-versus-leukaemia effect associated with rejection of the allograft.

4. Prediction of graft rejection by the monitoring of chimerism within lymphocyte subsets

Patients who receive reduced-intensity conditioning reveal persisting leukocytes of recipient genotype more commonly than patients who receive myeloablative conditioning. The higher incidence of mixed or recipient chimerism may be attributable both to cells of myeloid and lymphoid lineages (1). In patients who receive T-cell depleted grafts, there is a strong association with the presence of mixed or recipient chimerism within T-cells (CD3+) and NK-cells (CD56+). Detection of mixed chimerism within lymphocyte populations is associated with an increased risk of late rejection (1, 4). In most instances, serial analysis reveals a persistently high or an increasing recipient-specific allelic pattern prior to overt graft rejection (1,

4, 6). The correlation between the observation of mixed or recipient chimerism and graft rejection was shown to be higher for NK-cells than for T-helper (CD3+/CD4+) or T-suppressor (CD3+/CD8+) cells (1). Patients displaying recipient chimerism in CD56+ cells between days +14 and +35 appear to have an extremely high risk of graft rejection. By contrast, virtually all patients who experience late graft rejection show pure donor genotype within the myeloid (CD14+ and CD15+) cells during the same period (1). Hence, the observation of recipient chimerism within the CD56+ and CD3+ cell subsets is highly predictive for the occurrence of late graft-rejection. These findings underscore the importance of cell subset analysis during post-transplant chimerism testing.

Timely diagnosis of impending graft rejection is crucial for effective therapeutic intervention. In a recent study, the predictive potential of early leukocyte subset-specific chimerism for graft loss has been investigated in children undergoing allo-HSCT for treatment of malignant and non-malignant diseases after reduced-intensity or myeloablative conditioning. Monitoring of lineage-specific chimerism was performed upon first appearance of leukocyte counts amenable to cell sorting. The first chimerism analysis of T- and NK-cells performed at a median of 20 days after HSCT identified three different risk groups which were independent from the conditioning regimen: recipient chimerism (RC) levels in T-cells below 50% indicated a very low risk of rejection (1.4%), while high levels of RC (>90%) both in T- and NK-cells were associated graft loss in the majority of patients (90%) despite therapeutic interventions. Recipient chimerism >50% in T-cells and ≤90% in NK-cells defined an intermediate risk group in which timely immunotherapy frequently prevented rejection. Early analysis of T- and NK-cell chimerism can therefore be instrumental in the risk assessment and therapeutic management of imminent graft rejection (10). Key points are summarised below.

Key points

Commercial kits for standardised quantitative monitoring of chimerism based on STR PCR analysis will soon be available from Miltenyi Biotech, and may facilitate harmonisation of diagnostics between centres

Analysis of chimerism within specific leukocyte lineages can permit earlier assessment of impending complications such as graft rejection or disease relapse

Lineage-specific chimerism analysis of T- and NK-cells within the first three weeks post-transplant permits early risk assessment of impending graft rejection

References

1. Matthes-Martin S, Lion T, Haas OA et al. Lineage-specific chimaerism after stem cell transplantation in children following reduced intensity conditioning: Potential predictive value of NK cell chimaerism for late graft rejection. Leukemia 2003; 17: 1934–1942.

2. Liesveld JL, Rothberg PG. Mixed chimerism in SCT: Conflict or peaceful coexistence? Bone Marrow Transplant 2008; 42: 297–310.

3. Lawler M, McCann SR, Marsh JC et al. Serial chimerism analyses indicate that mixed haemopoietic chimerism influences the probability of graft rejection and disease recurrence following allogeneic stem cell transplantation (SCT) for severe aplastic anaemia (SAA): Indication for routine assessment of chimerism post SCT for SAA. Br J Haematol 2009; 144: 933–945.

4. Lion T, Daxberger H, Dubovsky J et al. Analysis of chimerism within specific leukocyte subsets for detection of residual or recurrent leukemia in pediatric patients after allogeneic stem cell transplantation. Leukemia 2001; 15: 307–310.

5. Bader P, Kreyenberg H, Hoelle W et al. Increasing mixed chimerism defines a high-risk group of childhood acute myelogenous leukemia patients after allogeneic stem cell transplantation where pre-emptive immunotherapy may be effective. Bone Marrow Transplant 2004; 33: 815–821.

6. Bader P, Kreyenberg H, Hoelle W et al. Increasing mixed chimerism is an important prognostic factor for unfavorable outcome in children with acute lymphoblastic leukemia after allogeneic stem-cell transplantation: Possible role for pre-emptive immunotherapy? J Clin Oncol 2004; 22: 1696–1705.

7. Lion T. Summary: Reports on quantitative analysis of chimerism after allogeneic stem cell transplantation by PCR amplification of microsatellite markers and capillary electrophoresis with fluorescence detection. Leukemia 2003; 17: 252–254.

8. Watzinger F, Lion T, Steward C. The RSD code: Proposal for a nomenclature of allelic configurations in SRT-PCR-based chimerism testing after allogeneic stem cell transplantation. Leukemia 2006; 20: 1448–1452.

9. Thiede C, Bornhäuser U, Brendel C et al. Sequential monitoring of chimerism and detection of minimal residual disease after allogeneic blood stem transplantation (BSCT) using multiplex PCR amplification of short tandem repeat-markers. Leukemia 2001; 15: 293–306.

10. Breuer S, Fritsch G, Daxberger H et al. Early recipient chimerism in the T- and NK-cell lineages is indicative of impending graft rejection in pediatric patients undergoing allogeneic hematopoietic stem cell transplantation. Leukemia 2011 Sep 16. doi: 10.1038/leu.2011.244. [Epub ahead of print].

Multiple Choice Questionnaire

To find the correct answer, go to http://www.esh.org/online-training/handbook/

1. **Early analysis of cell lineage-specific chimerism after allogeneic stem**

cell transplantation permits risk assessment of graft rejection. The following leukocyte lineages are of major importance in this context:
a) B-lymphocytes and plasma cells... ☐
b) Granulocytes and monocytes.. ☐
c) T-lymphocytes and natural killer (NK) cells .... ☐
d) Donor- and recipient-derived haematopoietic stem cells................. ☐

2. Impending relapse of leukaemia after allogeneic hHSCT may be revealed by the monitoring of chimerism. Which of the following findings is *not* suggestive of relapse?
a) Reappearance of recipient cells displaying the immunophenotype of the original leukaemia .... ☐
b) Increasing recipient chimerism within total leukocytes.................. ☐
c) Chimerism findings indicative of graft rejection....................... ☐
d) Increasing donor chimerism within total leukocytes .... ☐

* CHAPTER 17

Immunotherapy post-transplant

Inge Jedema, J.H. Frederik Falkenburg

1. Introduction

The use of immunosuppressive drugs including antibodies such as antithymocyte globulin (ATG) or anti-CD52 (alemtuzumab) in conditioning regimens preceding allo-HSCT is associated with delayed immune reconstitution, as is also the application of post-transplant immune suppression or removal of the T-cells from the graft to prevent GvHD. Since the immunological effect is the main therapeutic effect of allo-HSCT, this delayed immune reconstitution warrants the need for post-transplant immunotherapy strategies that can be applied early after the transplantation. This includes both therapeutic strategies to prevent or treat post-transplant infections by boosting the graft-versus-infection (GvL) reactivity and therapeutic strategies to prevent or treat active disease (relapse) by inducing profound graft-versus-tumour (GvT) reactivity in the absence of, or with limited, coinciding GvHD. Attempts to amplify GvL and GvT reactivities and to reduce GvHD reactivity are mainly based on timing and dosing of adoptive immunotherapy strategies and on the selection or depletion of specific cell types.

2. Immunotherapy for infections

2.1 Anti-viral immunity

In normal, immunocompetent individuals, viral infections are actively controlled by anti-viral immunity. This may comprise both the production of virus-specific antibodies by plasma cells and the generation and expansion of virus-specific T-cells. Antibodies may be especially effective in the prevention of viral infection of cells by capturing circulating viral particles. However, antibodies are unlikely to play an active role in the elimination of virus-infected cells. To obtain efficient, long-lasting anti-viral protection in individuals, the formation of virus-specific T-cell immunity is pivotal. These T-cells are capable of recognising peptides derived from the viral proteins which are presented in the HLA molecules of the virus-infected cells. During a primary virus infection, the T-cell response must be initiated from the naive T-cell compartment after priming by professional antigen presenting cells (APCs) presenting the relevant viral antigens. This will lead to the priming and expansion of virus-specific T-cells that are capable of controlling the viral infection. After the initial infectious episode, memory T-cells may persist, which can rapidly expand and react upon subsequent viral infections. Anti-viral T-cell immunity comprises both CD8 and CD4 positive T-cells. Virus-specific CD8 positive T-cells harbour the intrinsic potential to kill infected cells. This effector function is often accompanied by the production of pro-inflammatory cytokines including interferon (IFN)-γ, tumour necrosis factor (TNF)-α and interleukin (IL)-2. Although virus-specific

CD4 positive T-cells can exert a direct cytotoxic effect against virus-infected cells, their main function in the immunological cascade is thought to be a helper function. By the production of cytokines and their interaction with B-cells, the CD4 positive T-cells support the production of specific antibodies and the attraction and expansion of virus-specific CD8 positive T-cells. Therefore, effective antiviral immunity is mediated by the interplay between CD8 positive T-cells, CD4 positive T-cells and B-cells.

2.2 Viral infections after allogeneic stem cell transplantation
Following allo-HSCT a novel haematopoietic system of donor origin will reconstitute from the transplanted stem cells. This is a timely process, which is influenced by several factors including the age of the patient and the donor, the stem cell dose and source, and the pre-transplant conditioning. To avoid the occurrence of severe acute GvHD after the transplantation, post-transplant immune suppression is given or mature donor T-cells can be removed from the stem cell graft. Both strategies are associated with delayed post-transplant immune reconstitution in the patient, including the *de novo* formation of virus-specific T-cells from the transplanted stem cells. Moreover, due to the suppression and/or deletion of mature anti-viral donor T-cells from the stem cell graft, in the absence of autologous residual virus-specific T-cells, patients will be at risk for viral infections for a prolonged period after allo-HSCT. Although in all patients this anti-viral immunity will eventually reconstitute from the transplanted stem cells, late development of *de novo* immune responses often causes serious infectious complications early after transplantation in those situations where no mature anti-viral memory is either preserved in the recipient or transferred from the donor.

Viral infections are a major cause of morbidity and mortality after allo-HSCT. This mainly comprises infections with endogenous viruses including *Cytomegalovirus* (CMV), *Epstein-Barr virus* (EBV) and *Varicella zoster virus* (VZV), or *Adenovirus* (ADV) in children. Especially for CMV and EBV, the viral immune serological status of the patient and the stem cell donor are important risk factors for the incidence and severity of viral complications after the transplantation. The lowest risk is observed in seronegative patients transplanted with seronegative donors. In contrast, seropositive patients who receive a (T-cell depleted) stem cell graft from a seronegative donor have a higher risk for the development of severe post-transplant viral complications. Seropositive patients receiving a T-cell depleted stem cell graft from a seropositive donor are at intermediate risk for post-transplant infections, due to the possibility that low frequencies of protective virus-specific memory T-cells of donor or patient origin may be able to survive the conditioning or T-cell depletion therapies. Although viral reactivations can be treated with anti-viral drugs, long-lasting effective control is only achieved after development of anti-viral immunity.

To improve and/or accelerate the recovery of anti-viral immunity after allo-HSCT, different immunotherapeutic strategies have been explored. Since tolerance to donor cells is induced in the patient after allo-HSCT, adoptively transferred virus-specific donor T-cells may persist and mediate effective anti-viral control in the patient.

If anti-viral immunological memory is present in the donor (e.g. seropositive donors), the virus-specific T-cells are usually present at significant frequencies in peripheral blood of the donor. As described earlier, infusion of unselected mature donor T-cells (donor lymphocyte infusion, DLI) with or early after the transplant harbours a significant risk of inducing severe GvHD. Riddell et al. have pioneered the isolation and adoptive transfer of in vitro generated CMV-specific T-cell clones for viral control after allo-HSCT (1), and demonstrated the feasibility of this approach. However, broad clinical application required the development of novel strategies that can be applied under good manufacturing practice (GMP) conditions to allow rapid isolation of selected populations of virus-specific donor T-cells that are able to persist and mediate efficacy after adoptive transfer.

2.3 *In vitro* selection of CMV-specific memory T-cells

Especially for CMV-specific memory T-cells, extensive experience has been gained in recent years with various methods for *in vitro* selection. Virus-specific T-cells can be easily activated *in vitro* by stimulation of peripheral blood from virus-experienced donors with viral antigen. In earlier studies total viral lysates were used, but at present this uncontrolled product is not allowed in clinical grade production processes. For CMV, many HLA-class I binding peptides from the immunogenic CMV-derived proteins pp50, pp65 and immediate early antigen 1 (IE1) have been identified. Stimulation with these HLA-class I binding peptides results in the activation of only virus-specific CD8 positive T-cells. Since effective long-term anti-viral protection most likely requires the interplay between both CD8 and CD4 positive T-cells, more recently protein-spanning overlapping pools of longer (15mer) synthetic peptides have been used for the coordinated stimulation of virus-specific CD8 and CD4 positive T-cells. After stimulation, enrichment of the virus-specific T-cell populations can be achieved based on preferential expansion of the activated cells during subsequent *in vitro* culture. However, several studies have suggested that extensive *in vitro* expansion may be inversely correlated with the potential of the cells to survive and persist after adoptive transfer. Therefore, strategies have been developed to shorten the *in vitro* culture period. A very specific method is direct isolation of virus-specific T-cells based on their capacity to recognise and bind specific synthetic HLA-peptide multimeric complexes. These HLA-peptide multimers have been developed in different forms (e.g. tetramers, pentamers, streptamers), differing in the amount of HLA molecules in the complexes and the agents used for stabilisation of the complexes. These HLA-peptide multimers allow the selection of very pure populations of virus-specific T-cells using either flow cytometric cell sorting (FACS), based on fluorochromes bound to the HLA-peptide multimers, or magnetic bead separation (MACS) using magnetic beads coupled to the HLA-peptide multimers. However, since these HLA-peptide complexes are to date only available for a restricted number of, mainly class I, HLA molecules, this strategy is only suitable for the direct isolation of selected populations of CD8 positive virus-specific T-cells. To allow selection of broader populations of virus-specific T-cells, coordinated stimulations of both CD8 and CD4 positive virus-specific T-cells are performed using pools of long synthetic peptides derived from the immunogenic CMV proteins. Selection of the reactive T-cells has been performed based on markers for activated T-cells. This comprises FACS or MACS isolation based on the cell surface expression of an activation marker (e.g. CD154 (CD40L) or CD137 (4-1BB)) or MACS isolation based on the production of the cytokine IFN-γ using the IFN-γ capture system. In this system, the IFN-γ produced by the activated virus-specific T-cells is directly captured on the cell surface by specific monoclonal antibodies, followed by specific isolation of these cells using specific magnetic beads.

2.4 Adoptive transfer of CMV-specific T-cells to prevent or treat CMV reactivation or disease after allogeneic stem cell transplantation

Various clinical studies have been conducted to investigate the safety and efficacy of adoptive transfer of CMV-specific T-cells that have been selected *in vitro* using these different isolation strategies. In several studies, CMV-specific T-cells were applied in a prophylactic setting early (1–2 months) after transplantation to prevent the development of CMV disease. In other studies, CMV-specific T-cells were applied in a pre-emptive setting in patients with a positive CMV DNA load in peripheral blood (2). Adoptive transfer of CMV-specific T-cells has been used in a selected number of patients, in the treatment of active CMV disease (3). In the majority of patients expansion of CMV-specific T-cells was detected in peripheral blood after the adoptive transfer. This *in vivo* expansion of circulating virus-specific T-cells often coincided with clearance or prevention of development of a viral load. Intriguingly, adoptive transfer of extremely small cell numbers (1×10^3 cells/kg) appeared to be sufficient for the protective effect of the therapy. However, although the results obtained in these studies suggest the potential clinical efficacy of the adoptively transferred cells, controlled, randomised studies are necessary to really prove the role of the adoptively transferred cells. No adverse events related to the infusion of CMV-specific T-cells were reported in any of these studies.

2.5 Generation and adoptive transfer of EBV, ADV and *Aspergillus*-specific T-cells

Similar strategies have been used in a more limited number of studies to generate and adoptively transfer T-cells specific for EBV, ADV, or *Aspergillus*. EBV-specific T-cells have been applied to prevent or treat EBV-associated lymphoproliferative disorder (EBV-PTLD) or EBV-associated malignant lymphoma (4). Clinical responses have also been observed in these studies, in a significant number of patients, especially when the T-cells were applied in a prophylactic or pre-emptive setting. Treatment with ADV-specific T-cells has only been performed in a limited set of (mainly paediatric) patients who suffered from persisting ADV load after allo-HSCT that could not be cleared using pharmacological therapy. In the majority of these patients *in vivo* expansion of ADV-specific T-cells coincided by clearance of the viral load was observed. In Perugia, pathogen-specific CD4+ T-cell clones targeting CMV and *Aspergillus* were applied in patients after haploidentical transplantation, resulting in control of *Aspergillus* and CMV antigenaemia and infectious mortality (5). However, also in these studies there appeared to be an association between the adoptive transfer of the T-cells and the observed clinical effects but this requires confirmation in a randomised trial.

2.6 Immunotherapy to prevent or treat post-transplant infectious complications: Future strategies

Novel strategies under development comprise the generation of T-cell products targeting multiple pathogens, including CMV, EBV, and ADV (6). In the future also VZV, or other pathogens like *Aspergillus fumigatus* may be added as targets to this strategy. These multi-virus or multi-pathogen-specific T-cells may be derived from the original stem cell donor as outlined above, but there is also increasing clinical evidence that off-the-shelf products derived from unrelated third party healthy donors may be used to boost, at least temporarily, the anti-viral immunity in patients early after allo-HSCT. Future practice may include generation of large cell banks containing multi-virus-specific T-cell products with different HLA types. This would allow off-the-shelf application of fully or partially HLA-matched T-cell products when direct clinical intervention is warranted. Important to note is the potential GvHD risk associated with the adoptive transfer of HLA-mismatched virus-specific T-cells, due to the intrinsic chance of alloreactivity against non-self HLA molecules by these T-cells (7).

Another strategy that is currently being developed is the generation of virus-specific T-cell products from virus-inexperienced donors like seronegative adult stem cell donors and umbilical cord blood. In these situations the virus-specific T-cells are not present in the memory T-cell compartment, but must be primed and expanded from the naive T-cell compartment by stimulation with professional APC presenting the viral antigens, followed by selection or enrichment of the virus-specific T-cells.

This is a technically challenging strategy of which the success is influenced by several factors, including the extremely low frequencies of precursor T-cells directed against viral epitopes in the naive T-cell compartment. However, apparent successful strategies have been developed that allow the generation of virus-specific T-cell products for adoptive transfer from both seronegative adult donors (8) and umbilical cord blood (9), which will be or already have been translated into clinical practice.

Alternative strategies to induce or boost the anti-viral immunity post-transplant include vaccination of the stem cell donor or the patient with viral vaccines or adoptive transfer of autologous virus-specific T-cells harvested from peripheral blood of the patient prior to the transplant. Although strategies to vaccinate the donor or the patient are both being pursued at the moment, it is anticipated that the fully immunocompetent seropositive stem cell donor will be more capable of mounting an effective immune response after vaccination. In the situation of transplantation with an unrelated stem cell donor, this will probably raise ethical questions. Application of autologous of CMV-specific T-cells has been found to be feasible and effective for short-term anti-viral control. However, when an effective allo-response is induced post-transplant, these autologous virus-specific T-cells are likely to be eliminated by the alloreactive donor T-cells. Therefore, donor-derived anti-viral immunity will be required for long-term protection.

Several other strategies are being developed to preserve or boost post-transplant anti-viral immunity without the associated risk of GvHD, by infusion of donor T-cell populations depleted of potentially allo-reactive T-cells. In an ongoing study, patients are being treated with donor T-cell populations depleted of CD45RA expressing naive T-cells, based on the assumption that the anti-viral immunity is present in the CD45RA negative memory T-cell compartment, whereas the allo-reactive T-cells mediating the GvHD are mainly present in the naive compartment. Another strategy is the adoptive transfer of enriched populations of CD4 positive donor T-cells, obtained either by positive CD4 selection or CD8 depletion. Since under normal, non-inflammatory conditions, HLA-class II expression is mainly restricted to haematopoietic cells, application of CD4 enriched donor T-cell populations early after transplantation may result in protection from viral infections with a limited risk of inducing GvHD. In several non-randomised studies CD4 enriched donor T-cell populations have been safely applied (10) and a randomised study analysing the effect or prophylactic CD4 DLI at three months after T-cell-depleted allo-HSCT is currently applied in Leiden. Another strategy that is currently pursued in a clinical study is the generation of donor T-cell products depleted for potentially allo-reactive cells using a photodepletion strategy. In this strategy, T-cells activated by non-haematopoietic cells of the recipient are depleted using a light sensitive dye.

3. Immunotherapy for persistent or recurrent malignant disease after allogeneic stem cell transplantation

3.1 The post-transplant allo-response

Although stem cell donors are preferentially HLA-matched with the recipient, genetic differences between individuals caused by single nucleotide polymorphisms (SNPs) give rise to the formation of proteins that are differentially processed and presented as peptides on cells of the recipient and the donor. These so-called minor histocompatibility antigens (MiHA) have been described as targets for the allo-response of donor T-cells recognising cells of the recipient after allo-HSCT. Skewing of the immune response towards MiHA that are selectively expressed on haematopoietic cells of the patient may give rise to a specific graft-versus-tumour (GvT) response without coinciding GvHD. In contrast, when the immune response is directed against MiHA with a ubiquitous expression on both haematopoietic and non-haematopoietic cells of the recipient, severe GvHD may accompany the GvT response (11). Targeting of so-called tumour-associated antigens may also lead to a specific GvT without GvHD. These tumour-associated antigens like Wilm's tumor protein 1 (WT1), proteinase 3 (PR1), and preferentially expressed antigen in melanoma (PRAME) are self antigens that show over-expression in malignant cells of different origins. It is however questionable whether donor T-cells are not tolerised against these antigens in the fully HLA-matched allo-HSCT setting due to low expression in normal cells.

Since T-cells that reconstitute from the transplanted donor stem cells are educated in the immunological environment of the patient, these T-cells will likely be tolerised against patient-derived MiHA. Therefore, the most potent allo-response is induced when mature donor T-cells recognising MiHA expressed on cells of the recipient are adoptively transferred into the patient.

3.2 Donor lymphocyte infusion for the prevention or treatment of post-transplant disease

Infusion of unselected mature donor T-cell populations (DLI) has been broadly applied to prevent or treat post-transplant residual or recurring malignancy (12). Application of these unselected mature donor T-cell populations containing a broad spectrum of potentially allo-reactive T-cells at the time of the transplant or early (within 3 months) after the transplant often results in the induction of severe GvHD, even at dosages as low as 0.1×10^6 T-cells/kg. Delaying application to more than 6 months post-transplant of unselected DLI at dosages as high as $1–5 \times 10^6$ T-cells/kg has been found to be a feasible therapeutic strategy that is associated with a more limited risk of GvHD. This lower incidence of GvHD after delayed application of DLI may be explained by several factors including the absence of tissue damage by the conditioning and the resulting pro-inflammatory environment, and the limited homeostatic proliferation due to the immune recovery at later time points after the transplantation. Another factor likely to play an important role in the specificity of the immune response that is induced after delayed versus early application of DLI is the substitution of professional APCs in the recipient by cells of donor origin. As a result, the main cells of recipient origin that can elicit an immune response by the infused mature donor T-cells are likely to be the circulating malignant cells or professional APCs from donor origin cross-presenting recipient-specific antigens after engulfment of (apoptotic) tumor cells. This combination of factors probably skews the specificity of the immune response towards antigens expressed on the haematopoietic cells of the patient.

Although delayed application of unselected DLI can lead to the induction of profound GvT responses, this is certainly not the case in all patients. Especially patients with slowly progressing disease and a malignancy consisting of cells with an intrinsic APC phenotype, like chronic myeloid leukaemia (CML) in chronic phase, do benefit greatly from the GvT response after allo-HSCT and DLI. In patients with other relatively slowly progressing disease like multiple myeloma (MM) or chronic lymphocytic leukaemia (CLL) the highly variable APC function of the malignant cell is often likely to hamper the induction of a proper GvT response. In patients with more aggressive diseases like CML in accelerated phase or blast crisis, acute myeloid leukaemia (AML) and acute lymphoblastic leukaemia (ALL) the rapid progression of the disease and the time necessary for the immune response to be induced and amplified will significantly lower the therapeutic capacity of DLI. As a result, the application of unmodified DLI results in the induction of effective GvT responses in only 10–40% of the non-CML patients.

3.3 Strategies to increase the anti-tumour reactivity after donor lymphocyte infusion

Since the limited immunogenicity of especially the B-cell malignancies CLL, ALL and MM may hamper proper activation of the donor T-cells after DLI, various groups have explored the clinical safety and efficacy of pre-activated DLI. In these studies donor lymphocytes were activated *in vitro* using anti-CD3/anti-CD28 T-cell stimulation beads. This resulted in vigorous activation and polyclonal expansion of the donor T-cells, thereby increasing the total numbers as well as probably the activation threshold for secondary stimulation of potentially alloreactive T-cells. Indeed, GvT responses were observed after application of pre-activated DLI, coinciding with acceptable GvHD (13). Another non-specific way to increase the likelihood of developing an effective GvT response after DLI is the simultaneous treatment with the pro-inflammatory cytokine IFN-α.

In several clinical studies strategies have been explored to boost the GvT effect after DLI by using vaccination with either tumour-associated antigens (WT1, survivin, PR1), MiHA (HA-1), or disease-specific idiotype proteins. These strategies included vaccination with synthetic peptides, vaccination of dendritic cells (DCs) loaded with the specific antigens, and vaccination with DCs loaded with apoptotic malignant cells of the patients. Although increased frequencies of T-cells recognising the specific antigens have been observed in peripheral blood of the patients after vaccination, thus far no sustained overt clinical responses that could be attributed to the vaccination have been reported.

Besides T-cells, natural killer (NK) cells may also mediate a potent GvT response after allo-HSCT (14). Different strategies are being pursued to isolate and adoptively transfer either mature donor NK cells or NK cells in vitro expanded from donor CD34+ stem cells. Especially in the HLA mismatched allo-HSCT setting the alloreactive potential of donor NK cells may be most effectively exploited, due to the license to kill signal triggered by the absence of self HLA molecules on the (malignant) cells of the patient.

3.4 Suicide gene transduced T-cells as a safe treatment for early post-transplant relapses

As outlined above, application of mature donor T-cells with or early after allo-HSCT is associated with the induction of severe GvHD. This hampers the use of DLI for the prevention or treatment of relapses occurring early after the transplantation. Bonini et al. (15) pioneered the equipment of donor T-cells with the suicide gene TK via retroviral gene transfer technologies. These cells can be easily eliminated using ganciclovir treatment at the moment that they induce an undesired immune response in the GvHD direction. This strategy was found to be feasible and interestingly the infusion of TK-transduced T-cells appeared to augment and accelerate the reconstitution of non-TK-transduced donor cells, thereby reducing the immune compromised period.

3.5 Adoptive transfer of in vitro generated tumour-reactive donor T-cells

Adoptive strategy of in vitro generated tumor-reactive donor T-cells will be an elegant strategy to prevent or treat disease relapses or persistence early after transplantation. Since the normal haematopoiesis after allo-HSCT is of donor origin, treatment of patients with donor T-cells recognising with relative specificity antigens expressed on haematopoietic cells of the patient is anticipated to result in a specific GvT effect while preserving donor haematopoiesis in the patient, and to result in limited GvHD reactivity. Different strategies have been explored in the recent years and are being optimised to improve the *in vitro* selection and *in vivo* persistence and efficacy of the cells. Different groups have generated leukaemia-reactive T-cells by co-culture of donor T-cells with APCs generated from primary leukaemic blasts of the patient. Enrichment by preferential *in vitro* expansion or selection based on T-cell activation markers like IFN-γ production or expression of activation markers (e.g. CD154 and CD137) has been applied (16). In a limited number of patients these T-cells have demonstrated to be of potential clinical efficacy (17, 18), but larger clinical studies are necessary to prove the feasibility and efficacy of both the generation and the clinical effect of these cells. The discovery of an increasing number of MiHA allows the selection of those antigens that have selective expression on haematopoietic cells to be used as targets for the generation of tumour-reactive T-cells. These antigens can be used either *in vivo* vaccination strategies to boost post-transplant GvT reactivity or as an *in vitro* vaccine loaded on professional APC to generate leukaemia-reactive T-cells *in vitro*. Strategies have been developed to induce primary immune responses from the naive donor T-cell repertoire followed by subsequent isolation of the reactive cells either based on their cell surface expression of an activation marker (CD137) or production of IFN-γ, or based on the specificity of their TCR using HLA/peptide multimers (8). These strategies will be translated to clinical protocols shortly.

3.6 *In vitro* generation of tumour-reactive T-cells by redirection of T-cell reactivity using TCR gene transfer or introduction of chimeric antigen receptors
Anti tumour reactivity specific for MiHA can be transferred to other T-cells using retroviral gene transfer of the specific T-cell receptor (TCR) encoding genes (19). Different groups are about to test the clinical feasibility of donor T-cells equipped with gene-transferred TCRs against tumour-associated antigens (WT1, PRAME and several melanoma antigens) or against MiHA (HA-1). By introducing these TCRs in a population of donor T-cells with a defined specificity (e.g. virus-specific T-cells), a T-cell product with potent GvT reactivity but no GvHD reactivity can be generated. Non MHC-restricted chimaeric antigen receptors (CARs) combine antigen-specificity and T-cell activating properties in a single fusion molecule that is introduced into donor T-cells via gene transfer (20). T-cell survival is promoted by the addition of the cytoplasmic regions of CD3 zeta, CD28 and/or CD137 to the construct. Clinical studies using T-cells engineered with different CARs directed against for instance CD19 are currently being pursued.

References
1.   Walter EA, Greenberg PD, Gilbert MJ et al. Reconstitution of cellular immunity against cytomegalovirus in recipients of allogeneic bone marrow by transfer of T-cell clones from the donor. N Engl J Med 1995; 333: 1038–1044.

2. Einsele H, Roosnek E, Rufer N et al. Infusion of cytomegalovirus (CMV)-specific T-cells for the treatment of CMV infection not responding to antiviral chemotherapy. Blood 2002; 99: 3916–3922.

3. Feuchtinger T, Opherk K, Bethge WA et al. Adoptive transfer of pp65-specific T-cells for the treatment of chemorefractory cytomegalovirus disease or reactivation after haploidentical and matched unrelated stem cell transplantation. Blood 2010; 116: 4360–4367.

4. Bollard CM, Aguilar L, Straathof KC et al. Cytotoxic T lymphocyte therapy for Epstein-Barr virus+ Hodgkin's disease. J Exp Med 2004; 200: 1623–1633.

5. Perruccio K, Tosti A, Burchielli E et al. Transferring functional immune responses to pathogens after haploidentical hematopoietic transplantation. Blood 2005; 106: 4397–4406.

6. Hanley PJ, Shaffer DR, Cruz CR et al. Expansion of T-cells targeting multiple antigens of cytomegalovirus, Epstein-Barr virus and adenovirus to provide broad antiviral specificity after stem cell transplantation. Cytotherapy 2011; 13: 976–986.

7. Amir AL, D'Orsogna LJ, Roelen DL et al. Allo-HLA reactivity of virus-specific memory T-cells is common. Blood 2010; 115: 3146–3157.

8. Jedema I, van de Meent M, Pots J et al. Successful generation of primary virus-specific and anti-tumor T-cell responses from the naive donor T-cell repertoire is determined by the balance between antigen-specific precursor T-cells and regulatory T-cells. Haematologica 2011; 96: 1204–1212.

9. Hanley PJ, Cruz CR, Savoldo B et al. Functionally active virus-specific T-cells that target CMV, adenovirus, and EBV can be expanded from naive T-cell populations in cord blood and will target a range of viral epitopes. Blood 2009; 114: 1958–1967.

10. Meyer RG, Wagner EM, Konur A et al. Donor CD4 T-cells convert mixed to full donor T-cell chimerism and replenish the CD52-positive T-cell pool after alemtuzumab-based T-cell-depleted allo-transplantation. Bone Marrow Transplant 2010; 45: 668–674.

11. Falkenburg JH, van de Corput L, Marijt EW, Willemze R. Minor histocompatibility antigens in human stem cell transplantation. Exp Hematol 2003; 31: 743–751.

12. Kolb HJ. Graft-versus-leukemia effects of transplantation and donor lymphocytes. Blood 2008; 112: 4371–4383.

13. Porter DL, Levine BL, Bunin N et al. A phase 1 trial of donor lymphocyte infusions expanded and activated ex vivo via CD3/CD28 costimulation. Blood 2006; 107: 1325–1331.

14. Velardi A, Ruggeri L, Mancusi A et al. Natural killer cell allorecognition of missing self in allogeneic hematopoietic transplantation: A tool for immunotherapy of leukemia. Curr Opin Immunol 2009; 21: 525–530.

15. Ciceri F, Bonini C, Stanghellini MT et al. Infusion of suicide-gene-engineered donor lymphocytes after family haploidentical haemopoietic stem-cell transplantation for leukaemia (the TK007 trial): A non-randomised phase I-II study. Lancet Oncol 2009; 10: 489–500.

16. Jedema I, Meij P, Steeneveld E et al. Early detection and rapid isolation of leukemia-reactive donor T-cells for adoptive transfer using the IFN-gamma secretion assay. Clin Cancer Res 2007; 13: 636–643.

17. Falkenburg JHF, Wafelman AR, Joosten P et al. Complete remission of accelerated phase chronic myeloid leukemia by treatment with leukemia-reactive cytotoxic T lymphocytes. Blood 1999; 94: 1201–1208.
18. Warren EH, Fujii N, Akatsuka Y et al. Therapy of relapsed leukemia after allogeneic hematopoietic cell transplant with T-cells specific for minor histocompatibility antigens. Blood 2010; 115: 3869–3878.
19. Heemskerk MH, Hoogeboom M, Hagedoorn R et al. Reprogramming of virus-specific T-cells into leukemia-reactive T-cells using T-cell receptor gene transfer. J Exp Med 2004; 199: 885–894.
20. Sadelain M, Brentjens R, Riviere I. The promise and potential pitfalls of chimeric antigen receptors. Curr Opin Immunol 2009; 21: 215–223.

Multiple Choice Questionnaire

To find the correct answer, go to http://www.esh.org/online-training/handbook/

1. **The use of immunosuppressive drugs including antibodies such as antithymocyte globulin (ATG) or anti-CD52 (alemtuzumab) in conditioning regimens preceding the allogeneic stem cell transplantation is associated with an increased risk of disease relapses due to:**
   a) The higher incidence of graft rejection ☐
   b) Promotion of malignant cell proliferation ☐
   c) The depletion/suppression of donor T-cells mediating the allo-immune effect ☐
   d) The higher incidence of viral complications ☐

2. **CMV seropositive patients who receive a stem cell graft from a CMV seronegative donor have a high risk for the development of severe post-transplant viral complications because:**
   a) The donor T cells are infected with the CMV virus residing in the patient ☐
   b) The donor T-cell population does not contain CMV-specific memory cells ☐
   c) The donor T-cells are rejected by the patient ☐
   d) They are often resistant to conventional anti-viral therapy ☐

3. **Infusion of unselected mature donor T-cells with or early after allogeneic stem cell transplantation harbors a significant risk of inducing severe GvHD, because:**
   a) These T-cells are educated in the immunological environment of the donor ☐
   b) These T-cells are rejected by the immune system of the patient ☐
   c) These T-cells suppress recovery of normal B-cells in the patient ☐
   d) These T-cells delay the engraftment of the transplanted stem cells ☐

4. **Adoptive transfer of which cell population is unlikely to increase GvL reactivity after allogeneic stem cell transplantation?**
   a) Regulatory T-cells (T_{reg}) ☐
   b) Alloreactive NK cells ☐
   c) MiHA-specific $CD4^+$ T-cells ☐
   d) MiHA-specific $CD8^+$ T-cells ☐

5. **The optimal cell product for immunotherapy post-transplant contains a cell population with:**
   a) Short *in vivo* persistence ☐
   b) A broad reactivity against cells of the patient ☐
   c) Short telomeres ☐
   d) Defined antigen specificity ☐

CHAPTER 18

Indications for
and current practice of
allogeneic and autologous HSCT

Alois Gratwohl, Helen Baldomero, Anna Sureda

1. Introduction

In 1973 when EBMT was founded, HSCT was restricted to allogeneic bone marrow transplantation for acute leukaemias, aplastic anaemia and severe combined immunodeficiency (1). Since then it has evolved into a complex medical process using autologous or allogeneic stem cells from bone marrow, peripheral blood or cord blood from patients, family donors or unrelated volunteers (2). HSCT is supplemented today by donations of additional cells, such as donor lymphocyte infusions, natural killer cells, mesenchymal cells or others from the stem cell donor or a third party donor. It has expanded to the use of HSC for non-haematopoietic use and also the transplantation of non-haematopoietic stem cells. There have been major changes in indications, such as the rise and fall of autologous HSCT for breast cancer or of allogeneic HSCT for chronic myeloid leukaemia (CML), and in technology as illustrated by the change from bone marrow to peripheral blood, the rapid increase in use of unrelated donors and the introduction of reduced-intensity conditioning. It is apparent that some guidance is warranted, for transplant teams, hospital administrators, health care providers and also patients. It is evident that recommendations have to be given with caution in an ever-changing field when follow-up is lacking for recently introduced methods and long term observations relate to technologies no longer used today. EBMT has recognised this need and has published on a regular basis over the last two decades reports on indications for and current practice of HSCT in Europe for haematological disorders, solid tumours, immune disorders and inborn errors of metabolism for adults and children (Table 1A and 1B) (3). This chapter will review the basic concepts underlying current practice and give a view of likely future developments.

2. Health Technology Assessment considerations

Most countries are confronted today with rising health care costs. In any system based on the solidarity principle, tools are required to close the gap between increasing demands and limited health care budgets. Health Technology Assessment (HTA) is considered by many as such an instrument. It was introduced initially as an instrument to exclude harmful and ineffective procedures from reimbursement. It was soon expanded to include efficacy and efficiency, expressed as the gain in quality adjusted years of life (QALY) compared to other treatment approaches, primarily based on prospective randomised studies according to the principles of evidence-based medicine (4). HSCT has been subject of HTA questions in the past; and it is easy to predict that HSCT teams will be confronted increasingly with such assessments in the future. There are inherent difficulties in such a process. Few if any prospective randomised studies have established the role of HSCT unequivocally. Long term follow-up is essential since the inherent early mortality associated with

Table 1: Indications for HSCT by EBMT. Recommendations 2010

A. Adult patients

Disease	Disease stage	Donor type			
		HLA id sib	Matched unrelated	Mismatched donor	Auto
AML	CR1 (low risk)	CO	D	GNR	CO
	CR1 (intermediate risk)	S	CO	D	S
	CR1 (high-risk)	S	S	CO	CO
	CR2	S	S	CO	CO
	CR3, incipient relapse	S	CO	D	GNR
	M3 molecular persistence	S	CO	GNR	GNR
	M3 molecular CR2	S	CO	GNR	S
	REL or refractory disease	CO	D	D	GNR
ALL	CR1 (stand/intermed risk)	D	GNR	GNR	D
	CR1 (high-risk)	S	S	CO	D
	CR2 incipient relapse	S	S	CO	GNR
	REL or refractory disease	CO	D	D	GNR
CML	1st CP, failed imatinib	S	S	CO	D
	Accelerated phase, >1st CP	S	S	CO	D
	Blast crisis	CO	CO	CO	GNR
MF	Primary, secondary with intermediate or high Lille score	S	S	D	GNR
MDS	RA, RAEB	S	S	CO	GNR
	RAEB-t, sAML, CR1, CR2	S	S	CO	CO
	More advanced stages	S	CO	D	GNR
CLL	High-risk disease	S	S	D	CO
NHL					
DLBC	CR1 (intermed/high-risk at Dx)	GNR	GNR	GNR	CO
	Chemosensitive REL, ≥CR2	CO	CO	GNR	S
	Refractory disease	D	D	GNR	GNR
Mantle cell	CR1	CO	D	GNR	S
	Chemosensitive REL, ≥CR2	CO	D	GNR	S
	Refractory disease	D	D	GNR	GNR
LL, BL	CR1	CO	CO	GNR	CO
	Chemosensitive REL, ≥CR2	CO	CO	GNR	CO
	Refractory disease	D	D	GNR	GNR
Follicular	CR1 (intermed/high-risk at Dx)	GNR	GNR	GNR	CO
	Chemosensitive REL, ≥CR2	CO	CO	D	S
	Refractory disease	CO	CO	D	GNR

continue

A. Adult patients

Disease	Disease stage	Donor type			
		HLA id sib	Matched unrelated	Mismatched donor	Auto
NHL (cont.)					
T-cell NHL	CR1	CO	D	GNR	CO
	Chemosensitive REL, ≥CR2	CO	CO	GNR	D
	Refractory disease	D	D	GNR	GNR
Hodgkin's lymphoma					
	CR1	GNR	GNR	GNR	GNR
	Chemosensitive REL, ≥CR2	CO	CO	CO	S
	Refractory disease	D	D	GNR	CO
Nodular	CT1	GNR	GNR	GNR	GNR
Lymphocyte predominant	Chemosensitive REL, ≥CR2	GNR	GNR	GNR	CO
	Refractory disease	GNR	GNR	GNR	CO
Multiple myeloma		CO	CO	GNR	S
Primary amyloidosis		CO	CO	GNR	CO
SAA	Newly diagnosed	S	CO	GNR	GNR
	REL, refractory	S	S	CO	GNR
PNH		S	CO	CO	GNR
Solid tumours					
Breast cancer	Adjuvant high-risk	GNR	GNR	GNR	CO
	Metastatic respond	D	D	GNR	D/CO
Germ cell	Sensitive REL	GNR	GNR	GNR	CO
	3rd line refractory	GNR	GNR	GNR	S
Ovarian cancer	CR/PR	GNR	GNR	GNR	D
	Platinum sensitive REL	D	GNR	GNR	NO
Medulloblastoma	Post-surgery	GNR	GNR	GNR	D
Small cell lung	Limited stage	GNR	GNR	GNR	D
Renal cell ca	Metastatic, cytokine refr	CO	CO	GNR	NO
Soft cell sarcoma	Metastatic responsive	D	GNR	GNR	D
AID					
Immune cytopenias		CO	D	D	CO
Systemic sclerosis		D	GNR	GNR	CO
Rheumatoid arthritis		NO	GNR	GNR	CO
Multiple sclerosis		D	GNR	GNR	CO
Lupus erythematosus		D	GNR	GNR	CO
Crohn's disease		NO	GNR	GNR	CO
CIDP		NO	GNR	GNR	D

continue

B. Paediatric patients

Disease	Disease stage	Donor type			
		HLA id sib	Matched unrelated	Mismatched donor	Auto
AML	CR1, low risk	GNR	GNR	GNR	GNR
	CR1, high risk	S	CO	GNR	S
	CR1, very high risk	S	S	CO	CO
	CR2	S	S	S	S
	>CR2	CO	D	D	GNR
ALL	CR1, low risk	GNR	GNR	GNR	GNR
	CR1, high risk	S	S	CO	GNR
	CR2	S	S	CO	CO
	>CR2	S	S	CO	CO
CML	Chronic phase	S	S	D	GNR
	Advanced phase	S	S	CO	GNR
NHL	CR1, low risk	GNR	GNR	GNR	GNR
	CR1, high risk	CO	CO	GNR	CO
	CR2	S	S	CO	CO
HD	CR1	GNR	GNR	GNR	GNR
	1st REL, CR2	CO	D	GNR	S
MDS		S	S	D	GNR
Primary immunodeficiencies		S	S	S	NA
Thalassemia		S	CO	GNR	NA
Sickle cell anaemia, high risk		S	CO	GNR	NA
Aplastic anaemia		S	S	CO	NA
Fanconi anaemia		S	S	CO	NA
Blackfan-Diamond anaemia		S	CO	GNR	NA
CGD		S	S	CO	NA
Kostman's disease		S	S	GNR	NA
MPS-1H Hurler		S	S	CO	NA
MPS -1H Hurler-Scheie (severe)		GNR	GNR	GNR	NA
MPS -VI Maroteaux-Lamy		CO	CO	CO	NA
Osteopetrosis		S	S	S	NA
Other storage diseases		GNR	GNR	GNR	NA
Autoimmune disorders		GNR	GNR	GNR	CO
Germ cell tumour		GNR	GNR	GNR	CO
Ewing's sarcoma, high risk or >CR1		D	GNR	GNR	S
Soft tissue sarcoma, high risk or >CR1		D	D	GNR	CO
Neuroblastoma, high risk		CO	GNR	GNR	S
Neuroblastoma >CR1		CO	D	D	S
Wilms' tumour, >CR1		GNR	GNR	GNR	CO
Osteogenic sarcoma		GNR	GNR	GNR	D
Brain tumours		GNR	GNR	GNR	CO

The table provides graded recommendations for HSCT by indication, disease stage and donor type as published by EBMT in 2010 (see ref. 3). Grading is grouped into four categories: S: standard of care; CO: clinical option, can be carried out after careful assessment of risks and benefits; D: developmental; should be carried out only at accredited and experienced centres on IRB approved protocols; GNR: generally nor recommended. Donor type is subdivided into: HLA id sib: HLA identical sibling donor; matched unrelated: there is no uniformly accepted definition. A ≥10/10 antigen matched donor is unequivocally considered as matched. Mismatched donor: there is no uniformly accepted definition. A <8/8 antigen matched unrelated and a >1 antigen mismatched family donor is unequivocally considered as mismatched. Each team should have their own insitutional guidelines. Mismatched donor HSCT should be carried out only at accredited and experienced centres on IRB approved protocols. Auto: autologous HSCT. A syngeneic twin donor is generally considered as S for all indications except, by definition, congenital disorders. As discussed in the text, the table serves as starting point for risk adapted assessment

HSCT gives different outcomes early compared to late after treatment. Past analyses of patients with a donor vs no donor, specifically in AML, have integrated disease risks but not HSCT risks. Hence, the key questions to be asked for HTA will be whether HSCT for a given patient, with a given disease, at a given time point with the given donor with the planned transplant technique at the selected transplant centre will provide a better quality adjusted survival at lower costs than an alternative therapy. It is evident that the answer will not only depend on the disease indication or the donor type but might be different in different countries (5).

3. Current status (activity survey 2009)
EBMT has collected, analysed and regularly published since 1990 numbers of HSCT in Europe by indication, donor type and stem cell source (6). This gives an oversight, in a snapshot, of current practice and, when integrated into the previous reports, yields information on trends and permits predictions for the future. The report was initially introduced as a quality control instrument. Recently, the World Health Organization (WHO; *www.who.org*) has recognised in its guiding principles on organ, cell and tissue transplants the importance of an annual survey and defined data collection and data analysis as integral part of any therapy. The EBMT survey hence was expanded to a global survey by the Worldwide Network for Blood and Marrow Transplantation WBMT (5). Figure 1 illustrates the indications for allogeneic (1A) and autologous (1B) HSCT in Europe for the year 2009 as well as the donor types for allogeneic HSCT (1C) (2).

4. Macroeconomic factors associated with use of HSCT
Numbers of HSCT, distribution in indications and use of technologies vary between countries in absolute terms as well as by transplant rates, e.g. the number of transplants per number of inhabitants. This may in part relate to differences in prevalence of a disease entity, as exemplified by the haemoglobinopathies. Recent

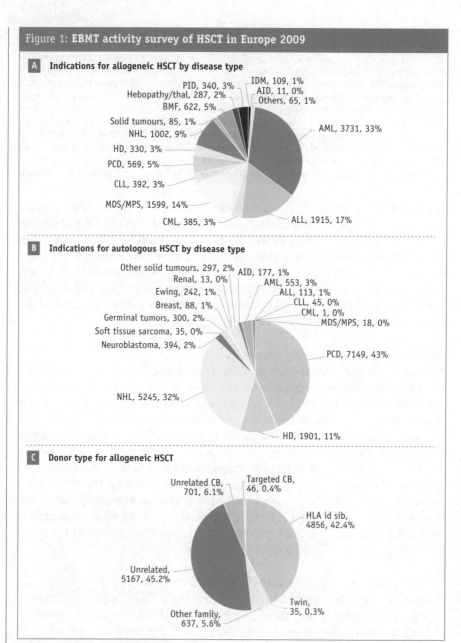

Figure 1: **EBMT activity survey of HSCT in Europe 2009**

A Indications for allogeneic HSCT by disease type

PID, 340, 3%
Hebopathy/thal, 287, 2%
BMF, 622, 5%
Solid tumours, 85, 1%
NHL, 1002, 9%
HD, 330, 3%
PCD, 569, 5%
CLL, 392, 3%
MDS/MPS, 1599, 14%
CML, 385, 3%
IDM, 109, 1%
AID, 11, 0%
Others, 65, 1%
AML, 3731, 33%
ALL, 1915, 17%

B Indications for autologous HSCT by disease type

Other solid tumours, 297, 2%
Renal, 13, 0%
Ewing, 242, 1%
Breast, 88, 1%
Germinal tumors, 300, 2%
Soft tissue sarcoma, 35, 0%
Neuroblastoma, 394, 2%
AID, 177, 1%
AML, 553, 3%
ALL, 113, 1%
CLL, 45, 0%
CML, 1, 0%
MDS/MPS, 18, 0%
PCD, 7149, 43%
NHL, 5245, 32%
HD, 1901, 11%

C Donor type for allogeneic HSCT

Unrelated CB, 701, 6.1%
Targeted CB, 46, 0.4%
HLA id sib, 4856, 42.4%
Unrelated, 5167, 45.2%
Twin, 35, 0.3%
Other family, 637, 5.6%

Reprinted with permission from (2)

studies have given more insight into the underlying macroeconomic mechanisms. Availability of resources (as expressed by gross national income per capita), governmental support (as expressed by governmental health care expenditures) and access to therapy (as expressed by team density) are key determinants for the establishment of a procedure in a given country. Availability of economical resources, evidence, external regulations and expectations of the physicians are the key factors (the 4 "E") for the diffusion of HSCT technology (5, 7). Hence HSCT, as any other therapy, is undertaken if the therapy is paid for, if there is some evidence for a benefit, if external regulations permit its use and if physicians and patients believe HSCT to be the best possible approach.

It is one of the major challenges for EBMT to provide such evidence by data collection and analysis and to harmonise external regulations between the competent national authorities in order to safeguard the financial basis of HSCT through the respective national HTA agencies. AHCTA, the Alliance for Harmonisation of Cellular Therapy Accreditation (*www.ahcta.org*) has undertaken the task to coordinate this harmonisation on a global level. Recent data give proof that the introduction of the quality management system JACIE (*www.jacie.org*) is indeed associated with better outcome of individual patients (8). Data show as well that teams in principle follow recommendations by EBMT (2).

5. Risk factors associated with outcome of HSCT

The outcome of HSCT is not erratic; its risk can be assessed with reasonable accuracy. Already twenty years ago, the EBMT risk score was introduced for patients with CML, the most frequent indication for an allogeneic HSCT at that time. It showed that patient age, disease stage, donor type and donor recipient gender combination each had an impact on outcome and that each of the five pre-transplant risk factors added to the overall risk (Table 2). Transplant-related mortality increased in a stepwise pattern with increasing risk score, and survival decreased correspondingly. Recent analyses confirmed that patients transplanted at an older age, in a more advanced disease stage, after a longer time interval from diagnosis (autologous and allogeneic HSCT) and with a donor other than an HLA identical sibling donor and a female donor for a male recipient (allogeneic HSCT) had uniformly a worse outcome than younger patients, transplanted still in early disease after a short time interval from diagnosis from an HLA identical sex-matched sibling donor (9, 10). The risk score was correlated with all three outcomes, non-relapse mortality, relapse risk and survival, for patients transplanted with any acquired haematological disease, with reduced or standard conditioning, with T-cell depleted or T-cell replete graft products and with bone marrow, peripheral blood or cord blood as stem cell source. Non-relapse mortality was always higher with a higher EBMT risk score,

Table 2: EBMT risk score definition and additional pre-transplant risk factors

Risk factor	Score points
Age of the patient, years	
<20	0
20–40	1
>40	2
Disease stage[1]	
Early	0
Intermediate	1
Late	2
Time interval from diagnosis to transplant, months[2]	
<12	0
>12	1
Donor type[3]	
HLA-identical sibling donor	0
Unrelated donor, other	1
Donor recipient sex combination[3]	
All other	0
Female donor, male recipient	1
Additional additive elements, not yet formally validated	**Add or deduct from score**
Patient CMV serostatus positive	1
Karnofsky performance score ≤80	1
Comorbidity score >3	1
Iron overload	1
For unrelated donors	
HLA matching ≥10/10 antigens	-1
Frequent haplotype/high probability to find a donor	-1

[1] See reference (9) for definitions according to main disease category. Disease stage does not apply for aplastic anaemia (score 0). [2] Does not apply for patients transplanted in first complete remission (score 0). [3] Does not apply for patients with autologous HSCT (score 0)

survival correspondingly lower with increasing score, regardless of the technology used. The score was validated for all teams regardless of their JACIE accreditation status and for teams in high, middle or low income countries defined by World Bank Category. These pre-transplant factors influenced risk in an additive way (8, 9). This holds true for other well described pre-transplant factors not captured with the EBMT score, such as CMV serostatus, comorbidity, performance score, degree of matching for unrelated donors or non-HLA polymorphisms. Their impact is not uniform and depends on the sum of the risks. Some factors become negligible with increasing risks, others predominant. Survival is worse for CMV seropositive patients compared to CMV seronegative patients in low- but not in very high-risk patients (risk score 5–7). Hence, the additional influence of CMV serostatus becomes negligible in high-risk patients (Figure 2). In contrast, a poor performance score has little additional negative effects in low-risk patients; it has a deleterious effect in patients with a high EBMT risk score. Similar analyses have indicated that the benefit of optimal matching in unrelated donor transplants is greatest in low-risk patients (10).

Pre-transplant risk assessment is essential to advise for or against HSCT and for choosing the adequate transplant technique. Conditioning intensity can be used to shift the balance between risks of transplant-related mortality and relapse. A wide variety of reduced-intensity conditioning (RIC) regimens has been introduced and almost one-third of all allogeneic HSCT is now performed with a RIC regimen. There are no data from prospective randomised studies but multiple retrospective comparative studies indeed show that early mortality is reduced with RIC regimens at the expense of a higher relapse rate with probably little impact on long-term survival. It might be advised for older patients with comorbidities and relative low-risk disease; *vice versa* standard conditioning should remain the therapy of choice for younger patients with no comorbidity and for those with high-risk disease.

6. Goal of recommendations and principles

Over the past twenty years EBMT has published on a regular basis recommendations on current practice and classified indications for HSCT as: 1. standard of care,

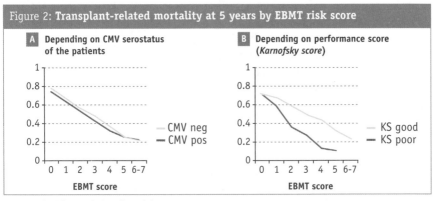

Figure 2: **Transplant-related mortality at 5 years by EBMT risk score**

A Depending on CMV serostatus of the patients
— CMV neg
— CMV pos
EBMT score

B Depending on performance score (*Karnofsky score*)
— KS good
— KS poor
EBMT score

Reprinted with permission from (9)

2. clinical option, 3. developmental and 4. generally not recommended (3). This has been proven useful for a long period and the principle still holds true. Recommendations do not imply, however, that a transplant should always be performed for a recommended indication nor that it should not be used for a non-recommended one. Risk assessment needs to be integrated. HSCT is never "the only chance for cure". It is always associated with the risk for early mortality. These years of life lost need to be recovered compared to a non-transplant treatment strategy. The latter have made considerable progress as well as illustrated by the introduction of tyrosine kinase inhibitors for CML, better supportive strategies in MDS, or gene therapy and enzyme replacement for congenital disorders. HSCT must therefore provide for the individual patient a better outcome than a non-transplant strategy, with better long-term survival and at a lower price. Hence, a patient with low-risk AML might be considered for allogeneic HSCT in first CR if he or she is CMV seronegative, has no comorbidity, is in optimal clinical condition and has a young HLA-matched sex identical donor. It should not be performed in first CR, if the same patient is a CMV positive male patient with iron overload and a matched sister as donor. Similarly, an older patient with refractory high risk AML, poor performance and high comorbidity score should not be submitted to HSCT; chances for success are too low to justify a transplant. The exception might be HSCT at an accredited institution with experience and an IRB approved protocol. Similar considerations hold true for all haematological malignancies, including lymphoma or myeloma; they hold true as well for the use of autologous HSCT. In addition, cost considerations might show that in a given country allogeneic HSCT with an optimal donor might be the most cost effective therapy for a young patient with a congenital disorder or a high-risk early malignancy, e.g. CML, MDS, myeloma or AML in first CR (5).

Such an approach has some far reaching consequences. Risk assessment is a continuous process, at predetermined time points, evaluating disease risk, response to therapy and transplant risk. It implies donor search (family donor and unrelated donor) and contact with the transplant team at diagnosis and discussion in an open dialogue with the patient, the donor and the family without prejudice. It can be achieved by close collaboration between transplant teams, non-transplant clinics and the respective authorities on a national level, optimally within the context of a quality management system.

7. Conclusions

The traditional HSCT "yes or no" indications list is just a starting point which has to be supplemented today by a risk-adapted approach. Each team is faced with the challenge to define its own strategic profile based on its expertise and accreditation status, in collaboration with its referring physicians, its neighboring transplant teams, its unrelated donor registry and its competent authorities. EBMT is faced with the challenge to define more precisely individual risk factors in their different contexts, to analyse more rapidly and more comprehensively HSCT outcome data in comparison to non-transplant strategies, in close collaboration with other international transplant registries and with non-transplant disease oriented groups. Better integration of the individual risk profiles into the decision process at the macroeconomic and microeconomic level will ultimately lead to a better selection of transplant patients. It will lead to earlier HSCT for one patient, but evidently also withhold a transplant procedure from another patient with a better outcome without HSCT or with a minimal chance for success. Such an individualised risk-based approach will ultimately lead to a better outcome for all patients and better utilisation of resources.

References

1. Thomas ED, Storb R, Clift RA, et al. Bone marrow transplantation. N Engl J Med 1975; 292: 895–902.
2. Baldomero H, Gratwohl M, Gratwohl A et al. The EBMT activity survey 2009: Trends over the past 5 years. Bone Marrow Transplant 2011; 46: 485–501.
3. Ljungman P, Bregni M, Brune M et al. Allogeneic and autologous transplantation for haematological diseases, solid tumours and immune disorders: Current practice in Europe 2009. Bone Marrow Transplant 2010; 45: 219–234.
4. Chalkidou K, Walley T. Using comparative effectiveness research to inform policy and practice in the UK HHS: Past, present and future. Pharmacoeconomics 2010; 28: 799–811.
5. Gratwohl A, Baldomero H, Aljurf M, Pasquini MC, Bouzas LF, Yoshimi A, Szer J, Lipton J, Schwendener A, Gratwohl M, Frauendorfer K, Niederwieser D, Horowitz M, Kodera Y; Worldwide Network of Blood and Marrow Transplantation. Hematopoietic stem cell transplantation: A global perspective. JAMA 2010; 303: 1617–1624.
6. Gratwohl A. Bone marrow transplantation activity in Europe 1990. Report from the European Group for Bone Marrow Transplantation (EBMT). Bone Marrow Transplant 1991; 8: 197–201.
7. Gratwohl A, Schwendener A, Baldomero H et al. Changes in use of hematopoietic stem cell transplantation; a model for diffusion of medical technology. Haematologica 2010; 95: 637–643.
8. Gratwohl A, Brand R, Niederwieser D, Baldomero H, Chabannon C, Cornelissen J et al, for the Joint Accreditation Committee (JACIE) of the International Society for Cellular Therapy (ISCT) and the European Group for Blood and Marrow Transplantation (EBMT) and the European Leukemia Net. Introduction of a quality management system and outcome after hematopoietic stem cell transplantation. J Clin Oncol 2011; 29: 1980–1986
9. Gratwohl A, Stern M, Brand R, Apperley J, Baldomero H, de Witte T et al, for the European

Group for Blood and Marrow Transplantation and the European Leukemia Net. Risk score for outcome after allogeneic hematopoietic stem cell transplantation: A retrospective analysis. Cancer 2009; 115: 4715–4726.

10. Gratwohl A. The EBMT risk score. Review. Bone Marrow Transplant 2011, june 6. Epub ahead of print.

Multiple Choice Questionnaire

To find the correct answer, go to http://www.esh.org/online-training/handbook/

1. **Which of the following risk factors is *not* included in the EBMT score to assess the risk for an allogeneic stem cell transplantation:**
   a) Age of the patient ☐
   b) Disease stage ☐
   c) Blood group of patient/donor ☐
   d) Type of donor ☐

2. **With respect to the EBMT activity survey, which one of the following statements is *not* correct:**
   a) The activity survey was started by the EBMT in 1990 and has the aims to collect indication, donor type and stem cell source of the stem cell transplant performed in Europe ☐
   b) The EBMT survey has recently been expanded to a global survey by the Worldwide Network for Blood and Marrow Transplantation ☐
   c) The initial purpose of this survey was to be a quality control instrument ☐
   d) As indicated by the survey performed in 2009, acute leukaemias are no longer the major indication for allogeneic stem cell transplantation because of the significant increase in the numbers of allogeneic procedures in lymphomas ☐

3. **Indicate the correct answer regarding the indications manuscript regularly published by EBMT:**
   a) In the manuscript, the indications to perform a haematopoietic stem cell transplantation are divided into: standard of care (S), clinical option (CO), developmental (D) and generally not recommended (GNR) ☐

b) Its main objective is to serve as an official document for commissioners and insurance companies .... ☐
c) This indications manuscript has not been modified since 2005 .... ☐
d) In the document, chronic myeloid leukaemia is still the major indication for allogeneic stem cell transplantation .... ☐

* CHAPTER 19

Indications for HSCT in adults

* 19.1

Acute myeloid leukaemia

Mohamad Mohty

1. Introduction

Acute myeloid leukaemia (AML) is a heterogeneous clonal disorder of haematopoietic progenitor cells which lose the ability to differentiate normally and to respond to normal regulators of proliferation. In younger patients, the incidence is 2 to 3 per 100,000, which rises to 13 to 15 per 100,000 in the seventh and eighth decade. The median age at presentation is approximately 68 years but the majority of data on AML treatment refer to younger patients (<60 years). Over the last few years, considerable knowledge has accumulated about the pathophysiology of adult AML, which has proved to be a highly heterogeneous disease in terms of phenotype, cytogenetics, and molecular abnormalities. Indeed, there has recently been an explosion in new prognostic factors in AML, which is driving the development of new therapeutic targets. However, at present, the use of continuous infusion cytarabine combined with anthracycline (the "3+7" regimen), is still the mainstay for induction therapy in most centres worldwide in younger and fit AML patients. Response rates for induction chemotherapy in the literature range from 50 to 80%. After induction, intensive consolidation chemotherapy, consisting of high dose cytarabine with or without other agents, is routinely employed as post-remission therapy. However, in many patient subgroups, the rate of post-remission leukaemia-free survival (LFS) remains rather poor when using chemotherapy alone. This is the reason why allogeneic HSCT represents one of the most widely used post-remission therapies in those patients who are eligible. According to the EBMT registry, AML represents the most frequent indication for allogeneic HSCT. The immune-mediated graft-versus-leukaemia (GvL) effect contributes greatly to the efficacy of allogeneic HSCT through reduction of disease relapse. Unfortunately, the benefit of allogeneic HSCT can be considerably offset by the complications of the procedure. Therefore, elderly patients - who represent the majority of AML patients - can rarely benefit from standard myeloablative conditioning (MAC) allogeneic HSCT because of an unacceptably high risk of procedure-related toxicity. This point is especially critical when considering AML in first complete remission (CR). Finally, most patients lack an HLA-matched sibling donor. These limitations have prompted the search over the last decade for alternative stem cell sources and for reduced-intensity conditioning (RIC) regimens to decrease allogeneic HSCT-related toxicities.

At present, the key issues being addressed in the clinical use of HSCT for adult AML include the following:

• Based on the novel molecular classifications of the disease, in what category of patients is allogeneic HSCT the therapy of choice?
• What is the role of autologous HSCT?
• What is the overall value of less toxic RIC regimens prior to allogeneic HSCT?

- What is the current role of alternative stem cell sources?
- What future developments might be expected to improve HSCT outcome?

2. Indications for allogeneic HSCT in adult AML

Until recently, the consensus reflected in treatment guidelines of most international cooperative groups was based on cytogenetic stratification into good-, intermediate-, and poor-risk AML. Young patients (age <60 or 65 years) with good-risk AML in first CR were recommended to undergo consolidation high-dose chemotherapy with or without autologous HSCT. Patients with poor-risk AML in first CR were most often recommended to undergo allogeneic HSCT, especially if an HLA-identical related donor was available. In contrast, due to conflicting results from different trials, there was no clear or preferred therapy for patients with intermediate-risk AML in first CR, with allogeneic HSCT, consolidation chemotherapy, or autologous HSCT being considered of equivalent benefit by many investigators.

With this background, several prospective trials were undertaken in the late 90s and early 2000s to clarify the role of allogeneic HSCT for AML in first CR. In these trials, treatment assignment was typically based on the "donor" versus "no-donor" principle, which is widely accepted as providing good-quality evidence of treatment effect in the field of allogeneic HSCT. In a systematic review and meta-analysis of these different prospective trials evaluating allogeneic HSCT versus non-allogeneic HSCT therapies for AML in first CR (1), 24 such trials were identified and the meta-analysis showed that compared with non-allogeneic HSCT, the hazard ratio of relapse or death with allogeneic HSCT for AML in first CR was 0.80. A significant benefit in LFS with allogeneic HSCT was documented for poor-risk (hazard ratio = 0.69) and intermediate-risk AML (hazard ratio = 0.76) but not for good-risk AML (hazard ratio = 1.06). Also, a significant overall survival benefit with allogeneic HSCT was documented for poor-risk and intermediate-risk AML, but not for good-risk AML. Overall, this meta-analysis confirmed that compared with non-allogeneic HSCT therapies, allogeneic SCT has significant LFS and overall survival benefit for intermediate- and poor-risk AML but not for good-risk AML in first CR.

A major complication associated with the use of a sibling donor versus sibling no-donor as a surrogate control arm in the absence of randomised studies, is that this method may be less valuable with the emergence of the use of HLA-matched unrelated donors, and the deferral of allogeneic HSCT to second CR for some patients. Also, one must acknowledge that cytogenetic and molecular risk profiling in adult AML is an evolving field and new patient subgroups are increasingly being identified, especially within the normal and intermediate-risk cytogenetic traditional group. The most recent prognostic molecular aberrations in adult AML and their therapeutic implications are summarised in Table 1. Based on these novel molecular

Table 1: Prognostic molecular aberrations in adult AML and their therapeutic implications

Aberration	Prognostic impact	ELN classification	Possible therapeutic considerations
KIT mutations in CBF AML	Unfavourable		Allogeneic HSCT or TKI-containing clinical trial
FLT3-ITD	Unfavourable, especially with high allelic ratio, larger size and C-terminal location	Intermediate	Allogeneic HSCT of FLT3 inhibitor-containing clinical trial
MLL-PTD	Unfavourable		Allogeneic HSCT or clinical trials with DNA methyltransferase or histone deacetylase inhibitors
High EVI1 expression of mutations	Unfavourable		Allogeneic HSCT or clinical trials with DNA methyltransferase or histone deacetylase inhibitors
IDH1 and IDH2 mutations	Unfavourable	Favourable	Undecided
NPM1 mutations but no FLT3-ITD	Favourable	Favourable	Consolidation chemotherapy
Biallelic C/EBP alpha mutations	Favourable		Consolidation chemotherapy
Low BAALC expression	Favourable, especially those with low ERG		Consolidation chemotherapy
WT1 mutation	Unfavourable		Undecided
Low global DNA methylation	-		Undecided
Increased genome-wide promoter methylation	-		Undecided; clinical trials with demethylating therapies

Adapted from (2). AML: acute myeloid leukaemia; ELN: European LeukemiaNet; CBF: core-binding factor; TKI: tyrosine kinase inhibitor; FLT3: FMS-like tyrosine kinase 3; ITD: internal tandem duplication; MLL: mixed lineage leukaemia; PTD: partial tandem uplication; EVI1: ecotropic virus integration site-1; IDH: isocitrate dehydrogenases; NPM1: nucleophosmin1; C/EBP alpha: CCAAT/enhancer binding protein alpha; ERG: ets erythroblastosis virus E26 oncogene homolog (avian); WT1: Wilms' tumour 1

features, one can further stratify AML outcomes within a defined cytogenetic risk group. For instance, Schlenk et al. (3) reported that for patients with cytogenetically normal AML (who would be classified as intermediate-risk), allogeneic HSCT was beneficial for those with FLT3 internal tandem duplication (FLT3-ITD) or, in the absence of FLT3-ITD, for those without mutations in NPM1 and CEBPA, whereas for the subgroup with mutations in NPM1 and without FLT3-ITD there was no apparent benefit to having a matched sibling donor. However, testing for such novel genetic lesions, as well as whole genome analyses, RNA and microRNA profiles which have the potential to further refine AML risk are not yet in routine clinical use in many transplant centres. Also, these molecularly defined entities have not yet been robustly evaluated for outcome of allogeneic HSCT, since the currently published molecular analyses have usually been done in highly selected subgroups of patients and in the context of retrospectively performed studies.

The ongoing prospective trials from different cooperative groups are currently testing the true value of these molecular entities, and firm conclusions are expected within the next 3 to 5 years.

3. Outcome of allogeneic HSCT from an HLA-matched related and unrelated donor

Allogeneic HSCT using an HLA-matched related donor is usually considered as the standard reference for any other transplant modality or stem cell source. The LFS benefit of allogeneic HSCT for AML in first CR using an HLA-matched related donor is shown in Table 2 for the most important and largest studies in the field. According to the EBMT registry, the most recent results for AML patients transplanted in first CR give a probability of LFS of approximately 55–60%. Results are continuously improving with respect to the past, with centres considering older patients for allogeneic HSCT. However, there is still a significant variation among centres depending on the type of patients transplanted and on the experience and economical context of the Centre. The relapse rate for patients transplanted with an HLA-identical sibling is approximately 20–25% for patients from the intermediate cytogenetic risk group.

For AML patients who lack a family donor, the recommendations for allogeneic HSCT are not consistent across studies. The use of HLA-matched unrelated donors is increasing worldwide thanks to the tremendous efforts of the donor registry network which encompasses now more than 17 million potential donors. Mature randomised studies are still lacking in this field, though many studies have suggested that the results of well-matched unrelated donor transplants can approach those of transplant using a HLA-identical sibling donor (4). The continuous improvement in HLA typing will allow for further improvement of non-relapse mortality (NRM) associated with the use of unrelated donors. Data from the EBMT registry (considering the limitation of the quality of data related to HLA typing in the registry) suggest a LFS rate around

Table 2: Relapse-free survival (RFS) benefit of allogeneic HSCT for AML in first complete remission

Source	No. of Patients		Hazard ratios (95% CI)
	Donor group	No-donor group	
Ferrant et al.	24	72	0.50 (0.30–0.85)
Cassileth et al.	54	29	0.84 (0.48–1.49)
Schiller et al.	28	54	0.88 (0.48–1.64)
Archimbaud et al.	27	31	0.69 (0.36–1.32)
Hewlett et al.	53	110	0.85 (0.58–1.27)
Sierra et al.	47	68	1.56 (0.95–2.57)
Harousseau et al.	88	134	0.94 (0.67–1.33)
Keating et al.	279	355	0.77 (0.63–0.94)
Slovak et al.	89	174	0.83 (0.58–1.19)
Suciu et al.	293	441	0.80 (0.64–1.00)
Jourdan et al.	182	290	0.75 (0.59–0.96)
Burnett et al.	419	868	0.81 (0.70–0.95)
Cornelissen et al.	326	599	0.77 (0.64–0.91)
Overall RFS benefit (fixed effects)	**1909**	**3225**	**0.80 (0.74–0.86)**

Adapted from (1)

45% for AML patients transplanted in first CR using a matched (at least 6/6) unrelated donor.

While the degree of HLA match significantly affects outcome, the timing and selection of patients for whom a search is initiated also has a significant impact on the final outcome, since AML is a highly proliferative disease which can relapse within a relatively short period despite achieving first CR. Most unrelated donor allogeneic HSCT are currently performed in patients with AML in first remission with poor risk features, in patients in second remission, and, most recently, in elderly patients with AML. The timing and kinetics of donor search is increasingly recognised as an important determinant for the ultimate outcome, prompting some centres to consider using the so-called alternative donors if a matched unrelated donor cannot be identified within a reasonable delay.

4. Role of allogeneic HSCT from alternative donors

Patients with AML lacking an HLA-matched related or unrelated donor, but who are transplant candidates, may benefit from a family mismatched donor (*haploidentical transplant*). The Perugia group has pioneered this strategy showing LFS rates of approximately 45–50% for patients receiving their transplant in remission (5). In the EBMT registry, LFS at 2 years was 48, 21 and 1% for patients with AML undergoing haploidentical transplantation in first CR, ≥CR2, and in non-remission (6). Despite these encouraging results, the haploidentical HSCT approach has been developed and evaluated in only a limited number of patients and centres to date. Inclusion of patients in clinical trials is highly desirable before it can be implemented in routine clinical practice on a broader scale. Laboratory data showed that the anti-leukaemic activity after haploidentical HSCT may rely on the possibility of a donor-versus-recipient NK cell alloreactivity (7).

Unrelated cord blood cell transplantation (UCBT) represents another alternative for allogeneic HSCT in adult AML. In comparison to healthy donors, the use of UCBT offers several advantages including:

• Less restrictive HLA compatibility requirements,
• Rapid time to transplant and
• Absence of risk for the donor.

The first large retrospective studies in this field were published in 2004 and have shown a favourable outcome associated with the use of UCBT in adult AML. Such a favourable outcome was confirmed in a more recent analysis which included 880 AML cases, (of which 76 were UCBT). This large retrospective study showed that LFS was similar regardless of HSC source (8). The latter report is the first analysis that shows similar LFS in recipients of 4–6/6 HLA-matched UCBT compared with 8/8 HLA-matched and 7/8 HLA-matched peripheral blood stem cells and bone marrow, confirming that UCBT is a possible alternative to 8/8 and 7/8 HLA-matched donors. However, NRM was higher after 4–6/6 HLA-matched UCBT than after 8/8 HLA-matched unrelated donor transplant, despite lower probabilities of acute and chronic GvHD. A major limitation to the use of UCBT is the availability of sufficient numbers of haematopoietic stem cells for haematopoietic recovery. Several strategies for reducing the period of neutropenia currently being explored might lead to lower early NRM and potentially improved LFS. These include the transplantation of two UCB units, *ex-vivo* expansion of CB cells to augment the number of HSC and progenitors in the UCB graft, co-infusion of T-cell depleted haploidentical PBPC to bridge the period of neutropenia, and the injection of UCB cells directly into the patient's bone marrow to reduce non-specific losses of HSCs, as well as improve homing of HSCs and progenitor cells (9).

5. Role of reduced-intensity conditioning (RIC) regimens

The development of so-called non-myeloablative or RIC regimens appears to decrease allogeneic HSCT-related toxicities. In contrast to standard dosed myeloablative allogeneic HSCT, RIC regimens are relatively well tolerated by patients with high-risk clinical features such as advanced age or associated co-morbidities. Nevertheless, in the context of adult AML, toxicity may represent only one aspect of the problem, since AML encompasses a group of diseases of varying chemosensitivity, raising concerns that significant reduction of the intensity of the conditioning may have a negative impact on long-term control of leukaemia. This concern is particularly relevant in patients with high-risk leukaemic features. Indeed, the importance of dose intensity has already been shown in myeloablative allogeneic HSCT. However, the beneficial effect of more intensive conditioning is associated with a reduced risk of relapse, but offset by an increased transplant-related toxicity. The latter may be even more complex since the relative benefit of myeloablation as part of the conditioning regimen also depends on the patient and disease status at the time of allogeneic HSCT (e.g. CR1 vs beyond CR1 or advanced disease) (reviewed in Blaise et al. (10)). Thus, investigators are currently faced with a dilemma on how to optimise the potential role of RIC allo-SCT in elderly patients with AML, while delivering minimal myeloablation and maximising allogeneic immunotherapy. Indeed, due to a reduced anti-leukaemia effect of the conditioning regimen, the procedure largely relies on the GvL effect of the alloreactive lymphocytes to eradicate residual leukaemia cells. Accordingly, the relapse rate after RIC has always been shown to be higher than after MAC. Also, the favourable immunological anti-leukaemia effect may be counterbalanced by the morbidity and mortality associated with late onset acute GvHD. Since several phase II studies strongly suggested that the morbidity and NRM after RIC are less than after MAC, many investigators have already raised the upper age limit for allogeneic HSCT in AML to 65–70 years. Indeed, the current NRM rates after RIC for AML range from 15 to 20% and relapse after transplant is the most frequent cause of death. Also, from a methodology point of view, the assessment of the overall benefit of RIC for AML must not only take into account disease status at the time of transplant, but also the global treatment strategy including any intensive chemotherapy received prior to transplantation, and the level of myeloablation delivered within the RIC regimen itself; it is important to distinguish between truly non-myeloablative regimens (e.g. 2 Gy TBI) and other RIC regimens. Other potential confounding factors are related to immunologic senescence in the elderly, which may lead to an increased incidence of infections, secondary tumours and autoimmune diseases.

In summary, reducing toxicity without compromising the GvL effect could be of significant benefit to many AML patients, but more intensive RIC regimens, despite the hazard of increased toxicity, may be necessary in others. Thus, the trade-off between dose intensity, toxicity, and disease control will need to be assessed for each individual patient. In addition, the specific roles of matched unrelated transplants from alternate stem cell sources are yet to be investigated. As well as reducing toxicity, the reduction of relapse rates after RIC while preserving patients' quality of life remains a major goal. The efficacy of RIC allogeneic HSCT against AML may be improved by *in vitro* generation of T-cell responses directed against defined minor histocompatibility antigens.

Another important challenge facing investigators is the regular and close monitoring of minimal residual disease (MRD), since the relapse risk may be determined by levels of occult residual disease. The serial use of lineage specific chimerism may also identify patients at risk of relapse, in whom therapeutic intervention may be indicated. Prophylactic use of systematic manipulated or non-manipulated DLI may be useful. Early administration of biologically targeted therapies, such as flt-3 or farnesyl transferase inhibitors, or vaccinations, after RIC may be an attractive strategy in certain biologically defined subgroups of patients. Alternatively, the testing of radio-immunotherapy to intensify the anti-leukaemic activity of the RIC regimen without increasing toxicity may be of interest. Radio-immunotherapy with isotopes targeting CD33, CD45 or CD66 can potentially allow intensification of anti-leukaemia therapy, and will likely prove useful when used in combination with standard chemotherapy in the treatment of AML before and after RIC allo-SCT. Also, the introduction of moderate to intensive dosages of iv busulfan, thiotepa, or melphalan in the conditioning regimen may help decreasing the risk of relapse while waiting for the GvL effect. These approaches are currently being tested in phase II studies.

Overall, based on the current results in different high-risk AML populations, it is reasonable to consider that RIC allogeneic HSCT represents a valid option for those AML patients with a matched related donor who are not eligible for standard myeloablative allo-SCT (11). The immune-mediated GvL effect is usually stronger than any other form of salvage chemotherapy. Eventually, the appropriate comparison of autologous HSCT or chemotherapy as consolidation therapies by donor/no donor studies should establish the definitive benefit and appropriate use of RIC allogeneic HSCT for AML.

6. Role of autologous HSCT

The role of autologous HSCT in AML is still controversial. Available data indicate that better outcome (less relapse) is achieved when cells are harvested after the second or third course of chemotherapy. Bone marrow is the preferred stem cell source. In general, the results of autograft for AML have remained constant over the last 10 years. There has been a reduction of NRM, probably due to better supportive therapy. In most studies, LFS ranges from 40 to 50% at 3 years. These results are encouraging, especially considering that autologous HSCT can be now offered to patients up to 65 years and beyond. Auto-HSCT produces durable second remission in 25–30% of patients with relapsed AML who achieved a second CR, but its low NRM is offset by a high relapse rate (12).

For a number of reasons, autologous HSCT activity for AML has declined in the last 5 years. The reasons lie in the fact that there has not been any improvement in methods of reducing relapse. Another drawback lies with the fact that no more than 50 to 60% of patients candidate for autologous HSCT actually reach the transplant. This has mainly been caused by early relapse of leukaemia, or the harvest of an insufficient graft. Currently, autologous HSCT is usually restricted to older AML patients, patients with APL in second molecular remission and younger patients lacking a sibling or unrelated donor. However, the picture may change in the future given the fact that the novel molecular and cytogenetic stratification methods may allow for identification of AML entities which could benefit from autografting as a post-remission therapy. Though MRD monitoring is more difficult than is the case in acute lymphoid leukaemia, the use of it represents an attractive tool for refining the global therapeutic strategy including the optimal use of autologous HSCT.

7. HSCT for primary induction failure

In AML, primary treatment failure is defined by failure to achieve CR after two courses of induction chemotherapy or by early relapse within 6 months from documented CR. For these patients, the chance to achieve a CR with further conventional chemotherapy, including the use of high-dose cytarabine, is 10–20% at best, and overall survival at 1 year is less than 10% with a median survival of 4 months only. A few historical studies suggested that allogeneic HSCT can rescue some of those patients, with LFS rates between 15 and 40%. Therefore, patients failing induction chemotherapy may still be considered candidates for an allogeneic HSCT.

Thus far, no prospective trial has been published which would allow a standard transplant approach to be defined for these refractory AML patients. The results achieved with the strategy developed by the Munich group of sequential FLAMSA (fludarabine, intermediate dose cytarabine, and amsacrine followed by TBI 4 Gy), cyclophosphamide, and anti-thymocyte globulin are among the most promising ones published so far (13). Outside clinical trials, and despite the relatively high risk of the procedure that may hamper the overall safety and success of the procedure, it is reasonable to discuss this salvage approach in individual patient cases, taking into account some important factors determining outcome (e.g. age, general status, kinetics of disease proliferation, cytogenetics, type of donor, level of HLA matching, etc.) so as to identify patients with a reasonable chance of long-term disease control.

8. Future perspectives and conclusion

In the last 5 years, there have been great advances in understanding AML biology through the use of new technologies. Novel disease-related prognostic markers that can impact significantly on AML classification, response to therapy, and survival are increasingly identified and validated in large series. This is particularly the case in the traditional "intermediate-risk" group where provisional new disease entities and therapeutic targets have been identified based on these studies. As therapy for AML advances, the importance of individual prognostic factors will need to be reassessed in light of new treatments. Most experts today consider that the effect of allogeneic HSCT needs to be re-assessed in specific biological subgroups taking account both the "classical" cytogenetic risk group classification and the wide variety of new molecular markers. In addition, the use of MRD assessment beyond consolidation chemotherapy provides an important new tool to identify patients in whom HSCT may be indicated (14). In parallel, the risks of the transplant toxicity can also be better assessed, based on patient (including comorbidity scores) and donor characteristics. In any case, for patients with high-risk features and beyond first CR, allo-HSCT remains the sole possibility of cure. In order to implement future strategies, every young patient with newly diagnosed AML should have the most comprehensive assessment of disease risk and should be considered for a donor search as soon as possible.

References

1. Koreth J, Schlenk R, Kopecky KJ et al. Allogeneic stem cell transplantation for acute myeloid leukemia in first complete remission: Systematic review and meta-analysis of prospective clinical trials. JAMA 2009; 301: 2349–2361.
2. Burnett A, Wetzler M, Lowenberg B. Therapeutic advances in acute myeloid leukemia. J Clin Oncol 2011; 29: 487–494.
3. Schlenk RF, Dohner K, Krauter J et al. Mutations and treatment outcome in cytogenetically normal acute myeloid leukemia. N Engl J Med 2008; 358: 1909–1918.
4. Flomenberg N, Baxter-Lowe LA, Confer D et al. Impact of HLA class I and class II high-

resolution matching on outcomes of unrelated donor bone marrow transplantation: HLA-C mismatching is associated with a strong adverse effect on transplantation outcome. Blood 2004; 104: 1923–1930.

5. Stern M, Ruggeri L, Mancusi A et al. Survival after T cell-depleted haploidentical stem cell transplantation is improved using the mother as donor. Blood 2008; 112: 2990–2995.

6. Ciceri F, Labopin M, Aversa F et al. A survey of fully haploidentical hematopoietic stem cell transplantation in adults with high-risk acute leukemia: A risk factor analysis of outcomes for patients in remission at transplantation. Blood 2008; 112: 3574–3581.

7. Velardi A, Ruggeri L, Mancusi A et al. Natural killer cell allorecognition of missing self in allogeneic hematopoietic transplantation: A tool for immunotherapy of leukemia. Curr Opin Immunol 2009; 21: 525–530.

8. Eapen M, Rocha V, Sanz G et al. Effect of graft source on unrelated donor haemopoietic stem-cell transplantation in adults with acute leukaemia: A retrospective analysis. Lancet Oncol 2011; 11: 653–660.

9. Rocha V, Broxmeyer HE. New approaches for improving engraftment after cord blood transplantation. Biol Blood Marrow Transplant 2010; 16: S126–132.

10. Blaise D, Vey N, Faucher C, Mohty M. Current status of reduced-intensity-conditioning allogeneic stem cell transplantation for acute myeloid leukemia. Haematologica 2007; 92: 533–541.

11. Mohty M, de Lavallade H, El-Cheikh J et al. Reduced intensity conditioning allogeneic stem cell transplantation for patients with acute myeloid leukemia: Long term results of a 'donor' versus 'no donor' comparison. Leukemia 2009; 23: 194–196.

12. Breems DA, Lowenberg B. Acute myeloid leukemia and the position of autologous stem cell transplantation. Semin Hematol 2007; 44: 259–266.

13. Schmid C, Schleuning M, Schwerdtfeger R et al. Long-term survival in refractory acute myeloid leukemia after sequential treatment with chemotherapy and reduced-intensity conditioning for allogeneic stem cell transplantation. Blood 2006; 108: 1092–1099.

14. Kronke J, Schlenk RF, Jensen KO et al. Monitoring of minimal residual disease in NPM1-mutated acute myeloid leukemia: A study from the German-Austrian Acute Myeloid Leukemia Study Group. J Clin Oncol 2011; 29: 2709–2716.

Multiple Choice Questionnaire

To find the correct answer, go to http://www.esh.org/online-training/handbook/

1. For good risk AML patients:

a) Allogeneic HSCT is always indicated .... ☐

b) Allogeneic HSCT is never indicated. .... ☐

c) Autologous HSCT is always indicated .... ☐

d) None of the above statements is correct .... ☐

2. **The meta-analysis of studies comparing chemotherapy, allo-transplant, and auto-transplant has shown better OS for allo-transplant in:**
   a) Poor-risk cytogenetic patients...... ☐
   b) Intermediate-risk patients...... ☐
   c) Favourable-risk patients...... ☐
   d) a+b...... ☐

3. **Good risk AML is characterised by involvement of which of the following genes?**
   a) FLT3-ITD...... ☐
   b) EVI-1...... ☐
   c) WT1...... ☐
   d) NPM1 alone...... ☐

4. **In case of a poor risk AML patient in CR2, what type of donor is most suitable for allogeneic HSCT?**
   a) Double cord blood units...... ☐
   b) Single cord blood unit...... ☐
   c) Haploidentical donor...... ☐
   d) All of the above options are valid ones...... ☐

5. **In the context of reduced intensity conditioning (RIC) for AML prior to allo-HSCT, which one of the following is correct?**
   a) NRM incidence ranges from 40 to 70%...... ☐
   b) Relapse after transplant is the most frequent cause of death...... ☐
   c) RIC allogeneic HSCT is never indicated for AML...... ☐
   d) Relapse incidence is lower than after standard myeloablative conditioning...... ☐

NOTES

*CHAPTER 19

Indications for HSCT in adults

*19.2
Acute lymphoblastic leukaemia

Mohamad Mohty

1. Introduction

In contrast to childhood acute lymphoblastic leukaemia (ALL), in which overall survival is more than 80% at 5 years, the outcome of adult ALL is disappointing, with an average survival of 35% in patients age 18 to 60 years. The poorer outcome of adult ALL compared with children relates to multiple factors, including a higher incidence of poor prognostic markers such as the Philadelphia chromosome and a lower incidence of favourable subtypes.

Because of the heterogeneity of the disease, adult ALL therapy requires a complex and highly diversified approach to treatment. Over the past 10 to 15 years, allogeneic HSCT has been increasingly proposed for adult ALL in first remission, and the use of matched unrelated and alternative donors has vastly increased the availability of the donor pool for ALL patients. However, the curative potential of allogeneic HSCT must be balanced against the problems associated with the procedure, namely non-relapse mortality, chronic GvHD and its corollary of long-term morbidity, late side effects and altered quality of life. Also, allogeneic HSCT must be assessed in relation to the improved outcome of chemotherapy treatments alone. Despite a significant amount of data and trials, reports from different cooperative groups differ in their conclusions, and indications for HSCT in first CR (whether autologous or allogeneic) are still not well-defined. A radical view may recommend that allogeneic HSCT should be performed in all patients with an HLA-matched donor, owing to the higher anti-leukaemic activity provided by the immune-mediated graft-versus-leukaemia (GvL) effect. However, another increasingly growing option is to reserve allogeneic HSCT for high-risk (HR) patients by identifying patients who have a chance of cure without HSCT. The evaluation of minimal residual disease (MRD) can without doubt improve significantly the definition of adult ALL risk class. One of the most debated topics in the treatment of adult ALL is which is the best consolidation approach for adults who attain first complete remission (CR) after intensive induction therapy.

2. Indications for allogeneic HSCT in adult ALL

Results of treatment for adult ALL (studies with >100 patients) according to HSCT strategy are summarised in Table 1. When interpreting outcome data derived from these trials, one should bear in mind that these studies are inherently different (various trial designs, different eligibility criteria, sample size, duration of follow-up, definition of risk factors etc.). Therefore, a measured understanding of the message in each of these studies is required when managing an individual patient case.

Most European ALL study groups define an indication for allogeneic HSCT in adult ALL patients with high risk (HR) features and unfavourable prognostic factors

Table 1: Results of treatment programs for adult ALL (studies with >100 patients) according to HSCT strategy

Study	Year	No of patients	Ages (years)		CR rate		Allogeneic HSCT strategy*	DFS	OS	HSCT realisation†	HSCT outcome (by intention)
			Median	Range	No	%					
CALGB 9111	1998	198	35	16-83	167	85	Ph+	46%, 3 y	50%, 3 y	-	-
SWOG 8417/8419	2001	353	32	15-84	218	62	-	25-32%, 5 y	35%, 8 y	-	-
NILG 08/96	2001	121	35	15-74	102	84	HR with donor; others to auto-HSCT or CHT	48%, 3 y	49%, 3 y	Allo 21 (29%), auto 28 (39%)	DFS donor 38% vs no donor 43% (p=NS)
JALSG 93	2002	263	31	15-59	205	78	All patients with donor and age <40	30%, 6 y	30%, 6 y	Allo 51 (25%)	-
Sweden	2002	153	42	16-82	131	86	HR; to auto-HSCT if no donor	30%, 5 y	28%, 5 y	Allo 26 (20%), auto 10 (8%)	-
GIMEMA 02/88	2002	767	28	12-60	627	82	HR with donor: Ph+, WBC >50	33%, 9 y	27%, 9 y	-	-
MDACC	2004	288	408	15-92	269	92	Ph+	38%, 5 y	38%, 5 y	-	-
EORTC ALL3	2004	340	33	14-79	253	74	All patients with donor and age <50; others CHT vs auto-HSCT	36%, 6 y	36%, 6 y	Allo 49 (19%)	DFS donor 38% vs no donor 37% (p=NS)
LALA 94	2004	922	33	15-55	771	84	HR with donor; others CHT vs auto-HSCT	30%, 5 y	36%, 5 y	Allo 145 (36%)§, auto 159 (41%)§	Ph-: DFS donor 45% vs no donor 18% (p=0.007)
GOELAL 02	2004	198	33	15-59	170	86	HR patients with donor and age <50; others auto-HSCT	NR	41%, 6 y	Allo 41 (24%), auto 91 (53%)	OS allo-HSCT 75% vs auto-HSCT 43% (p=0.002)
PETHEMA ALL-93	2005	222	27	15-50	183	82	HR; others CHT vs auto-HSCT	35%, 5 y	34%, 5 y	Allo 57 (31%), auto 31 (17%)	DFS donor 33% vs no donor 39% (p=NS)
GMALL 07	2007	713	34	15-55	635	89	HR allo or auto; others CHT	NR	54%, 5 y	SCT feasibility 70% (allo+auto)	-
MRC-ECOG	2008	1646 (Ph-)		15-64	1,484	90	All patients with donor and age <55; others CHT vs auto-HSCT	NR	39%, 5 y	Allo 320 (21%), auto 162 (11%)	OS donor 53% vs no donor 45% (p=0.01)
HOVON	2009	433	NR		288**		All patients with donor and age <55; others to auto-HSCT	NR	37%, 5 y	Allo 122 (42%), auto 126 (44%)	DFS donor 60% vs no donor 42% (p=0.01)

*Table 1: Legend. Adapted from Bassan R, Hoelzer D. J Clin Oncol 2011; 29: 532–543. CR: complete response; DFS: disease-free survival; OS: overall survival; CALGB: Cancer and Leukemia Group B; SWOG: Southwest Oncology Group; NILG: Northern Italy Leukemia Group (plus ongoing trial NILG-10, ClinicalTrials.gov Identifier NCT00795756); HR: high risk; SCT: stem cell transplantation; CHT: chemotherapy; NS: not significant; JALSG: Japan Adult Leukaemia Study Group; GIMEMA: Gruppo Italiano Malattie Ematologiche dell'Adulto; MDACC: MD Anderson Cancer Center; EORTC: European Organisation for the Research and Treatment of Cancer; LALA: Leucémie Aiguës Lymphoblastique de l'Adulte; GOELAMS: Groupe Ouest-Est des Léucemies Aigus et Maladies du Sang; NR: not reported; PETHEMA: Programa Espanol de Tratamiento en Hematologia; GMALL: German Multicenter Study Group for Adult ALL; MRC: Medical Research Council; ECOG: Eastern Cooperative Oncology Group; HOVON: Dutch-Belgian Cooperative Trial Group for Hematology/Oncology. *All patients: allo-HSCT applicable to all patients with potential compatible donor (genetic randomisation); or to selected risk groups as indicated (risk stratification criteria vary among studies); CHT (randomisation vs. auto-HSCT arm). †HSCT realisation = the % of eligible CR patients who actually received the planned HSCT. ‡DFS (when available) or OS. §Of 399 eligible patients. **CR patients satisfying SCT criteria*

associated with a survival probability of less than 40% with chemotherapy alone (http://www.leukemia-net.org). The prognostic models may differ between groups as well as the upper age limits. HR has traditionally been defined by certain characteristics of the patient and disease at time of diagnosis and before any therapy. The MRC UKALL XII/ECOG E2993 trial included presence of Philadelphia chromosome t(9;22), B-ALL with presenting white blood count (WBC) >30 x 10^9/L, and T-ALL with WBC >100 x 10^9/L as being high risk. Importantly, age >35 years was also considered-high risk disease. Another recent MRC/ECOG publication has also highlighted additional high-risk cytogenetic groups, which include t(4;11), t(8;14), low hypodiploidy, near triploidy, and a complex karyotype (1). However, in addition to the above disease-related risk factors, prognostic factors should be also used to estimate the risks of the HSCT procedure itself, such as patient age, donor characteristics, degree of HLA matching, etc. Bringing together the different risk estimates can allow for a more accurate definition of indications. In addition, scoring of comorbidities can assist decision-making with respect to the choice of the intensity of the conditioning regimen.

The largest prospective randomised adult ALL study (UKALL XII/ECOG 2993) employed a "biological randomisation" on a donor versus no-donor basis. The 443 patients with a donor, when compared to the 588 patients without a donor, had a superior event-free survival (EFS) of 50% versus 41% (p=0.009) and OS of 53% versus 45% (p=0.01) (2). Of importance, this benefit was primarily seen in the standard-risk patients OS, 62% for donor versus 52% for no-donor (p=0.02). In HR patients the increased OS did not reach statistical significance; OS was 40% for donor versus 36% for no-donor (p=0.6). This lack of difference in outcome between donor and no-donor patients in the higher-risk patients was related to a high NRM of 36% at

2 years for the HR patients compared to 20% at 2 years for the standard-risk patients. Furthermore, this difference was largely related to older age. Among HR patients, age over 35 was the only factor that could be shown to be independently responsible for the increased NRM (2).

The increasing use of MRD assessment beyond first consolidation chemotherapy provides an important new tool for defining indications for HSCT. Such a strategy was promoted by the GMALL, NILG, and PETHEMA groups (3, 4) who were able to show that even selected HR ALL patients who do not express the most adverse features (WBC >100, pre/pro/mature-T phenotype, very HR cytogenetics), benefit from chemotherapy programs without allogeneic HSCT if they are MRD negative. In MRD-positive patients, the success of allogeneic HSCT ranged from 35% to 60% again depending again on post-graft conversion to MRD-negative status. Thus, the impact of MRD on the allogeneic HSCT decision-process is not straightforward, since one may question both whether allogeneic HSCT is really recommended for patients with high MRD, since they are prone to a higher relapse rate after allogeneic HSCT, and whether allogeneic HSCT is justified in HR ALL patients who have achieved negative MRD status. Finally, it should be remembered that risk can be redefined, or at least modified, during treatment based on disease dynamics.

In contrast to the situation in first CR, there is general agreement that all patients in 2nd or later remission are candidates for allogeneic HSCT. This includes molecular relapse, defined as reappearance of MRD above 10^{-4}–10^{-3}. In advanced ALL, depending on donor availability and general condition, experimental allogeneic HSCT procedures (ideally within clinical trials) may be considered.

3. Outcome of allogeneic HSCT from an HLA-matched related and unrelated donor

According to the EMBT and CIBMTR registries, overall survival after allogeneic HSCT from an HLA identical sibling donor for adult ALL in 1st CR is around 50%. The cumulative incidences of relapse and NRM both range between 25% and 30%. Although NRM is strongly correlated with age, the upper age-limit for allogeneic HSCT has increased continuously over recent years, especially with the introduction of the so-called reduced-intensity conditioning (RIC) regimens. As expected, survival after allogeneic HSCT is poorer for patients in 2nd remission (around 30%) and with advanced disease (around 15%). The latter is mainly due to an increased incidence of disease relapse or progression.

The use of unrelated donors may extend the transplant option to those previously excluded on the basis of not having a suitable sibling donor. In the HLA-matched unrelated setting, survival in 1st CR is around 40–45% (5–7), with a lower relapse incidence, but higher NRM (around 30–40%) compared to the HLA-identical sibling setting. However, these data need to be interpreted appropriately as the studies suffer from the inherent selection bias that goes into assigning a patient to an unrelated transplant. Indeed, the patient eligibility criteria for such a procedure may be more restrictive than for a sibling transplant. Despite the increasing perception of a similar outcome between matched-related and unrelated donors, it is common practice in many transplant centres for there to be a discrepant approach in the institutional policy for selecting suitable patients.

In 2nd remission or beyond, HLA-matched unrelated allogeneic HSCT results in a long term survival around 28% and in advanced disease of around 10%, due to a higher relapse rate and higher NRM around 45% (8). Due to improved supportive care, refinement of HLA typing, and better donor selection, the results of allogeneic HSCT using unrelated donors are expected to further improve in the near future.

4. Role of allogeneic HSCT from alternative donors

At present, the use of haploidentical HSCT is still considered as an experimental approach in many transplant centres worldwide, and should be restricted to specialised centres and for disease beyond first CR. Such an approach should preferably be performed within clinical trials.

On the other hand, the current development of unrelated cord blood transplantation (UCBT) in adult ALL is mainly based on the wider paediatric experience in this field. In practice, applying UCBT in adults is limited by the cell dose: trials testing double UCBT or CB expansion are currently ongoing in order to overcome this major obstacle. Initial registry results for younger adults with ALL indicated that UCBT (single or double) can be considered as an alternative stem cell source, in very HR patients. In a more recent small series of 22 adult ALL patients (21 of 22 in CR), overall survival, NRM and relapse rates were 50%, 27% and 36% at 3 years, respectively (9).

5. Role of reduced-intensity conditioning regimens

In the standard myeloablative conditioning (MAC) setting, most regimens are based on total body irradiation (TBI) combined with cyclophosphamide or VP16. However, according to the EBMT registry, the use of reduced-toxicity myeloablative regimens (e.g. regimens using myeloablative doses of iv busulfan) is increasingly considered in many patients in order to avoid TBI-related short- and long-term toxicities. Also, RIC or non-myeloablative regimens are gaining popularity in elderly ALL patients (age >50 years) or in patients with significant comorbidities. A recent retrospective study from the EBMT assessed the outcome of 576 adult ALL patients aged ≥45 years, who received a RIC (n=127) or MAC (n=449) allogeneic

HSCT from an HLA-identical sibling while in CR. With a median follow-up of 16 months, at 2 years, the cumulative incidences of NRM and relapse incidence were 29% (MAC) versus 21% (RIC; p=0.03), and 31% (MAC) versus 47% (RIC; p <0.001), respectively. In a multivariate analysis, NRM was decreased in RIC recipients (p=0.0001, hazard ratio 1.98) whereas it was associated with higher relapse rate (p=0.03, hazard ratio 0.59). At 2 years, LFS was 38% (MAC) versus 32% (RIC; p=0.07). In multivariate analysis, the type of conditioning regimen (RIC vs MAC) was not significantly associated with leukaemia-free survival (p=0.23, hazard ratio 0.84), suggesting that RIC is a potential therapeutic option for ALL patients aged ≥45 years in CR, candidates for transplant, but not eligible for MAC (10).

6. Role and outcome of autologous HSCT

When allogeneic HSCT is precluded, high-dose therapy followed by autologous HSCT was considered as an alternative in some trials which randomly assigned patients between chemotherapy and autologous HSCT. Most randomised studies showed no difference for the comparison of chemotherapy versus autologous HSCT or even a significantly inferior outcome for autologous HSCT (2). In addition, most comparisons of allogeneic and autologous HSCT have shown an inferior outcome for autologous HSCT. According to available data, the overall survival of patients receiving autologous HSCT in 1st CR is around 40%. The major problem with autologous HSCT is the high incidence of relapse. Thus, post-transplant maintenance has been attempted, with some suggested benefit (11), but proved to be difficult to administer (12).

More recently, and though autologous HSCT remains a developmental approach for adult ALL according to EBMT recommendations, this strategy has gained a renewed interest among several investigators, especially for patients who were MRD negative (defined as MRD negativity of the patient as well as of autologous stem cells).

7. HSCT in Philadelphia chromosome positive ALL

Due to the poor outcome with intensive chemotherapy, in the pre-imatinib era, allogeneic HSCT has always been the treatment of choice for Philadelphia chromosome positive ALL (Ph+ ALL). The survival after allogeneic HSCT in first CR ranges between 27 and 65% (13). It is also well established that the relapse incidence is higher than in Ph-negative ALL, and the overall outcome is compromised by NRM due to the higher median age of Ph+ ALL patients. Nowadays the majority of patients with Ph+ ALL receive imatinib or other tyrosine kinase inhibitors (TKI) as front-line therapy. Treatment with TKIs allows for increased rate of CR and greater opportunity for patients to proceed to allogeneic HSCT, which remains the only curative option in those eligible patients. Despite the short follow-up, data from the EBMT registry suggests that the introduction of TKIs after the year 2007 within European centres has probably improved the outcome of adult Ph+ ALL patients eligible for allogeneic HSCT. Prospective evaluations are ongoing and further improvements would be expected in the next few years with the wider use of MRD assessment associated with TKI-based pre-emptive and/or maintenance strategies.

8. Comparisons of chemotherapy and HSCT based approaches in young adult ALL

The issue of the optimal management for young adults with ALL is a matter of considerable debate with reports by paediatric groups suggesting an apparently superior outcome for adolescents treated on paediatric regimens. This information is derived from comparative outcome data between patients treated on paediatric versus adult protocols, e.g. LALA-94 versus FRALLE-93 (14). Based on theses retrospective comparisons, many physicians are now using paediatric regimens in young adults up to the end of the third decade, with some phase II data already suggesting improved outcome in adults up to the age of 45 treated with paediatric protocols (15). However, it is important to emphasise that these protocols have been adopted for use in young adults rather than assessed for use in young adults using prospective trials. Furthermore, the age profiles of the teenagers and young adult patients in both groups are not entirely comparable. With these pitfalls in mind, and while waiting for the results of prospective controlled trials, there is insufficient evidence to conclude that allogeneic HSCT in first CR should be completely abandoned in this group of patients, particularly for those with HR disease.

9. Future perspectives and conclusion

An ever-growing body of evidence shows that the outcome after HSCT in adult ALL is influenced by the status of MRD before and after HSCT. Therefore MRD status must be considered both before and after HSCT, to decide on additional treatment either before HSCT in order to reduce tumour load or after HSCT to prevent relapse. The use of pre-emptive DLI immediately after allogeneic HSCT may be beneficial, especially in early relapse (preferably molecular relapse). In addition, amplification of the GvL effect may be one way to reduce the rate of relapse (e.g. by IL-2 activation) or using specific sensitisation prior to graft infusion. Post-HSCT maintenance therapy may also succeed in eradicating residual leukaemic cells. Monoclonal antibodies directed against antigens expressed by leukaemic cells (e.g. anti-CD20/22) may be less toxic and more efficient than chemotherapy. In Ph+ ALL post-transplantation treatment with imatinib or other TKIs (either up-front or after detection of MRD) increasingly appears to be a successful approach.

Great strides have been made over the past decades in defining the optimal role for allogeneic and autologous HSCT in adult patients with ALL. However, great attention needs to be given to the appropriate methodologies for each study to fully understand the importance of the data provided as well as the limitations.

At present, efforts are directed towards development of the optimal chemotherapy schedules/intensity and optimal integration of HSCT in the front-line strategy. Criteria for defining HR disease are being refined and would allow to better determine the optimal candidates and the timing of allogeneic HSCT. A low or negative MRD at time of HSCT is a pre-requisite for reduction of relapse incidence. Better donor selection, use of less toxic conditioning regimens, improved GvHD prophylaxis and supportive care, are key determinants for reducing NRM. Nevertheless, given the low incidence of adult ALL, reliable and definitive data can only be generated by well-designed and conducted large prospective studies that can only be achieved through a collaborative effort among national and international cooperative groups and across continents.

References

1. Moorman AV, Harrison CJ, Buck GA et al. Karyotype is an independent prognostic factor in adult acute lymphoblastic leukemia (ALL): Analysis of cytogenetic data from patients treated on the Medical Research Council (MRC) UKALLXII/Eastern Cooperative Oncology Group (ECOG) 2993 trial. Blood 2007; 109: 3189–3197.
2. Goldstone AH, Richards SM, Lazarus HM et al. In adults with standard-risk acute lymphoblastic leukemia, the greatest benefit is achieved from a matched sibling allogeneic transplantation in first complete remission, and an autologous transplantation is less effective than conventional consolidation/maintenance chemotherapy in all patients: Final results of the International ALL Trial (MRC UKALL XII/ECOG E2993). Blood 2008; 111: 1827–1833.
3. Raff T, Gokbuget N, Luschen S et al. Molecular relapse in adult standard-risk ALL patients detected by prospective MRD monitoring during and after maintenance treatment: Data from the GMALL 06/99 and 07/03 trials. Blood 2007; 109: 910–915.
4. Bassan R, Spinelli O, Oldani E et al. Improved risk classification for risk-specific therapy based on the molecular study of minimal residual disease (MRD) in adult acute lymphoblastic leukemia (ALL). Blood 2009; 113: 4153–4162.
5. Kiehl MG, Kraut L, Schwerdtfeger R et al. Outcome of allogeneic hematopoietic stem-cell transplantation in adult patients with acute lymphoblastic leukemia: No difference in related compared with unrelated transplant in first complete remission. J Clin Oncol 2004; 22: 2816–2825.
6. Dahlke J, Kroger N, Zabelina T et al. Comparable results in patients with acute lymphoblastic leukemia after related and unrelated stem cell transplantation. Bone Marrow Transplant 2006; 37: 155–163.

7. Marks DI, Perez WS, He W et al. Unrelated donor transplants in adults with Philadelphia-negative acute lymphoblastic leukemia in first complete remission. Blood 2008; 112: 426–434.

8. Fielding AK, Richards SM, Chopra R et al. Outcome of 609 adults after relapse of acute lymphoblastic leukemia (ALL); an MRC UKALL12/ECOG 2993 study. Blood 2007; 109: 944–950.

9. Bachanova V, Verneris MR, DeFor T et al. Prolonged survival in adults with acute lymphoblastic leukemia after reduced-intensity conditioning with cord blood or sibling donor transplantation. Blood 2009; 113: 2902–2905.

10. Mohty M, Labopin M, Volin L et al. Reduced-intensity versus conventional myeloablative conditioning allogeneic stem cell transplantation for patients with acute lymphoblastic leukemia: A retrospective study from the European Group for Blood and Marrow Transplantation. Blood 2010; 116: 4439–4443.

11. Bassan R, Lerede T, Di Bona E et al. Induction-consolidation with an idarubicin-containing regimen, unpurged marrow autograft, and post-graft chemotherapy in adult acute lymphoblastic leukaemia. Br J Haematol 1999; 104: 755–762.

12. Cornelissen JJ, van der Holt B, Verhoef GE et al. Myeloablative allogeneic versus autologous stem cell transplantation in adult patients with acute lymphoblastic leukemia in first remission: A prospective sibling donor versus no-donor comparison. Blood 2009; 113: 1375–1382.

13. Fielding AK, Goldstone AH. Allogeneic haematopoietic stem cell transplant in Philadelphia-positive acute lymphoblastic leukaemia. Bone Marrow Transplant 2008; 41: 447–453.

14. Boissel N, Auclerc MF, Lheritier V et al. Should adolescents with acute lymphoblastic leukemia be treated as old children or young adults? Comparison of the French FRALLE-93 and LALA-94 trials. J Clin Oncol 2003; 21: 774–780.

15. Huguet F, Leguay T, Raffoux E et al. Pediatric-inspired therapy in adults with Philadelphia chromosome-negative acute lymphoblastic leukemia: The GRAALL-2003 study. J Clin Oncol 2009; 27: 911–918.

Multiple Choice Questionnaire

To find the correct answer, go to http://www.esh.org/online-training/handbook/

1. Which post-transplantation strategy is likely to be most successful in Ph/BCR-ABL positive ALL (especially in case of positive minimal residual disease after transplant)?

a) A tyrosine kinase inhibitor such as imatinib .... ☐
b) Mercaptopurine/Methotrexate .... ☐
c) No treatment (to avoid toxicities) .... ☐
d) DLI only .... ☐

2. **Is RIC allogeneic HSCT an option in adult ALL?**
   a) Not at all .... ☐
   b) Generally preferable in younger patients due to lower toxicity .... ☐
   c) Within studies focussed on older patients and those
      with comorbidities .... ☐
   d) Studies showed no benefit for RIC in ALL .... ☐

3. **Concerning the results of allogeneic HSCT in adult ALL, which of the following statments is correct?**
   a) The use of unrelated or other alternative donors is usually
      contra-indicated in adult ALL .... ☐
   b) In the HLA-matched unrelated setting, survival in 1st CR is around
      40–45% .... ☐
   c) The use of cord blood cells is the graft source of choice in adult ALL .... ☐
   d) The use of haploindetical donors is not feasible in allogeneic HSCT
      for adult ALL .... ☐

4. **What are the results of autologous HSCT compared to chemotherapy in adult ALL?**
   a) The overall survival of patients receiving autologous HSCT in 1st CR
      is around 40% .... ☐
   b) The major problem with autologous HSCT in ALL is the high incidence
      of NRM .... ☐
   c) Overall survival is superior compared to allogeneic HSCT .... ☐
   d) Post-transplant maintenance after autologous HSCT for ALL proved
      to be easy to administer .... ☐

5. **What is the role of MRD assessment in adult ALL?**
   a) No role at all for MRD in adult ALL since this is a chemosensitive
      disease .... ☐
   b) MRD is useful only after allogeneic HSCT for detection of relapse .... ☐
   c) MRD status is increasingly considered both before and after allogeneic
      HSCT, to decide on additional treatment either before HSCT in order
      to reduce tumour load or after HSCT to prevent relapse .... ☐
   d) None of the above statements is correct .... ☐

NOTES

* CHAPTER 19

Indications for HSCT in adults

* 19.3
HSCT for myelodysplastic syndromes

Nicolaus Kröger

1. Introduction

The myelodysplastic syndromes (MDS) are a heterogeneous group of clonal stem cell disorders characterised by hypercellular bone marrow, peripheral cytopenias, and dysplastic features in blood and bone marrow. The clinical course of the disease varies from an indolent course over several years to a more rapid progression into secondary acute myeloid leukaemia. MDS is mainly diagnosed in elderly patients with an annual incidence of MDS over the age of 50 years of 4.9/100,000. The current WHO classification (2008) distinguishes the following MDS subtypes (Table 1).

Due to the variable course of the disease several risk scores have been developed. The most common risk classification is the International Prognostic Scoring System (IPSS) which was introduced by Greenberg in 1997 (Table 2) (1). This classification uses cytogenetic abnormalities, number of cytopenias, and blast count to distinguish 4 risk groups: low, intermediate I, intermediate II, and high-risk, which predict survival and the risk of AML evolution. Age was an additional prognostic factor for survival but not for AML evolution. The median survival time for patients in these four groups has been estimated at 5.7 years (low-risk), 3.5 years (intermediate I), 1.2 years (intermediate II), and 0.4 years (high-risk). Therefore intensive treatment strategies are predominantly used in patients with intermediate II and high-risk and in some cases also in patients with intermediate I risk.

The importance of transfusion dependency is included in a WHO prognostic scoring system (WPSS) and the increasing knowledge of different cytogenetic abnormalities will lead to an updated version of the IPSS in the near future.

2. Autologous stem cell transplantation

Due to the high relapse rate observed after chemotherapy alone, autologous stem cell transplantation has been applied as a post-remission therapy to reduce the risk of relapse. The major concerns about autologous stem cell transplantation are the probability of contamination of the graft and the feasibility of collecting a sufficient number of stem cells. However, it could be demonstrated by clonality analysis that polyclonal haematopoietic progenitor cells can be harvested in MDS patients and a sufficient number of haematopoietic progenitor cells can be collected in 50–70% of the MDS patients. Two large studies of autologous stem cell transplantation in MDS have been published. In a registry study of the EBMT including 79 patients with MDS who underwent autologous HSCT in first complete remission (2), the two year disease-free and overall survival were 34 and 39%, respectively, while non-relapse mortality and relapse rate were 19 and 64%, respectively. Age lower than 40 years was associated with a superior disease-free survival (39 vs 25%). More recently the EBMT reported a comparison between peripheral blood stem cells and bone marrow

Table 1: **Classification of MSD**

Disease	Blood findings	Bone marrow findings
Refractory cytopenias with unilineage dysplasia (RCUD) Refractory anaemia (RA) Refractory neutropenia (RN) Refractory thrombocytopenia (RT)	Unicytopenia or bicytopenia[1] No or rare blasts (<1%)[2]	Unilineage dysplasia: ≥10% of the cells in one myeloid lineage <5% blasts <15% of erythroid precursors are ring sideroblasts
Refractory anaemia with ring sideroblasts (RARS)	Anaemia No blasts	≥15% of erythroid precursors are ring sideroblasts Erythroid dysplasia only <5% blasts
Refractory cytopenia with multilineage dysplasia (RCMD)	Cytopenia(s) No or rare blasts (<1%)[2] No Auer rods <1 x 10⁹/L monocytes	Dysplasia in ≥10% of the cells in ≥ two myeloid lineages (neutrophil and/or erythroid precursors and/or megakaryocytes) <5% blasts in marrow No Auer rods ±15% ring sideroblasts
Refractory anaemia with excess blasts-1 (RAEB-1)	Cytopenia(s) <5% blasts[2] No Auer rods <1 x 10⁹/L monocytes	Unilineage or multilineage dysplasia 5-9% blasts[2] No Auer rods
Refractory anaemia with excess blasts-2 (RAEB-2)	Cytopenia(s) 5-19% blasts Auer rods ±[3] <1 x 10⁹/L monocytes	Unilineage or multilineage dysplasia 10-19% blasts Auer rods ±[3]
Myelodysplastic syndrome – unclassified (MDS-U)	Cytopenias ≤1% blasts[2]	Unequivocal dysplasia in less than 10% of cells in one or more myeloid cell lines when accompanied by a cytogenetic abnormality considered as presumptive evidence for a diagnosis of MDS and with <5% blasts
MDS associated with isolated del(5q)	Anaemia Usually normal or increased platelet count No or rare blasts (<1%)	Normal to increased megakaryocytes with hypolobated nuclei <5% blasts Isolated del(5q) cytogenetic abnormality No Auer rods

[1] *Bicytopenia may occasionally be observed. Cases with pancytopenia should be classified as MDS-U;*
[2] *If the marrow myeloblast percentage is <5% but there are 2-4% myeloblasts in the blood, the diagnostic classification is RAEB-1. Cases of RCUD and RCMD with 1% myeloblasts in the blood should be classified as MDS-U;* [3] *Cases with Auer rods and <5% myeloblasts in the blood and <10% in the marrow should be classified as RAEB-2*

Table 2: Risk-score according to the International MDS Workshop (IPSS)

Single factors

Prognostic factors	Score				
	0	0.5	1.0	1.5	2.0
Bone marrow blasts	<5%	5-10%	5-10%	11-20%	21-30%
Karyotype*	Low-risk	Intermediate risk	High-risk		
Involved cell lines**	0-1	2-3			

Risk groups

Prognostic factors	Score sum	Risk of malignant transformation***	Median time of survival
Low risk	0	>18	65 months
Intermediate 1 (Int 1)	0.5–1.0	8 years	40 months
Intermediate 2 (Int 2)	1.5–2.0	3 years	14 months
High risk	>2.5	0.5 years	5 months

*   Low-risk: Normal karyotype, -Y, 5q-, 20q-
     High-risk: Complex karyotype, anomalies of Chromosome 7
     Intermediate risk: All other aberrations.
** Number of involved cell lines (granulopoiesis, erythropoiesis, thrombopoiesis)
*** Time until development of AML (median)

as stem cell source for autologous transplantation in 336 patients. The engraftment after PBSC was faster in comparison to bone marrow, but the risk of relapse and the event-free survival were similar. However there was an interaction between age and source of stem cells indicating a more favourable outcome in younger patients if autologous peripheral blood cells were used.

In a prospective French trial 24 out of 45 patients who received induction chemotherapy underwent autologous stem cell transplantation (3). Haematological recovery occurred in all patients but no difference between PBSC and bone marrow with regard to the speed of engraftment could be observed. The median disease-free and overall survivals were 29 and 33 months, respectively. Table 3 shows results of selected trials investigating intensive chemotherapy followed by autologous stem cell transplantation in high-risk MDS.

In a multicentre study of the EORTC, EBMT, SAKK, and GIMEMA, 159 patients with MDS or sAML (secondary AML) received induction chemotherapy with anthracycline, cytosine arabinoside, and etoposide, to be followed by allogeneic stem cell transplantation, if an HLA-identical donor was available, or autologous stem cell transplantation if there was no donor. 69% of the patients with a donor actually

Table 3: Selected trials of autologous stem cell transplantation in MDS

Author	Patient	Median age	CR	Number of transplants	Outcome
de Witte, 1997 (2)	MDS (n=19) sAML (n=60)	39	79	79 (only CR patients selected for transplants)	DFS: 34% OS: 39%
Wattel, 1999 (3)	MDS (n=37) sAML (n=46)	45	51	24	DFS: 29 months OS: 33 months

received an allograft and 49% of those with no donor received an autograft. The 4 year event-free survival was 23% for patients with a donor and 22% for patients without a donor (4).

The EBMT also reported results of autologous stem cell transplantation in 65 patients with therapy-related MDS or AML. The non-relapse mortality was 12% and the cumulative incidence of relapse was 58%, resulting in a 3 year disease-free survival of 32% (5). Younger age of patients (<40 y) and complete remission at time of transplantation influenced the survival significantly. However, in the European transplant community autologous stem cell transplantation has only a negligible role in MDS and the number of autografts for MDS decreased from 105 in 2001 to less than 50 in 2007.

3. Syngeneic stem cell transplantation

Only one out of three hundred patients with MDS will have a syngeneic twin. Therefore, syngeneic stem cell transplantation can be performed only rarely. The EBMT reported results for 38 patients with MDS/sAML who received a syngeneic graft after standard myeloablative conditioning (6). The authors compared the result with 1444 patients who received stem cell transplantation from an HLA-identical sibling within the same time period. The engraftment after syngeneic transplantation was faster and the non-relapse mortality was lower (27% vs 38%). The relapse rate was only slightly higher after twin transplantation (39% vs 32%), resulting in a trend for improved disease free survival at 5 years (34% vs 28%).

4. Allogeneic stem cell transplantation

Despite improvement in treatment of MDS and the approval of novel drugs such as hypomethylating agents, the treatment strategy with the highest curative potential remains allogeneic stem cell transplantation. The numbers of allogeneic stem cell transplants are rapidly increasing in Europe. While 620 patients with MDS were transplanted in 2001, the number increased to 1194 in 2007. This increase is due to an increase in transplantation of older patients (>50 years) from 316 (in 2001) to 724 (in 2007) and to an increase of matched unrelated donors: from 233 (in 2001) to 679 (in 2007).

4.1 HLA-identical sibling donors

Disease-free survival between 29% and 40% were reported. The non-relapse mortality ranged between 37% and 50% and the relapse rate between 23% and 48% (7–12). Table 4 shows results from selected trials of allogeneic stem cell transplantation from HLA-identical siblings in MDS patients.

Patients with less advanced stage of MDS such as RA or RARS may benefit most from allogeneic stem cell transplantation, with a long-term disease-free survival of more than 50%. The outcome of patients with RAEB and RAEB-t is less favourable due to a higher relapse rate. The EBMT reported a 5-year relapse rate of 44% for RAEB and 52% for RAEB-t and the Fred Hutchinson Cancer Research Center (FHCRC) reported a 49% relapse rate for RAEB patients in comparison to only 4% for patients without any bone marrow blasts. Large studies from the EBMT and the IBMTR confirmed age and number of blasts as independent risk factors for lower survival rates. Cytogenetic abnormalities were also shown to be of importance to the outcome of allogeneic HSCT. The EBMT recently reported on the impact of cytogenetic status - classified according to IPSS - on outcome after allogeneic HSCT. In 692 patients a complete data set was available. The cytogenetic risk according to IPSS significantly influenced survival: 47% for good risk, 40% for intermediate risk, and 31% for high risk. The relapse rate was 34% for good risk, 35% for intermediate risk, and 57% for high risk cytogenetic status. In addition to age, cytogenetic risk score remained an independent prognostic factor for relapse and survival in multivariate analysis (13). Another study also investigated outcomes of allogeneic stem cell transplantation in 70 MDS patients according to IPSS cytogenetic risk score. The event-free survival for good, intermediate, and high risk cytogenetic subgroups was 51%, 40%, and 6%, respectively. While no difference in non-relapse mortality was seen, the relapse rates

Table 4: Allogeneic stem cell transplantation for MDS and sAML from HLA-identical sibling donors

Author	Patients	Median age (years)	DFS	Relapse (%)	Non-relapse mortality (%)
Anderson, 1993 (7)	93	30	40% (at 5 y)	29	44
Sutton, 1996 (8)	71	37	32% (at 7 y)	48	39
Runde, 1998 (12)	131	33	34% (at 5 y)	39	44
Nevill, 1998 (14)	60	40	29% (at 7 y)	42	50
de Witte, 2000 (9)	885	33	36% (at 3 y)	36	43
Sierra, 2002 (11)	452	38	40% (at 3 y)	23	37
Deeg, 2002 (10)	41	46	56% (at 3 y)	16	28

were 19% for good risk, 12% for intermediate, and 82% for high risk patients (14). These results suggested a major impact of cytogenetic abnormalities on outcome after allogeneic stem cell transplantation. Originally the IPSS scores were based on patients who did not receive cytoreductive therapy but recent reports suggest that IPSS scores may have also impact on survival after allogeneic stem cell transplantation. If classified according to IPSS, the 5 year disease-free survival was 60% for low and intermediate I risk, 36% for intermediate II risk, and 28% for high risk.

4.2 Alternative donors

Since most patients with MDS are lacking an HLA-identical sibling as stem cell donor, unrelated stem cell transplantation has been investigated. Table 5 shows results of selected trials investigating unrelated HSCT in patients with MDS.

The studies listed in Table 5 reported a high non-relapse mortality which was mostly influenced by age (15, 16). However the results have improved more recently due to a lower non-relapse mortality. The National Marrow Donor Program reported a relative risk for DFS of 1.43 for transplantation performed between 1988 and 1993 versus more recent transplantation (17). Additional further reduction of non-relapse mortality was observed after the introduction of targeted busulfan/cyclophosphamide conditioning (10). Unpublished results of the EBMT registry showed, for MDS transplantation in recent years, no difference in survival of unrelated stem cell transplantation in comparison to HLA-identical sibling transplantation after adjustment for age and disease status.

A retrospective study of the EBMT compared unrelated stem cell transplantation with autologous stem cell transplantation in patients in first complete remission. The disease-free survival was 50% for unrelated stem cell transplantation and 41% for autologous stem cell transplantation (p=0.01). The better survival of unrelated stem cell transplantation was due to a lower risk of relapse (24 vs 62%), despite the higher non-relapse mortality (38 vs 17%) (18).

Table 5: **Selected results of unrelated stem cell transplantation in patients with MDS/sAML**

Author	Patients	Median age	DFS	Relapse (%)	TRM (%)
Anderson, 1996 (15)	52	33	38% (at 2 y)	28	48
Arnold, 1998 (16)	118	24	28% (at 2 y)	35	58
Deeg, 2002 (10)	64	46	59% (at 2 y)	11	30
Castro-Malaspina, 2002 (17)	510	38	29% (at 2 y)	14	54

However, the success of unrelated stem cell transplantation depends on the degree of HLA matching: high resolution DNA matching for HLA-A, HLA-B and HLA-C and DRB1 alleles of donor-recipient HLA is associated with improved survival.

Alternative stem cell sources, such as cord blood or haplo-identical stem cell transplantation are being used increasingly for patients lacking a suitable donor, but comparative studies are so far lacking.

5. Timing of transplantation

The optimal timing of stem cell transplantation with MDS is still a matter of debate. To determine the optimal timing for an allograft in MDS-patients a multistate model was used to determine the relevance of IPSS scores and the expected outcome after transplantation (19). The results suggest that MDS patients with intermediate II and high risk have best survival if transplantation is performed immediately after diagnosis, while MDS patients with low or intermediate I risk score benefit most from allogeneic stem cell transplantation if the transplant is delayed until clear signs of progression occur. The weakness of the study is that only myeloablative transplantation and HLA-identical siblings were included, while age or comorbidity were not addressed.

6. Induction chemotherapy: yes or no?

Another issue of importance is the question of pre-transplant chemotherapy in patients with advanced MDS (high number of blasts). The impact of pre-transplant chemotherapy still remains controversial. A French trial of therapy-related MDS reported a substantially better outcome in those patients who achieved remission with pre-transplant chemotherapy (20). However, patients who failed to achieve remission after induction chemotherapy and underwent stem cell transplantation while not in CR had a worse outcome after transplantation than those who did not receive pre-transplant chemotherapy. These results suggest that the pre-transplant chemotherapy selects patients with an improved post-transplant outcome. Results from prospective randomised trials addressing this important issue are not available. A more recently investigated approach is performing induction chemotherapy followed immediately by the conditioning regimen and stem cell transplantation. A schedule of induction chemotherapy with fludarabine, amsacrine and high-dose cytosine arabinoside followed by a three-day rest and then TBI (4 Gy) and cyclophosphamide with or without anti-thymocyte globulin and stem cell transplantation with pre-emptive donor lymphocyte infusion has been used in patients with MDS (n=67) or sAML (n=90). The overall survival rate for the MDS patients at 10 years was 50% and was significantly higher than for patients with sAML (26%).

An alternative to chemotherapy is epigenetic modulation by biochemical modifications of chromatin without altering the sequence of DNA. Two DNA hypomethylating agents are available for patients with MDS: azacitidine (5-azacitidine) and decitabine (5-aza-2'-deoxycitidine), but only the former is approved in Europe. Both drugs are DNMT inhibitors that have demethylating effects. Azacitidine has been shown superiority regarding time to AML transformation and overall survival in randomised trials comparing it to best supportive care or other chemotherapeutic interventions (21). Only small phase II studies have investigated the feasibility of using azacitidine or decitabine as induction therapy prior to allogeneic stem cell transplantation and so the number of patients treated with hypomethylating agents before allogeneic stem cell transplantation is still limited and valid conclusions cannot be drawn.

7. Source of stem cells

A retrospective study of the EBMT compared bone marrow with peripheral blood stem cells as the stem cell source in HLA-identical sibling transplantation. MDS patients who received peripheral blood stem cells (PBSC) had a faster engraftment and a lower relapse rate resulting in improved disease-free survival compared to patients who received bone marrow. Furthermore, while the incidence of acute GvHD was similar between both groups, patients who received PBSC had a higher incidence of chronic GvHD (22). Similar results have been reported from the Seattle group with a 3-year DFS of 68% for PBSC transplant compared to 48% who received bone marrow.

8. Preparative regimen

As reported by the EBMT, most MDS patients received either a busulfan/cyclopho-sphamide-based (52%) or a TBI-based (44%) regimen. A report of the National Marrow Donor Program for unrelated stem cell transplantation reported a lower relapse rate and a better survival for patients with busulfan/cyclophosphamide conditioning in comparison to TBI regimen (17). Improved outcome using targeted busulfan/cyclopho-sphamide regimen has been reported by the Seattle group. They used a target level of busulfan (800–900 ng/mL) to avoid severe toxicity (10). Patients with RA/RARS had a 68% probability of disease-free survival after HLA-identical transplantation and of 70% if they received a graft from an unrelated donor. The non-relapse mortality was 12% at 100 days and 31% at 3 years, while relapse occurred in only 5%. For advanced patients with RAEB a 45% probability of disease-free survival after HLA-identical sibling transplantation and a 40% disease-free survival at 3 years after unrelated transplantation was reported.

Since cyclophosphamide is not stem cell toxic but contributes to non-haematological toxicity, attempts have been made to replace cyclophosphamide by fludarabine. Targeting busulfan in combination with fludarabine has been investigated in patients with myeloid malignancies. In 38 patients with MDS the non-relapse mortality at day 100 and 1 year was 7% and 24%, respectively. Further improvement in non-relapse mortality has been reported by using intravenous busulfan in combination with fludarabine, resulting in a non-relapse mortality of only 3% and 1 year (23).

Attempts to reduce the relapse rate by using an intensified regimen have been made by the Fred Hutchinson Cancer Center, evaluating the combination of busulfan (7 mg/kg), cyclophosphamide (120 mg/kg), and TBI (12 Gy) in advanced MDS (RAEB, RAEB-t, and CMML) patients. In comparison to an historical control group the relapse rate could be lowered (28% vs 54%), however this advantage was offset by a higher non-relapse mortality (68% vs 36%) resulting in a worse relapse-free survival (23% vs 30%). Even if cyclophosphamide was replaced by fludarabine in 50 patients with advanced MDS and sAML, the NRM was still very high at day 100 (38%) resulting in a disappointing overall survival of only 26% at 3 years. Therefore intensified conditioning regimens do not appear to be beneficial.

8.1 Non-myeloablative or reduced intensity regimen

The rationale to decrease the intensity is to shift tumour reduction or eradication of tumour cells from cytoreduction to an immunologically mediated graft-versus-tumour effect. Furthermore, reduction of the intensity will also reduce transplant-related toxicity and therefore transplant-related mortality. This approach would also allow transplantation of older patients and those who are not eligible for a standard myeloablative conditioning regimen.

Table 6 shows results of a selection of phase II studies investigating several reduced intensity conditioning regimens in patients with MDS or sAML. The most commonly used regimen is busulfan (8 mg/kg) in combination with fludarabine, with or without Campath or ATG. In 62 patients the Bu/Flu/Campath regimen has been investigated either with related or unrelated donors. The relapse-free survival was about 60% at 1 year and non-relapse mortality was 5% for related and 21% for unrelated stem cell transplantation (24).

Busulfan/fludarabine and ATG (for unrelated HSCT) was used in studies from the German Co-operative Transplant Study Group resulting in non-relapse mortality of 32%, a relapse incidence of 32%, and a disease-free survival of 38% at 3 years (25). Busulfan plus fludarabine without any T-cell depletion in HLA-identical sibling transplantation resulted in a low treatment related mortality of only 5% at 1 year and a disease-free survival of 66% at 1 year. The low-intensity approach with 2 Gy TBI ± fludarabine in 78 patients with MDS had a 25% TRM and an estimated 3 years disease-free survival of 20% (26). Another regimen included treosulfan, an alkylating agent, in combination with fludarabine and ATG for elderly patients with MDS and sAML. The median age was 60 years, and patients received stem cells from a related

Table 6: **Examples of reduced-intensity conditioning regimens in patients with MDS or sAML**

Author	Patients	Median age (years)	Conditioning regimen	DFS	Relapse (%)	NRM (%)
Ho, 2004 (24)	24	56	Bu (8 mg/kg) + Campath + Fludarabine	61% (at 1 y)	-	5
Ho (MUD), 2004 (24)	38	52	ditto	59% (at 1 y)	-	21
Kröger, 2003 (25)	37	55	Bu (8 mg/kg) Fludarabine ± ATG	38% (at 3 y)	32	32
Kröger, 2006 (27)	26	60	Treosulfan Fludarabine ± ATG	34% (at 2 y)	21	28
Stuart, 2003 (26)	78	59	2 Gy TBI ± Fludarabine	20% (at 3 y)	43	25

(n=6) or unrelated donor (n=20). No graft failure was observed and the day 100 non-relapse mortality was 28%. The relapse rate at 2 years was 21% resulting in a 2 year disease-free survival of 34% (27). The EBMT performed a retrospective study comparing dose-reduced (RIC) and standard conditioning in 836 patients with MDS who underwent HLA-identical sibling transplantation. They found a significantly lower incidence of treatment related mortality (p=0.015), but a significantly higher incidence of relapse (p=0.001) in the RIC group, resulting in comparable disease-free and overall survival rates in both groups (28). However it is of note that patients transplanted with reduced intensity conditioning were of higher age and often suffered from comorbidities and were therefore not eligible for a standard conditioning. For this reason the EBMT has started a randomised trial comparing standard and reduced intensity conditioning (*http://www.ebmt.org*).

9. Post-stem cell transplantation modifications
Besides improving the pre-transplant status of MDS patients by inducing clinical and cytogenetic remission, further approaches to reduce the risk of relapse after allogeneic stem cell transplantation involve post-transplant modifications.
1. Adoptive immunotherapy: donor-lymphocyte infusion. The experience of DLI in MDS patients is limited; complete remission rates of 14–22% have been reported, but most patients with complete remission also experienced severe acute and chronic GvHD.

2. Relapse or maintenance therapy with azacitidine. Efficacy of azacitidine for relapsing patients after allogeneic stem cell transplantation in combination with DLI was shown in a small phase II trial. The MD Anderson Cancer Center investigated azacitidine at doses between 8 and 24 mg/m² for five days given for one to four cycles as maintenance therapy in 40 high-risk MDS or AML patients. They observed no severe side effects and no impact of azacitidine on GvHD and chimerism. The recommended dose of azacitidine was 24 mg/m² x 5 for at least 4 cycles.

3. Vaccination and T-cell specific immunotherapy. The donor-derived haematopoietic and lymphopoietic system offers a platform for several immunologic based interventions after allogeneic stem cell transplantation to treat residual minimal disease and to prevent relapse. Leukaemia-specific antigens such as WT1, PR1, RHAMM or cancer testis antigens have been tested as peptide based vaccinations eliciting immunologic T-cell response and some clinical remission, however only a very few of the study population suffered from MDS.

10. Conclusions

Allogeneic HSCT is the treatment of choice for patients with advanced stage MDS who have a suitable donor. The outcome after allogeneic stem cell transplantation has improved progressively in recent years due to a continuous reduction in non-relapse mortality. Reduced-intensity conditioning (RIC) regimens have extended the use of allogeneic stem cell transplantation to patients up to the age of 70 years, but its role in the treatment of MDS patients remains to be determined.

Several questions remain to be solved by prospective studies such as the impact of pre-transplant chemotherapy in RAEB/RAEB-t patients or the comparison between reduced-intensity and standard myeloablative conditioning. Since age is no longer a limiting factor, comorbidity indices needed to be considered in new studies. New trials of allogeneic HSCT will incorporate new agents such as demethylating agents or histone-deacetylase-inhibitors either as induction to reduce blast count prior to transplantation or as a post-transplant strategy to prevent relapse.

References

1. Greenberg P, Cox C, Le Beau M et al. International scoring system for evaluating prognosis in myelodysplastic syndromes. Blood 1997; 89: 2079–2088.
2. De Witte T, van Biezen A, Hermans J et al. Autologous bone marrow transplantation for patients with myelodys plastic syndrome (MDS) or acute myeloid leukemia following MDS. Blood 1997; 90: 3853–3857.
3. Wattel E, Solary E, Leleu X et al. Groupe Français des Myélodysplasies (GFM) and Groupe Ouest-Est d'étude des Leucémies aiguës myéloïdes (GOELAMS). A prospective study of autologous bone marrow or peripheral blood stem cell transplantation after intensive chemotherapy in myelodysplastic syndromes. Leukemia 1999; 13: 524–529.

4.   Oosterveld M, Suciu S, Verhoef G et al. The presence of an HLA-identical sibling donor has no impact on outcome of patients with high-risk MDS or secondary AML (sAML) treated with intensive chemo-therapy followed by transplantation: Results of a prospective study of the EORTC, EBMT, SAKK and GIMEMA Leukemia Groups (EORTC study 06921). Leukemia 2003; 17: 859–868.

5.   Kröger N, Brand R, van Biezen A et al. Autologous stem cell transplantation for therapy-related acute myeloid leukemia and myelodysplastic syndrome. Bone Marrow Transplant 2006; 37: 183–189.

6.   Kröger N, Brand R, van Biezen A et al. Myelodysplastic Syndromes Subcommittee of the Chronic Leukaemia Working Party, European Blood and Marrow Transplantation Group. Stem cell transplantation from identical twins in patients with myelodysplastic syndromes. Bone Marrow Transplant 2005; 35: 37–43.

7.   Anderson JE, Appelbaum FR, Fisher LD et al. Allogeneic bone marrow transplantation for 93 patients with myelodysplastic syndrome. Blood 1993; 2: 677–681.

8.   Sutton L, Chastang C, Ribaud P et al. Factors influencing outcome in de-novo myelodysplastic syndromes treated by allogeneic bone marrow transplantation: A long-term study of 71 patients. Blood 1996; 88: 358–365.

9.   De Witte, Hermans J, Vossen J et al. Haematopoietic stem cell transplantation for patients with myelodysplastic syndromes and secondary acute myeloid leukaemias: A report on behalf of the Chronic Leukemia Working Party of the European Group for Blood and Marrow Transplantation (EBMT). Br J Haematol 2000; 110: 620–630.

10. Deeg HJ, Storer B, Slattery JT et al. Conditioning with targeted busulfan and cyclophosphamide for he mopoietic stem cell transplantation from related and unrelated donors in patients with myelodysplastic syndrome. Blood 2002; 100: 1201–1207.

11. Sierra J, Pérez WS, Rozman C et al. Bone marrow transplantation from HLA-identical siblings as treatment for myelodysplasia. Blood 2002; 100: 1997–2004.

12. Runde V, de Witte T, Arnold C et al. Bone marrow transplantation from HLA-identical siblings as first-line treatment in patients with myelodysplastic syndromes: Early transplantation is associated with improved outcome. Bone Marrow Transplant 1998; 21: 255–260.

13. Onida F, Brand R, van Biezen A et al. Impact of cytogenetics on outcome of patients with MDS or secondary AML undergoing allogeneic HSCT from HLA-identical siblings: A retrospective analysis of the EBMT-CLWP. Abstract in: Blood 2006 Nov 16; 108: 11 (abs).

14. Nevill TJ, Fung HC, Shepherd JD et al. Cytogenetic abnormalities in primary myelodysplastic syndrome are highly predictive of outcome after allogeneic bone marrow transplantation. Blood 1998; 92: 1910–1917.

15. Anderson JE, Anasetti C, Appelbaum FR et al. Unrelated donor marrow transplantation for myelodysplasia (MDS) and MDS-related acute myeloid leukemia. Br J Haematol 1996; 93: 59–67.

16. Arnold R, de Witte T, van Biezen A et al. Unrelated bone marrow transplantation in patients with myelodysplastic syndromes and secondary acute myeloid leukemia: An EBMT survey. Bone Marrow Transplant 1998; 21: 1213–1216.

17. Castro-Malaspina H, Harris RE, Gajewski J et al. Unrelated donor marrow transplantation for myelodysplastic syndromes: Outcome analysis in 510 transplants facilitated by the National Marrow Donor Program. Blood 2002; 99: 1943–1951.
18. Al-Ali KH, Brand R, van Biezen A et al. Myelodysplasias. A retrospective comparison of autologous and unrelated donor hematopoietic cell transplantation in myelodysplastic syndrome and secondary acute myeloid leukemia: A report on behalf of the Chronic Leukemia Working Party of the European Group for Blood and Marrow Transplantation (EBMT). Leukemia 2007; 21: 1945–1951.
19. Cutler CS, Lee SJ, Greenberg P et al. A decision analysis of allogeneic bone marrow transplantation for the myelodysplastic syndromes: Delayed transplantation for low-risk myelodysplasia is associated with improved outcome. Blood 2004; 104: 579–585.
20. Yakoub-Agha I, de la Salmonière P, Ribaud P et al. Allogeneic bone marrow transplantation for therapy-related myelodysplastic syndrome and acute myeloid leukemia: A long-term study of 70 pa-tients-report of the French Society of Bone Marrow Transplantation. J Clin Oncol 2000; 18: 963–971.
21. Silverman LR, Demakos EP, Peterson BL et al. Randomized controlled trial of azacitidine in patients with the myelodysplastic syndrome: A study of the cancer and leukaemia group B. J Clin Oncol 2002; 20: 2429–2440.
22. Guardiola P, Runde V, Bacigalupo A et al. Subcommittee for Myelodysplastic Syndromes of the Chronic Leukaemia Working Group of the European Blood and Marrow Transplantation Group. Retrospective comparison of bone marrow and granulocyte colony-stimulating factor-mobilized peripheral blood progenitor cells for allogeneic stem cell transplantation using HLA identical sibling donors in myelodysplastic syndromes. Blood 2002; 99: 4370–4378.
23. de Lima M, Couriel D, Thall PF et al. Once-daily intraveneous busulfan and fludarabine: Clinical and pharmacokinetic results of a myeloablative, reduced-toxicity conditioning regimen for allogeneic stem cell transplantation in AML and MDS. Blood 2004; 104: 857–864.
24. Ho AY, Pagliuca A, Kenyon M et al. Reduced intensity allogeneic haematopoietic stem cell transplantation for myelodysplastic syndrome and acute myeloid leukemia with multilineage dysplasia using Fludarabine, Busulphan, and Alemtuzumab (Campath-1H) (FBC) conditioning. Blood 2004; 104: 1616–1623.
25. Kröger N, Bornhäuser M, Ehninger G et al. German Cooperative Transplant Study Group. Allogeneic stem cell transplantation after fludarabine/busulfan-based reduced-intensity conditioning in patients with myelodysplastic sydrome or secondary acute myeloid leukemia. Ann Hematol 2003; 82: 336–342.
26. Stuart MJ, Cao TM, Sandmaier BM et al. Efficacy of non-myeloablative allogeneic transplant for patients with myelodysplastic syndrome (MDS) and myeloproliferative disorders (MPD) (except chronic myelogenous leukemia). Blood 2003; 102 (Part 1): 185a, #644 (abs).
27. Kröger N, Shimoni A, Zabelina T et al. Reduced-toxicity conditioning with treosulfan, fludarabine and ATG as preparative regimen for allogeneic stem cell transplantation

(alloSCT) in elderly patients with secondary acute myeloid leukemia (sAML) or myelodysplastic syndrome (MDS). Bone Marrow Transplant 2006; 37: 339–344.
28. Martino R, Iacobelli S, Brand R et al. Myelodysplastic Syndrome Subcommittee of the Chronic Leukemia Working Party of the European Blood and Marrow Transplantation Group. Retrospective comparison of reduced-intensity conditioning and conventional high-dose conditioning for allogeneic hematopoietic stem cell transplantation using HLA-identical sibling donors in myelodysplastic syndromes. Blood 2006; 108: 836–846.

Multiple Choice Questionnaire

To find the correct answer, go to http://www.esh.org/online-training/handbook/

1. **The median survival for MDS patients with intermediate 2 risk without transplantation is:**
   a) 48 months .... ☐
   b) 36 months .... ☐
   c) 24 months .... ☐
   d) 14 months .... ☐

2. **The 5 year disease-free survival after identical twin transplantation for MDS patients is:**
   a) 62% .... ☐
   b) 48% .... ☐
   c) 34% .... ☐
   d) 12% .... ☐

3. **In comparison to autologous transplantation, allogeneic stem cell transplantation from an unrelated donor results in:**
   a) Lower treatment-related mortality .... ☐
   b) Higher risk of relapse .... ☐
   c) Better overall survival .... ☐
   d) Lower toxicity .... ☐

4. **According to a retrospective EBMT study a reduced-intensity regimen, in comparison to standard myeloablative regimen, is associated with:**

a) Higher risk of relapse... ☐
b) Similar treatment-related mortality............................ ☐
c) Significantly more GvHD .... ☐
d) Significantly more graft failure............................... ☐

5. **The value of induction chemotherapy before transplantation in advanced MDS is:**
   a) Uncertain... ☐
   b) International standard .... ☐
   c) Proven only in young patients................................ ☐
   d) Based on karyotype... ☐

* CHAPTER 19

Indications for HSCT in adults

* 19.4

Chronic myeloid leukaemia and the myeloproliferative disorders

Jiri Pavlu, Jane Apperley

1. Chronic myeloid leukaemia

1.1 History and introduction

Chronic myeloid leukaemia (CML) was the first leukaemia described and the first to be characterised by a consistent chromosomal aberration, the 22q- or "Philadelphia" (Ph) chromosome, later identified as a reciprocal translocation, t(9;22), encoding the Bcr-Abl oncoprotein. Early descriptions of therapy included radiotherapy, introduced at the beginning of 20th century and later oral chemotherapy, in particular busulfan and hydroxycarbamide. These approaches could control the signs and symptoms of CML in chronic phase but could not prevent its inevitable transformation into a rapidly fatal chemoresistant blastic disease. The first treatment that eradicated the Ph-positive clone and induced cure was bone marrow transplantation, initially described in syngeneic twins and soon followed by procedures involving HLA-matched siblings and later unrelated donors.

Transplantation, once the treatment of choice for this disease, has been relegated to second, third and even fourth line treatment in parallel with the development of the targeted tyrosine kinase inhibitors (TKI). As more potent TKI move to first-line therapy, patients destined to respond poorly to these drugs are identified earlier and transplant will return to use as a second-line strategy.

1.2 Factors identified pre-transplant which affect outcome

The benefit of allo-HSCT is that it can provide cure, but the clear disadvantage is its association with considerable morbidity and mortality, which typically occur early post procedure. Outcome can be improved by better selection of those most likely to benefit. In this context the EBMT developed a risk score for patients with CML, based on five variables: donor type, disease phase, recipient age, donor/recipient gender combination, and interval from diagnosis to transplant, which together results in a score of 0–7 (Table 1) (2). Results of transplant are now highly predictable based on these five factors. It is worth remembering that the EBMT or "Gratwohl" score was developed in the mid-1990s and was based on 3142 patients transplanted between 1989 and 1996 (Figure 1A). With overall improvements in supportive care it would be reasonable to expect that a similar analysis performed on patients transplanted more recently would demonstrate improved results across all risk scores. However the analysis is complicated by the change in approach to management of CML. During the period of the original analysis, allo-HSCT was the treatment of choice for all patients. Since 2000 allo-HSCT has been replaced by imatinib as front-line therapy and hence the reasons for patients coming to transplant are not always clear from registry data. Although this should be

Table 1: **Pre-transplant factors affecting outcome (overall survival and transplant related-mortality) of allogeneic HSCT in chronic myeloid leukaemia**

Factor	Score
Disease phase	
Chronic phase	0
Accelerated phase or CP >1	1
Blast crisis	2
Age	
<20 years	0
20–40 years	1
>40 years	2
Stem cell source	
Sibling donor	0
Unrelated donor	1
Time from diagnosis to transplant	
<12 months	0
>12 months	1
Recipient-donor gender combinations	
Male into male	0
Male into female	0
Female into female	0
Female into male	1

compensated by the use of factors such as age at transplant, disease phase and time from diagnosis to transplant, some caution should be exercised in the interpretation of more recent results. Having said this, the analysis has been repeated recently for 8541 patients transplanted from 1996 to 2006 and confirmed improved outcome of 5 year overall survival across all risk scores by 5–10% (Figure 1B). In patients with scores of 3–7 the improvement has been a result of decreases in the rates of transplant related mortality (TRM), in those with lower risk scores, it is due to a combination of lower relapse rates (perhaps due to pre-emptive use of TKI) and a lower TRM.

Although these pre-transplant factors are known to affect outcome in all diseases, it is worth focusing specifically on the impact of disease phase in CML, in particular because one of the few problems of TKI therapy is that within the cohort of patients receiving transplants, the proportion transplanted in or after blast crisis has increased over time (Table 2). Allografts for CML were initially restricted to patients in advanced phase and improvements in survival came only when transplant was performed in the chronic phase. Data of 138 patients with CML transplanted between 1978 and 1982 and reported to the International Bone Marrow Transplant Registry

Figure 1: **Overall survival of CML patients after allo-HSCT according to EBMT risk score**

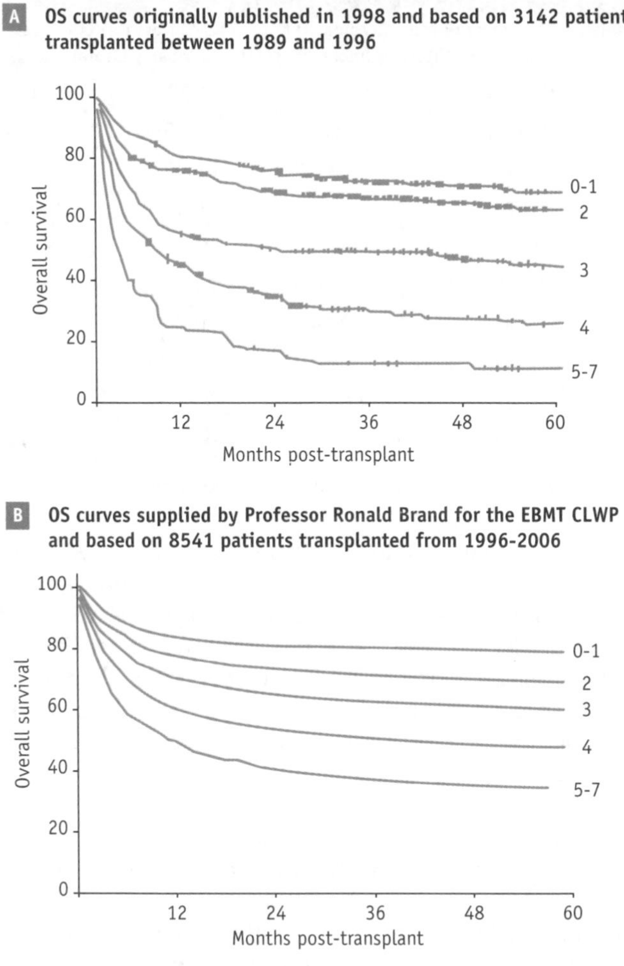
A
OS curves originally published in 1998 and based on 3142 patients transplanted between 1989 and 1996
Overall survival
100
80
60
40
20
0
12
24
36
48
60
Months post-transplant
0-1
2
3
4
5-7
B
OS curves supplied by Professor Ronald Brand for the EBMT CLWP and based on 8541 patients transplanted from 1996-2006
Overall survival
100
80
60
40
20
0
12
24
36
48
60
Months post-transplant
0-1
2
3
4
5-7

Modified from (2)

showed 3-year survivals of 63%, 56% and 16% for patients transplanted in the chronic, accelerated and blast phases respectively. Only 2 of 29 patients transplanted in chronic phase relapsed (7%) (3). The effect of disease phase on the outcome of transplantation has not changed over the years. To optimise the effect of allo-HSCT

Table 2: Change in proportion of patients transplanted in each disease phase from 1997-2006

Year of transplant	1st chronic phase Number (% total)	Acceleration Number (% total)	2nd or greater CP Number (% total)	Blast crisis Number (% total)
1997	763 (76)	139 (14)	54 (9)	51 (5)
1998	887 (74)	170 (14)	77 (10)	65 (5)
1999	954 (76)	174 (14)	78 (10)	56 (4)
2000	917 (80)	96 (8)	83 (10)	53 (5)
2001	646 (75)	72 (8)	99 (11)	47 (5)
2002	578 (68)	115 (13)	120 (14)	44 (5)
2003	424 (61)	107 (15)	118 (17)	47 (7)
2004	421 (63)	86 (13)	111 (17)	45 (7)
2005	369 (67)	64 (12)	76 (14)	41 (8)
2006	298 (60)	65 (13)	88 (18)	45 (9)

Data provided by Professor Ronald Brand on behalf of the EBMT CLWP

for a patient who has progressed to blast crisis, a second chronic phase should be achieved using TKI and/or conventional combination chemotherapy.

As the variable of disease phase was associated with higher relative risks than other variables in the model (2), Passweg et al. attempted to modify the score for patients in chronic phase for whom the decision of whether or not to transplant is most difficult. They found only one parameter with additional prognostic value, the Karnofsky performance score, but after inclusion the improvement over the original EBMT score was minimal (4).

1.3 Post-transplant factors affecting outcome

The major causes of morbidity and mortality during the early allo-HSCT period were infections and GvHD. In patients with CML the combination of cyclosporin and methotrexate gave good protection against GvHD without a significant increase in relapse and subsequently became a standard prophylactic regimen in most transplant centres.

The 1980s saw the introduction of T-cell depletion, first achieved by treating bone marrow *in vitro* with monoclonal antibodies and later by other *in vitro* techniques. This approach was effective in decreasing both the severity and frequency of GvHD, but was associated with a significantly higher frequency of graft failure. This was later overcome by increasing the intensity or immunosuppressive efficacy of conditioning, most elegantly achieved by the pre-transplant *in vivo* use of the same anti T-cell antibodies that were used for T-cell depletion of the graft. Unfortunately the widespread application of T-cell depletion soon revealed an increased relapse rate, which first became apparent in patients transplanted for CML (5). The increase in relapse rate led to many groups abandoning the use of T-cell depletion in sibling allografts for CML and often also in unrelated donor procedures. Others continued with its use and have reported good outcomes in sibling transplants, particularly following the introduction of donor lymphocyte infusions (DLI) (see later). As T cell-depletion delays immune reconstitution, infections are more common and CMV serological status is a significant predictor of overall survival with this transplantation technique. Although use of T-cell depletion in unrelated allo-HSCT showed shorter hospital stay and increased cost effectiveness compared to non T-cell depleted transplants, a clear survival advantage of this approach in CML has never been demonstrated.

1.4 Graft-versus-leukaemia and the use of donor lymphocyte infusions

Until the advent of T-cell depletion, relapse after allo-HSCT for chronic phase disease was rare: the increased incidence of relapse following T-cell depleted grafts and the ability of additional donor lymphocytes at the time of relapse to restore remission was proof of principle of the presence and importance of a graft-versus-leukaemia (GvL) effect.

Administration of DLI can re-induce remission in 60–90% of patients with CML transplanted in, and relapsing in, chronic phase. The use of escalating doses in case of persistent disease reduces the risk of GvHD (6). An EBMT study showed 69% 5-year survival in 328 of patients who received DLI for relapsed CML. DLI-related mortality was 11% and disease-related mortality was 20%. Some form of GvHD was observed in 38% of patients. Risk factors for developing GvHD after DLI were T-cell dose at first DLI, time interval from transplant to DLI and donor type. In a time-dependent multivariate analysis, GvHD after DLI was associated with a 2.3-fold increase in risk of death of compared with patients without GvHD (7).

Interestingly the introduction of DLI necessitated the development of new statistical methods. As the majority of relapsed patients could re-enter remission the method of calculation of LFS requires revision. One possible solution is the use of "current leukaemia-free survival" defined as the probability that a patient is alive and in remission at a given time after transplantation (8).

1.5 Minimal residual disease monitoring

The observation of an increased relapse rate following immunomodulation of the graft and the knowledge that DLI could restore durable remissions were the incentives to develop effective methods to identify small volumes of residual or recurrent disease so that treatment could be given promptly. In the 1980s conventional cytogenetics was the principal technique for detection of residual leukaemia. Reverse-transcriptase polymerase chain reaction (RT-PCR) assays were developed in the late 1980s and although these early assays were qualitative only they were useful in identifying early relapse post transplant. Modern quantitative RT-PCR (RQ-PCR) enabled the monitoring of early molecular relapse and the reliable prediction of cytogenetic and haematological disease. The technique, further sophisticated through real-time quantitative equipment, has become a standard tool for monitoring of CML responses to allo-HSCT and the TKI.

Many CML patients will remain RQ-PCR positive during the first three months after allo-HSCT, especially in the era of reduced-intensity preparative regimens. In patients who are at least four months post allo-HSCT one working definition of molecular relapse is one of the following:

a. BCR-ABL/ABL1 ratio higher than 0.02% in three samples a minimum of four weeks apart
b. Clearly rising BCR-ABL/ABL1 ratio in three samples a minimum of four weeks apart with the last two higher than 0.02%
c. BCR-ABL/ABL1 ratio higher than 0.05% in two samples a minimum of four weeks apart (9).

RQ-PCR values are not currently transferable between laboratories but this is the subject of a global collaboration to implement standardisation of molecular monitoring.

1.6 Reduced intensity conditioning

The recognition that much of the curative effect of allo-HSCT was due to the alloimmune effect has led to the development of reduced-intensity conditioning (RIC) regimens. This has enabled transplantation of older patients and those with comorbidities. Retrospective comparisons of the outcome of myeloablative and reduced-intensity approaches are always confounded by the fact that the two patient groups are not matched for factors (such as age, disease and co-morbidity) that are likely to affect the outcome directly. In CML an early attempt at a retrospective study showed a reduction in the early treatment-related mortality. However it failed to demonstrate significantly improved 3-year survivals in patients with EBMT scores of 0–2, though overall survival was improved in patients with scores of 3–5 (10).

Although RIC approaches with pre-emptive (based on chimerism) or early (based on molecular monitoring of MRD) use of DLI might have been predicted to be most effective in CML, the advent of the TKI prevented randomised studies of RIC versus myeloablative conditioning. However it has offered new possibilities for combinations of RIC regimens, TKI and cellular immunotherapy as TKI act synergistically with DLI.

1.7 Place of HSCT in current therapy

The introduction of the TKI into clinical practice dramatically changed the prognosis of the majority of patients with CML for the better and rightfully displaced HSCT from first-line therapy. With extended follow-up it appears that some 60% of patients can achieve excellent long-term disease control on imatinib and a small proportion may even be able to stop treatment without experiencing disease recurrence.

However this leaves a sizeable minority who fail to respond, lose an established response and/or are intolerant of the drug. Approximately half of this group will achieve or regain remission on one of the second generation TKI (2GTKI), bosutinib, dasatinib, nilotinib or ponatinib. The efficacy of these 2GTKI has led to their use as first line therapy and recently completed phase III studies suggest that approximately 80% of patients will achieve complete cytogenetic remissions within the first year, compared to 65% on imatinib. In addition the 2GTKI are at least as well-tolerated as imatinib. Based on these results dasatinib and nilotinib have both been licensed for use in newly diagnosed patients. Although not yet proven in clinical practice it is unlikely that a patient who fails to respond to a 2GTKI will respond to imatinib, such that transplant should be considered as second-line therapy for these individuals. Furthermore, a number of national and international study groups are now reporting that long-term response to imatinib can be predicted by the rate of fall of Bcr-Abl transcript levels (as measured by RQ-PCR at 3 and 6 months).

If a similar result can be substantiated for the 2GTKI it will be possible to identify the patient destined for transplant within the first year of diagnosis whilst still in chronic phase and return to a more measured approach to transplant.

Key points are summarised at the end of the chapter.

2. The myeloproliferative disorders

2.1 History and introduction

The myeloproliferative disorders comprise polycythaemia vera, essential thrombocythaemia, chronic eosinophilic leukaemia, mastocytosis and primary myelofibrosis. Although allogeneic HSCT can be used in all these conditions in specific circumstances, the only diseases for which HSCT is regularly employed are primary and secondary myelofibrosis.

Primary myelofibrosis is a Ph-negative clonal myeloproliferative disorder characterised by cytopenias, hepatosplenomegaly due to extramedullary haemopoiesis and constitutional symptoms. Myelofibrosis can also be secondary to advanced polycythaemia vera or essential thrombocythaemia. Relatively recently the V617F mutation in the Janus kinase 2 (JAK2) gene has been implicated in the pathogenesis of these disorders and is present in approximately 50%, 100% and 30% of primary myelofibrosis, polycythaemia vera and essential thrombocythaemia respectively. A number of JAK2 inhibitors are currently being trialled and although at least one of these, ruxolitinib, induces reductions in spleen size and constitutional symptoms in many patients, but the only curative treatment remains allogeneic HSCT.

The natural history of primary myelofibrosis is highly variable, with some patients having very prolonged survivals, rendering the decision regarding the timing of transplant most difficult. A number of groups have developed scoring systems for the prediction of survival duration of which the two most commonly used are the Lille (or Dupriez) score (11) and that of the International Working Group for Myelofibrosis Research and Treatment (IWG-MRT) (12). The Lille score uses the presence of none, one or two adverse factors (Hb <10 g/dL, white blood cell count <4 x 10^9/L or >30 x 10^9/L) at diagnosis to define low, intermediate and high risk groups with median survivals of 93, 26 and 13 months. The IWG-MRT classification identifies four risk groups, low, intermediate-1, intermediate-2 and high, depending on the presence of none, one, two or three or more adverse factors, namely age >65 years, Hb <10 g/dL, white blood cell count >25 x 10^9/L, >1% peripheral blood blasts and constitutional symptoms. The median survivals of low, int-1, int-2 and high risk patients are 135, 95, 48 and 27 months respectively. Whilst these scoring systems are undoubtedly valuable in determining the time of transplant, their prognostic value is maintained through transplant such that patients with poor risk disease at diagnosis also have a poor transplant outcome. Perhaps of more use in these difficult decisions is the knowledge that the acquisition of poor risk factors over time adversely affects survival (13) such that the risk-benefit of transplant can be assessed in a dynamic manner in individual patients.

HSCT for primary myelofibrosis was first reported almost simultaneously from London and Angers in 1989. Subsequent reports were infrequent and contained small numbers of patients but confirmed that transplant was feasible and potentially curative, despite considerable risks of graft failure, TRM and disease recurrence. In 1999 a joint manuscript from EBMT and the Fred Hutchinson Cancer Research Center (FHCRC) described 55 patients of median age 42 years (range 4–53) who underwent predominantly myeloablative HLA-identical sibling bone marrow transplants (14). The 5-year overall survival in sibling transplants was 54% with a TRM of 22%.

This study highlighted a common dilemma in transplant for chronic diseases, namely that poor outcome in terms of TRM and relapse is associated with more advanced disease, suggesting that HSCT should be performed as early as possible, but confounded in this disease by the excellent prognosis of low-risk disease managed without transplant.

2.2 Choice of conditioning regimen

A number of series of myeloablative allogeneic transplants were reported later (Table 3) and are remarkably consistent in their outcome with 3–5 year disease free survivals of 30–40% and 1 year procedural related mortalities of 30–50%. Although the factors affecting outcome after HSCT varied somewhat in these reports, most probably attributable to the relatively small numbers in each series, consistent findings conferring a poorer outcome included increasing age, a high Lille score at transplant, low Hb and/or red blood cell transfusion dependency, advanced fibrosis, abnormal cytogenetics and increasing HLA-disparity. Most recently the impact of the JAK2 mutation status on the outcome of transplant has shown that the presence of the mutation (as opposed to wild type JAK2) confers improvement in survival. The mutation status was available in 139 patients of whom 95 were JAK2V617F positive. The 5-year overall and disease free survivals were 70% and 50% in patients carrying the mutation compared to 44% and 32% in those with the wild type gene.

Given that the median age of onset of myelofibrosis is 65 years, it was logical that investigators would evaluate the role of reduced-intensity conditioning (RIC) with the first reports appearing in 2002. These early studies importantly confirmed the feasibility of RIC transplants in myelofibrosis, particularly with respect to durable engraftment, and with limited follow-up reported low TRM and excellent survival. Subsequent studies (Table 4) were not quite as encouraging with disease free survivals very similar to those of myeloablative transplants. As expected, TRM is a little lower but relapse rates are higher. At least two studies reporting large retrospective series have been unable to identify any impact of the conditioning regimen on disease free survival. Of course it is always important to remember that patients treated by myeloablative or RIC regimens are probably very different in terms of age and co-morbidity so comparisons should be made with caution. A recent study of 30 patients aged between 60 and 78 years showed encouraging 3-year overall and disease free survivals of 45 and 40% respectively (15) suggesting that RIC regimens can produce useful outcomes in older patients. The role of RIC transplant for younger patients remains a matter of debate and would be best addressed by a randomised study. Unfortunately due to the rarity of the disease in younger patients this is unlikely to happen.

Table 3: **Outcome of myeloablative HSCT for myelofibrosis as reported in larger series**

Study*	(1)	(2)	(3)	(4)	(5)	(6)	(7)	(8)
No.	55	25	56	20	17	23	27	46
Age (range) In years	42 (4–53)	49 (46–50)	43 (10–66)	45 (22–57)	43 (5–58)	47 (31–60)	38 (19–54)	47 (20–56)
Time: diagnosis to HSCT in mths	1.7 (2–266)	11 (5–36)	83 (3–312)	13 (3–180)	NA	NA	9 (1–287)	NA
Stem cell source MF/UD/MMF	49/3/3	13/10/2	31/20/5	13/4/3	12/4/1	13/10/0	19/6/2	28/18/0
Stem cells BM/PB	49/6	23/2	33/23	5/15	NA	14/9	12/15	29/17
Lille score L/I/H	13/42#	3/9/7	25/17/13	7/8/5	3/9/4	2/14/7	6/8/11	8/16/16
No. splenectomised	27/55	7/25	20/36	12/20	6/17	2/23	8/17	13/46
Graft failure %	2%	10%	3/56	10%	4%	7/23	0%	10%
aGvHD II-IV	60%	13/25	38/56	NA	3/16	78%	29%	43%
aGvHD III-IV	33%	4/25	12/56	3/20	0/16	NA	15%	NA
cGvHD all	27/45	10/17	31/54	6/20	9/16	NA	11/20	39%
cGvHD ext.	16/45	6/17	28/54	NA	1/16	94%	6/20	NA
OS	47%	41% at 2 yrs	58% at 3 yrs	39% at 3 yrs	63%	48% at 3 yrs	44% at 3 yrs	39% at 4 yrs
PFS	39%	37% at 2 yrs	NA	NA	NA	43% at 3 yrs	44% at 3 yrs	32% at 4 yrs
TRM	27%	48%	NA	NA	30%	48% at 3 yrs	41%	39% at 4 yrs
RI	36%	NA	NA	15%	NA	9% at 3 yrs	15%	29% at 4 yrs
Median follow-up (range) in mths	36 (6–223)	35 (5–125)	34 (6–139)	14 (1–113)	(1–188)		47 (19–95)	36 (4–90)

*(1) Guardiola, Blood 1999; 93: 2381–88; (2) Daly, BMT 2003; 32: 35–40; (3) Deeg, Blood 2003; 102: 3912–18; (4) Ditschkowski, BMT 2004; 34: 807–13; (5) Merup Br J Haem 2006; 135: 367–373; (6) Gupta, BMT 2009; 44: 317–20; (7) Stewart, BMT 2010; 45: 1587–93; (8) Robin, Br J Haem 2010; 152: 331–39. Where possible multiple reports involving the same patients have been omitted in favour of the largest and last report. MF: matched family donor; UD: unrelated donor; MMF: mismatched family donor; BM: bone marrow; PB: peripheral blood derived stem cells; Lille score L/I/H: Lille score low/intermediate/high (#) = intermediate and high reported together; No: splenectomised given as number of those evaluable; aGvHD: acute graft versus host disease grades II-IV and II-IV given as number of those evaluable or % cumulative incidence; cGvHD: chronic GvHD limited and extensive given as number of those evaluable or % cumulative incidence; OS: OS at 5 years unless otherwise indicated in parentheses; DFS: DFS at 5 years unless otherwise indicated in parentheses; TRM: TRM at 1 year unless otherwise indicated in parentheses; RI: relapse incidence at 3 years unless otherwise indicated in parentheses; NA: not available from reference source

Table 4: **Outcome of reduced-intensity conditioning HSCT for myelofibrosis as reported in larger series**

Study*	(1)	(2)	(3)	(4)	(5)	(6)	(7)	(8)	(9)	(10)
No.	21	10	6	23	10 3	24	23	46	16 2	30
Age (range) In years	54 (27-68)	58 (52-63)	51 940-56)	54 (38-74)	53 (32-68)	54 (40-64)	58 (39-9)	51 (24-670	56 (32-73)	65 (60-78)
Time: diagnosis to HSCT in mths	11 (1.5-168)	NA	25 (10-243)	NA	19 (3-276)	54 (4-365)	NA	31 (2-239)	50 (3-360)	NA
Stem cell source MF/UD/MMF	18/2 /1	7/3 /0	4/2 /0	12/11 /0	33/70 /0	12/12 /0	8/15 /0	30/14 /2	46/116 /0	15/15 /0
Stem cells BM/PB	3/18	NA	0/6	2/21	3/99	2/22	2/21	34/12	NA	1/29
Lille score L/I/H	0/13 /8	2/6 /2	0/3 /3	5/14 /4	17/55 /31	6/8 /10	1/12 /10	4/20 /22	35/91 /32	NA
No. splenectomised	3/14	0/10	1/6	3/23	14/ 102	9/13	9/23	28/46	20/ 162	3/30
Graft failure %	5%	0%	0%	22%	5%	13%	NA	NA	6%	10%
aGvHD II-IV	7/21	4/8	1/6	18%	26%	9/24	14/23	NA	15%	40%
aGvHD III-IV	2/21	1/8	0/6	NA	11%	3/24	5/23	NA	6%	155
cGvHD all	13/18	5/8	NA	NA	48%	12/17	14/20	NA	36%	45%
cGvHD ext.	8/18	4/8	NA	45% at 1 yr	26%	7/17	10/20	NA	20%	NA
OS	85%	90%	100% 16 mths	77% at 1 yr	67%	31% at 3 yrs	80% at 3 yrs	45%	62%	40% at 3 yrs
PFS	76%	NA	100% 16 mths	68% at 1 yr	51%	24% at 3 yrs	NA	NA	46%	40% at 3 yrs
TRM	10%	10&	0%	23%	16%	32% at 2 yrs	NA	24%	22%	13% at +100
RI	5%	NA	NA	9% at 1 yr	22%	46%	NA	46%	23%	30%
Median follow-up (range) in mths	31 (12-122)	55 (14-180)	16 (10-24)	50 (20-89)	33 (12-76)	15 (12-49)	29 (10-97)	46 (11-168)	19 (1-111)	22 1-69)

* (1) Rondelli, Blood 2005; 105: 4115–19; (2) Merup, Br J Haem 2006; 135: 367–73; (3) George, BMT 2008; 42: 567–68; (4) Gupta BMT 2009; 44: 317–20; (5) Kroger, Blood 2009; 114: 5264–70; (6) Stewart, BMT 2010; 45: 1587–93; (7) Snyder, BBMT 2010; 16: 281–86; (8) Bacigalupo BMT 2010; 45: 458–63; (9) Alchalby, Blood 2010; 116: 3572–81; (10) Samuelson, Br J Haem 2011; 153: 76–82.
For abbreviations see Table 3.

2.3 Role of splenectomy before transplant
The majority of patients with myelofibrosis have splenomegaly, sometimes massive, and the issue as to whether HSCT should be preceded by splenectomy is long-standing. Surgery in this group of patients is not without its hazards and mortality of splenectomy is of the order of 5–10%. The role of splenectomy in transplant for myelofibrosis was first addressed by Li et al, who compared the transplant outcomes in 11 splenectomised patients with those of 15 non-splenectomised individuals and showed faster engraftment but no survival advantage (16). Faster engraftment has been a relatively consistent finding in other series but has not conferred an improvement in outcome. Again it is important to remember that there may be a difference in outcome according to the size of the spleen. A recent study described a reduction in relapse incidence in patients whose spleens were greater than 22 cm (by ultrasound measurement) at the time of splenectomy compared to those with similarly sized spleens that were not removed prior to HSCT (17). Splenectomy, however, had no influence on disease recurrence in patients with smaller spleens. It would seem reasonable to restrict splenectomy to those with massive splenomegaly and no contra-indication to surgery.

2.4 Time to remission and the identification of recurrence
Bone marrow fibrosis can be slow to regress even after a successful transplant. There is an understandable reluctance to subject patients to regular trephine biopsies so data relating to the time to bone marrow remission is relatively limited. In the original EBMT report (14) complete remission of fibrosis was observed at 6 months with a range from 0.6 to 23 months. Kroger et al, reporting on a small sub-group (16 patients) within their larger series, reported that 69% and 93% had achieved complete remission or near complete remission by day 100 and one year respectively (18). Concern that RIC regimens might be less effective in disease control was suggested by Gupta et al. who reported a median time to loss of fibrosis of 167 days (range 127–383) in recipients of myeloablative procedures compared to 363 days (range 75–750) in those who received reduced-intensity regimens (19).

RQ-PCR for the JAK2 mutation has now been successfully applied to the identification of remission and disease recurrence post-transplant. Regular monitoring occurred in 63 patients carrying the mutation and showed that 45 of them became JAK2V617F negative at a median of 96 days (range 20-427). Seven of the remaining patients were treated with donor lymphocyte infusions. The achievement of RQ-PCR negativity was significantly associated with a reduction in the risk of relapse, and in particular that patients who remained JAK2V617F positive at 6 months were significantly more likely to relapse than those who were negative (20). Since the efficacy of DLI in patients failing to remit or relapsing after HSCT has been reported by a number of investigators it is likely that regular RQ-PCR monitoring for JAK2V617F will become a standard procedure after HSCT for myelofibrosis.

2.6 Place of HSCT in current therapy

Allogeneic stem cell transplantation is the only curative treatment for primary and secondary myelofibrosis.

Since this is a disease of the elderly, relatively few patients are candidates for transplant although encouraging results using reduced-intensity conditioning regimens have been recently reported, and offer the possibility of extending the age for consideration of intensive therapy.

At present it is not clear that reduced-intensity procedures offer any benefit over myeloablative conditioning in younger patients. The issue of splenectomy before transplant remains controversial.

The identification of the JAK2V617F mutation in the pathophysiology of many cases of myelofibrosis allows accurate monitoring of disease response and the possibility of early intervention with donor lymphocyte infusions for residual or recurrent disease. Key points are summarised below.

Key points

Allo-HSCT remains the only curative treatment for chronic myeloid leukaemia but due to continued concerns regarding transplant related mortality, has been replaced as first line treatment by the tyrosine kinase inhibitors (TKI). With the upfront use of the more potent TKI, allo-HSCT will become second-line therapy for selected patients with poor responses to second generation TKI

Transplant outcome in CML can be predicted using five pre-transplant factors (the EBMT score)

Transplant for CML should be accompanied by regular monitoring for minimal residual disease by RQ-PCR and treatment with donor lymphocytes or a TKI initiated for patients with easily detectable molecular, cytogenetic or haematological recurrence

Allo-HSCT remains the only curative treatment for myelofibrosis but the heterogeneity of the disease in terms of severity and duration of survival require careful selection of patients for transplant

RIC regimens offer the opportunity of allo-HSCT to older patients with myelofibrosis and/or those with co-morbidities. The role of RICT in younger patients is less clear

The role of splenectomy pre-transplant is controversial. It would be reasonable to offer splenectomy only to those patients with very large spleens and low risk of surgical mortality

Transplant for myelofibrosis should be accompanied by regular monitoring for minimal residual disease by RQ-PCR for JAK2V617F and intervention with donor lymphocytes for patients with easily detectable molecular recurrence

References

1. Pavlu J, Szydlo RM, Goldman JM, Apperley JF. Three decades of transplantation for chronic myeloid leukemia: What have we learned? Blood 2011; 117: 755–763.
2. Gratwohl A, Hermans J, Goldman JM et al. Risk assessment for patients with chronic myeloid leukaemia before allogeneic blood or marrow transplantation. Chronic Leukemia Working Party of the European Group for Blood and Marrow Transplantation. Lancet 1998; 352 :1087–1092.
3. Mcglave PB, Hurd DD, Ramsay NK et al. Successful treatment of chronic myelogenous leukemia with allogeneic bone-marrow transplantation. Exp Hematol 1982; 10: 18.
4. Passweg JR, Walker I, Sobocinski KA et al. Validation and extension of the EBMT Risk Score for patients with chronic myeloid leukaemia (CML) receiving allogeneic haematopoietic stem cell transplants. Br J Haematol 2004; 125: 613–620.
5. Apperley JF, Jones L, Hale G et al. Bone marrow transplantation for patients with chronic myeloid leukaemia: T-cell depletion with Campath-1 reduces the incidence of graft-versus-host disease but may increase the risk of leukaemic relapse. Bone Marrow Transplant 1986; 1: 53–66.
6. Mackinnon S, Papadopoulos EB, Carabasi MH et al. Adoptive immunotherapy evaluating escalating doses of donor leukocytes for relapse of chronic myeloid-leukemia after bone-marrow transplantation - Separation of graft-versus-leukemia responses from graft-versus-host disease. Blood 1995; 86: 1261–1268.
7. Chalandon Y, Passweg JR, Schmid C et al. Outcome of patients developing GVHD after DLI given to treat CML relapse: A study by the chronic leukemia working party of the EBMT. Bone Marrow Transplant 2010; 45: 558–564.
8. Craddock C, Szydlo RM, Klein JP et al. Estimating leukemia-free survival after allografting for chronic myeloid leukemia: A new method that takes into account patients who relapse and are restored to complete remission. Blood 2000; 96: 86–90.
9. Kaeda J, O'shea D, Szydlo RM et al. Serial measurement of BCR-ABL transcripts in the peripheral blood after allogeneic stem cell transplantation for chronic myeloid leukemia: an attempt to define patients who may not require further therapy. Blood 2006; 107: 4171–4176.
10. Crawley C, Szydlo R, Lalancette M et al. Outcomes of reduced-intensity transplantation for chronic myeloid leukemia: An analysis of prognostic factors from the Chronic Leukemia Working Party of the EBMT. Blood 2005; 106: 2969–2976.

11. Dupriez B, Morel P, Demory JL et al. Prognostic factors in agnogenic myeloid metaplasia: A report on 195 cases with a new scoring system. Blood 1996; 88: 1013–1018.
12. Cervantes F, Dupriez B, Pereira A et al. New prognostic scoring system for primary myelofibrosis based on a study of the International Working Group for Myelofibrosis Research and Treatment. Blood 2009; 113: 2895–2901.
13. Passamonti F, Cervantes F, Vannucchi AM et al. A dynamic prognostic model to predict survival in primary myelofibrosis: A study by the IWG-MRT (International Working Group for Myeloproliferative Neoplasms Research and Treatment). Blood 2010; 115: 1703–1708.
14. Guardiola P, Anderson JE, Bandini G et al. Allogeneic stem cell transplantation for agnogenic myeloid metaplasia: A European group for blood and marrow transplantation, Societe Francaise de Greffe de Moelle, Gruppo Italiano per il Trapianto del Midollo Osseo, and Fred Hutchinson Cancer Research Center collaborative study. Blood 1999; 93: 2831–2838.
15. Samuelson S, Sandmaier BM, Heslop HE et al. Allogeneic haematopoietic cell transplantation for myelofibrosis in 30 patients 60-78 years of age. Br J Haematol 2011; 153: 76–82.
16. Li ZH, Gooley T, Appelbaum FR, Deeg HJ. Splenectomy and hemopoietic stem cell transplantation for myelofibrosis. Blood 2001; 97: 2180–2181.
17. Bacigalupo A, Soraru M, Dominietto A et al. Allogeneic hemopoietic SCT for patients with primary myelofibrosis: A predictive transplant score based on transfusion requirement, spleen size and donor type. Bone Marrow Transplant 2010; 45: 458–463.
18. Kroger N, Thiele E, Zander A et al. Rapid regression of bone marrow fibrosis after dose-reduced allogeneic stem cell transplantation in patients with primary myelofibrosis. Exp Hematol 2007; 35: 1719–1722.
19. Gupta V, Kroger N, Aschan J et al. A retrospective comparison of conventional intensity conditioning and reduced-intensity conditioning for allogeneic hematopoietic cell transplantation in myelofibrosis. Bone Marrow Transplant 2009; 44: 317–320.
20. Alchalby H, Badbaran A, Zabelina T et al. Impact of JAK2V617F mutation status, allele burden, and clearance after allogeneic stem cell transplantation for myelofibrosis. Blood 2010; 116: 3572–3581.

Multiple Choice Questionnaire

To find the correct answer, go to http://www.esh.org/online-training/handbook/

1. **Which of the following pre-transplant risk factors does *not* adversely affect overall survival after a T-cell replete transplant for chronic myeloid leukaemia?**
   a) Increasing patient age . . . . ☐
   b) Recipient CMV seropositivity . . . . ☐
   c) Disease phase . . . . ☐

d) Stem cell source .... ☐

2. **Which of the following statements is *untrue*?**
   a) A tyrosine kinase inhibitor is the ELN recommended front-line treatment for CML .... ☐
   b) Donor lymphocyte infusions restore remissions in patients relapsing in chronic phase in more than 60% of patients .... ☐
   c) RQ-PCR positivity for BCR-ABL within 3 months of a reduced intensity transplant should be treated with donor lymphocyte infusions and/or a TKI .... ☐
   d) Graft versus host disease occurs in more than a third of patients receiving escalating doses of donor lymphocyte infusions .... ☐

3. **Which of the following parameters is *not* included in the IWG-MRT risk score?**
   a) Age >65 years .... ☐
   b) Haemoglobin <10 g/dL .... ☐
   c) White blood cell count <4 x 10^9/L .... ☐
   d) Constitutional symptoms .... ☐

4. **Which of the following statements is *untrue*?**
   a) The one year transplant related mortality of reduced intensity transplantation for myelofibrosis is less than 25% .... ☐
   b) Pre-transplant splenectomy is recommended for all patients with spleens exceeding 20 cm on ultrasound examination .... ☐
   c) Bone marrow fibrosis can take more than 12 months to resolve following allo-HSCT for myelofibrosis .... ☐
   d) Patients with JAK2V617F positive myelofibrosis have better overall survivals than patients with wild type JAK2 sequences .... ☐

5. **Compared to T-replete myeloablative transplants, T-cell depletion in allogeneic transplantation for CML is associated with all the following, *except* one:**
   a) An increased relapse rate .... ☐

b) An increased incidence of viral infections...................................☐
c) A higher rate of transplant-related mortality.............................☐
d) A reduced incidence of graft failure.......................................☐

* CHAPTER 19

Indications for HSCT in adults

* 19.5
Chronic lymphocytic leukaemia

Peter Dreger, Johannes Schetelig

1. Introduction

Both autologous and allogeneic HSCT are continuing to be explored for the treatment of chronic lymphocytic leukaemia (CLL). The annual numbers of allogeneic transplants (allo-HSCT) for CLL registered with the EBMT are steadily increasing, making this the most frequent indication for allo-HSCT among the lymphoma subtypes. In contrast, autologous transplantation numbers for CLL are steadily declining with fewer than 50 cases reported in 2009 (Figure 1).

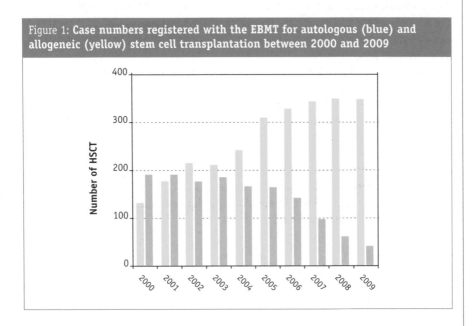

Figure 1: **Case numbers registered with the EBMT for autologous (blue) and allogeneic (yellow) stem cell transplantation between 2000 and 2009**

2. Indications

2.1 Allogeneic HSCT

In CLL, allo-HSCT is a possible treatment option for patients who have poor-risk disease as defined by the EBMT CLL Transplant Consensus (Table 1) (1). Although controlled trials are lacking, available evidence strongly suggests that allo-HSCT is currently the only therapy with curative potential in CLL. In contrast to conventional treatment, including purine analogue-rituximab combination regimens, it can provide long-term disease control even in patients with an unfavourable biological and clinical risk profile. Preliminary data suggest that in contrast to other haematopoietic

Table 1: Criteria for poor-risk disease according to the EBMT CLL Transplant Consensus (1)

- Non-response or early relapse (within 12 months) after purine analogue-containing therapy
- Relapse (within 24 months) after purine analogue **combination** therapy or treatment of similar efficacy (i.e. autologous stem cell transplantation)
- p53 deletion /mutation (del 17p13) requiring treatment

malignancies, such as myelodysplastic syndromes, in CLL allo-HSCT might overcome the adverse prognostic impact of genomic (e.g. TP53 lesions) as well as clinical (e.g. fludarabine resistance) factors. Thus, allo-HSCT may be offered to selected patients as a standard procedure (2).

Of paramount importance for the outcome of allo-HSCT in CLL is the appropriate timing of the transplant. Eligibility for allo-HSCT is usually defined by the quality of response to therapy, as defined by the first and second EBMT criteria. Therefore allo-HSCT is never indicated as part of the first-line treatment of CLL except for those few individuals who have del 17p and/or TP53 mutations and who require treatment (third EBMT criterion). However, large prospective studies of reduced intensity conditioning transplantation (RICT) uniformly show that in CLL the results of allo-HSCT are considerably impaired if the disease is not in remission at the time of transplant (3–5). Thus, allo-HSCT should be performed in a timely fashion, i.e. as soon as the EBMT criteria are met.

2.2 Autologous HSCT

Auto-HSCT, when used for consolidation in first or second remission, does not provide significant benefit over current chemo-immunotherapeutic standard treatments for CLL. Accordingly, there is no standard indication for auto- HSCT in CLL. It may be a clinical option, however, in individual situations, such as transformation (Richter's syndrome).

3. Conditioning regimens

There is no doubt that the crucial therapeutic principle of allo-HSCT in CLL is graft-versus-leukaemia (GvL) activity. Evidence for this derives from the observation that even in patients with the poorest-risk disease long-term clinical remissions can be observed after allo-HSCT but not with any other treatment modality, and from the fact that - in contrast to auto-HSCT or other intensive therapies - the incidence of relapse seems to decrease over time (6). In addition, the importance of GvL in CLL is indicated by a reduced relapse risk in the presence of chronic graft-versus-host disease (cGvHD) (7), an increased relapse risk associated with the use of

T-cell depletion (TCD) (8, 9), the efficacy of donor lymphocyte infusions (DLI) (8), and the kinetics of post allo-HSCT minimal residual disease (MRD) (see below). Altogether, there appears to be sound evidence that GvL activity represents the main contributor to durable disease control after allo-HSCT even in poor-risk CLL. Accordingly, long-term disease control can be achieved with a broad range of conditioning intensities. Current evidence is not sufficient to identify any single superior conditioning regimen. The most convincing data supporting allo-HSCT in CLL come from studies of RICT rather than from trials with traditional myeloablative allo-HSCT (10). However, impaired disease control associated with RIC as compared with more intensive conditioning cannot be excluded (6, 7). Thus the optimum choice of conditioning regimens may vary according to the individual situation. In the presence of comorbidity and chemosensitive disease RIC appear to be more appropriate, whereas high-intensity regimens might be preferable in younger patients with good performance status but poorly controlled disease (1). There is no evidence for any clinical benefit of T-cell depletion in CLL.

4. Outcome and role of allogeneic transplants in CLL

The risks of allo-HSCT in patients with CLL are mostly the general risks of transplant and are basically due to GvHD. Toxicity and mortality seem to be influenced by the type of conditioning regimen employed (10). With RIC, reported NRM risk at 4 years post-transplant ranges from 15 to 25% (3–5, 11, 12). As mentioned previously, long-term disease control due to a low rate of late recurrence has been observed in all published series irrespective of donor source and conditioning regimens. Accordingly, a considerable proportion of patients survive leukaemia-free after allo-HSCT, as illustrated by 5-year EFS and OS rates ranging from 30 to 70% in prospective RICT studies (3–5, 11, 12). In summary, cure seems to be possible in up to two-thirds of patients undergoing allo-HSCT for poor-risk CLL.

4.1 Outcome and role of unrelated and alternative transplants in comparison to HLA-identical sibling transplants in CLL

In prospective studies including both matched unrelated donors (UD) and sibling donors (3–5, 11, 12), as well as in a large EBMT registry study (6), significant outcome differences were not evident. Therefore in poor-risk CLL allo-HSCT from a well-matched UD is regarded as standard treatment similar to sibling transplants (1, 2). Transplants from partially matched or mismatched UD have been associated with significantly higher mortality in the EBMT registry study (hazard ratio 1.67) (6). However, with an OS probability of 38% at five years, outcome seems favourable when compared to the results of alternative treatment for patients with poor-risk CLL, justifying considering partially matched donor transplants as a clinical option in this risk group. Due to the rarity of the disease and the high average age, in CLL experience with haplo-identical transplants and cord blood transplants is very sparse to date.

4.2 Post-transplant minimal residual disease monitoring and immune intervention in CLL

In CLL, sensitive MRD quantification (i.e. 1 cell in 10^4 or less) can be obtained by PCR- or flow cytometry-based assays. The decline of the MRD level is often delayed and its close correlation with immune-relevant events strongly supports the assumption that GvL is the crucial contributor to tumour control in allo-HSCT. GvL-induced MRD negativity after allo-HSCT is sustained in the vast majority of cases and is highly predictive of freedom from relapse (5, 13).

Furthermore, in CLL quantitative MRD monitoring seems to be a valid instrument for sensitive guidance of pre-emptive immune interventions directed at disease eradication after allo-HSCT, such as the tapering of immunosuppression and the use of DLI (5). Whereas the published evidence strongly suggests that CLL is sensitive to timely pre-emptive immune intervention by modulation of systemic immunosuppression (5, 13, 14), DLI are less effective, in particular after T-replete allo-HSCT and in those patients who are treated with DLI for clinical progression/relapse (reviewed in (10)). Therefore, the best approach to post-transplant immunotherapy (including monoclonal antibodies and alternative B-depleting or immunomodulating agents, such as lenalidomide) in CLL requires further study (10).

5. Outcome and role of autologous transplants in CLL

Auto-HSCT for CLL was developed in the mid-1990s, before fludarabine was approved and before validated genomic prognostic markers were available. Based on favourable pilot data from single centre studies, the hypothesis was that high-dose treatment including myeloablative TBI could possibly cure the disease, in particular if administered early (8). Subsequent multicentre single-arm trials and longer follow-up, however, failed to demonstrate that permanent control of poor-risk CLL is possible with myeloablative auto-HSCT (8, 15, 16). Nevertheless, in the European multicentre studies from the UK (MRD pilot trial) and Germany/Austria (GLLSG CLL3 trial), the median progression free survival (PFS) of patients with CLL intended to undergo first-line auto-HSCT were encouraging at 54 and 68 months, respectively (15, 16).

Therefore, a prospective randomised trial comparing autografting with conventional treatment was performed as a European intergroup effort coordinated by the EBMT, in order to prove whether or not auto-HSCT could provide clinical benefit to patients with poor-risk CLL. Patients in first or second remission after conventional chemotherapy for symptomatic CLL were randomised to receive a consolidating auto-HSCT or just observation. Based on 229 patients enrolled, this trial showed that auto-HSCT indeed halved the relapse risk and doubled the time to CLL-specific retreatment, but failed to improve overall survival in comparison to chemotherapy alone (17). Moreover, an inter-trial comparison between the GCLLSG CLL3 study and the fludarabine, cyclophosphamide, rituximab (FCR) arm of the GCLLSG CLL8 study did not reveal a significant benefit of auto-HSCT in terms of time to retreatment (15).

Furthermore, even though there is no evidence that the incidence of treatment-related myelodysplastic syndromes and acute myeloblastic leukaemia (t-MDS/AML) after auto-HSCT for CLL exceeds the range reported for standard chemotherapy for B-cell lymphoma, these serious complications must be considered when weighing the benefits and risks of auto-HSCT versus alternative modalities.

In summary, auto-HSCT currently does not have a clearly defined role in the standard treatment algorithm for CLL.

6. Summary and perspectives

Allo-HSCT from related or unrelated donors can be highly effective in otherwise resistant CLL. Therefore it is regarded as a standard treatment option for eligible patients who fulfil accepted criteria for poor-risk disease. Allo-HSCT should be considered before the disease has advanced to a status of complete refractoriness to salvage therapy. Allo-HSCT for CLL should be performed within the frame of a research protocol whenever possible.

In contrast, auto-HSCT currently does not have a clearly defined role in the standard treatment algorithm for CLL.

References

1. Dreger P, Corradini P, Kimby E et al. Indications for allogeneic stem cell transplantation in chronic lymphocytic leukemia: The EBMT transplant consensus. Leukemia 2007; 21: 12–17.
2. Ljungman P, Bregni M, Brune M et al. Allogeneic and autologous transplantation for haematological diseases, solid tumours and immune disorders: Current practice in Europe 2009. Bone Marrow Transplant 2010; 45: 219–234.
3. Sorror ML, Storer BE, Sandmaier BM et al. Five-year follow-up of patients with advanced chronic lymphocytic leukemia treated with allogeneic hematopoietic cell transplantation after nonmyeloablative conditioning. J Clin Oncol 2008; 26: 4912–4920.
4. Brown JR, Kim HT, Li S et al. Predictors of improved progression-free survival after nonmyeloablative allogeneic stem cell transplantation for advanced chronic lymphocytic leukemia. Biol Blood Marrow Transplant 2006; 12: 1056–1064.

5. Dreger P, Döhner H, Ritgen M et al. Allogeneic stem cell transplantation provides durable disease control in poor-risk chronic lymphocytic leukemia: Long-term clinical and MRD results of the GCLLSG CLL3X trial. Blood 2010; 116: 2438–2447.
6. Michallet M, Sobh M, Milligan D et al. The impact of HLA matching on long-term transplant outcome after allogeneic hematopoietic stem cell transplantation for CLL: A retrospective study from the EBMT registry. Leukemia 2010; 24: 1725–1731.
7. Dreger P, Brand R, Milligan D et al. Reduced-intensity conditioning lowers treatment-related mortality of allogeneic stem cell transplantation for chronic lymphocytic leukemia: A population-matched analysis. Leukemia 2005; 19: 1029–1033.
8. Gribben JG, Zahrieh D, Stephans K et al. Autologous and allogeneic stem cell transplantation for poor risk chronic lymphocytic leukemia. Blood 2005; 106: 4389–4396.
9. Schetelig J, van Biezen A, Brand R et al. Allogeneic hematopoietic cell transplantation for chronic lymphocytic leukemia with 17p deletion: A retrospective EBMT analysis. J Clin Oncol 2008; 26: 5094–5100.
10. Delgado J, Milligan DW, Dreger P. Allogeneic hematopoietic cell transplantation for chronic lymphocytic leukemia: Ready for primetime? Blood 2009; 114: 2581–2588.
11. Schetelig J, Thiede C, Bornhauser M et al. Evidence of a graft-versus-leukemia effect in chronic lymphocytic leukemia after reduced-intensity conditioning and allogeneic stem-cell transplantation: The Cooperative German Transplant Study Group. J Clin Oncol 2003; 21: 2747–2753.
12. Delgado J, Thomson K, Russell N et al. Results of alemtuzumab-based reduced-intensity allogeneic transplantation for chronic lymphocytic leukemia: A British Society of Blood and Marrow Transplantation study. Blood 2006; 107: 1724–1730.
13. Farina L, Carniti C, Dodero A et al. Qualitative and quantitative polymerase chain reaction monitoring of minimal residual disease in relapsed chronic lymphocytic leukemia: Early assessment can predict long-term outcome after reduced intensity allogeneic transplantation. Haematologica 2009; 94: 654–662.
14. Moreno C, Villamor N, Esteve J et al. Clinical significance of minimal residual disease, as assessed by different techniques, after stem cell transplantation for chronic lymphocytic leukemia. Blood 2006; 107: 4563–4569.
15. Dreger P, Busch R, Stilgenbauer S et al. FCR vs autologous stem cell transplantation as first-line treatment for chronic lymphocytic leukemia: A comparison of two prospective studies of the GCLLSG [abstract]. Ann Oncol 2011; in press:
16. Milligan DW, Fernandes S, Dasgupta R et al. Autografting for younger patients with chronic lymphocytic leukaemia is safe and achieves a high percentage of molecular responses. Results of the MRC Pilot Study. Blood 2005; 105: 397–404.
17. Michallet M, Dreger P, Sutton L et al. Autologous hematopoietic stem cell transplantation in chronic lymphocytic leukemia: Results of European intergroup randomized trial comparing autografting versus observation. Blood 2011; 117: 1516–1521.

Multiple Choice Questionnaire

To find the correct answer, go to http://www.esh.org/online-training/handbook/

1. **Female patient, 53 years old, first diagnosis of CLL after known "elevated white blood count" over years, WBC 120 x 10⁹/L with no other laboratory abnormalities, no symptoms, no lymphadenopathy, stage Binet A. Which one of the following strategies should be recommended?**
   a) Further diagnostic procedures, e.g. bone marrow biopsy . . . . ☐
   b) No immediate intervention, observation of course . . . . ☐
   c) Chlorambucil . . . . ☐
   d) Fludarabine-cyclophosphamide followed by autologous stem cell
      transplantation . . . . ☐

2. **In which one of the following situations is allo-HSCT *not* worth considering?**
   a) Diagnosis of CLL with deletion 17p13 without symptoms in a 55-year
      old patient . . . . ☐
   b) Non-response of CLL to fludarabine in a 60-year old patient . . . . ☐
   c) Progressive disease 2 years after fludarabine-cyclophosphamide-
      rituximab in a 62-year old patient without siblings . . . . ☐
   d) Relapse of CLL in a 49-year old patient 18 months after auto-HSCT . . . . . ☐

3. **Which one of the following situations might be an indication for auto-HSCT?**
   a) Diagnosis of symptomatic CLL with deletion 17p13 in a 55-year old
      patient . . . . ☐
   b) Non-response of CLL to fludarabine in a 60-year old patient . . . . ☐
   c) CLL progression 2 years after fludarabine-cyclophosphamide-rituximab
      in a 62-year old patient . . . . ☐
   d) None of the above . . . . ☐

4. **Which one of the following statements is *not* correct?**
   a) In CLL, the sensitivity of MRD assessment using 4-colour flow
      cytometry cannot be higher than 1 tumour cell in 10,000 normal cells . . ☐

b) MRD negativity is frequently achieved after auto-HSCT for CLL and indicates cure .... ☐

c) MRD negativity after allo-HSCT for CLL often occurs only after immunomodulating manoeuvres, such as withdrawal of systemic immunosuppression or DLI .... ☐

d) MRD negativity one year after allo-HSCT for CLL indicates a favourable outcome .... ☐

5. **Female patient, 53 years old, refractory after salvage treatment with fludarabine, stage Binet C with 95% BM infiltration, night sweats, moderate lymphadenopathy. FISH karyotype del 11q22, del 17p13. Recommended strategy:**

a) Further diagnostic procedures, e.g. mutational status, ZAP70 .... ☐

b) Salvage fludarabine-cyclophosphamide-rituximab .... ☐

c) Salvage alemtuzumab, followed by allogeneic stem cell transplantation from an HLA-identical sibling or from a matched unrelated donor ...... ☐

d) Autologous transplantation .... ☐

NOTES

*CHAPTER 19

Indications for HSCT in adults

*19.6

Multiple myeloma

Jesús San-Miguel, José A. Pérez-Simón, M. Victoria Mateos

1. Introduction

Multiple myeloma (MM) is the most common plasma cell disorder with an incidence of 4–5 new cases per 100,000 individuals/year, which represents approximately 60,000 cases in Europe. Unfortunately, MM remains incurable with conventional chemotherapy. Nevertheless, the availability of new drugs, which target not only the PC but also the microenvironment, together with the well-established use of high dose chemotherapy is changing the prognosis of these patients.

2. Autologous stem cell transplant

High dose therapy (HDT) followed by autologous stem transplantation (ASCT) is considered the standard of care for young myeloma patients (<65–70 years). Accordingly, MM is currently the most common indication for ASCT in North America and Europe.

The availability of highly efficient novel agents is challenging the indication of ASCT as an upfront strategy, although these should probably be considered as complementary instead of alternative strategies. Here we will discuss: the optimal initial treatment regimens for remission induction and tumour debulking, the choice of conditioning regimen, the results of ASCT and the potential role of consolidation and maintenance treatments after ASCT. In the second part of the chapter we will analyse the role of allogeneic transplant for MM.

2.1 Induction treatment prior to ASCT

The combination of vincristine, doxorubicin, and dexamethasone (VAD) has long been the gold standard as a preparatory regimen for young newly-diagnosed MM patients who are candidates for ASCT, with partial response (PR) rates ranging between 52% and 63%, and CR rates from 3 to 13%. However, novel drug combinations have now been shown to be superior to VAD-like regimens for initial tumour reduction. Three randomised trials have compared thalidomide (T)-based regimens (TAD, TVAD or CTD) to VAD as initial therapy in transplant eligible patients, and have shown superiority for the three drug thalidomide combinations with approximately 80% ≥PR, including 10–20% CRs (Table 1, includes references). In contrast the efficacy of thalidomide plus dexamethasone (TDex) is in the range of that of VAD. In studies evaluating bortezomib (Bz) combination therapy, data from a French randomised trial comparing BzDex vs. VAD and the Hovon trial comparing BzAdriaDex vs. VAD show superiority for BZ regimens with ≥80 % PR and 10–30% CR. The Italian and Spanish groups have reported that the three drug combination BzTDex is significantly superior to TDex both before and after transplant and this triple combination appears to be also marginally superior to BzDex (Table 1) (1–5). Another efficient debulking

Table 1: Response obtained with novel induction regimens in randomised trials

Regimen	Patients	Response		Reference
		%>PR	(%CR + nCR)	
Thal-Dex vs Dex	470	63 vs 46	(7.7 vs 2.6)	Rajkumar, JCO 2008; 26: 2171–2177
TAD vs VAD	400	72 vs 54	(7 vs 3)	Lokhorst, Blood 2010; 115: 1113–1120
T+VAD vs VAD	230	81 vs 66		Zervas, Ann Oncol 2007; 18: 1369–1375
CTD vs CVAD	254	87 vs 75	(19 vs 9)	Morgan, ASH 2009 (abstr 352)
BzDx vs VA	486	82 vs 65	(15 vs 7)	Harousseau, JCO 2010; 28: 4926–4934
BzTD vs TD	256	94 vs 79	(32 vs 12)	Cavo, Lancet 2010; 376: 2075–2085
BzTD/TD/ChBz	173	80/66/78	(30/20/6)	Rosiñol, ASH 2010 (abstr 307)
BzAD vs VAD	300	83 vs 59	(5 vs 1)	Sonneveld, ASH 2010; 116: 40a
Len-Dex vs Len-dex	485	82 vs 71	(4 vs 2)	Rajkumar, Lancet 2010; 11: 29–37
Len-Dex vs Dex	198	85 vs 71	(22 vs 4)	Zonder, Blood 2010; 116: 5838–5841

T: thalidomide, Len: lenalidomide, C: cyclophosphamide, A: adriamycin, Bz: bortezomib, ChBz: chemotherapy plus Bz, D/Dex: high dose dexamethasone, dex: low dose dexamethasone

regimen is bortezomib-cyclophosphamide-dexamethasone (BzCycloDex). Regarding lenalidomide (Len), two large randomised studies have shown that the majority of patients (>85%) respond to LenDex induction, but probably a minimum of 6 cycles would be required to achieve a substantial number of CRs (6). Recent data using BzLenDex indicate that most patients (>90% achieve at least PR with over 30% CRs). Thalidomide or bortezomib combinations did not affect stem cell collection or granulocyte and platelet recovery post-transplant. Initial reports indicated a decrease in CD34+ cells harvested in patients treated with lenalidomide, but if collection is performed after no more than 3–4 cycles the number of stem cells are adequate for 1 or 2 transplants. In summary, current results show that with triple combinations such as BzTDex, BzLenDex or BzCycloDex >90% of MM patients will respond and 1/3 will achieve CR after 3-6 cycles, resulting in an optimal situation for ASCT.

2.2 Conditioning regimens

Melphalan 200 mg/m^2 is considered the gold standard conditioning regimen prior to autologous transplantation. The IMF randomised trial confirmed that patients receiving melphalan 200 mg/m^2 displayed a better median overall survival than patients treated with melphalan 140 mg/m^2 in combination with TBI (65 vs 45%

overall survival at 45 months). Other studies using intensification of the melphalan dose or addition of other alkylating agents have not demonstrated significant improvement either in terms of response rate or in outcome. The exception to this latter statement is the data recently reported by the Spanish group (7) showing that although the combination of busulfan and melphalan (BuMel) was equivalent to melphalan 200 mg/m² in terms of PFS during the first two years, subsequently the survival curves separated with a significant long-term benefit for the BuMel arm (PFS: 41 vs 31 months, p=0.009). This may be due to the potential effect of busulfan on myeloma progenitor cells. A randomised trial is ongoing in order to confirm these results. Several pilot studies are investigating the addition of bortezomib to melphalan, and although data is limited, the IFM group has reported a superior CR as compared to matched patients conditioned with melphalan alone (35 vs 11%) (8).

2.3 Autologous stem cell transplant results

High dose therapy (HDT) (usually based on melphalan 200 mg/m²) followed by ASCT prolonged overall survival (OS) as compared to standard dose therapy (SDT) in prospective randomised trials conducted by the French (IFM) and English (MRC) groups as well as in the Italian IMMSG trial, and there is evidence for >10 year survivorship in at least a subset of patients.

Nevertheless, the US study (SWOG 9321), the French MAG91 study and the Spanish PETHEMA-94 trial, although they confirmed the benefit of ASCT in terms of response and partially for event-free survival (EFS), did not find superiority in terms of survival as compared to SDT (Table 2, includes references). These discrepancies can be, at least in part, explained by:

Table 2: Randomised trials comparing high-dose therapy with conventional chemotherapy

	Patients	CR, %	EFS, mo	OS, mo	Reference
IFM 90	200	22/5+	28/18+	57/42+	Attal, NEJM 1996; 335: 91–97
MRC 7	401	44/9+	31/20+	55/42+	Child, NEJM 2003; 348: 1875–1883
IMMSG	194	25/7+	28/16+	58/43+	Palumbo, Blood 2004; 104: 3052–3057
MAG 91	190	36/20+	25/19+	47/47-	Fermand, JCO 2005; 23: 9227–9233
PETHEMA	185	30/11+	42/34-	67/65-	Blade, Blood 2005; 106: 3755–3759
USIG-9321	516	17/15-	25/21-	58/53-	Barlogie, JCO 2006; 24: 929–936

+ *statistically significant benefit for high-dose therapy; - no significant difference*

1. Differences in study design (the Spanish study randomised patients responding to initial therapy while, in the others, randomisation was performed up-front)
2. Differences in the conditioning regimens and, partially,
3. Differences in the intensity and duration of the chemotherapy arm (the dose of alkylating agents and steroids were higher in the SWOG and Spanish trials, which may explain why OS for conventionally treated patients was longer in these two studies as compared to the IFM and MRC trials).

In spite of these discrepancies, HDT with ASCT is currently considered as standard of care for younger patients in multiple myeloma, mainly based on the improved response rate and EFS.

In the setting of novel agents it is important to define whether or not ASCT enhances the response rates obtained with these new induction regimens. Table 3 summarises the CR or near CR rates before and after transplant in randomised studies using novel agents as induction therapy. All of them consistently showed an increase in CR following ASCT, with most trials showing CR figures that are at least double the CRs (Table 3, includes references). These data suggest that induction with novel agents and ASCT are complementary rather than alternative treatment approaches.

Regarding tandem ASCT, its use will decrease for two reasons:
1. According to IFM and Italian experience only patients achieving < very good partial response with the first transplant benefit from the second and
2. A similar benefit is obtained upon using thalidomide as consolidation/maintenance therapy. In contrast, there may be increasing use of a second transplant at relapse, providing that the duration of the response to the first transplant has lasted for more than 2–3 years.

Table 3: **Response before and after autologous stem cell transplant in randomised trials**

Induction regimen	% Complete responses and nCR		Reference
	Pre-ASCT	Post-ASCT(1st)	
TD	5	38	Cavo, Lancet 2010; 376: 2075–2085
TD	14	24	Rosiñol, Blood 2010; ASH (abstr 307)
TAD	4	31	Lokhorst, Blood 2010; 93: 127-7
BzDx	15	35	Harousseau, JCO 2010; 28: 4926–4934
BzTD	19	55	Cavo, Lancet 2010; 376: 2075–2085
BzTD	35	46	Rosiñol, Blood 2010; ASH (abstr 307)
BzAD	11	30	Sonneveld, Blood 2010; 116: 40a

2.4 Autologous stem cell transplant upfront or at relapse?

Some investigators, particularly USA based, consider that upfront transplants may be challenged by the optimal results obtained with "long-term" treatment with novel agent combinations (i.e. LenDex or BzLenDex) and they propose to reserve the ASCT for the time of relapse. In order to clarify this debate, several groups are testing these two alternatives through randomised trials. Nevertheless, until these results become available we consider that upfront ASCT should remain as the standard of care based on the following arguments:

1. During the initial phases of the disease the patient is more fit (both physically and psychologically) to tolerate intensive and repetitive therapies
2. ASCT is associated with a long treatment-free interval and excellent quality of life
3. ASCT is not more expensive than the costs of novel agents and
4. We know that relapses after ASCT are sensitive to treatment with novel agents, but it is not known how efficient high dose melphalan will be after long-term exposure to novel agents. Until this question is answered through the randomised trials we should not submit patients to uncontrolled alternative therapeutic approaches, unless the patient is reluctant to proceed to an upfront ASCT.

2.5 Consolidation and maintenance treatment after ASCT

The Arkansas group was the first to demonstrate the efficacy of consolidation and maintenance therapies through their total therapy programs (TTP 1 to 4), with up to 50% long term survivors (5). More recently, Ladetto et al. (9) have shown that the use of four consolidation cycles of BzTDex in patients in ≥VGPR after ASCT increases the CR rate from 15 to 49%, including 18% molecular remissions, an observation so far only reported with allogeneic transplant. The Italian randomised trial comparing VTD vs TD both as induction and consolidation in patients undergoing double ASCT has also confirmed the efficacy of consolidation; the quality of the response improved in 55% of patients, with a 5-log reduction in tumour burden by RQ-PCR (3).

Regarding maintenance, interferon and/or prednisone showed a prolongation of median survival by around 6 months, but due to their toxicity they have been abandoned. The availability of novel agents, particularly those in oral formulations (thalidomide and lenalidomide), has renewed the concept of maintenance in an attempt to prolong the duration of the responses after transplant. Six randomised trials (Table 4, includes references) have demonstrated the superiority of thalidomide maintenance (with or without prednisone) versus no maintenance or prednisone or interferon in terms of PFS, though only three of them showed an overall survival advantage. Moreover, in one of these trials an important concern was raised

Table 4: Thalidomide maintenance following autologous transplant: randomised trials

	Randomisation	N	Maintenance duration	Benefit on PFS	Benefit on OS	Reference
R	Thal+Pred Pred	234	12 months	yes	yes	Spencer, JCO 2009; 27: 1788–1793
R	Thal+Pamidronate Pamidronate None	597	until PD	yes	yes	Attal, Blood 2006; 108: 3289–3294
R	Thal None	668	until PD	yes	yes	Barlogie, N Eng J Med 2006; 354: 1021–1030 Barlogie, J Clin Oncol 2010; 28: 1209–1214
R	Thal IFN	556	until PD	yes	no	Lokhorst, Blood 2010; 115: 1113–1120
R	Thal None	820	until PD	yes	no	Morgan, ASH 2010 (abstr 623)
R	Thal+Pred None	332	until PD	yes	no	Stewart, ASH 2010 (abstr 39)

PD: progressive disease

about whether the continuous use of thalidomide may induce more resistant relapses. Moreover, the benefit of thalidomide maintenance for patients who are already in CR or for those with poor cytogenetics is not well established. Two large randomised trials (one conducted by the IFM and the other by the CALGB groups) are currently comparing the role of lenalidomide maintenance. The first conclusion is that the tolerability is much better than with thalidomide. In addition, a highly significant benefit in terms of PFS has been reported for lenalidomide maintenance arm in both trials (42 vs 22 months in the control arm) (10, 11). Although so far no benefit in overall survival has been observed, it is anticipated that based on the marked PFS benefit, a survival advantage may emerge with longer follow-up. Nevertheless, concern has recently been raised about the possibility of lenalidomide inducing secondary malignancies. A certain degree of precaution is therefore required with a need for long-term follow-up analysis and until these data become available maintenance treatment is not indicated outside of clinical trials (see Key points).

3. Allogeneic stem cell transplantation

Allogeneic stem cell transplantation (allo-HSCT) is a potentially curative treatment for multiple myeloma. Nevertheless, its role in the novel therapies era is debated due to its high morbidity and mortality.

3.1 Myeloablative conditioning

Early data on myeloablative conditioning can be extracted from the European Bone Marrow Transplantation (EBMT), the International Bone Marrow Transplantation Registry (IBMTR), and the Hutchinson Cancer Center registries (12–15). Transplant-related mortality (TRM) ranged in these studies from 40 to 49% and, for this reason myeloablative allo-HSCT was largely abandoned. Nevertheless, in patients who survived the procedure and achieved a complete response (CR), there were apparent plateaus in relapse-free survival (RFS) curves in the range of 34–39% at 5–6 years. The US Intergroup trial (S9321) demonstrated a progression-free survival (PFS) plateau of approximately 22% at 7 years in 36 patients undergoing allo-HSCT, which was higher as compared to 15% among patients who received auto-HSCT, in spite of a TRM of 53% in the former group (16). After 7 years of follow-up the OS rates were identical at 39% for both autologous and allogeneic recipients but, while the risk of relapse and death continued among patients undergoing ASCT, the OS curve for the allogeneic group reached a plateau. In a study performed by the Haemato-Oncology Foundation for Adults in the Netherlands (HOVON), ASCT was compared with semi-intensive treatment, but patients with an HLA-identical sibling donor could proceed to a partially T-cell–depleted myeloablative allo-HSCT (17). The TRM of the allo-HSCT patients exceeded 30% and PFS and OS were inferior compared to patients receiving auto-HSCT.

These data suggest that myeloablative allo-HSCT is a potentially curative treatment. However, due to the high TRM, myeloablative transplants are not currently considered as part of first-line treatment for MM while, in more advanced stages, other less toxic strategies, including reduced intensity conditioning (RIC) regimen may be more attractive. Nevertheless, this scenario may be changing. In this regard, the EBMT compared 334 patients who received transplants between 1983 and 1993 with 356 patients who received transplants between 1994 and 1998 (18) and described a marked reduction in TRM between the two time periods, with TRM at 2 years falling from 46 to 30%.

3.2 Reduced intensity conditioning

The Seattle group pioneered the strategy of an autologous transplantation followed by a RIC allograft based on the combination of low-dose TBI (2 Gy) plus fludarabine.

The same concept was piloted by Kroger et al. (19) using melphalan, fludarabine, and antithymocyte globulin (ATG). The Seattle group updated reports on 102 patients who received this treatment strategy with allo-HSCT from matched-related donors (20). The overall TRM was 18% at 1 year and the CR rate was 62%. With a median follow-up of 6.3 years the OS was 64% with a PFS of 36%.

The EBMT retrospectively compared RIC with standard myeloablative conditioning for allo-HSCT in MM (21). 196 patients conditioned with ablative regimens between 1998 and 2002, were compared with 320 patients undergoing RIC during the same time period. TRM was significantly lower for the RIC group. However, there was no statistical difference in OS. Furthermore, PFS was inferior for patients receiving RIC due to a higher relapse rate (54 vs 27%; p=0.001). The CIBMTR has carried out a similar analysis (22). A total of 1,211 patients undergoing allo-HSCT for MM between 1989 and 2005 were analysed in three cohorts based on year of allo-HSCT: 1989 to 1994 (n=346), 1995 to 2000 (n=285), and 2001 to 2005 (n=580). There was a decreasing use of myeloablative regimens over time (82 vs 62% vs 9%, respectively). Although the TRM at 5 years decreased in the most recent period (40 and 48 vs 29%), the OS was similar among the groups (30, 32, and 29 months), primarily because of increased risk of relapse in the latter cohort.

3.3 Prospective studies comparing ASCT followed by allo-RIC HSCT versus tandem ASCT as part of first-line therapy

Seven randomised trials addressing this question have been conducted (Table 5). All are based on biological randomisation, where patients with an HLA-identical sibling donor are assigned to ASCT followed by allo-RIC, while those without a donor are assigned to double ASCT.

In the French study, patients with an HLA-identical sibling donor and high-risk MM (defined by $\beta2$ microglobulin >3 mg/L and del ch 13 by fluorescent *in situ* hybridisation, FISH) were candidates for ASCT followed by allo-RIC with a conditioning regimen consisting of busulfan, fludarabine, and ATG and were compared with double ASCT. With a median follow-up of 56 months, no difference in EFS was observed (23). Moreover, there was a trend for a superior OS among patients undergoing double ASCT (median 48 vs 34 months, p=0.07) This study was, however, criticised for the inclusion of high dose ATG 12.5 mg/kg which might have negatively influenced on the GvM effect.

The Spanish PETHEMA trial found a trend for better PFS (p=0.08) for the allo-RIC arm, but did not observe a difference in EFS and OS between 25 patients treated with auto/allo-HSCT as compared to 85 receiving tandem ASCT, although higher CR rates after the allo-HSCT, were achieved (40 vs 11%; p=0.001) (24). In addition to the small number of patients, the interpretation of these results is difficult because

Table 5: Comparison trials of tandem autologous transplant with autologous + reduced intensity allograft

Trial (ref.)	Patients	CR + VGPR	TRM	DFS	OS
Garban (23)					
Auto Mel 200/220	219	33 + 18	5	0% at 5 y	44% at 5 y
Auto Mel 200	65	33 + 29	11	0% at 5 y	33% at 5 y
Allo Bu, Flu, ATG					
Bruno (25)					
Auto Mel 200	80	26 + NR	4	20% at 4 y	53% at 4 y
Auto Mel 200	82	55 + NR	10	42% at 4 y	75% at 4 y
Allo 2 Gy TBI		p=0.004	p<0.001	p=0.01	p=0.02
Rosignol (24)					
Auto Bu Mel-Mel, CBV	88	11 + 6	5	Med 26 mo	Med 57 mo
Auto Bu Mel-Mel	26	33 + NR	16	Med 19 mo	Med not reached
Allo Flu Mel 140					
Lokhorst (26)					
Auto Mel 200 + maintenance	141	42 + NR	NR	Med 30 mo	Med 60 mo
Auto Mel 200	126	45 + NR	14	Med 30 mo	Med 50 mo
Allo 2 Gy TBI					
Gahrton (27)					
Auto Mel 200	251	38 + NR	5	18% at 4 y	57% at 5 y
Auto Mel 200	107	43 + NR	13	35% at 4 y	65% at 5 y
Allo Flu Mel 140 + ATG					
Knop (28)					
Auto Mel 200	73	32 + NR	NR	NR	70% at 3 y
Auto Mel 200	126	59 + NR	16	NR	60% at 3 y
Allo Flu Mel 140 + ATG					

only patients not in CR or near CR after the first ASCT proceeded to the second transplant.

A multicentre Italian study (25) described a higher CR rate (55 versus 26%, p=0.004) and significantly longer PFS (36 versus 29 months, p=0.02), and OS (80 versus 54 months, p=0.01) among 82 patients with an HLA-identical sibling donor assigned to be treated with auto/allo-RIC HSCT as compared to 80 patients assigned to tandem ASCT arm. Critics of the study focused on the median OS of the ASCT patients, which was only 48 months, compared to >60 months in all the recently published prospective phase III auto-transplant studies.

The large US multicentre trial from the Blood and Marrow Transplant Clinical Trials Network (BMT CTN) comparing tandem ASCT with auto/allo-HSCT completed the targeted accrual in March 2007 with more than 150 patients biologically randomly assigned to the auto/allo-SCT group. The results from this study are expected to be released in the near future.

In the HOVON 54 study, patients with an HLA-identical sibling donor could proceed to allo-RIC. On the basis of an intention-to treat analysis, no difference in PFS and OS were found during an interim analysis that included 126 patients with a donor and 141 patients without a donor (26).

In the EBMT trial, PFS at 60 months was 35% for auto/allo-HSCT compared with 18% for tandem ASCT with OS of 65% and 57%, respectively (27). This trend for improved survival was seen in patients with or without deletion of chromosome 13. In the German DSMM V trial (28) inclusion was restricted to newly diagnosed patients with deletion 13q14 as determined by FISH. Allocation to either treatment arm was by availability of an HLA-matched donor. ATG was added to the conditioning in case of a MUD donor. Preliminary analysis showed a higher CR rate in 13q- subjects undergoing ASCT/allo-HSCT when compared to tandem ASCT (59 vs 32%; p=0.003). However, the projected OS at 3 years was 70% for double ASCT versus 60% for the auto/allo-HSCT patients (p=0.22). TRM at 2 years from allo-HSCT was only 12.7% even though 60% received MUD allo-HSCT.

3.4 Allo-HSCT in high-risk myeloma

Before the incorporation of novel therapies, the outcome of patients with poor prognostic features defined by cytogenetics (t4;14; t14;16; 17p-) was universally dismal. Currently, there is increasing evidence that bortezomib-based regimens are capable of overcoming at least some of the adverse prognostic outcomes (e.g. t(4;14)).

Schilling et al. (29) reported the outcome of reduced-intensity transplantation in 101 patients with a variety of cytogenetic abnormalities: 61% with del(13q14), 19% with t(4;14)(p16.3; q32), 16% with del(17p13), and 5% with t(14;16)(q32;q23). There were no differences in response rates nor in transplantation-related mortality, with the exception that patients with 17p13 deletions had a lower CR rate (7 vs 56%).

Rotta et al. (20) reported the Seattle Consortium experience in 102 patients completing auto/allo-HSCT. While β2 microglobulin >3.5 mg/L was a poor-risk factor, cytogenetic abnormalities were not predictive of outcome.

Given the small number of patients in these studies, it is uncertain whether reduced-intensity allogeneic transplants can overcome poor-risk indicators. However, it is conceivable that a full allo-HSCT may be considered in selected patients.

3.5 Allogeneic HSCT: Conclusions and future directions

Myeloablative allo-HSCT may cure a minority of patients, but is associated with a high TRM. Considering the improvement in TRM and the plateau in OS observed in several studies, myeloablative conditioning could be evaluated in well-designed prospective clinical trials. Non-myeloablative allo-HSCT in first-line therapy is associated with a lower TRM but a greater risk of relapse and convincing evidence is still lacking that allo-RIC improves survival as compared to autologous HSCT. Even when a late survival benefit is shown by the donor versus no donor comparisons, it may still be questionable if in the era of novel agents allo-RIC should be offered to patients in first-line therapy. Key points are summarised below.

In early first relapses, allo-HSCT is an attractive option within well-designed clinical trials. Future studies of allo-HSCT in myeloma should aim at improving the graft-versus-tumour effect while reducing the morbidity and mortality of allo-HSCT. Novel anti-MM agents in the post-allo setting may favour the GvM effect. However, exact mechanisms of action as well as the optimal timing and dosage of these agents after transplantation have yet to be determined. New strategies should be explored prospectively in selected groups of patients.

Key points

Induction regimens based on novel agents (i.e. Btz TD) are clearly superior to conventional VAD

New induction regimens and high dose melphalan should be considered complementary rather than alternative treatment approaches

Several randomised trials are comparing the value of ASCT upfront versus at first relapse. Until these results become available, the ASCT upfront should remain as the standard of care

Consolidation treatment (e.g. VTD) and maintenance therapy (mainly with lenalidomide) are associated with a significant prolongation in PFS, but they should still be considered as experimental approaches restricted to clinical trials

In the upfront setting, allogeneic transplant should be restricted to clinical trials, but could be offered to young patients relapsing within 1 year after and optimised induction followed by ASCT

The use of ASCT followed by allo-RIC is associated with lower relapse rate than tandem ASCT but higher mortality

The role of allogeneic transplant must be revisited in the era of novel agents

References

1. San-Miguel J, Harousseau JL, Joshua D et al. Individualizing treatment of patients with myeloma in the era of novel agents. J Clin Oncol 2008; 26: 2761–2766.
2. Stewart AK. Reduced-intensity allogeneic transplantation for myeloma: Reality bites. Blood 2009; 113: 3135–3136.
3. Cavo M, Tacchetti P, Patriarca F. et al. Bortezomib with thalidomide plus dexamethasone compared with thalidomide plus dexamethasone as induction therapy before, and consolidation therapy after double autologous stem-cell transplantation in newly diagnosed multiple myeloma: A randomized phase 3 study. Lancet 2010; 376: 2075–2085.
4. Harousseau JL, Attal M, Avet –Loiseau H et al. Bortezomib-dexamethasone is superior to vincristine-doxorubicin-dexamethasone as induction treatment prior to autologous stem cell transplantation in newly diagnosed multiple myeloma: Results of the IFM 2005-01 phase 3 trial. J Clin Oncol 28: 4926–4934, 2010.
5. Barlogie B, Attal M, Crowley J et al. Long-term follow-up of autotransplantation trials for multiple myeloma: Update of protocols conducted by the intergroupe francophone du myelome, southwest oncology group, and university of Arkansas for medical sciences. J Clin Oncol 2010; 28: 1209–1214.
6. Rajkumar SV, Jacobus S, Callander N et al. Lenalidomide plus high-dose dexamethasone versus lenalidomide plus low-dose dexamethasone as initial therapy for newly diagnosed multiple myeloma: An open-label randomized controlled trial. Lancet Oncol 2010; 11: 29–37.
7. Lahuerta JJ, Mateos MV, Martínez-López J et al. Busulfan 12 mg/kg plus melphalan 140 mg/m2 versus melphalan 200 mg/m^2 as conditioning regimens for autologous transplantation in newly diagnosed multiple myeloma patients included in the PETHEMA/GEM2000 study. Haematologica 2010; 95: 1913–1920.
8. Roussel M, Moreau P, Huynh A et al. Bortezomib and high-dose melphalan as conditioning regimen before autologous stem cell transplantation in patients with de novo multiple myeloma: A phase 2 study of the Intergroupe Francophone du Myelome (IFM). Blood 2010; 115: 32–37.
9. Ladetto M, Pagliano G, Ferrero S et al. Major tumor shrinking and persistent molecular remissions after consolidation with bortezomib, thalidomide, and dexamethasone in patients with autografted myeloma. J Clin Oncol 2010; 28: 2077–2084.
10. Attal M, Cristini C, Marti G et al. Lenalidomide maintenance after transplantation for myeloma. J Clin Oncol 2010; 28: 15s (suppl; abstr 8018).
11. McCarthy PL, Owzar K, Anderson KC et al. Phase III intergroup study of lenalidomide versus placebo maintenance therapy following single autologous stem cell transplant (ASCT) for multiple myeloma (MM): CALGB 100104. J Clin Oncol 2010; 28; 15s (suppl; abstr 8017).
12. Gahrton G, Tura S, Ljungman P et al. Allogeneic bone marrow transplantation in multiple myeloma. N Engl J Med 1991; 325: 1267–1273.
13. Gahrton G, Tura S, Ljungman P et al. Prognostic factors in allogeneic bone marrow transplantation for multiple myeloma. J Clin Oncol 1995; 13: 1312–1322.
14. Bensinger WI, Buckner CD, Anasetti C et al. Allogeneic marrow transplantation for multiple myeloma: An analysis of risk factors on outcome. Blood 1996; 88: 2787–2793.

15. Durie BG, Gale JP, Klein JP et al. Allogeneic transplants for multiple myeloma: An IBMTR analysis. Proc Am Soc Clin Oncol 1995; 15: 405 (abstr 1358).

16. Barlogie B, Kyle RA, Anderson KC et al. Standard chemotherapy compared with high-dose chemoradiotherapy for multiple myeloma: Final results of phase III US Intergroup trial S9321. J Clin Oncol 2006; 24: 929–936.

17. Lokhorst HM, Segeren CM, Verdonck LF et al. Partially T-cell-depleted allogeneic stem-cell transplantation for first-line treatment of multiple myeloma: A prospective evaluation of patients treated in the phase III study HOVON 24 MM. J Clin Oncol 2003; 21: 1728-1733.

18. Gahrton G, Svensson H, Cavo M et al. Progress in allogeneic bone marrow and peripheral blood stem cell transplantation for multiple myeloma: A comparison between transplants performed 1983-93 and 1994-98 at European Group for Blood and Marrow Transplantation centres. Br J Haematol 2001; 113: 209–216.

19. Kröger N, Schwerdtfeger R, Kieh M et al. Autologous stem cell transplantation followed by a dose-reduced allograft induces high complete remission rate in multiple myeloma. Blood 2002; 100: 755–760.

20. Rotta M, Storer BE, Sahebi F et al. Long term outcome of patients with multiple myeloma after autologous hematopoietic cell transplantation and nonmyeloablative allografting. Blood 2009; 113: 3383–3391.

21. Crawley C, Iacobelli S, Björkstrand B et al. Reduced-intensity conditioning for myeloma: Lower non relapse mortality but higher relapse rates compared with myeloablative conditioning. Blood 2007; 109: 3588–3594.

22. Kumar S, Shrestha S, Zhang M-J et al. Allogeneic stem cell transplantation (SCT) for multiple myeloma (MM) - what has changed? A CIBMTR analysis from 1989-2005. Blood 2009; 114 (abstr 52).

23. Moreau P, Garban F, Attal M et al. Long term follow-up results of IFM99-03 and IFM99-04 trials comparing nonmyeloablative allotransplantation with autologous transplantation in high-risk de novo multiple myeloma. Blood 2008; 112: 3914–3915.

24. Rosiñol L, Pérez-Simón JA, Sureda A et al. A prospective PETHEMA study of tandem autologous transplantation versus autograft followed by reduced intensity conditioning allogeneic transplantation in newly diagnosed multiple myeloma. Blood 2008; 112: 3591–3593.

25. Bruno B, Rotta M, Patriarca F et al. A comparison of allografting with autografting for newly diagnosed myeloma. N Engl J Med 2007; 356: 1110–1120.

26. Lokhorst H, Sonneveld P, van der Holt B et al. Donor versus no donor analysis of newly diagnosed myeloma patients included in the HOVON 50/54 study. Blood 2008; 112: 461 (abstr).

27. Gahrton G, Björkstrand B, Iacobelli S et al. Tandem autologous (ASCT)/allogeneic reduced intensity conditioning transplantation (RIC) with identical sibling donor versus ASCT in previously untreated multiple myeloma (MM): Long term follow up of a prospective controlled trial by the EBMT. Blood 2009; 114: 52 (abstr).

28. Knop S, Liebisch P, Hebart H et al. Allogeneic stem cell transplant versus tandem high-dose melphalan for front-line treatment of deletion 13q14 myeloma: An interim analysis

of the German DSMM V trial. Blood 2009; 114: 51 (abstr).

29. Schilling G, Hansen T, Shimoni A et al. Impact of genetic abnormalities on survival after allogeneic hematopoietic stem cell transplantation in multiple myeloma. Leukemia 2008; 22: 1250–1255.

Multiple Choice Questionnaire

To find the correct answer, go to http://www.esh.org/online-training/handbook/

1. **Which of the following statements about autologous stem cell transplant (ASCT) in myeloma patients is *not* correct:**
    a) Induction with novel agents and ASCT are complementary strategies rather than alternatives...☐
    b) Melphalan 200 mg/m² is the gold standard conditioning regiment prior to ASCT..☐
    c) Thalidomide and bortezomib do not affect stem cell collection..........☐
    d) All studies comparing high dose therapy followed by ASCT versus standard dose chemotherapy have demonstrated a benefit in overall survival for high dose therapy...☐

2. **Regarding the use of consolidation/maintenance therapy after ASCT, which statement is the correct one:**
    a) The administration of consolidation therapy with novel agent-based regimens is able to improve the quality of responses obtained after ASCT...☐
    b) Thalidomide as maintenance has been demonstrated to prolong progression-free survival...☐
    c) Lenalidomide as maintenance doubled progression-free survival as compared with placebo..☐
    d) All of the above are correct..☐

3. **Currently a controversial issue is the best time to perform an autologous transplant (ASCT) in MM patients. Which one of the following is *incorrect*?**
    a) So far ASCT upfront remains the standard of care......................☐

b) If the patient prefers to postpone the transplant until first relapse this can be an option .... ☐

c) Second transplant at relapse can be indicated if the duration of response after the first transplant lasted for more than 2–3 years .... ☐

d) All of the above are correct .... ☐

4. **Which one of the following statements is *incorrect*:**

a) The US Intergroup trial (S9321) demonstrated a progression-free survival (PFS) of approximately 22% at 7 years in patients undergoing allo-HSCT, compared to 15% among patients who received auto-HSCT .... ☐

b) The US Intergroup trial (S9321) reported 53% TRM for patients undergoing allo-HSCT .... ☐

c) In this trial OS at 7 years was 39% for both patients receiving allo-HSCT or auto-SCT .... ☐

d) For both autologous and allogeneic recipients the OS curve at 7 years reached a plateau .... ☐

5. **Among the following statements about autologous transplant followed by reduced intensity transplant, please choose the *incorrect* one:**

a) On the basis of an intention-to treat analysis, no difference in PFS and OS were found in the HOVON 54 study during an interim analysis that included 126 patients with a donor and 141 patients without a donor .... ☐

b) In the EBMT trial, PFS at 60 months was 35% for auto/allo-HSCT compared with 18% for tandem auto-SCT and OS 65% and 57%, respectively .... ☐

c) This trend for improved survival was only seen in patients with deletion 13 .... ☐

d) Schilling et al. reported the outcome of 101 patients undergoing reduced-intensity transplantations with a variety of cytogenetics abnormalities. There were no differences with the exception that patients with 17p13 deletions had a lower CR rate (7 vs 56%) .... ☐

* CHAPTER 19

Indications for HSCT in adults

* 19.7

Role of HSCT in primary amyloidosis

M. Teresa Cibeira, Jordi Esteve

1. Introduction

Immunoglobulin light chain (AL) amyloidosis is a misfolding protein disease with an incidence of 5–12 persons per million per year. In AL, clonal bone marrow plasma cells produce monoclonal light chains that misfold, leading to extracellular deposition of abnormal protein fibrils in tissues and organs, resulting in progressive organ failure and ultimately in death. Organs most frequently involved are kidney, heart, liver, autonomic and peripheral nervous system, gastrointestinal tract, and soft tissue. AL amyloidosis should be suspected in any patient with a compatible clinical syndrome and a monoclonal gammopathy detected by serum and/or urinary immunofixation or by bone marrow examination. Diagnosis of AL is based on the recognition of amyloid fibrils in a tissue biopsy, either of an involved organ or a surrogate site (such as abdominal fat, rectum or bone marrow). Classic Congo red staining (or electron microscopy) reveals amyloid deposition while immunohistochemical staining allows identification of the fibril precursor protein, which is a monoclonal light chain, in contrast to other types of amyloidosis (familial type, secondary amyloidosis, dialysis-associated and senile). Immunogold electron microscopy may also be useful and, more recently, laser microdissection with mass spectrometry (LMD/MS) and customised protein bioinformatics has proved to be a highly specific and sensitive test allowing definitive typing of amyloid deposits (1). Once the diagnosis has been confirmed, the degree of organ involvement must be determined in order to establish a treatment decision. Despite the usual low tumour burden characteristic of this disorder, AL is a poor-prognosis disease, with only a modest response pattern to standard chemotherapy. In contrast, intensive therapy with high-dose melphalan (HDM) and autologous stem cell transplantation (ASCT) produces a significant proportion of haematologic responses, followed by significant amelioration of organ damage in most responding patients. Unfortunately, this procedure is associated with an exceedingly high toxicity, due to the underlying organ dysfunction in this disease. It is possible that the use of novel agents for the treatment of AL, such as proteasome inhibitors or lenalidomide, may result in a higher response rate than standard non-intensive strategies, but their global impact in the natural history of the disease and their precise role in the management of the disease remains currently unknown.

2. Indications

Eligibility criteria for HDM/ASCT are variable depending on the transplanting centre and the dose of melphalan used as conditioning regimen. However, the usual eligibility criteria for HDM/ASCT with full dose melphalan (200 mg/m^2) include age ≤65 years, performance status 0 to 2, absence of significant clinical cardiac involvement (normal cardiac troponin concentration and left ventricular ejection fraction $\geq 45-50\%$), absence of severe orthostatic hypotension (i.e., systolic blood pressure ≥ 90 mm Hg), and diffusion lung capacity for carbon monoxide $>50\%$ (2). Renal failure has been commonly considered an exclusion criterion although some authors have reported that HDM/ASCT is also an effective treatment in selected patients with AL amyloidosis associated end-stage renal disease, with similar outcome in terms of morbidity and mortality to that observed in non-dialysis patients (3).

3. Stem cell mobilisation and collection

Stem cell mobilisation and leucapheresis in patients with AL is associated with unusual morbidity and with some reports of fatal events, due to the impaired organ function and subclinical cardiovascular impairment of these patients. A syndrome of hypoxia and hypotension has been described both during mobilisation with G-CSF and during the leucapheresis procedure itself, probably as a result of a capillary leak syndrome triggered by G-CSF, together with platelet activation during SC collection, and the release of inflammatory cytokines. Therefore, use of reduced doses of G-CSF (such as 10 µg/kg per day for 4 days) and careful monitoring during the leucapheresis procedure are important in order to avoid or correct immediately any sudden volume imbalance (hypovolemia or fluid overload) that may arise during the stem cell collection process. Despite this, Gertz et al. reported that 10% of patients transplanted in a highly experienced centre required a delay of at least 1 month to recover from stem cell collection, usually due to marked fluid retention in patients with moderate heart failure or severe nephrotic syndrome (4).

4. Conditioning regimen

Conditioning regimens in AL are based on high-dose melphalan. The usual melphalan dose is 200 mg/m², although a "risk-adapted" approach, with dose reduction to 140 mg/m², has been proposed in higher-risk patients in order to decrease transplant-related toxicity (5). No uniform criteria for selecting patients for reduced dose melphalan have been established. Proposed criteria for defining high-risk patients are age 61 to 70 years, poor performance status (score of 2), compensated cardiac failure or left ejection fraction between 40% and 45/50%, stem cell collection of 2 to <2.5 x 10⁶ CD34+ cells/kg, and increased creatinine level (higher than 1.5 or 2 mg/dL; 133–176.8 µmol/L) (6, 7). However, reduced melphalan dose has been associated with a decreased response rate in retrospective analyses conducted by the Mayo Clinic and Boston University groups (5, 6), although this observation has not been confirmed in other studies (8) and might be related to the poorer prognostic characteristics of the population receiving the reduced melphalan dose. An even lower dose of melphalan as conditioning regimen is being explored in a multi-centre study conducted by the Southwest Oncology Group (S 0115). In this study patients receive two cycles of modified high dose melphalan at 100 mg/m² and ASCT.

5. Results: response, long-term outcome and toxicity

The introduction of HDM/ASCT in the 1990s improved markedly the poor results obtained with standard chemotherapy in this disease. Published series from both single and multicentre studies showed haematologic complete response (CR) rates ranging from 16 to 40%, organ responses in 25 to 45% of patients, and a median overall survival of about 5 years (Table 1). In the recently updated experience of the Mayo Clinic group, with 434 patients transplanted from 1996 to 2010, the CR rate was almost 40% and organ response was obtained in approximately half of

Table 1: Summary of the outcome of patients with primary amyloidosis undergoing autologous stem cell transplantation, according to largest published series

Source	No. of pts	Overall response rate (CR)%	TRM (%)	Overall survival (%)
Boston (US) *Skinner et al, 2004 (6)*	277	NR (40) (30 by ITT)	13 (100-day)	60 (3-yr)
CIBMTR (multicentre) *Vesole et al, 2006 (9)*	107	32 (16)	18 (30-day) 27 (1-yr)	66 (1-yr) 56 (3-yr)
UK (multicentre) *Goodman et al, 2006 (10)*	92	64 (35)	23 (100-day)	50 (5-yr)
French Intergroup (MAG-IFM) *Jaccard et al, 2007 (11)*	50	49 (30)	24 (100-day)	45 (3-yr)
Mayo Clinic *Gertz et al, 2010 (4)*	434	75.8 (38.7)	10 (100-day)	Median not reached for patients in CR and 32 mos. for non-responders
Boston (US) *Cibeira et al, 2010 (12)*	421	NR (34.4)	11.4 (100-day)	86 (5-yr) for CR patients 58 (5-yr) for non-CR patients

CR: complete response; TRM: transplant-related mortality; NR: not reported; ITT intention to treat; CIBMTR: Center for International Blood and Marrow Transplant Research; UK: United Kingdom; MAG-IFM: Myélome Autogreffe-Intergroupe Francophone du Myélome

patients (4). The organ response rate is higher (78.6%) in the group of patients who achieve CR, according to the Boston group experience (12). In this setting, haematologic CR is defined as absence of monoclonal gammopathy by immunofixation electrophoresis of serum and urine, normal bone marrow biopsy (i.e. absence of kappa or lambda clonal plasma cells by immunohistochemistry) and, for those patients who were treated after the serum free-light chain (FLC) test became available, a normal serum immunoglobulin FLC ratio and concentration. Clinical (or organ) response is defined as improvement in at least one involved organ according to published consensus criteria (13). Although median time to achieve a haematological response is between 3–4 months, organ responses can take several months, up to 2 years, in some patients. On the other hand, relapses after CR occurred in 21 and 27% of patients in the long-term experience of the Boston and Mayo Clinic groups, respectively (4, 6). These combined results translate into a long-term survival beyond 10 years in approximately one quarter of all patients with AL amyloidosis treated with HDM/ASCT and half of those achieving haematologic CR (14).

Unfortunately, HDM/ASCT is associated with a remarkably high risk of morbidity and mortality in AL patients, with a transplant-related mortality (TRM) ranging from the 30–40% reported by some early multicentre series to a more acceptable 10–15% described in recent reports from experienced single centres (8, 14, 15) (Table 1). Moreover, a further decrease in TRM (5–7%) has been reported by the larger series of both the Mayo Clinic (7) and Boston groups (12) during recent years, as a result of both an improved selection of patients and better peri-transplant management. Cardiogenic shock, supraventricular tachyarrhythmias, gastrointestinal tract bleeding, and infections are the most frequent complications involved in procedure-related deaths during this phase. Infrequent causes such spontaneous splenic rupture or DMSO-triggered cardiac arrest have also been reported. Furthermore, acute renal insufficiency may develop immediately after melphalan conditioning in up to 18% of patients (16).

6. Prognostic factors

Several factors have been associated with transplant outcome in AL. Cardiac involvement, as defined by several methods such as the presence of congestive heart failure, thickened interventricular wall on ultrasonography or increased serum cardiac biomarkers, is invariably identified as an adverse prognostic factor. In this regard, measurement of serum cardiac troponins (cTnT, cTnI) and N-terminal pro-brain natriuretic peptide (NT-proBNP) provides a quantitative assessment of cardiac damage and wall strain in AL and are strong predictors of survival after HDM/SCT. Based on this, a cardiac staging system that allows the stratification of AL patients into three stages (I, II and III), depending on whether none, only one or both cardiac biomarkers are high, has been proposed by the Mayo group. Moreover, these three stages translate into a different outcome, with a median survival of 26.4, 10.5 and 3.5 months, respectively (17). The baseline level of FLC has also been identified as a prognostic factor, with an increased TRM in patients with higher pre-transplant levels (18). Concurrent renal failure and involvement of more than two organs, as a measure of disease extent, have also been associated with shorter survival after transplant. Although not being an initial prognostic factor, the degree of response achieved after transplant showed a striking correlation with long-term outcome, with a longer survival observed in patients who achieve CR (19). Of note, the strongest predictors of survival in a recently published large series were the cardiac stage and the achievement of complete response after transplant (4).

7. Role of HDM/ASCT in the management of the disease: comparison with other treatment approaches

Fewer than 5% of patients with AL amyloidosis survived for more than 10 years before the introduction of HDM/ASCT. Oral melphalan and prednisone (MP), the first effective regimen used in AL, modestly increased the median survival up to 18 months, but with almost no CR or reversal of organ dysfunction. Multiple alkylating agents did not show any benefit compared with standard MP. In this setting, a retrospective case-control study conducted by the Mayo Clinic group demonstrated a significant benefit of HDM/ASCT for patients younger than 70 years of age compared to non-transplant regimens (which mostly consisted of MP), with a 4-year survival of 71 versus 41%, respectively (15). However, this observation should be interpreted with caution since transplant candidates constitute a selected population with better prognosis. Recently, the combination of oral melphalan and pulse dexamethasone (MD) in selected patients has also resulted in high haematologic response rates (52 to 67%) as well as organ responses (39 to 48%) and a median survival of around 5 years (11, 20). This regimen was compared to HDM/ASCT in a randomised trial and outcomes were comparable (11), although some concerns regarding this multicentre study are the relatively small number of patients included (50 per arm), the fact that 26% of patients randomised to transplant did not receive the planned treatment, and, furthermore, the high TRM observed among transplanted patients (24%). On the other hand, there is a high long-term risk of myelodysplasia in AL patients treated with repeated courses of oral melphalan, up to 20% (21). Therefore, the relative benefit of these two approaches remains uncertain. Finally, promising results have been reported with regimens that include the so-called "new drugs" used in patients with myeloma, namely thalidomide, lenalidomide and/or bortezomib

(22). For example, there is a preliminary report of an impressive 80% haematologic response rate, including 42% complete responses, in a phase II trial using the combination MD with bortezomib. Of interest, an international clinical trial comparing MD and MD combined with bortezomib for newly diagnosed AL patients has recently started. Longer follow-up is needed in order to establish the definitive role of these drugs in the management of the disease.

8. Future perspective and conclusions

Given the relevance of achieving haematologic CR after HDM/ASCT in the outcome and survival of AL amyloidosis, several approaches have been proposed to increase the responses after this procedure. The Boston group conducted a trial of tandem transplants in patients not achieving CR after the first course, and observed an increase in the overall CR rate. Incorporation of novel agents in the pre-transplant setting (as induction or part of conditioning) or for consolidation/maintenance after transplant, is another treatment approach that should be investigated in the context of clinical trials. Allogeneic SCT using reduced-intensity conditioning has also been performed in a minority of patients, with the aim of exploiting a potential "graft-versus-amyloidosis" effect. Finally, the possibility of solid organ transplantation should be considered in selected patients: kidney transplant in patients with end-stage renal disease secondary to AL and in CR after HDM/ASCT, and heart transplant followed by HDM/SCT in patients with isolated or predominant advanced cardiac involvement.

In conclusion, HDM/ASCT results in haematologic and organ responses in a significant proportion of patients with AL, as well as a prolonged survival in responding patients. Unfortunately, this procedure is associated with a high TRM, although it has decreased to an acceptable 5–10% in the recent experience of single referral centres. Therefore, careful selection of patients and an experienced peri-transplant management are critical (Table 2). In this regard, a more refined assessment of cardiac involvement by means of cardiac staging system might contribute to a more accurate evaluation of patients prior to SCT. Nevertheless, the only randomised trial comparing HDM/ASCT with MD failed to show superiority for the intensive arm. As a result of this, the precise impact of transplant in the management of AL amyloidosis remains controversial and the target population remains to be clarified in further studies. Moreover, the potential improvement in the "control arm" (i.e., based on non-intensive therapy) with the introduction of newer agents such as immunomodulators (thalidomide, lenalidomide) or the proteasome inhibitor bortezomib, should be considered. Further prospective studies are therefore required to clarify the role of HDM/ASCT in AL.

Table 2: **Specific considerations regarding evaluation of autologous stem cell transplantation in patient with primary amyloidosis**	
Diagnostic accuracy	1. Demonstration of amyloid deposition (Congo Red staining) 2. Confirmation of primary origin (immunoglobulin light-chain amyloidosis, AL): • Presence of monoclonal light chain in amyloid fibril • (or) Detection serum/urine monoclonal light-chain • New methods: laser microdissection with mass spectrometry
Is the patient a candidate for HDM/ASCT?	1. Age up to 65–70 years 2. Adequate performance status (≤2) 3. Absence of limiting organ damage: • Significant cardiac involvement (no CHF, high troponin level, and/or LVEF <45%) • Severe orthostatic hypotension • DLCO >50% • Severe renal failure (ASCT to be considered only in highly specialised referral centres)
Assessment of risk factors	1. Assessment of amyloid deposition: • Number of involved organs (renal, cardiac, hepatic, gastrointestinal, peripheral & autonomic neuropathy, soft tissue) • Serum free-light chain (FLC) measurement 2. Assessment of cardiac involvement: • Determination of cardiac biomarkers (cTnT, cTnI, NT-proBNP) • Echocardiogram (interventricular wall thickness)
Recommended care during procedure	1. Monitoring during stem cell mobilisation and collection 2. Risk-adapted conditioning: • Standard dose: melphalan 200 mg/m^2 • Reduced dose (if concurrent risk factors): melphalan 140 mg/m^2 3. Careful post-transplant management • Close monitoring of cardio-vascular function • Prevention of mucosal & gastrointestinal bleeding: specific platelet transfusional policy (maintain >50 x 10^9/L)
Adequate assessment of post-transplant response	1. Haematologic response: • CR: negative serum & urine immunofixation, normal FLC ratio and <5% plasma cells in bone marrow • PR: 50% reduction of serum M component, urine light chain & FLC 2. Organ response. Re-assessment of pre-transplant involved organ: • Renal (24-hour urinary protein, creatinine level) • Heart (functional class, septal thickness, ejection fraction) • Liver (alkaline phosphatase, liver size) • Nerve (nerve conduction)

CHF: cardiac heart failure; LVEF: left ventricular ejection fraction

References

1. Vrana JA, Gamez JD, Madden BJ et al. Classification of amyloidosis by laser microdissection and mass spectrometry-based proteomic analysis in clinical biopsy specimens. Blood 2009; 114: 4957–4959.
2. Merlini G, Seldin DC, Gertz MA. Amyloidosis: Pathogenesis and new therapeutic options. J Clin Oncol 2011; 29: 1924–1933.
3. Sanchorawala V, Quillen K, Finn KT et al. High-dose melphalan and autologous stem cell transplantation in AL amyloidosis and monoclonal immunoglobulin deposition disease associated end-stage renal disease requiring dialysis. Blood (ASH Annual Meeting Abstracts), Nov 2010; 116: 3553.
4. Gertz MA, Lacy MQ, Dispenzieri A et al. Autologous stem cell transplant for immunoglobulin light chain amyloidosis: A status report. Leuk Lymphoma 2010; 51: 2181–2187.
5. Gertz MA, Lacy MQ, Dispenzieri A et al. Risk-adjusted manipulation of melphalan dose before stem cell transplantation in patients with amyloidosis is associated with a lower response rate. Bone Marrow Transplant 2004; 34: 1025–1031.
6. Skinner M, Sanchorawala V, Seldin DC et al. High-dose melphalan and autologous stem-cell transplantation in patients with AL amyloidosis: An 8-year study. Ann Intern Med 2004; 140: 85–93.
7. Gertz MA, Lacy MQ, Dispenzieri A et al. Trends in day 100 and 2-year survival after auto-SCT for AL amyloidosis: Outcomes before and after 2006. Bone Marrow Transplant 2010; published on October 11, 2010, as DOI 10.1038/bmt-2010-234.
8. Perfetti V, Siena S, Palladini G et al. Long-term results of a risk-adapted approach to melphalan conditioning in autologous peripheral blood stem cell transplantation for primary (AL) amyloidosis. Haematologica 2006; 91: 1635–1643.
9. Vesole DH, Perez WS, Akasheh M et al. High-dose therapy and autologous hematopoietic stem cell transplantation for patients with primary systemic amyloidosis: A Center for International Blood and Marrow Transplant Research Study. Mayo Clin Proc. 2006; 81: 880–888.
10. Cibeira MT, Sanchorawala V, Seldin DC et al. Outcome of AL amyloidosis after high-dose melphalan and autologous stem cell transplantation: Long-term results in a series of 421 patients. Blood 2011; 118: 4346–4352.
11. Jaccard A, Moreau P, Leblond V et al; Myélome Autogreffe (MAG) and Intergroupe Francophone du Myélome (IFM) Intergroup. High-dose melphalan versus melphalan plus dexamethasone for AL amyloidosis. N Engl J Med 2007; 357: 1083–1093.
12. Cibeira MT, Sanchorawala V, Seldin DC et al. Outcome of patients with AL amyloidosis who do not achieve hematologic complete response after treatment with high dose melphalan and autologous transplantation: Results in a series of 421 patients. Blood (ASH Annual Meeting Abstracts) 2010; 116: 2394.
13. Gertz MA, Comenzo R, Falk RH et al. Definition of organ involvement and treatment response in immunoglobulin light chain amyloidosis (AL): A consensus opinion from the 10th International Symposium on Amyloid and Amyloidosis, Tours, France, 18-22 April 2004. Am J Hematol 2005; 79: 319–328.
14. Sanchorawala V, Skinner M, Quillen K et al. Long-term outcome of patients with AL amyloidosis treated with high-dose melphalan and stem-cell transplantation. Blood 2007; 110: 3561–3563.

15. Dispenzieri A, Kyle RA, Lacy MQ et al. Superior survival in primary systemic amyloidosis patients undergoing peripheral blood stem cell transplantation: A case-control study. Blood 2004; 103: 3960–3963.

16. Leung N, Slezak JM, Bergstralh EJ et al. Acute renal insufficiency after high-dose melphalan in patients with primary systemic amyloidosis during stem cell transplantation. Am J Kidney Dis 2005; 45: 102–111.

17. Dispenzieri A, Gertz MA, Kyle RA et al. Serum cardiac troponins and N-terminal pro-brain natriuretic peptide: A staging system for primary systemic amyloidosis. J Clin Oncol 2004; 22: 3751–3757.

18. Dispenzieri A, Lacy MQ, Kartzmann JA et al. Absolute values of immunoglobulin free light chains are prognostic in patients with primary systemic amyloidosis undergoing peripheral blood stem cell transplantation. Blood 2006; 107: 3378–3383.

19. Gertz MA, Lacy MQ, Dispenzieri A et al. Effect of hematologic response on outcome of patients undergoing transplantation for primary amyloidosis: Importance of achieving a complete response. Haematologica 2007; 92: 1415–1418.

20. Palladini G, Russo P, Nuvolone M et al. Treatment with oral melphalan plus dexamethasone produces long-term remissions in AL amyloidosis. Blood 2007; 110: 787–788.

21. Gertz MA, Lacy MQ, Lust JA et al. Long-term risk of myelodysplasia in melphalan-treated patients with immunoglobulin light-chain amyloidosis. Haematologica 2008; 93: 1402–1406.

22. Cohen AD, Comenzo RL. Systemic light-chain amyloidosis: Advances in diagnosis, prognosis and therapy. Hematology 2010 (American Society of Hematology Education Program Book); 287–294.

Multiple Choice Questionnaire

To find the correct answer, go to http://www.esh.org/online-training/handbook/

1. **Concerning the diagnosis of immunoglobulin light chain (AL) amyloidosis, which of the following is the correct answer?**
    a) A monoclonal light chain is rarely detected in serum ....☐
    b) Diagnosis of AL relies exclusively on Congo red positivity..............☐
    c) Congo Red and immunohistochemical staining must be performed in the involved organ ....☐
    d) Laser microdissection with mass spectrometry has been considered the gold standard for amyloid typing ....☐

2. **Which one of the following is *not* an exclusion criterion for high-dose melphalan with autologous stem cell transplant (HDM/ASCT)?**
    a) Age over 70 years........................☐

b) Renal insufficiency ☐
c) Significant clinical cardiac involvement ☐
d) Severe orthostatic hypotension ☐

---

3. **Which one of the following statements is *not* true regarding response after high-dose melphalan with autologous stem cell transplant (HDM/ASCT)?**
   a) Haematologic response assessment is based on serum and urine immunofixation and serum free light chain measurement ☐
   b) HDM/ASCT results in a significant rate of organ responses, which is higher in the group of patients who achieve haematologic complete response ☐
   c) Organ responses are always observed in the early period post-transplant, i.e., no longer than 3 months ☐
   d) In a large series, long-term survival beyond 10 years was 53% for those patients achieving haematologic CR ☐

---

4. **Concerning transplant related-mortality in patients with AL undergoing HDM/ASCT, indicate the correct answer:**
   a) It is exceedingly high, between 30–40% ☐
   b) It has decreased to less than 5% in the recent years as a result of better selection of patients and peri-transplant management ☐
   c) Stem cell mobilisation and leucapheresis in patients with AL are associated with unusual morbidity and occasional fatal events ☐
   d) It is correlated with cardiac staging system but not with baseline levels of free-light chain ☐

---

5. **Which of the following complications can be observed in AL patients undergoing autotransplant?**
   a) Frequent gastrointestinal bleeding ☐
   b) DMSO-triggered cardiac arrest ☐
   c) G-CSF induced respiratory failure during mobilisation ☐
   d) All the previous have been reported in this setting ☐

NOTES

* CHAPTER 19

Indications for HSCT in adults

* 19.8
HSCT for non-Hodgkin's lymphoma

Harry C. Schouten, Anna Sureda

1. Introduction

Malignant lymphomas consist of a wide array of different diseases (see Table 1) with a huge variation in prognosis; however, they all originate from missteps in the developing immune system. Classically they can be classified as diseases with a very indolent behaviour, where wait-and-see approaches seem to result in a similar outcome as active treatment, and more aggressive types where cure can be achieved in a significant proportion of patients with standard chemotherapy (see Table 1). The diagnosis and treatment of patients with these malignancies have been hampered by several issues: the median age at diagnosis is generally over 60 years while clinical trials mainly deal with younger patients. Also, classifications of these malignancies have changed over the decades making interpretations of clinical studies sometimes difficult. The results of many phase II studies based on dose intensity (like MACOP-B, ProMace-MOPP, etc.), were ultimately disappointing when applied in a randomised clinical trial which showed that "good-old" CHOP was at least equivalent in outcome. This study also challenged the conception of the dose response curve in large cell lymphoma. But an important change has resulted from the introduction of monoclonal antibodies as part of lymphoma treatment, with impressive improvements in outcome, making the interpretation of clinical studies before 2000 difficult. Nonetheless the first support for high dose therapy in malignant lymphoma came from this time period.

2. Development of the human immune system

A short introduction to the development of the normal immune response is important to understand the enormous variation in malignant lymphomas. Early B- and T-cell development occurs in the bone marrow, where B-cell precursors start a process resulting in the production of the BCR-complex (B-cell receptor-complex), consisting of two heavy and two light chains. As a result of VDJ recombination various V, D and J genes can cluster together resulting in a large variation of different VDJ complexes, where some may be autoreactive or non-functional and subsequently deleted by apoptosis. The next maturation step occurs in the germinal centre of the lymph node, where two other processes take place. The first of these is called somatic hypermutation; various mutations can take place in the B-cells making them better or worse-fitting to the antigen-resulting in further development (in case of a good fit) or, again, apoptosis in case of a bad fit. The third and final step is class switch mutation where changes will occur in the heavy chain constant region resulting in the switch from e.g. IgM to IgG or IgA class. These three radical processes can result in various mistakes which may not be corrected by innate guardians and so may result in a rich variety of diseases, either at an immature level (before or after VDJ recombination) or at the more mature level of somatic hypermutation or class switch (Table 2).

Table 1: Subtypes of non-Hodgkin's lymphoma (WHO Classification)	
Precursor B-cell tumour	Precursor B-lymphoblastic leukaemia/lymphoma*
Mature B-cell tumours	B-cell chronic lymphocytic leukaemia/small lymphocytic lymphoma+
	B-cell prolymphocytic leukaemia+
	Lymphoplasmacytic lymphoma+
	Splenic marginal zone B-cell lymphoma+
	Hairy cell leukaemia+
	Plasma cell myeloma/plasmocytoma+
	Extranodal marginal zone B-cell lymphoma of the MALT type+
	Nodal marginal zone B-cell lymphoma (= monocytoid B cells)+
	Follicular lymphoma+
	Mantle cell lymphoma++
	Diffuse large B-cell lymphomas (including mediastinal large B-cell lymphoma and primary effusion lymphoma)*
	Burkitt's lymphoma*
Precursor T-cell tumour	Precursor T-lymphoblastic leukaemia/lymphoma*
Mature T-cell tumours	T-cell prolymphocytic leukaemia+
	T-cell granular lymphocytic leukaemia*
	Aggressive NK cell leukaemia*
	Adult T-cell lymphoma/leukaemia (HTLV-1 positive)*
	Extranodal NK/T-cell lymphoma, nasal type*
	Enteropathy-type T-cell lymphoma*
	Hepatosplenic gamma-delta T-cell lymphoma*
	Subcutaneous panniculitis-like T-cell lymphoma*
	Mycosis Fungoides/Sezary syndrome+
	Anaplastic large cell lymphoma, T/null cell, primary cutaneous*
	Anaplastic large cell lymphoma, T/null cell, primary systemic*
	Peripheral T-cell lymphoma, not otherwise characterised*
	Angioimmunoblastic T-cell lymphoma*

aggressive; + indolent; ++ indolent but more rapidly progressive

Table 2: B-cell malignancies in relation to B-cell maturation		
Process	**Pre/post**	**Example of B-cell malignancy**
VDJ recombination	Pre	Acute leukaemias
	Post	Unmutated CLL
Somatic hypermutation	Pre	Mantle cell lymphoma
	Post	Follicular lymphoma GC DLBCL
Class switch		Mutated CLL ABC DLBCL

GC: germinal centre; DLBCL: diffuse large B-cell lymphoma; ABC: activated B-cell

Although the maturation process in T-cells level is less well-defined, VDJ-hypermutation- and class switch problems do not occur in T-cells and this may explain the lower likelihood of mistakes and, therefore, the lower frequency of T-cell malignancies.

3. Follicular lymphoma

About one third of all lymphomas have a follicular histology. These malignant lymphomas are characterised by an indolent clinical behaviour and a relatively long median survival of more than 8 years. In addition, it is clear that standard chemotherapy does not prolong survival, when compared with a wait and see policy. Prognostic factors like those included in the International Follicular Lymphoma Prognostic Index (FLIPI) are able to define better or less favourable subgroups but up to now it is not completely clear whether this is helpful in designing treatment policies which will lead to improved overall survival (OS) in follicular lymphoma.

Although median survival is long, cure is generally not achievable, so there is a need to design treatment policies with curative potential. This has lead to the exploration of high dose therapy followed by autologous transplantation (auto-HSCT) in relapsed patients.

Several phase II studies have been published, all showing a promising long survival after high dose therapy, also with the suggestion of cure, although in almost all studies follow up was still too short to be sure of this conclusion, and also these studies did not include a comparative treatment arm. In addition, with current follow-up data, harm in these patients is not unlikely due to the observed incidence of myelodysplasia and secondary leukaemias. Randomised studies are therefore urgently needed.

3.1 First line treatment

The promising results in phase II studies plus the very low toxicity when using peripheral blood as a stem cell source led several groups to introduce high dose therapy as part of first line treatment. Data from several randomised studies are available (1–4). None of these studies showed an improved survival, although some showed improved EFS (Table 3). In a very recent meta-analysis Al Khabori et al. concluded that there was no improvement of OS applying high dose therapy as part of initial treatment (5). Subgroup analyses in the studies revealed that patients with a better performance status and a limited number of nodal areas involved did better and that achieving a molecular remission after transplant, as expected, has a favourable prognostic impact. However, with current follow-up there is already some evidence of an increased incidence of secondary malignancies, which is not reflected in EFS or PFS but will most likely negatively influence OS.

Most of these studies were performed in the pre-rituximab era making it difficult to extrapolate to the current situation, where monoclonal antibodies are generally part of the first line or later therapy. However, the Italian study (4) was done in the rituximab era, with comparable outcome and not showing a survival advantage. Data on allogeneic transplantation (allo-HSCT) in first line treatment are very scarce. Based on the favourable outcome with the currently available treatment options allo-HSCT in first line is generally not recommended (Table 4).

3.2 Second line and later treatment

Based on the promising results from the phase II studies, also in relapsed follicular lymphoma, a randomised study was performed (6) comparing chemotherapy with high dose therapy, with an additional question whether *in vitro* purging of the stem cell graft could favourably influence EFS and OS. Although this study suffered from insufficient accrual, reducing the power of the conclusions, there was a significant improvement of PFS and OS comparing the combined transplant arms with chemotherapy. There was no difference between purging and not purging.

Table 3: **Randomised studies in first line follicular lymphoma**		
Author	**EFS/PFS**	**OS**
Gyan (1)	PFS	= OS
Sebban (2)	= EFS	= OS
Lenz (3)	PFS	OS?
Ladetto (4)	EFS	= OS

EFS: event-free survival; PFS: progression-free survival; OS: overall survival

Table 4: EBMT recommendations for HSCT in non-Hodgkin's lymphoma

Disease	Disease status	Sibling donor	Allogeneic		Autologous
			Well-matched Unrelated	mm unrelated >1 Ag mm related	
Follicular B-cell NHL	CR1 (intermediate/high IPI at diagnosis)	GNR/III	GNR/III	GNR/III	CO/I
	Chemosensitive relapse; ≥CR2	CO/II	CO/II	D/III	S/I
	Refractory	CO/II	CO/II	D/II	GNR/II
Diffuse large B-cell lymphoma	CR1 (intermediate/high IPI at dx)	GNR/III	GNR/III	GNR/III	CO/I
	Chemosensitive relapse; ≥CR2	CO/II	CO/II	GNR/III	S/I
	Refractory	D/II	D/II	GNR/III	GNR/II
Mantle cell lymphoma	CR1	CO/II	D/III	GNR/III	S/II
	Chemosensitive relapse; ≥CR2	CO/II	D/II	GNR/III	S/II
	Refractory	D/II	D/II	GNR/III	GNR/II
Lymphoblastic lymphoma and Burkitt's lymphoma	CR1	CO/II	CO/II	GNR/III	CO/II
	Chemosensitive relapse; ≥CR2	CO/II	CO/II	GNR/III	CO/II
	Refractory	D/III	D/III	GNR/III	GNR/III
T-cell NHL	CR1	CO/II	D/II	GNR/III	CO/II
	Chemosensitive relapse; ≥CR2	CO/II	CO/II	GNR/III	D/II
	Refractory	D/II	D/II	GNR/III	GNR/III

Adapted from (7)

However, this study was performed in the pre-rituximab era making it difficult to extrapolate to the current situation where almost every patient is pre-treated with rituximab. A European study (Lym-1) assessed the questions whether the addition of rituximab to achieve *in vivo* purging leads to improved results, however, data are not yet available. A French retrospective analysis shows that relapsed patients treated with rituximab-containing therapy did much better than in the past, but the best results were obtained by the combination of rituximab-containing therapy followed by auto-HSCT (8). Several phase II studies with a long follow-up show a plateau in progression-free survival after auto-HSCT, suggesting cure (9, 10).

Histologic transformation to an aggressive lymphoma is a well-described event in the natural history and clinical course of patients with follicular lymphoma with a prevalence of up to 60%. Generally this event is accompanied by a very poor prognosis. This has led to the application of high-dose therapy in these patients with transformed follicular lymphoma, with variable results (11–18). No data from randomised studies are available. The general conclusion may be that auto-HSCT has a favourable impact in these patients, especially when they are chemosensitive and, if possible, in complete clinical remission at time of transplant.

Allogeneic transplantation has also been applied in second or later remissions, with myeloablative conditioning and more recently also using reduced intensity conditioning. The high treatment-related mortality after myeloablative conditioning reduced its applicability in patients with follicular lymphoma because of their relatively long natural survival. However, reduced intensity conditioning reversed this negative influence, resulting in a potentially greater benefit. The basis for the use of allo-HSCT was the observation of a graft-versus-lymphoma effect in follicular lymphoma (19–25). The general consensus is that allo-HSCT in follicular lymphoma is a potentially curative treatment option. Whether allo-HSCT should be reserved for patients relapsing after auto-HSCT or should replace autologous transplantation is a matter of debate and should be seen in relation to TRM. Current recommendations are shown in Table 4. Allo-HSCT may also be used in patients with transformed lymphoma; however, the limited available data are disappointing.

A novel approach is the application of radio-labelled monoclonal antibodies as part of the pre-transplant conditioning in auto-HSCT. Its use and publication is currently limited to phase II studies, however, data are encouraging.

Data on stem cell transplantation should be viewed in perspective of what can currently be achieved using combined chemo-immunotherapy. One of the important studies which may be used as a comparator for the results of transplantation is an EORTC-HOVON study (26), which showed an improved survival when comparing CHOP plus rituximab with CHOP resulting in an OS of 85% at three years in patients with relapsed lymphoma. Another issue to be taken into consideration is the increasing suggestion that after high dose therapy the incidence of secondary myelodysplasia and leukaemia is increased, not only when applied as second or later line therapy (27) but also when used as part of first-line treatment (28).

4. Other low grade lymphomas

Several subtypes of lymphoma other than follicular lymphoma have an indolent behaviour. As a result of the great number of these lymphoma subtypes and the relatively good prognosis, the numbers of patients treated with intensive therapies are limited. Recently EBMT studies have been completed and published in Waldenström's disease with encouraging results (29, 30). HSCT should probably not be used in end stage patients.

4.1 Diffuse large B-cell lymphoma
The first data showing evidence of the value of high dose therapy in DLBCL are derived from the Parma study in relapsed patients with intermediate and high-grade lymphoma (which is more or less comparable what nowadays is called DLBCL) (31). This randomised study showed an improved survival after auto-HSCT in patients with relapsed lymphoma who were chemosensitive to reinduction chemotherapy according to the DHAP schedule. From later follow-up, we also have learned that transplantation in first line was of value, but not in later remissions and using subgroup analysis it was shown that patients with a low IPI-score did not benefit (31).
Based on these data, high dose therapy followed by auto-HSCT is now standard therapy in chemosensitive relapsed DLBCL.

4.1.1 First line therapy
As a result of the successful data from the Parma study several study groups have started randomised trials assessing the value of high-dose therapy followed by auto-HSCT as part of first line therapy. The majority of these studies did not show any impact on EFS or OS. In a subsequent meta-analysis (32) high dose therapy treated patients did not do better than standard dose treated patients (difference not significant), and patients with low- and low-intermediate risk according to IPI did significantly worse after high dose therapy compared with standard therapy.
One has to realise that these patients were almost all treated in the pre-rituximab era. As the addition of rituximab to standard CHOP has much improved outcomes one can question the role of high-dose therapy in first line DLBCL.

4.1.2 Relapsed DLBCL lymphoma
As discussed above in chemosensitive relapsed patients autologous transplantation is standard of care. Several approaches are possible to improve on the current data in relapsed DLBCL. Better patient selection may result in better outcome of the selected patients but does not influence the outcome of the total group of relapsed patients. Early data suggest that patients with a PET-negative remission before transplant have a better outcome. However, in patients not fulfilling this criterion, outcome is not so poor that they should be excluded from this treatment option. Other ways of improving outcome are alternative reinduction approaches aiming for

more responding patients who would then be eligible for high-dose therapy. Currently, there is no convincing evidence that chemotherapy schedules other than DHAP result in better outcome. However, the addition of monoclonal antibodies to salvage chemotherapy has resulted in higher response rates with better outcomes. This study included virtually no patients treated with monoclonal antibodies in first line. Nowadays almost all relapsed patients have been pre-treated with rituximab in first line making the observations from the Coral trial relevant, which shows that patients relapsing within one year after rituximab-containing chemotherapy do very poorly, even after auto-HSCT. As shown in other trials, patients with a relapse after more than 12 months have a good outcome after auto-HSCT (33).

Several groups have analysed the impact of adding radio-labelled monoclonal antibodies to the pretransplant conditioning. No comparative trials have been published yet, but further exploration is warranted and promising.

Based on the positive data in other haematological malignancies and the suggestion that there may be a graft-versus-lymphoma effect in DLBCL based on the achievement of cure in patients relapsed after auto-HSCT several groups have employed allogeneic transplantation. Initially myeloablative and more recently non-myeloablative conditioning (34–37) were used resulting in promising outcomes, also as salvage treatment having failed auto-HSCT. Current recommendations are shown in Table 4.

5. Mantle cell lymphoma

Mantle cell lymphoma (MCL) is a unique subtype of B-cell non-Hodgkin's lymphoma characterised by the chromosomal translocation t(11;14)(q13;q32) and nuclear cyclin D1 over-expression in the vast majority of cases. Most patients present with advanced stage disease, often with extra-nodal dissemination, and may pursue an aggressive clinical course. Patients with a mantle cell lymphoma have a prognosis intermediate between indolent and aggressive lymphomas. In a randomised trial, comparing auto-HSCT with interferon, Dreyling et al. reported very promising results; an improved PFS was observed (38). A very large trial (however only phase II) from Scandinavia described 160 consecutive, untreated patients younger than 66 years, treated with dose-intensified induction immunochemotherapy including high-dose cytarabine. Responders received high-dose chemotherapy with BEAM or BEAC (carmustine, etoposide, cytarabine, and melphalan/cyclophosphamide) with rituximab-*in vivo* purged autologous stem cell support. Overall and complete response was achieved in 96 and 54%, respectively. The 6-year overall, event-free, and progression-free survival were 70, 56, and 66%, respectively, with no relapses occurring after 5 years (39). These observations led to the inclusion of cytarabine and auto-HSCT in standard first line care. This modality is also applicable in patients over 65 years with results similar to younger patients (40). The promising results using allogeneic transplantation in other subtypes of non-Hodgkin's lymphoma has also led to its application in mantle cell lymphoma (41). Although non-relapse mortality may be significant (up to 41%) OS can be up to 50–60% at 3–6 years. Also, it was observed that donor-lymphocyte infusions could induce an anti-tumour effect. Current recommendations are shown in Table 4.

6. T-cell NHL

T-cell lymphomas form a very heterogeneous group of diseases with a great variation in clinical behaviour and outcome. Its incidence is much lower than the B-cell lymphomas (approximately 10% of all lymphoma patients), which explains the absence of published randomised studies. The largest published study (42), although not randomised, showed an improved survival in those patients receiving auto-HSCT in first line, as compared with those who did not. Patients with the anaplastic large cell lymphoma variant can be divided into alk-positive and alk-negative groups, where alk-negativity is correlated with a worse outcome. In these patients autografting in first line may be considered.

Experience with allogeneic transplantation in T-cell lymphomas is also limited. Data on myeloablative and non-myeloablative transplants are available suggesting a graft versus lymphoma effect in T-cell NHL with PFS and OS of 81 and 64% at three years (43), 53 and 57% at 5 years (44), 53 and 59% (45). This has led to the start of a randomised study organised by the German High-Grade Lymphoma Group comparing autologous and allogeneic transplantation in first-line patients with T-cell NHL. We will have to wait several years for the first results.

Recently EBMT studies have been completed and published on patients with angio-immunoblastic T-cell lymphoma, with encouraging results (46, 47). If applied HSCT should probably not be used in end stage patients.

Limited data are available on allo-HSCT in *Mycosis fungoides* and Sèzary syndrome suggesting efficacy; however, no comparative data are available (48).

In a publication dealing with adult T-cell leukaemia/lymphoma (ATLL) subtypes Tanosaki et al. observed OS and PFS at 3 years of 36 and 31% (49).

Based on this fragmented data no good recommendations can be made, although the data support that transplantation may be an option for selected patients (Table 4).

7. Other aggressive lymphomas

Burkitt and lymphoblastic lymphomas are also very rare diseases, 1 and 2% of all lymphomas, respectively. There is a significant overlap with acute leukaemias for lymphoblastic lymphomas, and a significant subset of Burkitt's lymphoma presents as a mature B acute lymphoblastic leukaemia. In addition, in many cases it is difficult to discriminate between Burkitt's lymphoma and Burkitt-like lymphoma, making published data on Burkitt's lymphoma without histological review difficult to interpret.

It is generally accepted that in the first line treatment of Burkitt's lymphoma the outcome with cyclophosphamide containing therapy (like CODOX-M/IVAC or similar) leads to excellent results. Some poor-risk patients may benefit from high-dose therapy followed by auto-HSCT (50). In a registry study Sweetenham et al. (51) observed that especially patients with relapsed disease benefitted from high-dose therapy. Also for lymphoblastic lymphoma the data are too scarce to come to firm conclusions. Phase II data are available supporting high-dose therapy. A small randomised EBMT study (52) shows a trend of improved progression-free survival after autologous transplantation, but no overall survival. A registry study, performed by Peniket (53), did not provide much evidence of a graft versus lymphoma effect in Burkitt but showed a lower relapse rate in lymphoblastic lymphoma. Current recommendations are shown in Table 4.

8. Conclusions

Significant improvement has been achieved in the treatment of the various sub-types of non-Hodgkin's lymphoma. Several standard indications now can be identified, as done by the EBMT (6). However, we have to realise that with increasing knowledge of the immune system, (intra)cellular pathways and more effective monoclonal antibodies the whole picture may need reframing in the next few years.

References

1. Gyan E, Foussard C, Bertrand P et al. High-dose therapy followed by autologous purged stem cell transplantation and doxorubicin-based chemotherapy in patients with advanced follicular lymphoma: A randomized multicenter study by the GOELAMS with final results after a median follow-up of 9 years. Blood 2009; 113: 995–1001.
2. Sebban C, Mounier N, Brousse N et al. Standard chemotherapy with interferon compared with CHOP followed by high-dose therapy with autologous stem cell transplantation in untreated patients with advanced follicular lymphoma: The GELF-94 randomized study from the Groupe d'Etude des Lymphomes de l'Adulte (GELA). Blood 2006; 108: 2540–2544.
3. Lenz G, Dreyling M, Schiegnitz E et al. Myeloablative radiochemotherapy followed by autologous stem cell transplantation in first remission prolongs progression-free survival in follicular lymphoma: Results of a prospective, randomized trial of the German Low-Grade Lymphoma Study Group. Blood 2004; 104: 2667–2674.
4. Ladetto M, De Marco F, Benedetti F et al. Prospective, multicenter randomized GITMO/IIL trial comparing intensive (R-HDS) versus conventional (CHOP-R) chemoimmunotherapy

in high-risk follicular lymphoma at diagnosis: The superior disease control of R-HDS does not translate into an overall survival advantage. Blood 2008; 111: 4004–4013.

5. Al Khabori M, de Almeida JR, Guyatt GH et al. Autologous stem cell transplantation in follicular lymphoma: A systematic review and meta-analysis. J Natl Cancer Inst 2012; 104: 18–28. Epub 2011 Dec 21.

6. Schouten HC, Qian W, Kvaloy S et al. High-dose therapy improves progression-free survival and survival in relapsed follicular non-Hodgkin's lymphoma: Results from the randomized european CUP trial. J Clin Oncol 2003; 21: 3918–3927.

7. Ljungman P, Bregni M, Brune M et al. Allogeneic and autologous transplantation for haematological diseases, solid tumours and immune disorders: Current practice in Europe 2009. Bone Marrow Transplant 2010; 45: 219–234.

8. Sebban C, Brice P, Delarue R et al. Impact of rituximab and/or high-dose therapy with autotransplant at time of relapse in patients with follicular lymphoma: A GELA study. J Clin Oncol 2008; 26: 3614–3620.

9. Gerlinger M, Rohatiner AZS, Matthews J et al. Surveillance investigations after high-dose therapy with stem cell rescue for recurrent follicular lymphoma have no impact on management. Haematologica 2010; 95: 1130–1135.

10. Kornacker M, Stumm J, Pott C, Dietrich S et al. Characteristics of relapse after autologous stem-cell transplantation for follicular lymphoma: A long-term follow-up. Ann Oncol 2009; 20: 722–728.

11. Bastion Y, Brice P, Haioun C et al. Intensive therapy with peripheral blood progenitor cell transplantation in 60 patients with poor-prognosis follicular lymphoma. Blood 1995; 86: 3257–3262.

12. Bastion Y, Sebban C, Berger F et al. Incidence, predictive factors, and outcome of lymphoma transformation in follicular lymphoma patients. J Clin Oncol 1997; 15: 1587–1594.

13. Berglund A, Enblad G, Carlson K et al. Long-term follow-up of autologous stem-cell transplantation for follicular and transformed follicular lymphoma. Eur J Haematol 2000; 65: 17–22.

14. Chen CI, Crump M, Tsang R et al. Autotransplants for histologically transformed follicular non-Hodgkin's lymphoma. Br J Haematol 2001; 113: 202–208.

15. Foran JM, Apostolidis J, Papamichael D et al. High-dose therapy with autologous haematopoietic support in patients with transformed follicular lymphoma: A study of 27 patients from a single centre. Ann Oncol 1998; 9: 865–869.

16. Friedberg JW, Neuberg D, Gribben JG et al. Autologous bone marrow transplantation after histologic transformation of indolent B cell malignancies. Biol Blood Marrow Transplant 1999; 5: 262–268.

17. Williams CD, Harrison CN, Lister TA, et al. High-dose therapy and autologous stem-cell support for chemosensitive transformed low-grade follicular non-Hodgkin's lymphoma: A case-matched study from the European Bone Marrow Transplant Registry. J Clin Oncol 2001; 19: 727–735.

18. Brice P, Simon D, Bouabdallah R, et al. High-dose therapy with autologous stem-cell transplantation (ASCT) after first progression prolonged survival of follicular lymphoma patients included in the prospective GELF 86 protocol. Ann Oncol 2000; 11: 1585–1590.

19. Bloor AJ, Thomson K, Chowdhry N et al. High response rate to donor lymphocyte infusion after allogeneic stem cell transplantation for indolent non-Hodgkin lymphoma. Biol Blood Marrow Transplant 2008; 14: 50–58.

20. Vigouroux S, Michallet M, Porcher R et al. Long-term outcomes after reduced-intensity conditioning allogeneic stem cell transplantation for low-grade lymphoma: A survey by the French Society of Bone Marrow Graft Transplantation and Cellular Therapy (SFGM-TC). Haematologica 2007; 92: 627–634.

21. Thomson KJ, Morris EC, Milligan D et al. T-cell-depleted reduced-intensity transplantation followed by donor leukocyte infusions to promote graft-versus-lymphoma activity results in excellent long-term survival in patients with multiply relapsed follicular lymphoma. J Clin Oncol 2010; 28: 3695–3700.

22. Rezvani AR, Storer B, Maris M et al. Nonmyeloablative allogeneic hematopoietic cell transplantation in relapsed, refractory, and transformed indolent non-Hodgkin's lymphoma. J Clin Oncol. 2008; 26: 211–217.

23. Armand P, Kim HT, Ho VT et al. Allogeneic transplantation with reduced-intensity conditioning for Hodgkin and non-Hodgkin lymphoma: Importance of histology for outcome. Biol Blood Marrow Transplant 2008; 14: 418–425.

24. Hari P, Carreras J, Zhang MJ et al. Allogeneic transplants in follicular lymphoma: Higher risk of disease progression after reduced-intensity compared to myeloablative conditioning. Biol Blood Marrow Transplant 2008; 14: 236–245.

25. Khouri IF, McLaughlin P, Saliba RM et al. Eight-year experience with allogeneic stem cell transplantation for relapsed follicular lymphoma after nonmyeloablative conditioning with fludarabine, cyclophosphamide, and rituximab. Blood 2008; 111: 5530–5536.

26. van Oers MHJ, Klasa R, Marcus RE et al. Rituximab maintenance improves clinical outcome of relapsed/resistant follicular non-Hodgkin lymphoma in patients both with and without rituximab during induction: Results of a prospective randomized phase 3 intergroup trial. Blood 2006; 108: 3295–3301.

27. Rohatiner AZS, Nadler L, Davies AJ et al. Myeloablative therapy with autologous bone marrow transplantation for follicular lymphoma at the time of second or subsequent remission: Long-term follow-up. J Clin Oncol 2007; 25: 2554–2559.

28. Lenz G, Dreyling M, Schiegnitz E et al. Moderate increase of secondary hematologic malignancies after myeloablative radiochemotherapy and autologous stem-cell transplantation in patients with indolent lymphoma: Results of a prospective randomized trial of the German Low Grade Lymphoma Study Group. J Clin Oncol 2004; 22: 4926–4933.

29. Kyriakou C, Canals C, Cornelissen JJ et al. Allogeneic stem-cell transplantation in patients with Waldenstrom macroglobulinemia: Report from the Lymphoma Working Party of the European Group for Blood and Marrow Transplantation. J Clin Oncol 2010; 28: 4926–4934.

30. Kyriakou C, Canals C, Sibon D et al. High-dose therapy and autologous stem-cell transplantation in Waldenstrom macroglobulinemia: The Lymphoma Working Party of the European Group for Blood and Marrow Transplantation. J Clin Oncol 2010; 28: 2227–2232.

31. Blay J, Gomez F, Sebban C et al. The International Prognostic Index correlates to survival in patients with aggressive lymphoma in relapse: Analysis of the PARMA trial. Parma Group. Blood 1998; 92: 3562–3568.

32. Greb A, Bohlius J, Trelle S et al. High-dose chemotherapy with autologous stem cell support in first-line treatment of aggressive non-Hodgkin lymphoma - results of a comprehensive meta-analysis. Cancer Treat Rev 2007; 33: 338–346.

33. Gisselbrecht C, Glass B, Mounier N et al. Salvage regimens with autologous transplantation for relapsed large B-cell lymphoma in the rituximab era. J Clin Oncol 2010; 28: 4184–4190.

34. van Kampen RJ, Canals C, Schouten HC et al. Allogeneic stem-cell transplantation as salvage therapy for patients with diffuse large B-cell non-Hodgkin's lymphoma relapsing after an autologous stem-cell transplantation: An analysis of the European Group for Blood and Marrow Transplantation Registry. J Clin Oncol 2011; 29: 1342–1348.

35. Freytes CO, Zhang M-J, Carreras J et al. Outcome of lower-intensity allogeneic transplantation in non-Hodgkin lymphoma after autologous transplant failure. 2011, Submitted.

36. Thomson KJ, Morris EC, Bloor A et al. Favorable long-term survival after reduced-intensity allogeneic transplantation for multiple-relapse aggressive non-Hodgkin's lymphoma. J Clin Oncol 2009; 27: 426–432.

37. Rezvani AR, Norasetthada L, Gooley T et al. Non-myeloablative allogeneic haematopoietic cell transplantation for relapsed diffuse large B-cell lymphoma: A multicentre experience. Br J Haematol 2008; 143: 395–403.

38. Dreyling M, Hiddemann W. Current treatment standards and emerging strategies in mantle cell lymphoma. Hematology Am Soc Hematol Educ Program 2009: 542–551.

39. Geisler CH, Kolstad A, Laurell A et al. Long-term progression-free survival of mantle cell lymphoma after intensive front-line immunochemotherapy with in vivo-purged stem cell rescue: A nonrandomized phase 2 multicenter study by the Nordic Lymphoma Group. Blood 2008; 112: 2687–2693.

40. Jantunen E, Canals C, Attal M et al. Autologous stem-cell transplantation in patients with mantle cell lymphoma beyond 65 years of age: A study from the European Group for Blood and Marrow Transplantation (EBMT). Ann Oncol 2011. Epub doi: 10.1093/annonc/mdr035.

41. Cook G, Smith GM, Kirkland K et al. Outcome following reduced-intensity allogeneic stem cell transplantation (RIC AlloSCT) for relapsed and refractory mantle cell lymphoma (MCL): A study of the British Society for Blood and Marrow Transplantation. Biol Blood Marrow Transplant 2010; 16: 1419–1427.

42. Reimer P, Rudiger T, Geissinger E et al. Autologous stem-cell transplantation as first-line therapy in peripheral t-cell lymphomas: Results of a prospective multicenter study. J Clin Oncol 2009; 27: 106–113.

43. Corradini P, Dodero A, Zallio F et al. Graft-versus-lymphoma effect in relapsed peripheral T-cell non-Hodgkin's lymphomas after reduced-intensity conditioning followed by allogeneic transplantation of hematopoietic cells. J Clin Oncol 2004; 22: 2172–2176.

44. Le Gouill S, Milpied N, Buzyn A et al. Graft-versus-lymphoma effect for aggressive T-cell lymphomas in adults: A study by the Societe Francaise de Greffe de Moelle et de Therapie Cellulaire. J Clin Oncol 2008; 26: 2264–2271.

45. Shustov AR, Gooley TA, Sandmaier BM et al. Allogeneic haematopoietic cell transplantation

after nonmyeloablative conditioning in patients with T-cell and natural killer-cell lymphomas. Br J Haematol 2010; 150: 170–178.

46. Kyriakou C, Canals C, Finke J et al. Allogeneic stem cell transplantation is able to induce long-term remissions in angioimmunoblastic T-cell lymphoma: A retrospective study from the lymphoma working party of the European group for blood and marrow transplantation. J Clin Oncol 2009; 27: 3951–3958.
47. Kyriakou C, Canals C, Goldstone A et al. High-dose therapy and autologous stem-cell transplantation in angioimmunoblastic lymphoma: Complete remission at transplantation is the major determinant of Outcome-Lymphoma Working Party of the European Group for Blood and Marrow Transplantation. J Clin Oncol 2008; 26: 218–224.
48. Duarte RF, Canals C, Onida F et al. Allogeneic hematopoietic cell transplantation for patients with mycosis fungoides and Sezary syndrome: A retrospective analysis of the Lymphoma Working Party of the European Group for Blood and Marrow Transplantation. J Clin Oncol 2010; 28: 4492–4499.
49. Tanosaki R, Uike N, Utsunomiya A et al. Allogeneic hematopoietic stem cell transplantation using reduced-intensity conditioning for adult T cell leukemia/lymphoma: Impact of antithymocyte globulin on clinical outcome. Biol Blood Marrow Transplant 2008; 14: 702–708.
50. van Imhoff GW, van der Holt B, MacKenzie MA et al. Short intensive sequential therapy followed by autologous stem cell transplantation in adult Burkitt, Burkitt-like and lymphoblastic lymphoma. Leukemia 2005; 19: 945–952.
51. Sweetenham JW, Pearce R, Taghipour G et al. Adult Burkitt's and Burkitt-like non-Hodgkin's lymphoma-outcome for patients treated with high-dose therapy and autologous stem-cell transplantation in first remission or at relapse: Results from the European Group for Blood and Marrow Transplantation. J Clin Oncol 1996; 14: 2465–2472.
52. Sweetenham JW, Santini G, Qian W et al. High-dose therapy and autologous stem-cell transplantation versus conventional-dose consolidation/maintenance therapy as postremission therapy for adult patients with lymphoblastic lymphoma: Results of a randomized trial of the European Group for Blood and Marrow Transplantation and the United Kingdom Lymphoma Group. J Clin Oncol 2001; 19: 2927–2936.
53. Peniket AJ, Ruiz de Elvira MC, Taghipour G et al. An EBMT registry matched study of allogeneic stem cell transplants for lymphoma: Allogeneic transplantation is associated with a lower relapse rate but a higher procedure-related mortality rate than autologous transplantation. Bone Marrow Transplant 2003; 31: 667–678.

Multiple Choice Questionnaire

To find the correct answer, go to http://www.esh.org/online-training/handbook/

1. Standard treatment of T-cell NHL consists of:
   a) CHOP-containing chemotherapy .... ☐

b) CVP ☐
c) R-CHOP ☐
d) R-CVP ☐

2. **Standard treatment in chemosensitive patients with relapsed large cell NHL should include:**
   a) Allogeneic transplantation ☐
   b) Autologous transplantation ☐
   c) Alemtuzumab only ☐
   d) Rituximab only ☐

3. **Mantle cell NHL can be cured in more than 70% of patients using:**
   a) ARA-C containing chemotherapy ☐
   b) High-dose therapy followed by autologous transplantation ☐
   c) High-dose therapy followed by allogeneic transplantation ☐
   d) None of these ☐

4. **Which statement on patients with relapsed diffuse large B-cell lymphoma is most appropriate?**
   a) Second-line chemotherapy will not result in cure ☐
   b) Outcome is independent of first-line therapy containing rituximab or not ☐
   c) Rituximab is effective in purging the stem cell graft ☐
   d) PET positivity at transplant is a not a good predictor of outcome ☐

5. **Which statement on patients with Burkitt's lymphoma is most appropriate?**
   a) These lymphomas have a T-cell phenotype ☐
   b) Autologous stem cell transplantation should be part of first-line therapy ☐
   c) Allogeneic stem cell transplantation should be part of first-line therapy ☐
   d) Intensive cyclophosphamide-containing chemotherapy is the treatment of choice ☐

* CHAPTER 19

Indications for HSCT in adults

* 19.9
HSCT for Hodgkin's lymphoma in adults

Anna Sureda, Harry C. Schouten

1. Introduction

Newly diagnosed patients with advanced stage Hodgkin's lymphoma (HL) have an excellent prognosis as the vast majority of them can be cured with initial treatment (1). In contrast, the prognosis of patients relapsing after first-line therapy with either combination chemotherapy (CT) or CT followed by radiotherapy (RT) remains poor in many cases. In most of these cases, high-dose chemotherapy and autologous stem cell transplantation (auto-HSCT) is nowadays considered to be the treatment of choice. Current recommendations for HSCT in Hodgkin's disease are summarised in Table 1.

Table 1: **Current indications for HSCT in HL. Recommendations from the EBMT**				
	auto-HSCT	**HLA matched Sib**	**Well-matched URD/1 Ag mm Sib**	**mm URD/>1 Ag mm Sib**
CR1	GNR/I	GNR/III	GNR/III	GNR/III
Sens R/≥ CR2	S/I	CO/II	CO/II	CO/II
Refract Dis	CO/II	D/II	D/II	GNR/II

From Bone Marrow Transplantation, 2010. S: Standard; D: Developmental; CO: Clinical option; GNR: Generally not recommended; mm: Mismatched. Levels of Evidence: I, II, III

2. Autologous stem cell transplantation in refractory/relapsed Hodgkin's lymphoma

2.1 Autologous stem cell transplantation for relapsed Hodgkin's lymphoma

The use of auto-HSCT is now considered the standard of care for relapsed HL patients (2). In several phase II studies, auto-HSCT has been shown to produce between 30 to 65% long-term disease-free survival (DFS) in selected patients with refractory and relapsed HL (3–9). Two randomised trials showed significant benefit in freedom from treatment failure (FFTF) for auto-HSCT over conventional CT for relapsed disease (10, 11). The results of these trials have resulted in the recommendation of auto-HSCT at time of first relapse for even the most favorable patients, although salvage RT can offer an effective treatment for selected subsets of patients with relapsed or refractory HL.

2.1.1 Randomised trials

The first randomised trial of transplant for relapsed disease was from the British National Lymphoma Investigation comparing auto-HSCT with BEAM to mini-BEAM without autologous transplantation (10) in patients with active HL, for whom conventional therapy had failed. Twenty patients were assigned treatment with BEAM plus auto-HSCT and 20 mini-BEAM. All had been followed up for at least 12 months. Five BEAM recipients died (2 from causes related to auto-HSCT and 3 from disease progression) compared with 9 mini-BEAM recipients (all disease progression). Both 3-year EFS and PFS showed significant differences in favor of BEAM plus auto-HSCT (p=0.025 and p=0.005, respectively). There were no differences in OS. This trial was prematurely closed as recruitment became increasingly difficult because patients refused randomisation and requested an auto-HSCT.

In the second randomised trial, which was performed by investigators of the German Hodgkin's disease Study Group (GHSG), 161 patients between 16 and 60 years of age with relapsed HL were randomly assigned two cycles of Dexa-BEAM and either two further courses of Dexa-BEAM or high-dose BEAM (11). Only patients with chemosensitive disease after two courses of Dexa-BEAM proceeded to further treatment. Of the 117 patients with chemosensitive relapse there was a significant improvement in 3-year FFTF for patients undergoing auto-HSCT compared to 4 cycles of Dexa-BEAM (55% vs 34%, p=0.019). With a median follow-up of 39 months (range 3–78), the 3-year FFTF was significantly better for patients treated with BEAM, regardless of whether first relapse had occurred early (<12 months) (41% vs 12% p=0.007) or late (>12 months) (75% vs 44%, p=0.02). There was no statistically significant difference in OS for any subgroup of patients. The absence of differences in OS might be partly due to the fact that about one-third of the patients receiving conventional salvage CT received an auto-HSCT after further relapse.

In order to improve the results of auto-HSCT in this setting, the GHSG has employed a sequential high dose CT prior to the intensive procedure (12). Treatment started with two cycles of DHAP to reduce tumour burden. Patients achieving a CR or PR subsequently received a high-dose CT program with cyclophosphamide (4 g/m^2 iv), methotrexate (MTX) (8 g/m^2 iv), vincristine (1.4 mg/m^2 iv) and etoposide (2 g/m^2 iv). Patients were then autografted using BEAM. Response rate after the final evaluation was 80%. With a median follow up of 40 months (range 3–84), FFTF and OS for patients with early relapse were 62 and 78%, respectively and for patients with late relapse, 63% and 79%, respectively. The promising results coming from this phase II trial, prompted the GHSG to develop a prospective phase III clinical trial looking at relapsed patients with HL being treated either with the conventional salvage approach (DHAP x two cycles plus auto-HSCT with BEAM) vs DHAP plus high-dose sequential protocol plus auto-HSCT. Somewhat unexpectedly, there were no significant differences in terms of PFS, FFTF and OS between both arms (13). Length of treatment was significantly longer, protocol violations higher and mean administered total dose of chemotherapy lower in the experimental group.

2.2 Autologous stem cell transplantation in primary refractory disease

The prognosis of patients with primary refractory disease (PRD) is extremely poor. Nevertheless, and as opposed to non-Hodgkin lymphoma (NHL), where chemo-refractory patients are not salvaged by transplant, there seems to be a general consensus that even patients who fail first- and second-line CT may still enjoy a 20–30% chance of cure with auto-HSCT.

In the EBMT analysis published by Sweetenham et al. (14), 175 HL patients with PRD were presented; actuarial 5-year PFS and OS were 32% and 36%, respectively. In the ABMTR analysis on 122 patients undergoing auto-HSCT after an induction failure (IF) (15), actuarial probabilities at 3 years were 38% and 50% for PFS and OS, respectively. Lazarus et al. (15) found that the presence of B symptoms at diagnosis as well as Karnofsky status at auto-HSCT correlated with survival and that the absence of these 2 factors was associated with an excellent 2-year survival of 87%. In the EBMT analysis (15), patients receiving more than one line of CT before transplantation did worse, both in terms of OS and PFS.

The GELTAMO Cooperative Group presented the results of 62 patients treated with an auto-HSCT for an IF (16). One-year transplant related mortality (TRM) was 14%. Response rate at 3 months after auto-HSCT was 52% [CR in 21 patients (34%), PR in 11 patients (18%)]. Actuarial 5-year TTF and OS were 15 and 26%, respectively. The presence of B symptoms at auto-HSCT was the only adverse prognostic factor significantly influencing TTF. The presence of B symptoms at diagnosis, MOPP-like regimens as first line therapy, bulky disease at auto-HSCT and ≥2 lines of therapy before auto-HSCT adversely influenced OS.

Fermé et al. reported on 157 patients with either IF, PR of less than 75%, or relapse after doxorubicin-based chemotherapy ± RT (17). All patients received MINE as second-line therapy followed by auto-HSCT with BEAM as the preparative regimen. The 5-year OS rates were 30% for patients with IF versus 72% for patients with <75% PR and 76% for patients with relapsed disease following first-line therapy. Of the 101 patients who went on to transplant, the 5-year FFTF rate for patients with a response to MINE was 64% versus 25% for those not responding to MINE. Of the 64 patients with IF, 40 responded to second- or third-line salvage therapy and 32 of these patients went on to transplant. Of the 24 patients not responding to salvage, 9 went on to transplant, only 1 of whom achieved a CR with auto-HSCT.

Finally, the Memorial Sloan Kettering Cancer Center group summarised the long-term outcome of 75 consecutive patients with biopsy-confirmed HL at the completion of primary therapy (18). All patients underwent standard-dose salvage therapy followed by involved field RT (IFRT). Patients without progression went on to receive high-dose etoposide, cyclophosphamide and either total lymphoid irradiation (if no prior RT) or carmustine (if prior RT) followed by bone marrow or peripheral stem cell rescue. Seven patients were excluded from transplant because of progression on standard salvage therapy and had a 4 months median survival. Patients with less than a 25% decrease with standard salvage therapy (n=27) had a 10-year EFS of 17 versus 60% for those with at least a 25% decrease to standard second-line therapy (n=48).

2.3 How to improve results after an auto-HSCT? The role of PET

The impact of auto-HSCT in the long-term outcome of patients with relapsed/refractory HL is not the same in all subgroups of patients. Several authors have retrospectively analysed prognostic factors at first relapse with independent impact on the results of auto-HSCT. In this sense, time to relapse (<12 months vs ≥12 months), extranodal disease at relapse, advanced stage and anaemia at relapse, B symptoms and refractory disease were found by different authors of clinical importance. More recently, the role of PET has also been analysed in the autologous transplant setting: in a group of 101 patients with both NHL and HL, both FDG-PET positivity after 2 cycles of chemotherapy and clinical risk score were independent prognostic factors for failure-free survival after auto-HSCT (19). The group from the MD Anderson indicated that pre-transplant positive PET/Gallium scans were able to predict poor outcome after auto-HSCT in patients with relapsed/refractory HL (20).

In order to improve results after auto-HSCT, both new monoclonal antibodies (SGN-35) and histone deacetylase inhibitors (OLDH568, panobinostat) are being tested in prospective clinical trials as maintenance therapy in order to prevent relapse in those patients with high-risk relapsed HL being treated with an auto-HSCT.

3. Allogeneic stem cell transplantation in refractory/relapsed Hodgkin's lymphoma

3.1 Myeloablative conditioning and allo-HSCT in Hodgkin's lymphoma

The first reports on allogeneic stem cell transplantation (allo-SCT) in patients with HL with two larger registry-based studies published in 1996 gave disappointing results. Gajewski et al. analysed 100 HL patients allografted from HLA-identical siblings and reported to the International Bone Marrow Transplant Registry (IBMTR) (21). The 3-year-rates for OS, DFS, and the probability of relapse were 21, 15 and 65%, respectively. The major problems after transplantation were persistent or recurrent disease or respiratory complications, which accounted for 35% to 51% of deaths. A case-matched analysis including 45 allografts and 45 autografts reported to the EBMT was performed by Milpied et al. (22). They did not find significant differences in actuarial probabilities of OS, PFS, and relapse rates between allo-SCT and auto-HSCT (25%, 15%, 61% vs 37%, 24%, 61%, respectively). The actuarial TRM at 4 years was significantly higher for allografts than for autografts (48% vs 27%, p=0.04). Although the poor results after myeloablative conditioning could at least partly be explained by the very poor-risk features of many individuals included in these early studies, the high procedure-related morbidity and mortality prevented the widespread use of allo-HSCT.

3.2 Reduced-intensity conditioning and allo-HSCT in Hodgkin's lymphoma
Since the first clinical experiences that suggested that allo-HSCT after a nonmyeloablative conditioning (RIC allo-HSCT) might represent an interesting alternative to classical allo-HSCT, a number of reports have addressed the question whether RIC allo-HSCT might also work for patients with HL. Although the overall number of patients with HL treated with allo-HSCT has remained low in comparison to other haematological malignancies, the percentage of patients with refractory and relapsed HL who received a RIC allo-HSCT has been growing steadily in Europe over the last years (Figure 1).

3.3 Comparison of myeloablative and reduced-intensity conditioning prior to allo-HSCT in relapsed and refractory Hodgkin's lymphoma
The Lymphoma Working Party (LWP) has performed the only analysis reported so far which compares outcomes after reduced-intensity or myeloablative conditioning in patients with HL (23). Ninety-seven patients with HL were allografted after RIC

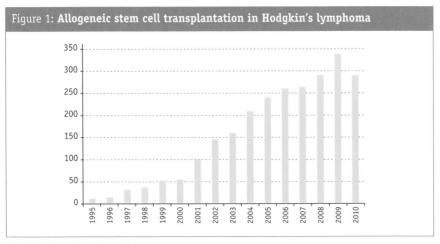

Figure 1: **Allogeneic stem cell transplantation in Hodgkin's lymphoma**

EBMT Database (1995–2010)

and 93 patients were allografted after a conventional regimen. A previous auto-HSCT was more frequent in the RIC allo-HSCT group (59% vs 41%, p=0.03) as was the use of peripheral blood stem cells (82% vs 56% p <0.001). Non-relapse mortality was significantly decreased in the RIC allo-HSCT group [HR 2.43 (95%CI 1.48–3.98), p <0.001]. PFS and OS were also better in the reduced intensity group [HR 1.28 (95% CI 0.92–1.78), p=0.1 and HR 1.62 (95% CI 1.15–2.28), p=0.005]. The development of chronic GvHD (cGvHD) significantly decreased the incidence of relapse after transplantation, suggesting a graft vs Hodgkin effect, which translated into a better PFS and OS. This analysis indicates that RIC allo-HSCT is able to significantly reduced TRM after transplantation and improves the long-term outcome of relapsed and refractory patients treated with an allograft. This reduction in TRM has been one of the leading factors contributing to the significant increment in the numbers of RIC allo-HSCT performed in this setting in Europe (Figure 2).

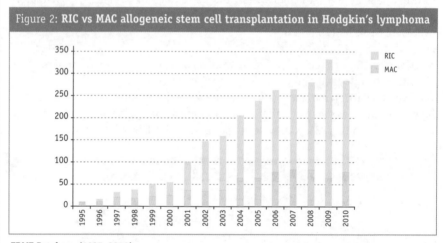

Figure 2: **RIC vs MAC allogeneic stem cell transplantation in Hodgkin's lymphoma**

EBMT Database (1995–2010)

3.4 Current studies of reduced-intensity allo-HSCT in relapsed/refractory HL
The largest cohort of patients treated with RIC allo-HSCT in HL was recently reported by the LWP of the EBMT (24) (n=285). Median time from diagnosis to allo-SCT was 41 (4–332) months. Patients had received an average of four lines of prior therapy (1–8) and 288 patients (77%) had failed one or two ASCT. At the time of allo-SCT, 47 patients (17%) were in CR, 123 patients (43%) had chemosensitive disease and 115 patients (40%) had chemoresistant disease or untested relapse. One hundred and seventy two patients (63%) were allografted from a matched sibling donor (MRD),

94 (33%) from a matched unrelated donor (MUD), and 19 from a mismatched donor (7%). Grade II-IV acute GvHD (aGvHD) was reported in 27% of patients and cGvHD in 40% of patients at risk. The 100-day TRM was 12% but increased to 20% at 12 months, and to 22% at three years; it was significantly worse for patients with chemoresistant disease. Two-year PFS was 29% and again significantly worse for patients with chemoresistant disease (p <0.001). The development of cGvHD was associated with a higher TRM and a trend to a lower relapse rate. In a landmark analysis the development of either acute or chronic GvHD by 9 months post-transplant was associated with a significantly lower relapse rate, supporting the existence of a graft vs Hodgkin effect.

The MD Anderson Cancer Center updated their experience (25) in 58 patients. Forty-eight (83%) patients had received a prior auto-HSCT. Disease status at RIC allo-HSCT was sensitive relapse (n=30) or refractory relapse (n=28). The conditioning regimen employed was fludarabine (125–130 mg/m² over 4–5 days), melphalan (140 mg/m² iv over 2 days) (FM) and antithymocyte globulin (thymoglobulin 6 mg/kg over 3 days) was added for the 14 most recent MUD transplants. Cumulative 100-day and 2-year TRM were 7% and 15%, respectively. Fourteen patients (24%) received a total of 25 (range 1-5) donor leukocyte infusions (DLI) for disease progression/relapse. Five of them (35%) received CT as well, and nine (64%) developed aGvHD after the DLI. Projected 2-year OS and PFS were 64% and 32%, with 2-year projected disease progression at 55%. There was no statistically significant difference between MRD and MUD transplants with regard to OS, PFS and disease progression. There was a trend for the response status prior to allo-HSCT to favourably impact PFS (p=0.07) and disease progression (p=0.049), but not OS (p=0.4).

Forty patients with relapsed or refractory HL treated with the combination of fludarabine (150 mg/m²) and melphalan (140 mg/m²) were analysed by the Spanish group (26). GvHD prophylaxis consisted of cyclosporin A (CsA) and MTX. Twenty patients were allografted in resistant relapse and 38 patients received haematopoietic cells from a MRD. One-year TRM was 25%. aGvHD developed in 18 patients (45%) and cGvHD in 17 (45%) of the 31 evaluable patients. Extensive cGvHD was associated with a trend to a lower relapse rate (71% vs 44% at 24 months, p=0.07). The response rate three months after RIC allo-HSCT was 67%. Eleven patients received DLI for relapse or persistent disease. Six patients (54%) responded. OS and PFS were 48% and 32% at 2 years, respectively. Refractoriness to CT was the only adverse prognostic factor for both OS and PFS.

Investigators from Seattle reported their results in relapsed/refractory HL patients (27). Thirty-eight patients had a MRD, 24 a MUD and 28 a HLA-haploidentical related donor. The patients received 2 Gy total body irradiation (TBI) alone (n=17) or in combination with fludarabine (90 mg/m²) and immunosuppression consisted of mycophenolate mofetil (MMF) and CsA. All patients were heavily pre-treated with a median of five prior regimens administered. 92% of the patients had failed a previous auto-HSCT. Prior to RIC allo-HSCT 22 patients were in CR, 30 in PR, 9 had relapsed disease, and 29 had refractory disease. TRM was significantly lower in those patients being allografted from a HLA-haploidentical donor. Relapse risk was also lower in haploidentical recipients.

Peggs et al. explored the effects of *in vivo* T-cell depletion with alemtuzumab followed by fludarabine (150 mg/m^2) and melphalan (140 mg/m^2) in multiply-relapsed patients; 90% of them had failed a previous autograft (28). At transplant, 8 patients were in CR, 25 patients were in PR, one patient was in untested relapse, and 15 patients had refractory disease. Thirty-one patients were allografted from a MRD and 18 from MUDs. All patients engrafted, grade II-IV aGvHD occurred in 16% of patients, 14% developed cGvHD before DLIs. Nineteen patients received DLIs for progression (n=16) or mixed chimerism (n=3). Nine patients (56%) showed a response, which was significantly associated with, acute and/or extensive cGvHD. Non-relapse mortality was 16% at 730 days. Projected 4-year OS and PFS were 56% and 39%, respectively.

Finally, the results of a multicentre phase II prospective study on the role of RIC allo-HSCT were presented at ASH 2010 (29). Ninety-two HL patients with an HLA identical sibling or a MUD were treated with two courses of salvage chemotherapy. Seventy-eight patients (85%) who showed at least stable disease were eligible to receive a RIC allo-HSCT; all 14 patients with chemorefractory disease died from progressive lymphoma. Most allografted patients had failed a prior autologous transplantation (86%); 50 patients were allografted with chemosensitive and 28 with resistant disease; MUDs were used in 23 patients. Fludarabine (150 mg/m^2 iv) and melphalan (140 mg/m^2 iv) were used as conditioning regimen and CsA plus MTX as GvHD prophylaxis. Non-relapse mortality was 8% at 100-days and 15% at 1-year. Relapse was the major cause of failure. PFS was 48% at 1-year and 24% at 4-years. cGvHD was associated with a lower relapse incidence and a better PFS. Patients allografted in CR had a significantly better outcome. OS was 71% at 1-year and 43% at 4-years.

No definitive information is available with respect to the best conditioning protocol or the impact of T-cell depletion in this setting. If one accepts that attempting an effective graft-versus-HL reaction may require several months, preventing early progression by administering a vigorous conditioning regimen remains an essential goal still to accomplish. In this sense, the combination of a more intensive preparative regimen, the BEAM protocol together with a profound T-cell depletion with alemtuzumab as aGvHD prophylaxis has demonstrated to be associated with sustained donor engraftment, a high response rate, minimal toxicity (NRM 7.6%) and a low incidence of GvHD (30). The two analyses presented by the LWP of the EBMT also strengthen this argument. The use of TBI-based RIC protocols significantly increased disease progression after RIC allo-HSCT in Robinson's analysis (24) and TBI-based conditioning regimens also emerged as an adverse prognostic factor for disease progression after transplant, PFS and OS in the comparative analysis between conventional and RIC protocols (23).

3.5 Graft-versus-Hodgkin effect

Evidence of a graft-vs-HL effect comes from two main sources: the demonstration that the development of acute or chronic GvHD after allo-HSCT is associated with a lower relapse rate and the clinical information coming from studies of DLI. Relapse rate is significantly lower in those patients developing GvHD after transplantation. This fact was already indicated by single centre analysis including small numbers of patients (25, 26, 28) but also by larger retrospective analyses such as those performed by the LWP of the EBMT. The development of either acute or chronic GvHD by 9 months after transplant was associated with a lower relapse rate in Robinson's analysis (24). The development of aGvHD alone did not reduce the relapse rate but was associated with a significantly higher TRM and a lower PFS and OS. In contrast, the development of cGvHD alone was associated with a trend to lower relapse rate, but a significantly higher TRM and no impact on OS or PFS. In the comparative analysis between conventional allo-HSCT and RIC allo-HSCT the development of cGvHD after transplantation significantly reduced relapse rate after transplant and improved PFS in those patients presenting with this complication (23). The most direct evidence for a graft versus malignancy effect comes from observations relating to disease responses to DLI. Peggs et al. (31) have recently summarised the outcomes of 76 consecutive patients with multiply relapsed or refractory HL who underwent allogeneic transplantation that incorporated *in vivo* T-cell depletion. DLI was administered in a dose-escalating fashion to 22 patients for mixed chimerism (median time of first dose, 9 months post-transplantation) and to 24 patients for relapse. Three-year donor lymphocyte-related mortality was 7%, relating mainly to the induction of GvHD. Nineteen (86%) of 22 patients receiving donor lymphocytes for mixed chimerism converted to full donor status. Four-year relapse incidence was 5% in these 22 patients compared with 43% in patients who remained relapse free but full donor chimeras at 9 months post-transplantation (p=0.0071). Nineteen (79%) of 24 patients receiving donor lymphocytes for relapse responded (14 CR, 5 PR). Four-year OS from relapse was 59% in recipients of donor lymphocytes, contributing to a 4-year OS from transplantation of 64% and a 4-year current PFS of 59% in all 76 patients. These data are the most demonstrative up to now about the potential for allogeneic immunotherapy with donor lymphocytes both to reduce relapse risk and to induce durable antitumour responses in patients with HL after allo-HSCT that incorporates *in vivo* T-cell depletion. Unfortunately, these results have not been reproduced in the non-T-cell depleted setting.

3.6 How to improve the results of allo-HSCT?

Relapse rate is the major cause of failure for those patients with relapsed/refractory HL being considered candidates for such an approach. There are several possible ways to address this issue, including better patient selection, especially regarding chemosensitivity of the tumour. Disease status at the time of allo-HSCT is the most important prognostic factor for the long-term outcome of this procedure. Only those patients in CR or very good PR should be considered adequate candidates for an allo-HSCT, at least with current protocols. For this reason, new salvage strategies to try to put patients into a better response should be sought. Pre-transplant PET does not seem to have a prognostic impact on either OS or PFS after allo-HSCT but PET was able to diagnose relapse after allo-HSCT earlier than conventional computed tomography, allowing earlier application of DLI (32, 33). Therefore, the role of PET should be further explored in this setting.

Modulation of the intensity of the conditioning regimen can also result in a lower relapse rate after allo-HSCT. Low-dose TBI containing regimens seem to be associated with a high relapse rate in the RIC-allo setting (23, 24). New drugs with potential antitumour activity against HL but with a safe profile are being currently tested by different groups. It may be possible to augment the intensity of the conditioning regimen without significantly modifying NRM taking into consideration the population of patients that are considered candidates for an allo-HSCT and the fact that GvT effect is not as potent as in low-grade lymphoproliferative disorders.

Finally, the "so called" maintenance strategy currently being explored in the auto-HSCT setting can also be evaluated in the context of allogeneic transplants.

References

1. Diehl V, Franklin J, Pfreundschuh M et al. Standard and increased-dose BEACOPP chemotherapy compared with COPP-ABVD for advanced Hodgkin's disease. N Engl J Med 2003; 348: 2386–2395.
2. Ljungman P, Bregni M, Brune M et al. Allogeneic and autologous transplantation for haematological diseases, solid tumours and immune disorders: Current practice in Europe 2009. Bone Marrow Transplant 2010; 45: 219–234.
3. Reece DE, Barnet MJ, Connors JM et al. Intensive chemotherapy with cyclophosphamide, carmustine, and etoposide followed by autologous bone marrow transplantation for relapsed Hodgkin's disease. J Clin Oncol 1991; 9: 1871–1879.
4. Chopra R, McMillan AK, Linch DC et al. The place of high dose BEAM therapy and

autologous bone marrow transplantation in poor-risk Hodgkin's disease. A single center 8-year study of 155 patients. Blood 1993; 81: 1137–1145.

5. Nademanee A, O'Donell MR, Snyder DS et al. High-dose chemotherapy with or without total body irradiation followed by autologous bone marrow and/or peripheral blood stem cell transplantation for patients with relapsed and refractory Hodgkin's disease: Results in 85 patients with analysis of prognostic factors. Blood 1995; 85: 1381–1390.

6. Bierman PJ, Anderson JR, Freeman MB et al. High-dose chemotherapy followed by autologous hematopoietic rescue for Hodgkin's disease patients following first relapse after chemotherapy. Ann Oncol 1996; 7: 151–156.

7. Caballero MD, Rubio V, Rifón J et al. BEAM chemotherapy followed by autologous stem cell support in lymphoma patients: Analysis of efficacy, toxicity and prognostic factors. Bone Marrow Transplant 1997; 20: 451–458.

8. Sureda A, Arranz R, Iriondo A et al. Autologous stem cell transplantation for Hodgkin's disease: Results and prognostic factors in 494 patients from the GEL/TAMO Spanish Cooperative Group. J Clin Oncol 2001; 19: 1395–1404.

9. Reece DE, Connors JM, Spinelli JJ et al. Intensive therapy with cyclophosphamide, carmustine, etoposide ± cisplatin, and autologous bone marrow transplantation for Hodgkin's disease in first relapse after combination chemotherapy. Blood 1995; 83: 1193–1199.

10. Linch DC, Winfield D, Goldstone AH et al. Dose intensification with autologous bone-marrow transplantation in relapsed and resistant Hodgkin's disease: Results of a BNLI randomized trial. Lancet 1993; 341: 1051–1054.

11. Schmitz N, Pfistner B, Sextro M et al. Aggressive conventional chemotherapy compared with high-dose chemotherapy requiring autologous haemopoietic stem cell transplantation for relapsed chemosensitive Hodgkin's disease: A randomised trial. Lancet 2002; 359: 2065–2071.

12. Josting A, Sieniawski M, Glossmann JP et al. High-dose sequential chemotherapy followed by autologous stem cell transplantation in relapsed and refractory aggressive non-Hodgkin's lymphoma: Results of a multicenter phase II study. Ann Oncol 2005; 16: 1359–1365.

13. Josting A, Müller H, Borchmann P et al. Dose intensity of chemotherapy in patients with relapsed Hodgkin's lymphoma. J Clin Oncol 2010; 28: 5074–5080.

14. Sweetenham JW, Carella AM, Taghipour G et al. High dose therapy and autologous stem cell transplantation for adult patients with Hodgkin's disease who fail to enter remission after induction chemotherapy: Results in 175 patients reported to the EBMT. J Clin Oncol 1999; 17: 3101–3109.

15. Lazarus HM, Rowlings PA, Zhang M-J et al. Autotransplants for Hodgkin's disease in patients never achieving remission: A report from the Autologous Blood and Marrow Transplant Registry. J Clin Oncol 1999; 17: 534–545.

16. Constans M, Sureda A, Terol MJ et al. Autologous stem cell transplantation for primary refractory Hodgkin's disease: Results and clinical variables affecting outcome. Ann Oncol 2003; 14: 745–751.

17. Fermé C, Mounier N, Diviné M et al. Intensive salvage therapy with high-dose

chemotherapy for patients with advanced Hodgkin's disease in relapse or failure after initial chemotherapy: Results of the Groupe d'Études des Lymphomes de l'adulte H89 trial. J Clin Oncol 2002; 20: 467–475.

18. Moskowitz CH, Kewalramani T, Nimer SD et al. Effectiveness of high dose chemoradiotherapy and autologous stem cell transplantation for patients with biopsy-proven primary refractory Hodgkin's disease. Br J Haematol 2004; 124: 645–652.

19. Schot BW, Zijlstra JM, Sluiter WJ et al. Early FDG-PET assessment in combination with cloinical risk scores determines prognosis in recurrent lymphomas. Blood 2007; 109: 486–491.

20. Jabbour E, Hosing C, Ayers G et al. Pretrasplant positive positron emission tomography/gallium scans predict poor outcome in patients with recurrent/refractory Hodgkin's lymphoma. Cancer 2007; 109: 2481–2489.

21. Gajewski JL, Phillips GL, Sobocinski KA et al. Bone marrow transplants from HLA-identical siblings in advanced Hodgkin's disease. J Clin Oncol 1996; 14: 572–578.

22. Milpied N, Fielding AK, Pearce RM et al. Allogeneic bone marrow transplant is not better than autologous transplant for patients with relapsed Hodgkin's disease. J Clin Oncol 1996; 14: 1291–1296.

23. Sureda A, Robinson S, Canals C et al. Reduced-intensity conditioning compared with conventional allogeneic stem-cell transplantation in relapsed or refractory Hodgkin's lymphoma: An analysis from the Lymphoma Working Party of the European Group for Blood and Marrow Transplantation. J Clin Oncol 2008; 26: 455–462.

24. Robinson S, Sureda A, Canals C, et al. Reduced intensity allogeneic stem cell transplantation for Hodgkin's lymphoma: Identification of prognostic factors predicting outcome. Haematol 2008; 94: 230–238.

25. Anderlini P, Saliba R, Acholonu S et al. Reduced-intensity allogeneic stem cell transplantation in relapsed and refractory Hodgkin's disease: Low transplant-related mortality and impact of intensity of conditioning regimen. Bone Marrow Transplant 2005; 35: 943–951.

26. Alvarez I, Sureda A, Caballero MD et al. Non-myeloablative stem cell transplantation is an effective therapy for refractory or relapsed Hodgkin's lymphoma: Results of a Spanish prospective cooperative protocol. Biol Blood Marrow Transplant 2006; 12: 172–183.

27. Burroughs LM, O'Donnell PV, Sandmaier BM et al. Comparison of outcomes of HLA-matched related, unrelated, or HLA-haploidentical related hematopoietic cell transplantation following nonmyeloablative conditioning for relapsed or refractory Hodgkin lymphoma. Biol Blood Marrow Transplantation 2008; 14: 1279–1287.

28. Peggs KS, Hunter A, Chopra R et al. Clinical evidence of a graft-versus-Hodgkin's-lymphoma effect after reduced-intensity allogeneic transplantation. Lancet 2005; 365: 1934–1941.

29. Sureda A, Canals C, Arranz R et al. Allogeneic stem cell transplantation after reduced-intensity conditioning in patients with relapsed or refractory Hodgkin's lymphoma: Results of the HDR-Allo Study, a prospective clinical trial by the Grupo Español de Linfomas/Trasplante de Médula Ósea (GEL/TAMO) and the Lymphoma Working Party of the European Group for Blood and Marrow Transplantation. Haematol (in press).

30. Faulkner RD, Craddock C, Byrne JL et al. BEAM-alemtuzumab reduced-intensity allogeneic stem cell transplantation for lymphoproliferative diseases: GVHD, toxicity, and survival in 65 patients. Blood 2004; 103: 428–434.
31. Peggs KS, Kasvani I, Edwards N et al. Donor lymphocyte infusions modulate relapse risk in mixed chimeras and induce durable salvage in relapsed patients after T-cell-depleted allogeneic transplantation for Hodgkin's lymphoma. J Clin Oncol 2011; 29: 971–978.
32. Hart DP, Avivi I, Thomson KJ et al. Use of 18F-FDG positron emission tomography following allogeneic transplantation to guide adoptive immunotherapy with donor lymphocyte infusions. Br J Haematol 2005; 128: 824–829.
33. Lambert JR, Bomanju JB, Pegas KS et al. Prognostic role of PET scanning before and alter reduced-intensity allogeneic stem cell transplantation for lymphoma. Blood 2010; 115: 2763–2768.

Multiple Choice Questionnaire

To find the correct answer, go to http://www.esh.org/online-training/handbook/

1. **Regarding the indications of haematopoietic stem cell transplantation in patients with Hodgkin's lymphoma, please identify the correct answer:**
   a) Autologous stem cell transplantation is a clinical option in patients in first complete remission and high-risk features at diagnosis . . . . ☐
   b) Autologous stem cell transplantation still is the standard of care in patients with Hodgkin's lymphoma in first chemosensitive relapse . . . . . . ☐
   c) The results of autologous stem cell transplantation in patients with primary refractory disease have significantly improved over the last 10 years . . . . ☐
   d) Allogeneic stem cell transplantation has no role in patients with relapsed Hodgkin's lymphoma . . . . ☐

2. **Regarding autologous stem cell transplantation in patients with relapsed Hodgkin's lymphoma, please identify the correct answer:**
   a) The use of BEAM as a conditioning regimen significantly improves the long term outcome of these patients as compared to the CBV combination . . . . ☐
   b) A tandem autologous stem cell transplantation has been associated with an exceedingly high non-relapse mortality when applied in high-risk patients . . . . ☐

c) As opposed to what happens in the first line setting, the use of PET before the autologous procedure does not allow discriminating patients into different prognostic groups ☐

d) Although autologous stem cell transplantation is indicated in patients in chemosensitive first relapse, not all patients do equally well after the procedure ☐

3. **Regarding the role of allogeneic stem cell transplantation in relapsed Hodgkin's lymphoma, please identify the *incorrect* answer:**
    a) Conventional allogeneic stem cell transplant has been associated with a very high non-relapse mortality ☐
    b) Reduced intensity conditioning regimens have become very popular in recent years ☐
    c) The intensity of the conditioning regimen does not matter in Hodgkin lymphoma patients; the relevant aspect is to decrease non-relapse mortality ☐
    d) Refractory patients do significantly worse with allogeneic stem cell transplantation than those patients with sensitive disease ☐

4. **Regarding the role of stem cell transplantation in patients with primary refractory disease, please identify the correct answer:**
    a) Primary refractory disease does not exist nowadays due to the generalised use of more intensive first-line protocols ☐
    b) Those patients with primary refractory disease but responding to salvage chemotherapy do significantly better than those with truly primary refractory disease ☐
    c) Autologous stem cell transplantation does have the same non-relapse mortality in primary refractory patients than in those being autografted with sensitive disease ☐
    d) The increase in the intensity of the conditioning regimen has led to significant improvement in the results of autologous stem cell transplantation in this subgroup of patients ☐

5. **Regarding the role of reduced intensity allogeneic stem cell transplantation in relapsed Hodgkin's lymphoma, please indicate the *incorrect* answer:**

a) The use of low dose TBI conditioning regimens seems to increase the relapse rate after allogeneic stem cell transplantation . . . . ☐

b) In children and adolescents, the use of myeloablative conditioning regimen is associated with a better progression free survival in the long-term because of a decreased relapse rate and no significant increase on non-relapse mortality in relation to reduced intensity conditioning protocols . . . . ☐

c) The use of Campath-1H as graft-versus-host-disease prophylaxis significantly increases the relapse rate in multiply relapsed Hodgkin's lymphoma patients . . . . ☐

d) The use of allogeneic stem cell transplantation in patients relapsing after an autologous stem cell transplant does not seem to improve the long-term outcome in relation to other standard therapies . . . . ☐

* CHAPTER 19

Indications for HSCT in adults

* 19.10

Solid tumours in adults

Marco Bregni

1. Introduction

In the years 2005–2010, more than 10,000 transplants in adults with solid tumours were reported to EBMT. These included 9897 (95.3%) autologous transplants (auto-SCT) and 485 (0.7%) allogeneic transplants (allo-SCT) (Table 1 and Table 2). The most frequent indications for auto-SCT were: germ cell tumours, Ewing family tumours (EFT)/PNET, medulloblastoma and breast cancer (Table 3). Allo-SCT, though less utilised in this period compared to previous years, particularly for epithelial tumours, is however used for neuroblastoma, Ewing family tumours/primitive neuroectodermal tumours (EFT/PNET) and rhabdomyosarcoma (Table 4).

Table 1: Numbers of autologous transplants in adults with solid tumours reported to the EBMT Registry 2005–2010	
Year	Autologous
2005	1899
2006	1817
2007	1613
2008	1620
2009	1552
2010	1396
Total	9897

Updated on June 1, 2011

Table 2: Numbers of allogeneic transplants in adults with solid tumours reported to the EBMT Registry 2005–2010	
Year	Allogeneic
2005	127
2006	87
2007	64
2008	65
2009	85
2010	57
Total	485

Updated on June 1, 2011

Table 3: **Most important indications (more than 50 transplants) for autologous transplants in adult solid tumours, 2005–2010**

Indication	Numbers	Percentage
Germ cell tumours*	2665	27.0
Ewing family tumours/PNET**	1853	18.7
Medulloblastoma	1067	10.8
Breast	721	7.3
Ovarian	235	2.4
Rhabdomyosarcoma	226	2.3
Wilms tumour	155	1.6
Osteosarcoma	115	1.2
Choriocarcinoma	105	1.1
Bone sarcoma (excluding Ewing/PNET)	78	0.8

*Includes the following: Germ cell tumour (40), seminoma (41), embryonal carcinoma (42), teratocarcinoma-yolk sac tumour (43), testicular (44), germ cell tumour, extragonadal (45), choriocarcinoma (46), mixed tumour without seminoma (47), mixed tumour with seminoma (48). **Includes: PNET (30), Ewing sarcoma (31), CNS, including CNS PNET (34), Ewing sarcoma/PNET, extra-skeletal (37), Ewing sarcoma/PNET, skeletal (38). Numbers refer to EBMT MED-B codes*

Table 4: **Most important indications for allogeneic transplants in adult solid tumours, 2005–2010**

Indication	Numbers	Percentage
Neuroblastoma	142	29.3
Ewing family tumours/PNET	56	11.5
Rhabdomyosarcoma	62	12.8
Breast carcinoma	39	8.0
Renal cell carcinoma	44	9.1
Ovarian carcinoma	14	2.9

2. Autologous transplant

2.1 Small-cell lung cancer

Leyvraz et al. (1), on behalf of the EBMT Solid Tumours Working Party (STWP), have recently reported a prospective multicentre phase III study of conventional dose chemotherapy (CDC) with ifosfamide, carboplatin and etoposide (ICE) vs high-dose chemotherapy (HDC) with stem cell support in patients with limited or extensive small-cell lung cancer (SCLC). The trial did not demonstrate any advantage of HDC for 3-year survival rates (18 and 19% in the HDC and ICE arms, respectively), nor in overall or complete response rates. Some limitations of the study may have accounted for the lack of favourable results. The study had a much lower than expected accrual rate (145 instead of the 360 originally planned patients were enrolled over an 8-year period), and the initial trial design had to be altered to include interim analyses. The trial allowed inclusion of a heterogeneous study population and patients with limited and extensive disease were enrolled. Eight percent of patients in the HDC arm died of therapy-related toxicity, a rate that would be considered unacceptable today. Thirty of 74 (40%) patients in the HDC arm either never started or failed to complete the protocol treatment.

It is likely that the role of dose intensification with stem cell support, including less toxic chemotherapy regimens, deserves further evaluation in patients with SCLC, considering also that no real advance has been made over the last 20 years in the treatment of this type of cancer.

2.2 Germ cell tumours

The numbers of transplants in patients with germ cell tumours (GCT) has been essentially stable over recent years (Table 5). Salvage treatment of patients with metastatic GCT who fail first-line chemotherapy is controversial. The introduction of high-dose chemotherapy (HDC) in the 1990s demonstrated for the

Table 5: **Numbers of autologous transplants for germ cell tumours reported to the EBMT Registry 2005–2010**

Year	GCT
2005	479
2006	495
2007	357
2008	440
2009	450
2010	444
Total	**2665**

Updated on June 1, 2011

first time constant and reproducible survival rates of approximately 30% even in patients with adverse prognostic factors. Over the next 15 years these data were confirmed (2). Others have questioned the role of HDC in the first salvage setting and argued that HDC represents an overtreatment for the majority of patients who might fare equally well with conventional-dose salvage chemotherapy (CDC). To help in the choice of an optimal strategy, the International Prognostic Factor Study Group recently performed a large retrospective data collection on 1984 patients from major centres worldwide, and identified seven prognostic factors with independent impact on survival rates after first-salvage treatment (3). This same database generated information on patients who experienced progression after at least three cisplatin-based cycles and were treated with either cisplatin-based CDC or carboplatin-based HDC chemotherapy. Patients could reliably be classified into five prognostic categories based on prior prognostic classification, from very low to very high risk. Within each of the five categories, the progression-free survival (PFS) and overall survival (OS) after CDC and HDC were compared using the Cox model. Overall, 773 patients received CDC, and 821 patients received HDC. Both treatment modalities were used with similar frequencies within each prognostic category. In low-risk patients, no difference in OS was observed between the two treatment groups, but in all other prognostic groups both PFS and OS were superior for HDC (4).

This retrospective analysis suggests a benefit for HDC given as intensification of first salvage treatment in male patients with GCT, and supports the prospective efforts that are underway to address the issue of HDCT versus CDCT in an international prospective randomised phase III trial (TIGER Trial).

2.3 Breast cancer
The results of metanalyses from the EBMT STWP and the MD Anderson Cancer Center of prospective randomised trials of high-dose chemotherapy in adjuvant and in advanced breast cancer have been presented on several occasions (5, 6). The main reason for this joint effort was that high-dose chemotherapy with autologous transplantation for high-risk primary breast cancer (i.e., node-positive disease) and for metastatic breast cancer had not shown prolongation of survival in individual trials but these had limited power to show any overall benefit or benefits within subsets. In the adjuvant study, individual patient data from 15 randomised trials that compared high-dose chemotherapy (HDC) with standard-dose chemotherapy (SDC) have been assembled (5). Prospectively defined primary endpoints were relapse-free survival and overall survival. After a median follow-up of six years, the results show that HDC prolonged relapse-free survival (hazard ratio [HR] 0.87; 95% CI 0.81–0.94; p=0.0001) but not overall survival (HR 0.95; 95% CI 0.87–1.02;

p=0.16). Overall survival was not statistically different by treatment arm in any of the subgroups except for women with HER2-negative disease, for whom there was a 21% reduction in the risk of death (p=0.009). However, HER2/neu was determined in only a fraction of patients (1695/6210, 27%), and the high rate of missing data did not allow for the conclusion that HDC was superior to CDC in this subset. In addition, HER2 determination in the 1990s was not standardised; the definition of "triple negative" tumours is today based on molecular characteristics, and is hardly comparable with that reported in the studies; moreover, the introduction of the anti-HER2 monoclonal antibody, trastuzumab, has radically changed the outcome of HER2-positive patients, in both the advanced and adjuvant settings. Also, the higher treatment-related mortality of HDC in the 1990s may have contributed to this negative result: of 89 total deaths attributed to toxicity, 72 (6.0%) occurred among the 1207 deaths in the HDC arms, and 17 (1.4%) occurred among the 1261 deaths in the control arms. In an additional analysis excluding patients whose deaths were attributed to toxicity, the hazard ratio for OS was favourable to HDC (0.90; 95% CI: 0.83–0.99; p=0.011) after adjusting for trial, age, hormone receptors, and the number of positive lymph nodes. Finally, the high-dose chemotherapy regimens were heterogeneous in terms of dose intensity, some being less "intense" than conventional dose therapy. By utilising appropriate statistical methods, an increasing summation dose intensity was associated with a statistically significant reduction in the risk of both disease recurrence (for one unit increase: HR=0.86, 95% CI: 0.80–0.92, p <0.0001) and death (HR=0.92, 95% CI: 0.85–1.00, p=0.039). In conclusion, the data do not support a superior outcome of high-dose chemotherapy in high-risk primary breast cancer: the issue of a HDC effect in subsets such as HER2-negative tumors is likely to remain unresolved, and the decision to use HDC in selected young patients with HER2-negative disease and high nodal burden is currently left to the clinical judgment of the caring physician.

The effects of HDC in metastatic breast cancer were assessed by the metanalysis of six randomised trials (6). The primary analysis of overall survival was a log rank test comparing high-dose versus standard-dose chemotherapy. The effect of high-dose chemotherapy on overall survival was not statistically different: median 2.16 versus 2.02 years, p=0.077. A statistically significant advantage in progression-free survival (median 0.91 versus 0.69 years) did not translate into a survival benefit. Subset analyses found little evidence to support the use of HDC in any patient group. In this metanalysis the small sample size of the individual trials (total 866 patients), the different regimens utilised, and the biologic heterogeneity of the patients (e.g., HER2, hormone receptor status) precluded the identification of an advantage in OS of HDC.

3. Allogeneic transplant

3.1 Colorectal cancer

Thirty-nine patients with metastatic colorectal cancer (mCRC) were treated with five different fludarabine-based RIC regimens within the prospective Phase I EBMT STWP-02 study, as reported by Aglietta et al. (7). The disease status at transplant was progressive disease (PD) in 31 patients (80%), stable disease (SD) in 6 (15%), and partial response (PR) in 2 (5%). The patients had received a median of 2 lines of chemotherapy, including oxaliplatin and irinotecan. All patients engrafted (median donor T-cell chimerism of 90% at day +60). Transplant-related morbidities were limited. Grades II-IV acute graft-versus-host disease (aGvHD) occurred in 14 patients (35%) and chronic GvHD (cGVHD) in 9 patients (23%). Transplant-related mortality occurred in 4 patients (10%). The best tumour responses were: 1 complete response (CR) (2%), 7 PR (18%), and 10 SD (26%), giving an overall disease control in 18 of 39 patients (46%). Responses occurred by a median of 90 days, and were observed irrespective of disease status at transplant (SD or PD), chimerism status or conditioning regimen. Patients who had a clinical response after transplant had a longer survival compared to non-responders (log rank test p=0.00018), even if the small numbers do not allow a firm conclusion. It is fair to say that allogeneic HCT after RIC is feasible in mCRC, even in progressing disease and in heavily pretreated patients; the data suggest that a graft-versus-mCRC exists, also based on a previous paper from the same group (8) showing induction of carcinoembryonic antigen (CEA)-specific T-cells in 3 of 3 patients concomitant with GvHD onset. The clinical results are difficult to compare with today's standard practice, in which new targeted treatments have been introduced (e.g. bevacizumab, cetuximab, panitumumab).

3.2 Renal cell cancer

Long-term survival is an infrequent occurrence in metastatic renal cell cancer (RCC), even if managed with new antiangiogenic drugs. In a series of 25 patients with cytokine-refractory clear-cell renal cell cancer (RCC) treated by reduced intensity conditioning transplant (RICT) (9), some of whom were included in retrospective analysis of the STWP (10), 5 patients survived more than 5 years. Three variables were correlated with survival in multivariate analysis, i.e. C-reactive protein, number of infused CD34+ cells and disease status after transplant. However, this study does not resolve questions that are still unanswered after more than 10 years of research in RCC transplantation, i.e.: does the GvT effect still occur after anti-angiogenic (i.e. TKI, VEGF) and/or mTOR inhibition therapies? Is there a therapeutic window for allograft after first- or second-line therapies for RCC? Can we envisage non-toxic clinical strategies for adoptive immunotherapy in RCC? The answer will likely come from well-designed studies with the combination of allograft with targeted therapies, and their associated disease control- and immune-effects.

3.3 Ovarian cancer
Although preliminary results suggest that allo-HSCT for advanced ovarian cancer (OC) is feasible, the low patient numbers in previous studies means that these had limited ability to evaluate any possible benefit. A retrospective multicentre study from Bay et al. (11) included 30 patients with OC allografted between 1995 and 2005 in EBMT centres. Prior to transplant, patients were in complete response (n=1), partial response (n=7), stable disease (n=11) or had progressive disease (n=13). An objective response (OR) was observed in 50% (95% CI: 33–67) of patients and this occurred in 3 patients following the development of aGvHD. The cumulative incidence of cGvHD was 34% (95% CI: 18–50). Transplant-related mortality rates were 7 and 20% at day 100 and at 1 year, respectively. With a median follow-up of 74.5 months (range 16–148), the median progression free survival (PFS) was 6 months and median overall survival (OS) was 10.4 months. Patients who developed cGvHD following allo-SCT had a significant improvement in OS compared to those who did not (17.6 vs 6.5 months, p=0.042). However, PFS was not significantly improved in patients who developed cGvHD (12 versus 3.7 months, p=0.81). Allo-HSCT in OC induces graft-versus-OC effects, whose clinical relevance remains to be shown in larger prospective trials.

3.4 Ewing tumours (ET)
The existence of a clinically relevant graft-versus-tumour effect in patients with ET after allo-HSCT is still a matter of debate: evidence for a graft-versus-Ewing tumour effect (GvETE) is solely deduced from case reports. In order to understand better the outcome of patients with advanced ET (AET) undergoing allo-HSCT and the optimal transplant regimen, data from 87 AET paediatric and adult patients treated with allo-HSCT from the European Group for Blood and Marrow Transplantation, Pediatric Registry for Stem Cell Transplantation, Asia Pacific Blood and Marrow Transplantation and MetaEICESS registries were retrospectively analysed by Thiel et al. (12). Fifty patients received reduced-intensity (RIC, group A) and 37 patients received high-intensity conditioning (HIC, group B). Sixty-three of 87 (72%) patients received grafts from either HLA-matched related or HLA-matched unrelated donors, whereas 24 of 87 (28%) patients received either haploidentical or otherwise HLA-mismatched grafts. The median overall survival was 7.9 months (±1.24, 95% CI: 5.44–10.31) for group A and 4.4 months (±1.06, 95% CI: 2.29–6.43) for group B patients (p=1.3). Death from complications (DOC) occurred in 4 of 50 (0.08) and

death from disease (DOD) in 33 of 50 (0.66) in group A and in 16 of 37 (0.43) and 17 of 37 (0.46) in group B patients, respectively. DOC incidence was decreased (p <0.01) and DOD/relapse increased (p <0.01) in group A compared with group B. HLA mismatch was not generally associated with GvETE. These data suggest an absence of a clinically relevant GvETE with current protocols.

4. Concluding remarks

We conclude that autologous transplant is a valuable strategy in young adults for indications similar to those of a paediatric population (e.g. EFT/PNET), and those with germ cell tumours, in particular in the setting of salvage treatment, and is now not indicated for epithelial tumours, for which the introduction of new molecularly targeted therapies have changed the approach to therapy, without however substantially altering the clinical course of the disease (e.g., triple-negative breast cancer, ovarian cancer, SCLC). Allogeneic transplant has been utilised as adoptive immunotherapy in the period 2000–2005 for epithelial solid tumours such as renal cancer, ovarian cancer, and colorectal cancer, but has been virtually abandoned in the last five years. The most compelling reasons for this are the considerable toxicity and transplant-related mortality of allo-SCT, even in its reduced-intensity version, and the poor design of prospective studies. The most promising advances in this field will come from the association of allo-SCT with molecularly targeted agents, taking advantage of their disease control- and immune-properties.

Key points

Autologous transplant is currently utilised for several solid tumours, and is standard indication for relapsed germ cell tumours

In the adjuvant setting in breast cancer, the EBMT/MDA metanalysis has shown that high-dose chemotherapy with autologous transplant increases disease-free survival, but not overall survival

Allogeneic transplant is utilised in neuroblastoma, EFT/PNET, rhabdomyosarcoma

Pilot studies of allografting have been conducted in renal cancer, colorectal cancer and ovarian cancer

The graft-versus-tumour effect of allografting has been offset by high transplant-related mortality, even with reduced-intensity conditioning

A promising area of research is the combination of allograft with molecularly targeted therapies

References

1. Leyvraz S, Pampallona S, Martinelli G et al. A threefold dose intensity treatment with ifosfamide, carboplatin, and etoposide for patients with small cell lung cancer: A randomized trial. J Natl Cancer Inst 2008; 100: 533–541.
2. Einhorn LH, Williams SD, Chamness A et al. High-dose chemotherapy and stem-cell rescue for metastatic germ-cell tumors. N Engl J Med 2007; 357: 340–348.
3. International Prognostic Factor Study Group, Lorch A, Beyer J et al. Prognostic factors in patients with metastatic germ cell tumors who fail cisplatin-based first-line chemotherapy. J Clin Oncol 2010; 28: 4906–4911.
4. Lorch A, Bascoul-Mollevi C, Kramar A et al. Conventional-dose versus high-dose chemotherapy as first salvage treatment in male patients with metastatic germ cell tumors: Evidence from a large international database. J Clin Oncol 2011; 29: 2178–2184.
5. Berry DA, Ueno NT, Johnson MM et al. High-dose chemotherapy with autologous stem cell support as adjuvant therapy in breast cancer: Overview of 15 randomized trials. J Clin Oncol 2011; 29: 3214–3223.
6. Berry DA, Ueno NT, Johnson MM, et al. High-dose chemotherapy with autologous hematopoietic stem cell transplantation in metastatic breast cancer: Overview of six randomized trials. J Clin Oncol 2011; 29: 3224–3231.
7. Aglietta M, Barkholt L, Schianca FC et al. Reduced-intensity allogeneic hematopoietic stem cell transplantation in metastatic colorectal cancer as a novel adoptive cell therapy approach. The European Group for Blood and Marrow Transplantation experience. Biol Blood Marrow Transplant 2009; 15: 326–335.
8. Carnevale-Schianca F, Cignetti A, Capaldi A et al. Allogeneic nonmyeloablative hematopoietic cell transplantation in metastatic colon cancer: Tumor-specific T cells directed to a tumor-associated antigen are generated in vivo during GVHD. Blood 2006; 107: 3795–3803.
9. Bregni M, Bernardi M, Servida P et al. Long-term follow-up of metastatic renal cancer patients undergoing reduced-intensity allografting. Bone Marrow Transplant 2009; 44: 237–242.
10. Barkholt L, Bregni M, Remberger M et al. Allogeneic haematopoietic stem cell transplantation for metastatic renal carcinoma in Europe. Ann Oncol 2006; 17: 1134–1140.
11. Bay JO, Cabrespine-Faugeras A, Tabrizi R et al. Allogeneic hematopoietic stem cell transplantation in ovarian cancer-the EBMT experience. Int J Cancer 2010; 127: 1446–1452.
12. Thiel U, Wawer A, Wolf P et al. No improvement of survival with reduced- versus high-intensity conditioning for allogeneic stem cell transplants in Ewing tumor patients. Ann Oncol 2011; 22: 1614–1621.

Multiple Choice Questionnaire

To find the correct answer, go to http://www.esh.org/online-training/handbook/

1. **The high-dose therapy approach to small cell lung cancer (SCLC) results in:**
   a) Prolongation of overall survival (OS) in all subsets.....................☐
   b) Prolongation of OS in limited-stage disease ....☐
   c) No effect on OS...☐
   d) OS benefit only in relapsed disease.................................☐

2. **High-dose chemotherapy with autologous transplant in germ cell tumours (GCT):**
   a) Is a standard therapy in first-line high-risk disease.....................☐
   b) Appears to be superior to standard-dose chemotherapy in second-line, except than for low-risk patients.....................................☐
   c) Is utilised in third-line only.......................................☐
   d) Is never used in GCT..☐

3. **According to the EBMT-MDA metanalysis on phase III studies of adjuvant high-dose chemotherapy in primary breast cancer:**
   a) Compared to standard-dose chemotherapy, high-dose chemotherapy prolongs disease-free survival but not overall survival...................☐
   b) High-dose chemotherapy is uniformly more intense than standard-dose therapy in adjuvant studies of breast cancer...........................☐
   c) There is no difference in outcome in different HER2 subsets treated with high-dose chemotherapy...☐
   d) The treatment-related mortality of standard-dose chemotherapy and high-dose chemotherapy are approximately superimposable.........☐

4. **Allogeneic transplant in solid tumours is indicated in:**
   a) Metastatic colorectal cancer.......................................☐
   b) Ovarian cancer, only with reduced-intensity conditioning ....☐
   c) Clear-cell renal cancer..☐
   d) None of the above...☐

5. **Transplant-related mortality in allogeneic transplant for solid tumours:**
   a) Is higher than that reported for haematological diseases .... ☐
   b) Is comparable to that reported for haematological diseases .... ☐
   c) Is in the range of 3–5% .... ☐
   d) Is mostly related to fungal infections .... ☐

* CHAPTER 19

Indications for HSCT in adults

* 19.11
Autoimmune diseases

John A. Snowden, Riccardo Saccardi, Dominique Farge

1. Introduction

Autoimmune diseases (ADs) are a heterogeneous group of diseases affecting 5–8% of the population. The vast majority are controlled, at least in the short term, with established treatments aimed at either immunosuppression or replacement of deficiency (such as type 1 diabetes) or even organ transplantation at time of end-stage organ failure. The side effects of chronically administered immunosuppressive treatment may compound the overall picture and a proportion of autoimmune disease patients develop progressive disability with shortened life expectancy in severely affected patients.

On the background of animal and clinical data, consensus indications for the use of HSCT to treat severe ADs were first published in 1997 (1). Since then patients have been considered for HSCT when fulfilling the following criteria:

1. Diagnosed with an AD severe enough to have an increased risk of mortality or advanced and irreversible disability;
2. The AD must be unresponsive to conventional treatments;
3. HSCT should be undertaken before irreversible organ damage so that significant clinical benefit can be achieved.

Today, more than 2000 patients worldwide (EBMT, CIBMTR, Asian registry) have received an HSCT for an AD alone (Table 1). In the EBMT database, with 1291 patients registered, the most commonly transplanted diseases are multiple sclerosis (MS), systemic sclerosis (SSc), Crohn's disease (CD) and systemic lupus erythematosus (SLE), coming from over 215 transplant centres in 30 countries. Prevalence of female sex and young age reflects the natural distribution of the diseases. The introduction of new biotherapies has resulted in a decrease of activity in HSCT in some diseases, particularly inflammatory arthritis. Long-lasting responses were obtained in all disease categories with an overall adjusted transplant related mortality (TRM) being 7±3% at three years, directly related to the type of AD disease (SLE at higher risk), the year of transplant (with a learning curve) and the intensity of conditioning (HSCT patients had a higher risk of TRM but lower probability of disease progression) (2). Running in parallel with the evolving panorama of "biological" treatments for AD,

Table 1: **Overview of data reported to the EBMT database (June 2011)**	
Patients	1291
Transplant procedures	1325
Centres/Countries	215
Autografts/Allografts	1234 (93%)/90 (7%)
Median age at transplant (yrs)	35 (<1–76)
Male/Female	39/61%

evidence for the clinical utility of HSCT in severe AD has gradually accumulated over the last 15 years with retrospective database analyses and prospective phase I/II studies (3, 4). The mechanism of action has not been fully elucidated but studies support initial immunosuppression with evidence of subsequent thymic reprocessing or increased regulatory T-cell activity in all types of ADs (5).

2. The EBMT Guidelines for HSCT in ADs

In 2011, the EBMT AD Working Party (ADWP) produced new consensus guidelines and recommendations for both haematologists and autoimmune disease specialists with a referral practice or who are planning local trials (6). These new guidelines aim to harmonise practice and provide a balance between safety and efficacy. Where possible prospective clinical trial activity with non-interventional or phase II-III studies is encouraged, but the rarity of some AD diseases may necessitate individual decisions to be taken by multidisciplinary teams. To ensure safety and quality, HSCT in AD should only be performed in European centres accredited by JACIE (or equivalent) with the necessary close liaison between HSCT and AD specialists, along with the appropriate facilities and experience in selecting and managing AD patients for HSCT. Long-term data reporting recommendations are also made with respect to specific aspects of the HSCT procedure, including patient selection, stem cell collection, graft manipulation, conditioning regimens and supportive care (6). Comprehensive cardiopulmonary screening and pre-transplant evaluation of heart, lung, kidney and gastrointestinal function are critically important and patients with advanced end organ disease should be excluded. The combination of cyclophosphamide and G-CSF, which protects against disease flare, has been the most commonly used HSC mobilisation regimen, although careful assessment and monitoring is recommended. Among the many conditioning regimens reported, the ADWP recommends cyclophosphamide 200 mg/kg with polyclonal or monoclonal anti-T-cell serotherapy generally, with cyclophosphamide 120 mg/kg, fludarabine 150 mg/kg and anti-T-cell serotherapy as an alternative in paediatric patients and BEAM + anti-T-cell serotherapy in multiple sclerosis specifically. Given the high associated TRM in ADs, "high intensity" or myeloablative conditioning regimens, including irradiation (e.g. TBI) at any dose, should be restricted to the clinical trial setting.

After HSCT, all patients should remain under the direct combined care of the transplant and the AD specialists for at least the first 100 days post transplant, and then on a quarterly basis for the first 2 years even if clinically stable. Thereafter joint annual review as a minimum is recommended. Long-term annual data reporting, including late effects, of all AD patients after HSCT to registries is a minimum recommendation (6).

In the following paragraphs clinical results and indications for the major ADs will be overviewed.

3. Multiple sclerosis

MS is the most frequent chronic inflammatory demyelinating disease, with a prevalence of 1 of 700 adults. MS may be categorised into relapsing-remitting (RR-MS) secondary progressive (SP-MS), a primary progressive form (PP-MS) and a rapidly evolving malignant (or Marburg) form. Various immunomodulators, such as glatiramer-acetate and interferon-β and more recently, the oral sphingosine 1 phosphate receptor agonist fingolimod, are used as first-line treatments and have proved considerably more effective than interferon-β in delaying progression of disability. Second-line treatments are mitoxantrone and the monoclonal antibody natalizumab. Nontheless (7) subsets of non-responders are recognised, necessitating the use of long-term immunosuppression. In this context, MS is the most frequent diagnosis for which HSCT has been used, and the majority of patients have SP-MS. In 2006, a retrospective analysis of 183 patients in the EBMT database (99 secondary progressive (SP), 19 primary progressive and 41 relapsing forms (RR), reported that 63% did not progress in their disability after a median follow-up of 42 months. TRM was 5%, with most deaths occurring before 2000, after which TRM has been minimal.

Most of the MS HSCT patients worldwide have been conditioned with the BEAM + ATG schedule. More aggressive regimens, including busulfan or the association of graft manipulation and serotherapy resulted in a higher toxicity without any advantage in terms of relapse prevention or disability progression. Cyclophosphamide and ATG conditioning has been used for autologous HSCT in early relapsing-remitting patients with low toxicity, but increased relapse rate. A better outcome in RR over SP forms, including sustained improvement of the disability, has been recently reported in single centre experiences, best explained by targeting the inflammatory phase of the disease before neurodegeneration has become established (6).

The ADWP updated guidelines recommend autologous HSCT for MS patients with RR-MS with high inflammatory activity who are rapidly deteriorating despite the use of at least one or more lines of treatment. Patients with rapidly deteriorating "malignant" MS are also suitable candidates. Although the majority of MS patients reported in the literature have SP-MS, autologous HSCT is appropriate in this phase only when some inflammatory activity (clinically or at MRI) is still present. Except for "malignant" forms, patients who have lost the ability to walk should not be treated with HSCT. BEAM + anti T-cell serotherapy is recommended as conditioning (6).

4. Systemic sclerosis

SSc is a rare AD of unknown origin, with an incidence of 1 in 100,000 and is characterised by skin and visceral (lung, gastrointestinal, cardiovascular and renal) fibrosis secondary to excessive collagen deposition (8). Limited (lcSSc) and diffuse cutaneous (dcSSc) forms can be distinguished by the extent of skin and organ involvement and autoantibody profile (9, 10). Rapidly progressing dcSSc within the first 4 years after disease onset, observed in 10–20% of cases is a life-threatening disease with 3–5 years survival between 50–80% (11–13). SSc patients benefit only marginally from prolonged oral cyclophosphamide, the only treatment with some proven efficacy (14, 15).

In the most severe form of dcSSc, registry analyses, case reports and pilot studies have confirmed rapid and sustained clinically relevant improvement after HSCT. Notably, autologous HSCT induced a major regression of SSc dermal fibrosis, confirmed by histological analysis, which had not hitherto been reported with any other treatment in SSc (16, 17). Prolonged follow-up of patients up to 7 years confirmed sustained improved functional status, fall in skin score and stabilisation of lung function, whereas death from disease progression was strikingly lower compared to the 5-year mortality rate estimated at 30% in such severe SSc patients (4, 16). An early steep learning curve with high toxicity led to careful consideration of patient selection, and consequent reduction in TRM. These results were the basis for the ASTIS trial comparing HSCT (Cy, ATG and CD34 selected graft) versus monthly intravenous pulse Cy 750 mg/m^2 for 12 months, which has now completed recruitment and is awaiting initial analysis in 2012. Other studies elsewhere have included the single centre ASSIST study, run by the Chicago group, which has recently completed recruitment, and the radiation based SCOT trial in North America, which continues to accrue.

The revised guidelines recommend autologous HSCT for dcSSc, ideally in the context of a multicentre clinical trial, but it may be considered as treatment for selected patients with early diffuse SSc with a modified Rodnan skin score ≥15 *plus* major organ involvement in respiratory, cardiovascular, or renal systems. Comprehensive cardiopulmonary screening and pre-transplant evaluation of heart, lung, kidney and gastrointestinal function is critically important to exclude patients at high risk of TRM (6).

5. Systemic lupus erythematosus

SLE is a heterogeneous chronic AD with a prevalence of 40–50/100,000, predominantly affecting females (>85%). The outcome of active severe SLE due to kidney, lung, heart or brain involvement has improved in adults and children with early diagnosis and new immunosuppressive agents combined with overall tighter control of blood pressure and infections (18). Response rates to standard first-line therapy with the classical NIH regimen (19, 20) or the Eurolupus regimen (21) vary according to extent of visceral involvement, ethnic origin and socio-economic profile, but even with modern treatments, around 5–15% of patients with SLE evolve towards end stage disease, and 10–15% die within 10 years. In severe SLE patients, refractory to conventional immunosuppressive therapies, autologous HSCT has been shown to achieve sustained clinical remissions in around half of patients with qualitative immunological changes (22, 23) not seen with other forms of therapy. In this high risk population, TRM has been significant in multicentre (as opposed to single centre) settings, and highlights the need for careful patient selection and recognition of the intrinsic immune suppression and other risks associated with advanced SLE well as the need for further clinical studies (24, 25).

In the revised guidelines, autologous HSCT is recommended in SLE ideally in the context of a multicentre clinical trial, but may be considered as treatment for carefully selected subpopulations of SLE patients early in their disease course. Such patients should have reliably predicting poor-prognostic factors. In view of the relatively high progression rate and TRM, the ASTIL phase IIb trial has been designed for patients with severe refractory SLE who have failed at least 6 months of best standard local therapy to examine the efficacy of autologous HSCT as induction therapy followed by maintenance therapy by mycophenolate mofetil.

6. Crohn's disease

CD is a chronic inflammatory bowel disease (IBD) with a prevalence of around 0.1% affecting both adults and children. Despite the major recent progress in the treatment of CD, based on corticosteroids, immunosuppressors and biologics, some patients fail all available therapies, including immunosuppressants (thiopurines, methotrexate) and biologic therapies (mainly anti-TNF monoclonal antibodies). Surgery may be considered as an option in many cases, but may lead to short bowel syndrome or to a definitive stoma, which may be refused by the patient. There is a growing body of data supporting the application of autologous HSCT as treatment in the subset of CD patients in whom the disease runs an aggressive course with progressive tissue damage with potentially reduced life expectancy. Autologous HSCT has been investigated in several phase II studies with encouraging responses, some prolonged, although a progressive incidence of relapse with long-term follow up is recognised (22). In Europe, the EBMT sponsored ASTIC trial which randomised patients between early and delayed autologous HSCT has recently completed recruitment and awaits follow-up for full analysis. The ADWP recommends autologous HSCT ideally in the context of a multicentre clinical trial, but on an individual basis may currently be considered for patients with active CD refractory to immunosuppressants and biological treatments, or unacceptable risks of surgical management (26).

7. Other diseases

In rheumatoid arthritis and juvenile idiopathic arthritis (JIA), EBMT analyses have enabled statements to be made regarding outcomes of HSCT (27, 28). The majority of patients have benefited. TRM in RA was minimal but more substantial in JIA. However, the advent of biological therapy over the last decade has generated a variety of alternative treatment options for resistant patients. In the case of extremely rare patients for whom there is no alternative option, HSCT may still be considered after detailed multidisciplinary review (6).

Likewise, although enrolment onto a prospective clinical trial or prospective non-interventional study is highly recommended, whenever possible, patients with other rare indications such as severe vasculitis (29) and chronic inflammatory demyelinating polyneuropathy (CIDP) (30) may be individually considered for treatment as a "clinical option" (see Table 2).

New-onset type 1 diabetes (T1D) (31) and refractory coeliac disease (at high risk of enteropathy associated T cell lymphoma) (32) potentially respond, but experience of autologous HSCT has been relatively recent and the ADWP recommendation is that patients should only be treated on an IRB/REC approved prospective clinical trials (6).

Table 2: Distribution of diagnosis in the EBMT database

Multiple sclerosis	472	**Haematological diseases**	72
Connective tissue diseases	400	ITP	25
SSc	267	Evan's syndrome	17
SLE	98	AIHA	14
PM-DM	16	Other	16
Sjögren's syndrome	3		
Antiphospholipid syndrome	3	**Vasculitis**	34
Other/Unknown	13	Wegener's granulomatosis	9
Arthritis	165	Behcet's disease	7
Rheumatoid arthritis	86	Takayasu's arteritis	2
Juvenile chronic arthritis:		Microscopic polyarteritis nodosa	2
- Systemic JIA	46	Classical polyarteritis nodosa	1
- Other JIA	18	Churg-Strauss syndrome	2
- Polyarticular JIA	10	Other/Unknown	11
Psoriatic arthritis	3		
Other	2	**Other neurological**	34
Inflammatory bowel disease	66	Myasthenia gravis	5
Crohn's disease	58	Other/Unknown	29
Ulcerative colitis	4	**Insulin dependent diabetes**	10
Other	4	**Other/Unknown**	38

PM-DM: polymyalgia/dermatomyositis

8. Allogeneic and syngeneic HSCT

Despite the theoretical attraction of immune replacement and the graft versus autoimmune effect, allogeneic HSCT has been used infrequently in the treatment of AD. The TRM risk far outweighs the risks of severe ADs, and therefore, allogeneic HSCT for AD are rarely justified except if an underlying haematological malignancy is coexisting with the autoimmune disease, as recommended originally in 1997 (33). Today, allogeneic HSCT has mostly been used in the context of immune cytopenia, predominantly in the paediatric setting, with encouraging results in terms of relapse-free outcome. Patients who received an allogeneic HSCT showed a sustained response in 33% of the cases reported to the EBMT database (34).

In exceptional circumstances allogeneic HSCT may be considered for patients with refractory ITP, AIHA and Evans' syndrome. Well matched unrelated allogeneic HSCT should be limited to the paediatric setting, but matched sibling allogeneic HSCT may be considered in patients up to 50 years of age with refractory cytopenias. Bone marrow or umbilical cord blood are recommended as graft source for allogeneic HSCT in autoimmune cytopenia. If no HLA matched sibling donor is available, or if an adult is over 50 years of age, autologous HSCT is recommended.

In other diseases, experience is limited to individual case reports in SSc, SLE, vasculitis and RA and no recommendations other than clinical trial enrolment in a clinical trial. As the risks of syngeneic HSCT approximate to those of autologous HSCT, it may be considered as an alternative in those rare patients who have an identical twin, providing donor welfare is given high priority.

9. Conclusions

In 2011, the major indications for HSCT for severe ADs are MS, SSc, SLE and CD, all ADs where a significant subset of patients with unsatisfactory responses to both conventional and new immunomodulating treatments can be carefully identified (see Key Points). In contrast, the demand for treatment of resistant inflammatory arthritis with autologous HSCT has declined dramatically in the era of biological treatments. HSCT units will receive referrals from AD specialists of complex patients in whom inflammatory activity persists despite conventional treatment. In SSc and CD patients, there is the prospect of phase III trial data becoming available in the next 2 years to answer definitive questions, but, in other AD patients, individual decisions need to be made in a multidisciplinary setting. The revised guidelines aim to assist with this approach at the same time as encouraging both clinical trial activity and harmonisation of practice for non-interventional and more meaningful registry based analysis. The aim is to update these in 2 years to incorporate the anticipated final results of phase III studies and other developments which will help clarify the place of HSCT in AD.

Key points

HSCT has been used clinically in the last 15 years to treat severe ADs and may achieve major responses in severe ADs where other treatments have failed

Evolving numbers of patients have been incorporated into the EBMT and other registries which have enabled retrospective studies whilst prospective phase I/II/III studies have been performed concurrently

Revised guidelines and recommendations from the EBMT ADWP have summarised clinical practice, patient selection, data management, and planning for prospective clinical trials and non-interventional studies

Patients must show a poor risk prognosis in terms of either survival or severe disability, after having failed 1-2 lines of approved treatments. Irreversible, end-stage organ failure is an exclusion criterion

Principal current indications for HSCT in ADs include MS, SSc, SLE and CD, although definitive phase III data is awaited. Treatment decisions are a balance of benefit and risk and must be multidisciplinary in order to incorporate full consideration of alternative non-HSCT approaches to treatment

Acknowledgements
The Authors are indebted to Manuela Badoglio for helpful assistance with data management.

References

1. Tyndall A, Gratwohl A. Blood and marrow stem cell transplants in autoimmune disease. A consensus report written on behalf of the European League Against Rheumatism (EULAR) and the European Group for Blood and Marrow Transplantation (EBMT). Br J Rheumatol 1997; 36: 390–392.
2. Gratwohl A, Passweg J, Bocelli-Tyndall C et al. Autologous hematopoietic stem cell transplantation for autoimmune diseases. Bone Marrow Transplant 2005; 35: 869–879.
3. Hough RE, Snowden JA, Wulffraat NM. Haemopoietic stem cell transplantation in autoimmune diseases: A European perspective. Br J Haematol 2005; 128: 432–459.
4. Farge D, Labopin M, Tyndall A et al. Autologous hematopoietic stem cell transplantation for autoimmune diseases: An observational study on 12 years' experience from the European Group for Blood and Marrow Transplantation Working Party on Autoimmune Diseases. Haematologica 2010; 95: 284–292.
5. Kapoor S, Wilson AG, Sharrack B et al. Haemopoietic stem cell transplantation-an evolving treatment for severe autoimmune and inflammatory diseases in rheumatology,

neurology and gastroenterology. Hematology 2007; 12: 179–191.

6. Snowden J, Saccardi R, Allez M et al. on behalf of the EBMT Autoimmune Disease (ADWP) and Paediatric Diseases (PDWP) Working Parties. Haematopoietic stem cell transplantation (HSCT) in severe autoimmune diseases: Updated guidelines of the European Group for Blood and Marrow transplantation (EBMT). Bone Marrow Transplant 2011 Oct 17. doi: 10.1038/bmt.2011.185. [Epub ahead of print; open access.]

7. Miller DH, Khan OA, Sheremata WA et al. A controlled trial of natalizumab for relapsing multiple sclerosis. N Engl J Med 2003; 348: 15–23.

8. Gabrielli A, Avvedimento EV, Krieg T. Scleroderma. N Engl J Med 2009; 360: 1989–2003.

9. Ferri C, Valentini G, Cozzi F et al. Systemic sclerosis: Demographic, clinical, and serologic features and survival in 1,012 Italian patients. Medicine (Baltimore) 2002; 81: 139–153.

10. Abraham DJ, Varga J. Scleroderma: from cell and molecular mechanisms to disease models. Trends Immunol 2005; 26: 587–595.

11. Nihtyanova SI, Tang EC, Coghlan JG et al. Improved survival in systemic sclerosis is associated with better ascertainment of internal organ disease: A retrospective cohort study. QJM 2010; 103: 109–115.

12. Domsic RT, Rodriguez-Reyna T, Lucas M et al. Skin thickness progression rate: A predictor of mortality and early internal organ involvement in diffuse scleroderma. Ann Rheum Dis 2011; 70: 104–109.

13. Ioannidis JPA, Vlachoyiannopoulos PG, Haidich A-B et al. Mortality in systemic sclerosis: An international meta-analysis of individual patient data. Am J Med 2005; 118: 2–10.

14. Tashkin DP, Elashoff R, Clements PJ et al. Cyclophosphamide versus placebo in scleroderma lung disease. N Engl J Med 2006; 354: 2655–2666.

15. Nannini C, West CP, Erwin PJ, Matteson EL. Effects of cyclophosphamide on pulmonary function in patients with scleroderma and interstitial lung disease: A systematic review and meta-analysis of randomized controlled trials and observational prospective cohort studies. Arthritis Res Ther 2008; 10: R124.

16. Vonk MC, Marjanovic Z, van den Hoogen FHJ et al. Long-term follow-up results after autologous haematopoietic stem cell transplantation for severe systemic sclerosis. Ann Rheum Dis 2008; 67: 98–104.

17. Verrecchia F, Laboureau J, Verola O et al. Skin involvement in scleroderma-where histological and clinical scores meet. Rheumatology (Oxford) 2007; 46: 833–841.

18. Fiehn C, Hajjar Y, Mueller K et al. Improved clinical outcome of lupus nephritis during the past decade: Importance of early diagnosis and treatment. Ann Rheum Dis 2003; 62: 435–439.

19. Illei GG, Austin HA, Crane M et al. Combination therapy with pulse cyclophosphamide plus pulse methylprednisolone improves long-term renal outcome without adding toxicity in patients with lupus nephritis. Ann Intern Med 2001; 135: 248–257.

20. Contreras G, Pardo V, Leclercq B et al. Sequential therapies for proliferative lupus nephritis. N Engl J Med 2004; 350: 971–980.

21. Houssiau FA, Vasconcelos C, D'Cruz D et al. Immunosuppressive therapy in lupus nephritis: The Euro-Lupus Nephritis Trial, a randomized trial of low-dose versus high-dose intravenous cyclophosphamide. Arthritis Rheum 2002; 46: 2121–2131.

22. Burt RK, Traynor A, Statkute L et al. Nonmyeloablative hematopoietic stem cell transplantation for systemic lupus erythematosus. JAMA 2006; 295: 527–535.
23. Alexander T, Biesen R, Jacobi A et al. Systemic lupus erythematosus. Target criteria for treatment. Z Rheumatol 2009; 68: 23–29.
24. Farge D, Passweg J, van Laar JM et al. Autologous stem cell transplantation in the treatment of systemic sclerosis: Report from the EBMT/EULAR Registry. Ann Rheum Dis 2004; 63: 974–981.
25. Jayne D, Passweg J, Marmont A et al. Autologous stem cell transplantation for systemic lupus erythematosus. Lupus 2004; 13: 168–176.
26. Burt RK, Craig RM, Milanetti F et al. Autologous nonmyeloablative hematopoietic stem cell transplantation in patients with severe anti-TNF refractory Crohn disease: Long-term follow-up. Blood 2010; 116: 6123–6132.
27. Snowden JA, Passweg J, Moore JJ et al. Autologous hemopoietic stem cell transplantation in severe rheumatoid arthritis: A report from the EBMT and ABMTR. J Rheumatol 2004; 31: 482–488.
28. Wulffraat NM, van Rooijen EM, Tewarie R et al. Current perspectives of autologous stem cell transplantation for severe Juvenile Idiopathic Arthritis. Autoimmunity 2008; 41: 632–638.
29. Daikeler T, Kötter I, Bocelli Tyndall C et al. Haematopoietic stem cell transplantation for vasculitis including Behcet's disease and polychondritis: A retrospective analysis of patients recorded in the European Bone Marrow Transplantation and European League Against Rheumatism databases and a review of the literature. Ann Rheum Dis 2007; 66: 202–207.
30. Mahdi-Rogers M, Kazmi M, Ferner R et al. Autologous peripheral blood stem cell transplantation for chronic acquired demyelinating neuropathy. J Peripher Nerv Syst 2009; 14: 118–124.
31. Couri CEB, Oliveira MCB, Stracieri ABPL et al. C-peptide levels and insulin independence following autologous nonmyeloablative hematopoietic stem cell transplantation in newly diagnosed type 1 diabetes mellitus. JAMA 2009; 301: 1573–1579.
32. Tack GJ, Wondergem MJ, Al-Toma A et al. Auto-SCT in refractory celiac disease type II patients unresponsive to cladribine therapy. Bone Marrow Transplant 2010. Available at: http://www.ncbi.nlm.nih.gov/pubmed/20818442. Last accessed april 20, 2011.
33. Tyndall A, Gratwohl A. Blood and marrow stem cell transplants in auto-immune disease: A consensus report written on behalf of the European League against Rheumatism (EULAR) and the European Group for Blood and Marrow Transplantation (EBMT). Bone Marrow Transplant 1997; 19: 643–645.
34. Passweg JR, Rabusin M, Musso M et al. Haematopoetic stem cell transplantation for refractory autoimmune cytopenia. Br J Haematol 2004; 125: 749–755.

Multiple Choice Questionnaire

To find the correct answer, go to http://www.esh.org/online-training/handbook/

1. **How many patients have received HSCT for an autoimmune disease in the past ten years?**
   a) 100–500 patients ☐
   b) 500–1000 patients ☐
   c) 1000–3000 patients ☐
   d) More than 3000 patients ☐

2. **Which are the main indications for HSCT among ADs?**
   a) Autoimmune cytopenia ☐
   b) Rheumatoid arthritis ☐
   c) Systemic lupus erythematosus and vasculitis ☐
   d) Systemic sclerosis and multiple sclerosis ☐

3. **Which is the current transplant related mortality in autologous stem cell transplantation for autoimmune disease?**
   a) <1% ☐
   b) 3–10% ☐
   c) 10–20% ☐
   d) 20–30% ☐

4. **Which of the following criteria is *not* an indication for HSCT?**
   a) Patients diagnosed with a AD severe enough to have an increased risk of mortality or advanced and irreversible disability ☐
   b) ADs not responsive to conventional treatment ☐
   c) Young patients at diagnosis ☐
   d) Advanced disease without irreversible severe organ damage ☐

5. **Which is the prevalent source of HSCs for transplantation in ADs?**
   a) PBSCs mobilised by cyclophosphamide and G-CSF ☐
   b) PBSCs mobilised by G-CSF alone ☐
   c) Bone marrow ☐
   d) Cord blood ☐

* CHAPTER 19

Indications for HSCT in adults

* 19.12

Aplastic anaemia and paroxysmal nocturnal haemoglobinuria

Judith Marsh, Carlo Dufour
with major contribution from Andrea Bacigalupo,
Antonio Risitano, Mahmood Aljurf, Regis de Latour,
on behalf of the EBMT Severe Aplastic Anaemia Working Party (SAAWP)

1. Aplastic anaemia

1.1 Diagnosis

The diagnosis of severe aplastic anaemia (SAA) is based on the following findings: a bone marrow biopsy with <25% cellularity plus at least two of the following:
- Reticulocytes <1% or ≤60 x 10^9/L
- Platelets <20 x 10^9/L
- Neutrophils <0.5 x 10^9/L.

If neutrophils are <0.2, AA is defined as very severe (VSAA). In non severe (NSAA), neutrophils are <0.5 x 10^9/L. Analysis of glycosyl-phosphatidylinositol (GPI)-anchored proteins, such as CD55 and CD59 by flow cytometry, is recommended as a sensitive and quantitative test for paroxysmal nocturnal haemoglobinuria (PNH). The most common differential diagnosis is hypocellular myelodysplastic syndrome (MDS), see Figure 1. Inherited AA is the main differential diagnosis in children but may present in adults. Fanconi anaemia is excluded by the DEB or MMN test on cultured peripheral blood lymphocytes. Dyskeratosis congenita can be identified through a known mutation (DKC1, TERC, TERT, TINF2) but probably many mutations are as yet unknown. Along with measuring telomere length, this is not currently available as a routine clinical service in many centres (Figure 1) (1, 2).

1.2 Treatment indications

HLA-identical sibling HSCT is indicated as first line treatment for SAA patients <50 years old.

Immunosuppressive therapy (IST) is indicated for:
1. Transfusion dependent NSAA
2. SAA <50 years old who lack an HLA-identical sibling and
3. SAA >50 years old.

First choice IST is horse ATG (ATGAM) with cyclosporin (CSA). In the absence of horse ATG, rabbit ATG may be considered despite a lower response rate compared with horse ATG (3, 4) (see also section on Immunosuppressive therapy). Unrelated donor (UD) HSCT is indicated after failure of one course of IST in patients <65 years old, but may be considered earlier in the absence of horse ATG or in the presence of infection where HSCT would offer the best chance of rapid neutrophil recovery. See the complete treatment algorithm for SAA (1) at: *http://www.ebmt.org/5WorkingParties/AAWP/wparties-aa3.html*.

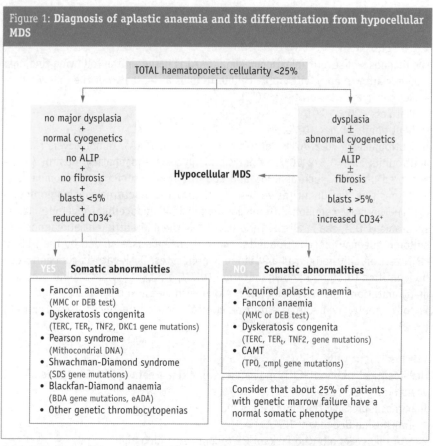

Figure 1: **Diagnosis of aplastic anaemia and its differentiation from hypocellular MDS**

TOTAL haematopoietic cellularity <25%

no major dysplasia
+
normal cyogenetics
+
no ALIP
+
no fibrosis
+
blasts <5%
+
reduced CD34+

Hypocellular MDS ←

dysplasia
±
abnormal cyogenetics
±
ALIP
±
fibrosis
+
blasts >5%
+
increased CD34+

YES **Somatic abnormalities**

- Fanconi anaemia
  (MMC or DEB test)
- Dyskeratosis congenita
  (TERC, TER$_t$, TNF2, DKC1 gene mutations)
- Pearson syndrome
  (Mithocondrial DNA)
- Shwachman-Diamond syndrome
  (SDS gene mutations)
- Blackfan-Diamond anaemia
  (BDA gene mutations, eADA)
- Other genetic thrombocytopenias

NO **Somatic abnormalities**

- Acquired aplastic anaemia
- Fanconi anaemia
  (MMC or DEB test)
- Dyskeratosis congenita
  (TERC, TER$_t$, TNF2, gene mutations)
- CAMT
  (TPO, cmpl gene mutations)

Consider that about 25% of patients with genetic marrow failure have a normal somatic phenotype

Cytogenetic abnormalities are seen in at least 10% of patients with otherwise typical aplastic anaemia, for example, trisomy 6 and trisomy 8. Therefore, they do not necessarily mean the diagnosis is MDS

1.3 HLA-identical sibling transplantation

1.3.1 Candidates for HLA-identical sibling HSCT

Allogeneic HSCT is the only available potentially curative treatment option for SAA. This should be the upfront therapeutic option of choice for patients <50 years old with SAA and for older patients who have failed previous IST. Currently, the expected 5-years survival of patients less than 20 years old receiving HLA-identical sibling HSCT as the primary treatment modality for is 88%, between 21 and 50 years it is 72% and above 50 years 43% (WPSAA 2010) (5, 6).

1.3.2 Conditioning regimens

Cyclophosphamide 200 mg/kg (CY 200) remains the standard conditioning regimen for SAA. The addition of ATG to CY 200 has been demonstrated to promote excellent engraftment and long term outcome (7). In a non-randomised trial, this combination resulted in a lower incidence of GvHD and improved survival compared to historical controls who received CY only conditioning (7, 8). A prospective randomised trial involving 134 patients did not show a significant benefit from the addition of ATG, but the study was underpowered (9) and a recent large registry based analysis has shown that survival of patients receiving ATG was significantly superior to that of patients not given ATG (84% vs 74%); in addition patients receiving ATG had a significantly lower risk of acute and chronic GvHD (10).

We would therefore recommend using ATG in association with CY because of the beneficial effect on engraftment and the reduced risk of GvHD. Whether fludarabine-containing regimens will improve the outcome of patients 30 years of age and older remains to be proven in prospective trials. One possible conditioning regimen would be CY 120 mg/kg, fludarabine (FLU) 120 mg/m^2 and either ATG or alemtuzumab (11, 12). A similar approach may be considered for patients aged 30–40 years.

Prevention of graft failure can be accomplished by the use of other more intense conventional conditioning regimens, including radiation-based regimens, but these are associated with higher transplant-related morbidity and mortality in a disease where the primary goal of transplantation is to secure adequate and durable engraftment only and where there is no malignancy that needs to be eradicated by high dose chemo-radiotherapy and no requirement for a graft versus malignancy effect (5).

1.3.3 Stem cell source

Unmanipulated bone marrow should be used as the stem cell source for all patients with AA, as the use of peripheral blood stem cells is associated with an increased risk of chronic GvHD. Despite the earlier engraftment with the use of peripheral blood stem cells, a joint EBMT/CIBMTR retrospective analysis suggests inferior outcome with the use of PBSC in this disease, particularly in young patients (13). A survival advantage for bone marrow graft was also confirmed in a more recent report in all age groups (14). These data do not support the current trend of increasing use of peripheral blood stem cells as a graft source in this disease. A bone marrow stem cell dose of at least 3 x 10^8 MNC/kg or 2 x 10^6 CD34/kg should be given, as a low stem cell dose increases the risk of graft failure (15), and small aliquots of marrow should be used at each aspiration to maximise the progenitor cell content. Peripheral blood is an alternative stem cell source if there is a contraindication to a bone marrow harvest, if the donor is unwilling to donate bone marrow, or in case of second transplants after graft failure.

1.3.4 Post-transplantation immunosuppression

Adequate post-transplantation immunosuppression is important, not only for the prevention of GvHD, but also to secure adequate suppression of the host immune system and thus to prevent graft rejection. The combination of CSA and short course methotrexate (MTX) should be considered the standard post-transplantation immunosuppression after ATG-based conditioning regimens. In a prospective randomised trial comparing CSA + MTX with CSA alone, the one year transplant-related mortality rates for patients given CSA/MTX or CSA alone were 3% and 15%, respectively (14). The 5-year probability of survival was 94% in the CSA/MTX group and 78% for those in the CSA alone group. There are limited data on the use of other immunosuppressive agents including the use of mycophenolate mofetil (MMF) in the presence of renal impairment, for example. Slow tapering of CSA should be carried out, usually after 9 months, with careful follow-up of chimerism and blood counts to avoid late graft failure.

1.4 Unrelated donor HSCT

1.4.1 Introduction

The outcome of UD HSCT has significantly improved, especially in the last 10 years (16, 17). Overall survival is in excess of 75%, and for some patient subgroups >80%. Better donor selection by high resolution HLA typing, better supportive care, and new conditioning regimens have all contributed to improved outcomes.

The improvement has been so dramatic, that the overall treatment strategy of patients with acquired SAA is changing: UD transplants are now considered after failing one course of IST. Currently UD transplants may be considered as first-line in children.

1.4.2 Donor selection

Centres are either matching for A, B, C and DRB1 at the allelic level, looking for 8/8 matched donors (18) or also for DQ, looking for a 10/10 match. In addition HLA mismatches can be classified as permissive or non-permissive (19, 20). In the recent EBMT analysis we showed an effect of mismatching (<8/8 vs 8/8 match) only for patients prepared with FLU-CY and ATG (FCA), but not for patients receiving FCA supplemented with low dose total body irradiation 2 Gy (FCA-TBI) (20). In general an 8/8 (A, B, C and DRB1) matched donor would be ideal, but a 7/8 match would probably be also acceptable if low-dose TBI is used.

1.4.3 Conditioning regimen

There is currently agreement on the combination of FLU-CY and ATG as the conditioning regimen in UD HSCT for acquired AA (17, 21). Low dose TBI, 2Gy or 3Gy, was added following the Japanese and USA studies (22, 23). The dose of CY was originally set at 300 mg/m^2 x 4 (17, 21). This was associated with a significant risk of rejection, so the current recommendation is to increase the dose of CY to 120 mg/kg. The WPSAA currently recommends FLU 30 mg/m^2 x 4, CY 30 mg/kg x 4 and ATG. TBI (2Gy) can be added on day -1 for patients aged >14 years, but can be considered also for children sensitised after numerous blood transfusions. Alemtuzumab has been reported to yield encouraging results with a very low incidence of chronic GvHD and can be considered as a substitute for ATG (12).

1.4.4 GvHD prophylaxis
Prophylaxis of GvHD is conventional CSA with low dose MTX on days +1, +3, +6, +11; the use of ATG or alemtuzumab in the conditioning regimen prevents severe acute and chronic GvHD.
In the EBMT study acute GvHD grade II-IV was low (18%) and chronic GvHD was more frequent, as expected, when TBI 2 Gy was added to FCA (50 vs 27%) (21): this was particularly true when peripheral blood was used as a source of stem cells. The risk of extensive chronic GvHD is 3% for BM and 20% for peripheral blood (PB).

1.4.5 Stem cell source
A recent EBMT analysis of 451 UD transplants performed with BM stem cells show a 10 year overall survival of 67% compared to 48% for 153 UD PBSCT (p <0.0001) (unpublished data). Therefore, as for sibling transplants, BM is the favoured stem cell source.

1.4.6 Interval from diagnosis to HSCT
The most relevant predictor of outcome is the interval between diagnosis and transplant, with a relative risk of death of 4.4, if the transplant was delayed beyond 2 years (21). All of the rejection-related deaths were in patients grafted beyond 2 years. For patients grafted within 2 years the actuarial 5-year survival is overall 87%, and 92% for patients (n=24) grafted since 2004 (20).

1.4.7 Graft failure
The cumulative incidence of graft failure was 17% in the EBMT study (20). Regarding predictors of graft failure, patients with a longer interval from diagnosis to transplant (>2 years) had a trend for a higher risk of graft failure (22%) compared to patients grafted <1 year (12%) or between 1-2 years from diagnosis (14%) (p=0.3). The median number of infused nucleated cells was 4.5 x 10^8/kg vs 4.24 x 10^8/kg for patients with or without sustained engraftment. Graft failure was seen in 1/10 (10%) peripheral blood transplants vs 15/88 (17%) bone marrow transplants.

1.4.8 EBV infection

In the EBMT study (21), the cumulative incidence of EBV lymphoproliferative disorder (LPD) was 4%. The current WPSAA recommendation is to monitor EBV-DNA weekly in patients undergoing UD HSCT with ATG in the conditioning regimen. There are two different strategies to prevent EBV-LPD: one is to treat pre-emptively patients showing an increase in EBV-DNA, above a given cut-off (1,000 copies/105 mononuclear cells, or 10,000 copies/mL) (24). The second strategy is to use prophylactic rituximab on day +5 (25). Prophylactic rituximab may also reduce the risk of GvHD. EBV may be less of a problem when alemtuzumab is used instead of ATG (12).

1.4.9 Outcome

Survival has overall improved from 29% in the decade 1981–1990, to 44% in the decade 1991–2000, to 67% in the decade 2001–2010. Using a conditioning regimen (FCA or FCA-TBI), the actuarial 10 year survival was overall 75%, and 83% for patients grafted since 2004 (Figure 2B) (21).

1.5 Alternative donor HSCT

The management of patients without a matched sibling or unrelated bone marrow donor, and who have failed at least course of IST, is not straightforward.

1.5.1 Cord blood transplantation

Unrelated cord blood transplantation (CBT) has become a widely accepted treatment for haematological malignancies, but there have been fewer studies on CBT in SAA. Small series and recent larger studies have reported some success, but with a high incidence of graft failure (26–28).

The Japan Cord Blood Network reported 31 patients undergoing single UCBT, with a median age of 27.9 years (range 0.8–72.7). Sustained engraftment was seen in only 17 patients. Survival at 2 years was 41 and 20% for patients aged >40 yr. Favourable outcome factors were conditioning with FLU, CY and TBI, and the absence of ATG (26). In a more recent but smaller retrospective study from Tokyo using FLU, melphalan and 4Gy TBI, observed successful engraftment in 11/12 patients and one late graft failure at 3 years, despite relatively low stem cell dose. Survival at 3 years was 83% (28). Due to a greater similarity of HLA types among the Japanese populations, many more recipients can find a suitable CB unit compared to other countries.

From a retrospective EUROCORD/EBMT study of 71 patients, median age 13 years (range 2–68), 3 year overall survival was 38%. Better engraftment and survival was observed when a pre-freezing total nucleated cell count >3.9 x 10^7/kg was infused (45%

Figure 2: **Effect of year of transplant on outcome of unrelated donor HSCT**

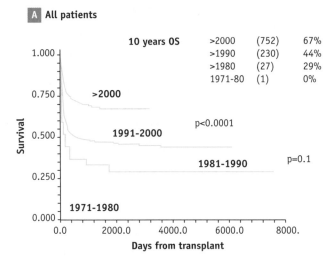

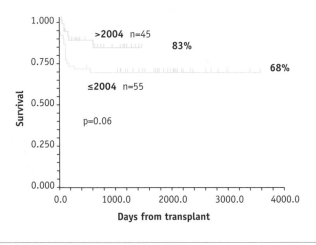

Data from the EBMT SAAWP registry

survival and 58% neutrophil recovery). Grade II-IV acute GvHD was 20%, with 15% limited and 18% extensive chronic GvHD. Infection was the major cause of death (38%) and graft failure (32%) (29).

The optimal conditioning regimen for CBT in SAA is uncertain, but should comprise a FLU-based RIC regimen. The current protocol from the French Society for SCT SAA and CBT uses FLU, CY, ATG and 2Gy TBI. In view of the high graft failure rate, a higher CB stem cell dose is recommended than that for haematological malignancies (30), and units evaluated also on the basis of CD34 and CFU dose whenever possible. The French group recommend a combined frozen TNC for two units should be >5 x 10^7/kg with no more than 2 mismatches between them and the patient (based on low resolution matching at class I (HLA-A and -B) and high resolution matching at class II (HLA-DRB1). Pre-transplant, patients should be screened for HLA antibodies, as workers in Japan have shown that HLA antibodies directed against the corresponding antigens expressed on the cord unit(s) increase the risk of delayed neutrophil and platelet recovery and graft failure after CBT (31).

1.5.2 Haploidentical HSCT
Related haploidentical HSCT is an attractive approach as there is a 50% chance that a sibling is a potential donor. Also, any patient shares a haplotype with one of their biological parents and any of their children. As with CBT, haploidentical HSCT carries a high risk of rejection, and in contrast to CBT, a high risk of severe GvHD. There have been only anecdotal successful reports in children with SAA. One small study used G-CSF mobilised CD34+-selected HSC with FLU 180 mg/m², CY 200 mg/kg and TLI 800 cGy in two patients who both had sustained donor engraftment and no chronic GvHD. One patient had grade I acute GvHD. The third patient who was conditioned with busulfan, CY 120 mg/kg, and FLU 180 mg/m², rejected the graft and died 4 months following a second HSCT (32).

A new approach from the Johns Hopkins group in haematological malignancies has been to use a non-myeloablative conditioning regimen pre-HSCT with high dose CY given on days +3 and +4 post HSCT to prevent GvHD (33). The same group evaluated this in three patients with haemolytic PNH who also had sickle cell disease. CY 14.5 mg/kg/day was given on days -6 to -5, FLU 30 mg/m²/day on days -6 to -2 followed by 2Gy TBI on day -1. On days +3 and +4, CY 50 mg/kg was given, along with MMF and tacrolimus. One patient with fungal sepsis just prior to HSCT died on day +8, but rapid and sustained donor engraftment with no GvHD occurred in the other two patients (34). Further studies using this approach in SAA are warranted.

1.5.3 Immunosuppressive therapy
Current standard first line treatment in Europe for patients, who lack an HLA-

identical family donor, is combined IST with ATG plus CSA. This combination therapy, using horse ATG, provides an overall response rate of 60–70% (35–37). After the withdrawal from the market in 2007 of horse ATG (hATG, Lymphoglobuline®), centres had to use rabbit ATG (Thymoglobuline®) as first line IST. Unfortunately, results obtained with rabbit ATG as first line IST have been discouraging. In the USA, the horse preparation (ATGAM) continues to be used, with similar success rates to Lymphoglobuline®.

The prospective randomised study from NIH, Bethesda showed a far better survival for ATGAM (85%) compared to rabbit ATG (about 55%) and a significantly higher response rate in the horse (69%) compared to the rabbit group (35%; p = 0.0017) (38). Similar results were obtained from a study of the EBMT Severe Aplastic Anemia Working Party (SAAWP), where survival was lower in patients treated upfront with Thymoglobuline® (68%) compared to matched historical controls treated with Lymphoglobuline® (86%), p = 0.009. HSCT-free survival was significantly higher with horse ATG (76%) compared to rabbit ATG (52%; p = 0.002) (39).

Other retrospective studies (40–42) confirmed a better outcome with horse ATG over rabbit ATG. Much fewer studies showed equivalent results between the two preparations (43, 44) and no study has demonstrated superiority of rabbit ATG over horse ATG.

The EBMT SAAWP currently advises that horse ATG (ATGAM) is first line IST for patients ineligible for HLA-identical sibling HSCT. If horse ATG (ATGAM) is not available, it would be reasonable to consider treatment with rabbit ATG even if response rates are lower, rather than no treatment at all (4). However, a lower dose of rabbit ATG (for example, 2.5 mg/kg/day for 5 days) than previously used should be considered on account of a high risk of infection using 3.75 mg/kg/day for 5 days. Alternative IST options include CSA alone. There are only limited data on using alemtuzumab as first line IST in AA (45). Early unrelated donor HSCT using FLU-based conditioning regimens may also be an option in view of improved outcomes.

G-CSF was originally given with ATG and CSA, and for up to 3 months after ATG, to help reduce infection-related mortality which was the primary cause of death (in around 30% of patients). Concerns were raised regarding the increased risk of late clonal diseases after IST regimens containing G-CSF. In this respect data are controversial. One study indicates a significantly higher hazard of MDS/AML associated with the use of G-CSF and a significantly worse outcome of relapse in G-CSF treated patients (46). However, prospective randomised trials showed that the combination of G-CSF plus ATG and CSA reduces the risk of relapse after IST and does not increase the occurrence of MDS/AML (47, 48). The recent prospective controlled study from the SAAWP (49) showed that G-CSF, while not affecting OS, event-free survival, response rate, mortality or relapse occurrence, increased the neutrophil count and reduced infections and days of hospitalisation in the first 3 months of treatment. Moreover, patients on G-CSF achieving neutrophils $\geq$0.5 x 10^9/L by day +30 on G-CSF were significantly more likely to achieve response compared to those who did not.

After failure of first line IST, in the absence of a suitably HLA matched unrelated donor (second choice option), patients can receive another course of IST, using rabbit ATG instead of horse ATG, if horse ATG (ATGAM) is not available. Prior to 2007, rabbit ATG given as second line IST after failure to respond to horse ATG resulted in 30–77% response rate (50, 51).

Alemtuzumab has been used in advanced AA patients who in more than 50% of cases achieved partial or complete, although often not a durable response. Viral infections were not especially frequent but regular monitoring of EBV and CMV viral DNA is recommended (45). Data are lacking on the use of alemtuzumab as first line IST in AA, but the results of a prospective randomised study using alemtuzumab or hATG (ATGAM) or rATG, are awaited from NIH. Responses have been reported using daclizumab (anti IL-2R antibody) in NSAA (52). Anecdotal long-term response was reported with anti TNF-α, though experience is still very limited (53). Other IST options include CY 50 mg/kg/day iv for five days without HSCT rescue resulting in 62 and 48% OS and EFS, respectively, in patients non responsive or refractory to 2 or 3 courses of IST (54). However, the infection risk was very high (49%) and often lethal, associated with prolonged pancytopenia after treatment, so there is less enthusiasm for this approach in Europe.

2. Paroxysmal nocturnal haemoglobinuria

2.1 Introduction

PNH is a rare haematological disorder due to the clonal expansion of abnormal haematopoietic stem cell(s), carrying a mutation in the *PIG-A gene*. PNH can arise *de novo*, or in the setting of acquired aplastic anaemia. Patients with the classical form of PNH tend to have a large percentage of PNH cells by flow cytometry, an elevated reticulocyte count, a normocellular bone marrow, and markedly elevated levels of lactate dehydrogenase (LDH). Their clinical picture is dominated by haemolysis and related manifestations and symptoms. Patients with acquired AA often have small populations of PNH cells and represent an overlap between AA and PNH (AA/PNH); they usually present with more severe peripheral cytopenias, a hypocellular bone marrow, a low reticulocyte count (not adequate for the Hb level), normal to mildly elevated levels of LDH. Thrombosis events can occur in both classic and AA/PNH and represent the main prognosis factor (55).

2.2 Non-transplant therapy: eculizumab and SAA

Recent studies in classic PNH have focused on inhibiting the complement cascade. Eculizumab is a humanised anti-complement component 5 (C5) monoclonal antibody (56), which inhibits C5 cleavage and prevents downstream assembly of the membrane attack complex. Eculizumab has proven highly effective in controlling intravascular haemolysis in PNH patients, leading to reduced transfusion requirement, haemoglobin stabilisation and resolution of all haemolysis-related symptoms (57, 58). The sustained control of intravascular haemolysis results in transfusion-independence in about half of the patients, with an excellent safety profile and negligible side effects (all patients need to be vaccinated against *Neisseria meningitidis*). In addition, eculizumab has proven effective in reducing the risk of thromboembolic events (59). Given that thrombosis (together with complications of marrow failure) is the main cause of death of PNH patients, it is expected that eculizumab should result in a remarkable improvement of survival, as recently shown in a preliminary analysis of a UK PNH patient cohort (60). Eculizumab should thus be offered as first treatment to all symptomatic classic PNH patients. Conversely, patients who meet criteria for severe AA with or without a PNH clone are currently managed with either HSCT or IST depending on the age of the patient and the availability of a suitable HLA-matched related donor (61).

2.3 HSCT for PNH: indications and results

HSCT has proven effective in eradicating the abnormal PNH clone, possibly leading to definitive cure of PNH (62–64); however, morbidity and mortality remain a major limitation. Large prospective studies of BMT for PNH are limited due to the rarity of the disease, and most case series suffer from obvious selection bias (65). There are to date only 2 registry studies. The Centre for International Blood and Marrow Transplant Registry (CIBMTR) reported the outcome of 57 consecutive allogeneic HSCT for PNH reported between 1978 and 1995 (66). The 2-year probability of survival in 48 recipients of HLA-identical sibling transplants was 56% (95% confidence interval 49–63%), and the median follow-up was 44 months. The most common causes of treatment failure were inadequate engraftment (n=7) and infections (n=3). Sixteen were grafted for PNH/AA. The incidence of acute GvHD of grade II or more was 34%, and chronic GvHD was 33%. A recent retrospective study from the GITMO on 26 PNH patients (4 AA/PNH) transplanted between 1998 and 2006 showed a 10-year survival of 57%. Acute and chronic GvHD were 42% (grade III-IV 12%) and 50% (extensive in 16%), respectively. In this series, TRM was higher in RIC transplants (63%, n=11) in comparison to myeloablative transplants (26%, n=15), possibly because more sick patients received a RIC regimen (however the RIC group included a higher number of UD transplants) (67).

The place of RIC regimens is still open (68) as well as the feasibility of HSCT from an unrelated donor (69, 70).

The most difficult task today is to identify PNH patients who could benefit from HSCT (61, 71). The main indication for BMT for PNH patients is concomitant AA, making the AA treatment algorithm described above applicable to all AA/PNH patients as well. Eculizumab has no effect on the underlying stem cell abnormality and should not be used in this indication. Refractoriness to transfusions and life-threatening thrombosis were also indications to BMT in the past, but today they represent indications for anti-complement treatment, with the exception of countries where eculizumab is not yet available. However, given that eculizumab is not a curative treatment and that clinical benefit may be heterogeneous, HSCT remains a worthy second-line therapy for the few patients not achieving a good response to eculizumab. As for AA, clonal evolution to MDS or even AML is a rare but possible occurrence in PNH; HSCT (either from sibling or UD) is the treatment of choice.

The role of BMT in PNH still carries a number of open issues, which can only be answered in large studies (71). The places of RIC regimens as well as UDs are still uncertain. Based on available data, AA/PNH patients should be treated as non-PNH AA patients; thus, the conditioning should be CY/ATG for sibling transplants, and FLU-based RIC for UD HSCT (to be performed as in case of failure of IST) (21). In contrast, classic, non-hypoplastic, PNH patients receiving HSCT should benefit from a myeloablative conditioning (e.g. busulfan-based) (72); however, RIC regimens (FLU-based) (68) may be appropriate for patients with relevant comorbidities or of older age. The most important issue, when and in whom a transplant should be performed, has never been addressed mainly because a prospective trial comparing alternative treatment strategies is impossible in such a rare disease. The EBMT SAAWP and the French PNH Registry are currently running a joint retrospective study comparing the outcome of all HSCT performed in Europe with the natural history of PNH (in the pre-eculizumab era). The results from this study will guide the future treatment strategy for PNH patients according to the specific disease presentation and complications.

References

1. The complete treatment algorithm for SAA (prepared by EBMT SAAWP) (http://www.ebmt.org/5WorkingParties/AAWP/wparties-aa3.html).
2. Marsh JCW, Ball SE, Cavenagh J, Darbyshire P, Dokal I, Gordon-Smith EC, AJ Keidan AJ, Laurie A, Martin A, Mercieca J, Killick SB, Stewart R, Yin JAL. British Committee for Standards in Haematology (BCSH). Guidelines for the diagnosis and management of aplastic anaemia. Br J Haematol 2009; 147: 43–70.

3. Scheinberg P, Wu CO, Scheinberg P et al. A randomized trial of horse versus rabbit antithymocyte globulin in severe acquired aplastic anemia. Blood (ASH Annual Meeting Abstracts) 2010; 116: LBA-4.

4. European Blood and Marrow Transplant Group Severe Aplastic Anaemia Working Party, writing committee: Dufour C, Bacigalupo A, Socie G, Tichelli A, Risitano AM, Schrezenmeier H, Locasciulli A, Aljurf M, Oneto R, Passweg JR, Marsh JCW. Replacement of horse ATG with rabbit ATG for treatment of aplastic anaemia: A backward step? Lancet (Comment) 2011, in press.

5. Armand P, Antin JH. Allogeneic stem cell transplantation for aplastic anemia. Biol Blood Marrow Transplant 2007; 13: 505–516.

6. Bacigalupo A, Brand R, Oneto R et al. Treatment of acquired severe aplastic anemia: Bone marrow transplantation compared with immunosuppressive therapy – The European Group for Blood and Marrow Transplantation experience. Semin Hematol 2000; 37: 69–80.

7. Storb R, Etzioni R, Anasetti C et al. Cyclophosphamide combined with antithymocyte globulin in preparation for allogeneic marrow transplants in patients with aplastic anemia. Blood 1994; 84: 941–949.

8. Storb R, Leisenring W, Anasetti C et al. Long-term follow-up of allogeneic marrow transplants in patients with aplastic anemia conditioned by cyclophosphamide combined with antithymocyte globulin (letter). Blood 1997; 89: 3890–3891.

9. Champlin RE, Perez WS, Passweg JR et al. Bone marrow transplantation for severe aplastic anemia: A randomized controlled study of conditioning regimens. Blood 2007; 109: 4582–4585.

10. Bacigalupo A, Socie G, Schrezenmeier H et al. Matched sibling transplants for aplastic anemia: Survival advantage for marrow vs peripheral blood transplants in all age groups. Blood 2010; 116: Abstract 523.

11. Maury S, Bacigalupo A, Anderlini P et al. Improving outcome of patients older than 30 years receiving HLA-identical sibling HSCT for severe acquired aplastic anemia using fludarabine-based conditioning: A comparison with conventional conditioning regimen. Haematologica 2009; 94: 1312–1315.

12. Marsh JC, Gupta V, Lim Z et al. Alemtuzumab with fludarabine and cyclophosphamide reduces chronic graft versus host disease after allogeneic stem cell transplantation for acquired aplastic anemia. Blood 2011; 118: 2351–2357.

13. Schrezenmeier H, Passweg JR, Marsh JCW et al. Worse outcome and more chronic GVHD with peripheral blood progenitor cells than bone marrow in HLA-matched sibling donor transplants for young patients with severe acquired aplastic anemia. Blood 2007; 110: 1397–1400.

14. Locatelli F, Bruno B, Zecca M et al. Cyclosporin A and short-term methotrexate versus cyclosporin A as graft versus host disease prophylaxis in patients with severe aplastic anemia given allogeneic bone marrow transplantation from an HLA-identical sibling: Results of a GITMO/EBMT randomized trial. Blood 2000; 96: 1690–1697.

15. Islam MS, Anoop P, Datta-Nemdharry P et al. Implications of CD34+ cell dose on clinical and haematological outcome of allo-SCT for acquired aplastic anaemia. Bone Marrow Transplant 2010; 45: 886–889.

16. Maury S, Balere-Appert ML, Chir Z, Boiron JM, Galambrun C, Yakouben K, et al. French Society of Bone Marrow Transplantation and Cellular Therapy (SFGM-TC). Unrelated stem cell transplantation for severe acquired aplastic anemia: Improved outcome in the era of high-resolution HLA matching between donor and recipient. Haematologica 2007; 92: 589–596.

17. Bacigalupo A, Locatelli F, Lanino E, Marsh J, Socié G, Maury S, et al. Severe Aplastic Anemia Working Party of the European Group for Blood and Marrow Transplantation. Fludarabine, cyclophosphamide and anti-thymocyte globulin for alternative donor transplants in acquired severe aplastic anemia: A report from the EBMT-SAA Working Party. Bone Marrow Transplant 2005; 36: 947–950.

18. Lee SJ, Klein J, Haagenson M et al. High-resolution donor-recipient HLA matching contributes to the success of unrelated donor marrow transplantation. Blood 2007; 110: 4576–4583.

19. Takakazu K, Yasuo M, Keitaro M, Koichi K, Hidetoshi I, Hiroh S, Shunichi K, Takeo J, Yoshihisa K, and Takehiko S, for The Japan Marrow Donor Program. High-risk HLA allele mismatch combinations responsible for severe acute graft-versus-host disease and implication for its molecular mechanism. Blood 2007; 110: 2235–2241.

20. Crocchiolo R, Zino E, Vago L, Oneto R, Bruno B, Pollichieni S, Sacchi N, Sormani MP, Marcon J, Lamparelli T, Fanin R, Garbarino L, Miotti V, Bandini G, Bosi A, Ciceri F, Bacigalupo A, Fleischhauer K; Gruppo Italiano Trapianto di Midollo Osseo, Cellule Staminali Ematopoietiche (CSE) e Terapia Cellulare; Italian Bone Marrow Donor Registry. Nonpermissive HLA-DPB1 disparity is a significant independent risk factor for mortality after unrelated hematopoietic stem cell transplantation. Blood 2009; 114: 1437–1444.

21. Bacigalupo A, Socié G, Lanino E, Prete A, Locatelli F, Locasciulli A, Cesaro S, Shimoni A, Marsh J, Brune M, Van Lint MT, Oneto R, Passweg J; Severe Aplastic Anemia Working Party of the European Group for Blood and Marrow Transplantation. Fludarabine, cyclophosphamide, antithymocyte globulin, with or without low dose total body irradiation, for alternative donor transplants, in acquired severe aplastic anemia: A retrospective study from the EBMT-SAA working party. Haematologica 2010; 95: 976–982.

22. Deeg HJ, Amylon ID, Harris RE et al. Marrow transplants from unrelated donors for patients with aplastic anemia: Minimum effective dose of total body irradiation. Biol Blood Marrow Transplant 2001; 7: 208–215.

23. Kojima S, Matsuyama T, Kato S et al. Outcome of 154 patients with severe aplastic anemia who received transplants from unrelated donors: The Japan Marrow Donor Program. Blood 2002; 100: 799–803.

24. Coppoletta S, Tedone E, Galano B et al. Rituximab treatment for Epstein-Barr virus DNAemia after alternative-donor hematopoietic stem cell transplantation. Biol Blood Marrow Transplant 2011;17: 901–907.

25. Dominietto A, Tedone E, Soracco M et al. In vivo B-cell depletion with rituximab for alternative donor hemopoietic SCT. Bone Marrow Transplant 2011 Apr 4. [Epub ahead of print].

26. Mao P, Zhu Z, Wang H et al. Sustained and stable hematopoietic donor-recipient mixed

chimerism after unrelated cord blood transplantation for adult patients with severe aplastic anemia. Exp Haematol 75: 430–435, 2005.

27. Chan KW, McDonald L, Lim D et al. Unrelated cord blood transplantation in children with idiopathic severe aplastic anemia. Bone Marrow Transplant 42: 589–595.

28. Yoshimi A, Kojima S, Taniguchi S, et al. for the Japan Cord Blood Bank Network (JCBBN). Unrelated cord blood transplantation for severe aplastic anemia. Biol Blood and Marrow Transplant 2008; 14: 1057–1063.

29. de Latour RP, Purtill D, Ruggeri A et al. Influence of nucleated cell dose on overall survival of unrelated cord blood transplantation for patients with severe acquired aplastic anemia: A study by Eurocord and the Aplastic Anemia Working Party of the European Group for Blood and Marrow Transplantation. Biol Blood Marrow Transplant 2010; 17: 78–85.

30. Avery S, Shi W, Lubin M et al. Influence of infused cell dose and HLA match on engraftment after double-unit cord blood allografts. Blood 2011; 117: 3277–3285.

31. Takanashi M, Atsuta Y, Fujiwara K et al. The impact of anti-HLA antibodies on unrelated cord blood transplantation. Blood 2010; 116: 2839–2846.

32. Woodard P, Cunningham JM, Benaim E et al. Effective donor lymphohematopoietic reconstitution after haploidentical CD34+-selected hematopoietic stem cell transplantation in children with refractory severe aplastic anemia. Bone Marrow Transplant 2004; 33: 411–418.

33. O'Donnell PV, Luznik L, Jones RJ et al. Non-myeloablative bone marrow transplantation from partially mismatched related donors using post transplant cyclophosphamide. Biol Blood Marrow Transplant 2002; 8: 377–386.

34. Brodsky RA, Luznik L, Bolaños-Meade J et al. Reduced intensity HLA-haploidentical BMT with post transplantation cyclophosphamide in nonmalignant hematologic diseases. Bone Marrow Transplant 2008; 42: 523–527.

35. Locasciulli A, Oneto R, Bacigalupo A et al. Outcome of patients with acquired aplastic anemia given first line bone marrow transplantation or immunosuppressive treatment in the last decade: A report from the European Group for Blood and Marrow Transplantation (EBMT). Haematologica 2007; 92: 11–18.

36. Bacigalupo A, Bruno B, Saracco P et al. Antilymphocyte globulin, cyclosporine, prednisolone, and granulocyte colony-stimulating factor for severe aplastic anemia: An update of the GITMO/EBMT study on 100 patients. European Group for Blood and Marrow Transplantation (EBMT) Working Party on Severe Aplastic Anemia and the Gruppo Italiano Trapianti di Midollo Osseo (GITMO). Blood 2000; 95: 1931–1934.

37. Rosenfeld S, Follmann D, Nunez O, Young NS. Antithymocyte globulin and cyclosporine for severe aplastic anemia: Association between hematologic response and long-term outcome. JAMA 2003; 289: 1130–1135.

38. Scheinberg P, Wu CO, Scheinberg P et al. A randomized trial of horse versus rabbit antithymocyte globulin in severe acquired aplastic anemia. Blood (ASH Annual Meeting Abstracts). 2010; 116: LBA.

39. Marsh J, Socie G, Tichelli A, Bacigalupo A, Risitano AM, Schrezenmeier H, Sedgwick P, Oneto R, Barrois A, Passweg J on behalf of the EBMT Severe Aplastic Anaemia (SAA) Working Party. Prospective phase II pilot study of rabbit antithymocyte globulin with ciclosporin

for patients with acquired aplastic anaemia and matched pair analysis with patients treated with horse ATG and ciclosporin. Bone Marrow Transplant 2011; 46: (S1): 208.

40. Atta EA, Dias SP, Marra VLN, de Azevedo, AM. Comparison between horse and rabbit antithymocyte globulin as first line treatment for patients with severe aplastic anemia: A single centre retrospective study. Ann Hematol 2010; 89: 851–859

41. Halkes CJM, Brand A, von dem Borne PA et al. Increasing the dose of rabbit-ATG does not lead to a higher response rate in the first-line treatment of severe aplastic anaemia. Bone Marrow Transplant 2011; 46: S90–S389. doi:10.1038/bmt.2011.48.

42. Saracco P, Lorenzati A, Oneto R et al, on behalf of the AIEOP Bone Marrow Failure Study Group. Italian registry of pediatric acquired aplastic anaemia: A retrospective study. Bone Marrow Transplant 2011; 46: S90-S389. doi:10.1038/bmt.2011.48.

43. Vallejo C, Montesinos P, Rosell A et al. Comparison between lymphoglobuline- and thymoglobuline-based immunosuppressive therapy as first-line treatment for patients with aplastic anemia. Blood 2009; 114: 3194a.

44. Afable MG, Shaik M, Sugimoto Y et al. Efficacy of rabbit antithymocyte globulin in severe aplastic anemia. Haematologica 2011; 96: 1269–1275.

45. Risitano AM, Selleri C, Serio B, Torelli GF, Kulagin A, Maury S, Halter J, Gupta V, Bacigalupo A, Sociè G, Tichelli A, Schrezenmeier H, Marsh J, Passweg J, Rotoli B; on behalf of the Working Party Severe Aplastic Anaemia (WPSAA) of the European Group for Blood and Marrow Transplantation (EBMT). Alemtuzumab is safe and effective as immunosuppressive treatment for aplastic anaemia and single-lineage marrow failure: A pilot study and a survey from the EBMT WPSAA. Br J Haematol 2010; 148: 791–796.

46. Sociè G, Mary JY, Schrezenmeier H et al. Granulocyte-stimulating factor and severe aplastic anemia: A survey by the European Group for Blood and Marrow Transplantation. Blood 2007; 109: 2794–2796.

47. Teramura M, Kimura A, Iwase S et al.Treatment of severe aplastic anemia with antithymocyte globulin and cyclosporin A with or without G-CSF in adults: A multicenter randomized study in Japan. Blood 2007; 110: 1756–1761.

48. Gluckman E, Rokicka-Milewka R, Hann I et al. Results and follow-up of a phase III randomized study of recombinant human- granulocyte stimulating factor as support for immunosuppressive therapy in patients with severe aplastic anaemia. Br J Haematol 2002; 119: 1075–1082.

49. Tichelli A, Schrezenmeier H, Socié G, Marsh J, Bacigalupo A, Dührsen U, Franzke A, Hallek M, Thiel E, Wilhelm M, Höchsmann B, Barrois A, Champion K, Passweg JR. A randomized controlled study in patients with newly diagnosed severe aplastic anemia receiving antithymocyte globulin (ATG), cyclosporine, with or without G-CSF: A study of the SAA Working Party of the European Group for Blood and Marrow Transplantation. Blood 2011; 117: 4434–4441.

50. Scheinberg P, Nunez O, Young N. Re-treatment with rabbit antithymocyte globulin and ciclosporin for patients with relapsed or refractory severe aplastic anaemia. Br J Haematol 2006; 133: 622–627.

51. Di Bona E, Rodeghiero F, Bruno B, Gabbas A, Foa P, Locasciulli A, Rosanelli C, Camba L, Saracco P, Lippi A, Iori AP, Porta F, De Rossi G, Comotti B, Iacopino P, Dufour C,

Bacigalupo A. Rabbit antithymocyte globulin (r-ATG) plus cyclosporine and granulocyte colony stimulating factor is an effective treatment for aplastic anaemia patients unresponsive to a first course of intensive immunosuppressive therapy. Gruppo Italiano Trapianto di Midollo Osseo (GITMO). Br J Haematol 1999; 107: 330–334.

52. Sloand EM, Olnes MJ, Weinstein B et al. Long-term follow-up of patients with moderate aplastic anemia and pure red cell aplasia treated with daclizumab. Haematologica 2010; 95: 382–387.

53. Dufour C, Giacchino R, Ghezzi P et al. Etanercept as a salvage treatment for refractory aplastic anemia. Pediatr Blood Cancer 2009; 52: 522–525.

54. Brodsky RA, Chen AR, Dorr D et al. High dose cyclophosphamide for severe aplastic anemia: Long-term follow-up. Blood 2010; 115: 2136–2141.

55. de Latour RP, Mary JY, Salanoubat C, Terriou L, Etienne G, Mohty M, Roth S, de Guibert S, Maury S, Cahn JY, Socié G, French Society of Hematology, French Association of Young Hematologists. Paroxysmal nocturnal hemoglobinuria: Natural history of disease subcategories. Blood 2008; 112: 3099–3106.

56. Rother RP, Rollins SA, Mojcik CF et al. Discovery and development of the complement inhibitor eculizumab for the treatment of paroxysmal nocturnal hemoglobinuria. Nat Biotechnol 2007; 25: 1256–1264.

57. Hillmen P, Young NS, Schubert J et al. The complement inhibitor eculizumab in paroxysmal nocturnal hemoglobinuria. N Engl J Med 2006; 355: 1233–1243.

58. Brodsky RA, Young NS, Antonioli E et al. Multicenter phase III study of the complement inhibitor eculizumab for the treatment of patients with paroxysmal nocturnal hemoglobinuria. Blood 2008; 114: 1840–1847.

59. Hillmen P, Muus P, Dührsen U et al. Effect of the complement inhibitor eculizumab on thromboembolism in patients with paroxysmal nocturnal hemoglobinuria. Blood 2007; 110: 4123–4128.

60. Kelly RJ, Hill A, Arnold LM et al. Long term treatment with eculizumab in paroxysmal nocturnal hemoglobinuria: Sustained efficacy and improved survival. Blood 2011; 117: 6786–6792.

61. Young NS, Scheinberg P, Calado T. Aplastic anemia. Curr Opin Hematol 2008; 15: 162–168.

62. Szer J, Deeg J, Witherspoon R, et al. Long-term survival after marrow transplantation for paroxysmal nocturnal hemoglobinuria with aplastic anemia. Ann Intern Med 1984; 101: 193–195.

63. Antin JH, Ginsburg D, Smith BR et al. Bone marrow transplantation for paroxysmal nocturnal hemoglobinuria: Eradication of the PNH clone and documentation of complete lymphohematopoietic engraftment. Blood 1985; 66: 1247–1250.

64. Bemba M, Guardiola P, Gardret L et al. Bone marrow transplantation for paroxysmal nocturnal haemoglobinuria. Br J Haematol 1999; 105 :366–368.

65. Matos-Fernandez NA, Abou Mourad YR, Caceres W, Kharfan-Dabaja MA. Current status of allogeneic hematopoietic stem cell transplantation for paroxysmal nocturnal hemoglobinuria. Biol Blood Marrow Transplant 2009; 15: 656–661.

66. Saso R, Marsh J, Cevreska L et al. Bone marrow transplants for paroxysmal nocturnal haemoglobinuria. Br J Haematol 1999; 105: 366–368.

67. Santarone S, Bacigalupo A, Risitano AM, Tagliaferri E, Di Bartolomeo E, Iori AP, Rambaldi A, Angelucci E, Spagnoli A, Papineschi F, Tamiazzo S, Di Nicola M, Di Bartolomeo P. Hematopoietic stem cell transplantation for paroxysmal nocturnal hemoglobinuria: long-term results of a retrospective study on behalf of the Gruppo Italiano Trapianto Midollo Osseo (GITMO). Haematologica 2010; 95: 983–988.
68. Takahashi Y, McCoy JP Jr., Carvallo C et al. In vitro and in vivo evidence of PNH cell sensitivity to immune attack after nonmyeloablative allogeneic hematopoietic cell transplantation. Blood 2004; 103: 1383–1390.
69. Hegenbart U, Niederwieser D, Forman S et al. Haematopoietic cell transplantation from related and unrelated donors after minimal conditioning as curative treatment modality for severe paroxysmal nocturnal hemoglobinuria. Biol Blood Marrow Transplant 2003; 9: 689–697.
70. Woodard P, Wang W, Pitts N et al. Successful unrelated donor bone marrow transplantation for paroxysmal nocturnal hemoglobinuria. Bone Marrow Transplant 2001; 27: 589–592.
71. Brodsky RA. Stem cell transplantation for paroxysmal nocturnal hemoglobinuria. Haematologica 2010; 95: 855–856.
72. Raiola AM, Lint Van, Lamparelli T et al. Bone marrow transplantation for paroxysmal nocturnal hemoglobinuria. Haematologica 2000; 85: 59–62.

Multiple Choice Questionnaire

To find the correct answer, go to http://www.esh.org/online-training/handbook/

1. **Which one of the following statements about the diagnosis of aplastic anaemia (AA) is *not* correct?**
   a) Is based on both peripheral blood and bone marrow findings............☐
   b) Bone marrow aspirate findings are sufficient and a biopsy is not essential...☐
   c) Hypocellular MDS is a common differential diagnosis in older patients ..☐
   d) Fanconi anaemia may occur in adults...☐

2. **Which one of the following statements about HLA-matched sibling HSCT is *not* correct?**
   a) Is not indicated for young patients with non-severe AA who are transfusion independent ....☐
   b) Is indicated as first line treatment for severe AA in patients up to the age of 50 years ....☐

c) Irradiation should be included as part of the conditioning regimen to reduce the risk of graft rejection .... ☐

d) High dose cyclophosphamide 200 mg/kg is a standard part of the conditioning regimen for young patients .... ☐

3. **Which one of the following statements about unrelated donor HSCT is *not* correct?**

a) Is indicated after failure to respond to at least two courses of immunosuppressive therapy .... ☐

b) Recent studies indicate on overall survival of at least 75% .... ☐

c) Fludarabine is recommended as part of the conditioning regimen .... ☐

d) Graft rejection occurs in around 10–20% of patients .... ☐

4. **Which one of the following is correct about the use of G-CSF in the treatment of AA?**

a) Is one of the options for first line treatment of AA .... ☐

b) Does not improve the response rate to ATG and cyclosporin .... ☐

c) Results in improved survival after ATG and cyclosporin .... ☐

d) Is routinely recommended after ATG and cyclosporin treatment .... ☐

5. **Regarding PNH, which of the following is *not* correct?**

a) Small PNH clones are rarely found in patients with AA .... ☐

b) HSCT for PNH is associated with a significant risk of GvHD .... ☐

c) HSCT is not indicated as first line treatment for uncomplicated haemolytic PNH .... ☐

d) The monoclonal antibody eculizumab (Soliris®) is not a curative treatment for PNH .... ☐

* CHAPTER 20

HSCT for children and adolescents

---

* 20.1
Acute myeloid leukaemia

Giorgio Dini, Stefano Giardino

1. Introduction

The prognosis of acute myeloid leukaemia (AML) in children has significantly improved over the past two decades: with intensive chemotherapy 80–90% of children achieve complete remission (CR) and 30–70% are cured if they receive post induction chemotherapy (1). Hence, HSCT is not recommended as frontline therapy for good-risk patients with AML (2).

2. Indications

Matched related donor (MRD) transplantation in CR1 represents an attractive option for children with high-risk (HR) AML (3) as it was proven to be more efficient than chemotherapy in a number of comparative studies, with event-free-survival (EFS) ranging from 55 to 72%. However, since approximately 60% of children lack an MRD, the pros and cons of alternative approaches must be carefully weighed on a case-by-case basis. Recently, the European Group for Blood and Marrow Transplantation (EBMT) published indications for HSCT in all diseases, including AML. These are shown in Table 1 (4).

Table 1: Indications for HSCT for children with acute myeloid leukaemia

Disease	Status	Sibling donor	Well matched unrelated/ 1 Ag related	Mismatched unrelated/ >1 Ag related	Auto-HSCT
AML	CR1 low-risk	GNR	GNR	GNR	GNR
	CR1 high-risk	S	CO	GNR	S
	CR1 very high-risk	S	S	CO	GNR
	CR2	S	S	S	S
	>CR2	CO	D	D	GNR

S: standard of care; generally indicated in suitable patients. CO: clinical option; can be carried out after careful assessment of risks and benefits. D: developmental; further trials are needed. GNR: generally not recommended. NA: not applicable. CR1, 2: first, second complete remission. Ag: antigen. This classification does not cover patients for whom a syngeneic donor is available

3. Conditioning regimens

Most teams currently use non-TBI-containing regimens for patients transplanted for AML in either first or subsequent remission. Busulfan and cyclophosphamide (BU-Cy) are the most commonly administered drugs, and in the majority of cases are supplemented with melphalan (5).

Because TBI was found to have no favourable impact on EFS in children undergoing HSCT for AML in first complete remission, and because of its deleterious late effects, it should no longer be administered to this subset of patients. Currently, fractionated TBI-containing regimens are being employed by some groups in selected advanced cases (6).

Treosulphan, a structural analogue of busulfan, has recently begun to be used in the preparative therapy of paediatric recipients of allogeneic HSCT for several malignant (including AML) and non-malignant diseases. Data show that conditioning regimens containing treosulphan and fludarabine are well-tolerated and yield encouraging results with minimal treatment-related-mortality (TRM) (7).

4. Role and outcome of autologous transplant
In the recent past, autologous HSCT (auto-HSCT) has been widely used as consolidation treatment after induction therapy in children with HR AML in CR1 or CR2 who lack an MRD. However, the results of paediatric studies comparing auto-HSCT to chemotherapy and autologous versus allogeneic HSCT are conflicting. It is currently believed that auto-HSCT (with *in vitro* purging) as consolidation therapy in patients in CR1 does not represent a valid alternative to multi-drug chemotherapy in the low risk group or to allo-HSCT (from MRD or UD) in higher risk groups. Data concerning adults confirm that performing early allo-HSCT led to better overall results than auto-HSCT, especially for younger patients or for those with bad/very bad risk cytogenetics (8).

Further randomised clinical trials are needed to address the pivotal clinical question of whether auto-HSCT is better than chemotherapy or allograft as consolidation treatment for childhood AML in first CR.

4.1. Open questions and future directions in auto-HSCT
Use of peripheral blood progenitor cells. Peripheral blood progenitor cells (PBPCs) are not often used for autologous HSCT in children with AML. This is mainly due to the difficulty in collecting adequate amounts of circulating haematopoietic progenitor cells, and also the lack of a clear benefit that is observed in this subset of children when PBPCs are used to accelerate the recovery of haematopoiesis.

Role of haematopoietic growth factors. The beneficial impact of haematopoietic growth factors on myeloid recovery in children undergoing autologous HSCT for AML has not been proven, and given the cost of these cytokines, their use in this subset of patients should be avoided.

In vitro purging. In vitro purging is associated with reduced RR (p=0.04) (5). These data (5) suggest that *in vitro* purging should be performed before carrying out autologous transplantation in childhood AML. Delayed platelet engraftment is one of the drawbacks that may be observed.

5. Role and outcome of HLA-identical sibling transplant
Several randomised trials have shown the statistically significant superiority of MRD

HSCT as compared to all other options. This, in turn, is correlated with longer periods of "quality of life time" (3). In a recent, single-centre, retrospective study involving 55 children given MRD HSCT for CR1 AML, the 5-year probability of survival was 74%, whereas the 5-year probability of relapse was 26% (10). None of the patients who developed acute GvHD relapsed, confirming a graft versus leukaemia (GvL) effect following allogeneic HSCT for AML. Better EFS among the older children receiving a higher dose of TBI was observed in this study. This issue was recently confirmed by a review of the literature comparing various TBI regimens (11).

6. Role and outcome of unrelated donor (UD) transplant
There is an absolute indication for UD HSCT in infant AML and in children with FAB M 7 AML, who stand a very poor chance of being cured by chemotherapy or by autologous HSCT. FAB M 0 or M 6 represent more controversial indications. Timing in the identification of a suitable donor constitutes a limiting factor for this subset of patients.
As compared to Unrelated Cord Blood Transplantation (UCBT), UD HSCT has shown a similar incidence of grade III-IV acute GvHD and a higher incidence of chronic GvHD, while 2 year overall survival is similar (12).
A recent study from the USA has shown that the 5-year EFS of children given an 8/8 allele matched UD HSCT is similar to results obtained with a 1 or 2 antigen mismatched UCBT. TRM is slightly higher and relapse rate is lower after a 2 antigen mismatched UCBT (13).

7. Role and outcome of cord blood transplant
Eurocord recently reported that the EFS of children with AML in CR 1 and in CR 2 is 57 and 47%, respectively, while the RR is 10% in CR1 and 23% in CR2. The main prognostic factors are disease stage and number of infused cells (14).

8. Role and outcome of haploidentical transplants
The results reported by the Perugia Group in patients with AML undergoing haploidentical HSCT showed that NK cells have an impressive effect on alloreactivity. In fact, no relapses occurred among the patients transplanted from haploidentical donors with a KIR mismatch in the GvL direction, suggesting that the haploidentical option may play a role in the early phase of treatment for very high-risk AML patients. *In vitro* studies have confirmed that alloreactive NK clones exert a potent cytotoxic activity against the leukaemic cells taken from patients with CML and AML (15). More recently, several paediatric teams have begun to investigate the use of haploidentical HSCT in children with no other allogeneic donor options, or with an

urgent need to proceed to transplant. Preliminary results confirm that the outcome of children in remission is similar to what can be achieved by using other donor stem cell sources (16).

9. Role and outcome of transplant for AML in relapse or primary induction failure

HSCT represents the only chance of being cured for children who are refractory to initial or reinduction chemotherapy and for relapsing children.

Patients with primary induction failure who undergo transplantation have the best prognosis if they are transplanted as soon as possible, which suggests that HSCT should be considered early on in patients resistant to initial induction chemotherapy. Indeed, additional chemotherapy could result in toxicity that might limit the success of transplantation.

Five risk factors associated with better outcome have been used to establish a prognostic scoring system for children who undergo transplantation while in relapse. These are CR1 duration >6 months, absence of blasts in the blood, an available MRD, performance score >90%, and standard-risk cytogenetics. Higher-risk patients had a 3-year survival of 6%, whereas 3-year survival for lower-risk patients was 42%. The type of conditioning regimen, GvHD prophylaxis, and graft source does not affect outcome (17).

10. Graft-versus-leukaemia effect and role of donor lymphocyte infusion

The role of GvL activity in the eradication of AML is not fully known. Early reports from the Centre for International Blood and Marrow Transplant Research (CIBMTR) suggested that AML patients who developed GvHD had a lower relapse rate (18). Studies on post-remission therapy in AML have consistently reported a decreased incidence of relapse after allogeneic transplantation as compared with autologous transplantation. The evidence that T-cell depletion increases relapse in AML patients following transplantation is relatively weak. The outcomes of patients receiving T-cell-depleted transplants in AML are similar to those infused with T-cell-replete haematopoietic stem cells. This contrasts with reports on CML patients in whom T-cell depletion led to higher relapse rates. On the other hand, the success of non-myeloablative transplantation for AML supports the importance of GvL activity in AML. Long-term remissions of 15–30% have been reported in patients who were transplanted following non-myeloablative conditioning despite active advanced leukaemia (19). Relapse rates are lower in patients developing chronic GvHD (20). The most recent comprehensive assessment of donor lymphocyte infusion (DLI) in AML was conducted by the European Group for Blood and Marrow Transplantation and was published in 2007 (21). In this retrospective analysis, 399 patients with AML in first haematological relapse following transplantation were evaluated. One hundred and seventy-one patients received DLI as part of their treatment, whereas 228 did not. In this study, patients receiving DLI with or without additional stem cell products in the absence of immunosuppression were included in the DLI group. Estimated survival at 2 years was higher in the 171 patients receiving DLI compared with the 228 patients who did not receive DLI (21 vs 9%), despite the fact that a smaller number of patients in the DLI group went on to second allogeneic HSCT compared with the non-DLI group (13 vs 33). After adjusting for all the clinical variables in the two groups, several factors emerged that appeared to be associated with improved outcome. These included younger patient age (p <0.008), relapse occurring more than 5 months following transplantation (p <0.0001), and DLI administration (p <0.04).

A multi-centre study in children with AML showed that despite early DLI, relapse was still significantly more frequent in patients with increasing mixed chimaerism (MC) than it was in patients with complete chimerism (CC), low-level MC (i.e. low level of host cells) or decreasing MC. Patients with increasing MC who received early DLI showed a significantly higher probability of EFS than patients with increasing MC who did not undergo immunological intervention. These results demonstrate that paediatric AML patients with increasing MC are at highest risk of relapse, and that early DLI can prevent relapse in these patients (22).

11. A treatment algorithm

A suitably matched UD (8/8 or 10/10 allele matched) can usually be located within 4 to 6 weeks for children with the most common haplotypes who lack an MRD. Alternative treatment options should be offered to children with rare HLA types, and a decision should be made as to whether to reduce the matching requirements or to select another type of therapy, such as UCBT or haploidentical HSCT. A matched or 1 antigen mismatched CB unit containing more than 3×10^7 mononuclear cells should be considered equivalent to an 8/8 allele matched UD. The decision should be made based on the urgency of the HSCT. Haploidentical HSCT should be offered if no donors and no CB units with the above mentioned characteristics are available. Some teams consider haploidentical HSCT the second option when an acceptable unrelated donor is not available.

Acknowledgements
G Dini thanks V Perricone for revising the manuscript.

References

1. Creutzig U, Ritter J, Schellong G for the AML-BFM Study Group. Identification of two risk groups in childhood acute myelogenous leukemia after therapy intensification in study AML-BFM-83 compared with study AML-BFM-78. Blood 1990; 75: 1932–1940.
2. Gibson BE, Wheatley K, Hann IM et al. Treatment strategy and long-term results in paediatric patients treated in consecutive UK AML trials. Leukemia 2005; 19: 2130–2138.
3. Woods WG, Neudorf S, Gold S et al. A comparison of allogeneic bone marrow transplantation, autologous bone marrow transplantation, and aggressive chemotherapy in children with acute myeloid leukaemia in remission: A report from the Children's Cancer Group. Blood 2001; 97: 56–62.
4. Ljungman P, Bregni M, Brune M et al. for the European Group for Blood and Marrow Transplantation. Allogeneic and autologous transplantation for haematological diseases, solid tumours and immune disorders: Current practice in Europe 2009. Bone Marrow Transplant 2010; 45: 219–234.
5. Vettenranta K on behalf of the Pediatric Diseases Working Party of the EBMT. Current European practice in pediatric myeloablative conditioning. Bone Marrow Transplant 2008; 41: S14–S17.
6. Nemecek ER, Gooley TA, Woolfrey AE et al. Outcome of allogeneic bone marrow transplantation for children with advanced acute myeloid leukemia. Bone Marrow Transplant 2004; 34: 799–806.
7. Nemecek ER, Guthrie KA, Sorror ML et al. Conditioning with treosulfan and fludarabine followed by allogeneic hematopoietic cell transplantation for high-risk hematologic malignancies. Biol Blood Marrow Transplant 2011; 17: 341–350.
8. Suciu S, Mandelli F, de Witte T et al. for the EORTC and GIMEMA Leukemia Groups. Allogeneic compared with autologous stem cell transplantation in the treatment of patients younger than 46 years with acute myeloid leukemia (AML) in first complete remission (CR1): An intention-to-treat analysis of the EORTC/GIMEMA AML-10 trial. Blood 2003; 102: 1232–1240.
9. Locatelli F, Labopin M, Ortega J et al. Factors influencing outcome and incidence of long-term complications in children who underwent autologous stem cell transplantation for acute myeloid leukaemia. Blood 2003; 101: 1611–1619.
10. Willemze AJ, Geskus RB, Noordijk et al. HLA-identical haematopoietic stem cell transplantation for acute leukaemia in children: Less relapse with higher biologically effective dose of TBI. Bone Marrow Transplant 2007; 39: 1–9.
11. Kal HB, Loes van Kempen-Harteveld M, Heijenbrok-Kal MH et al. Biologically effective dose in total-body irradiation and hematopoietic stem cell transplantation. Strahlenther Onkol 2006; 182: 672–679.
12. Hwang WY, Samuel M, Tan D et al. A meta-analysis of unrelated donor umbilical cord blood transplantation versus unrelated donor bone marrow transplantation in adult and pediatric patients. Biol Blood Marrow Transplant 2007; 13: 444–453.
13. Eapen M, Rubinstein P, Zhang MJ et al. Outcomes of transplantation of unrelated donor umbilical cord blood and bone marrow in children with acute leukaemia: A comparison study. Lancet 2007; 369: 1947–1954.

14. Gluckman E, Rocha V on behalf of Eurocord and Paediatric WP of EBMT. Indications and results of cord blood transplant in children with leukaemia. Bone Marrow Transplant 2008; 41: S80–S82.
15. Aversa F, Tabilio A, Velardi A et al. Transplantation of high-risk acute leukemia with T-cell-depleted stem cells from related donor with one fully mismatched HLA haplotype. N Engl J Med 1998; 339: 1186–1193.
16. Marks DI., Khattry N, Cummins M et al. Haploidentical stem cell transplantation for children with acute leukaemia. Br J Haematol 2006; 134: 196–201.
17. Duval M, Klein JP, Wensheng H et al. Hematopoietic stem-cell transplantation for acute leukemia in relapse or primary induction failure. J Clin Oncol 2010; 28: 3730–3738.
18. Soiffer RJ. Donor lymphocyte infusions for acute myeloid leukaemia. Best Pract Res Clin Haematol 2008; 21: 455–466.
19. Baron F, Maris MB, Sanmaier BM et al. Graft-versus-tumor effects after allogeneic hematopoietic cell transplantation with nonmyeloablative conditioning. J Clin Oncol 2005; 23: 1993–2003.
20. Alyea EP, Kim HT, Ho V et al. Impact of conditioning regimen intensity on outcome of allogeneic hematopoietic cell transplantation for advanced acute myelogenous leukemia and myelodysplastic syndrome. Biol Blood Marrow Transplant 2006; 12: 1047–1055.
21. Schmid C, Labopin M, Nagler A et al. Donor lymphocyte infusion in the treatment of first haematological relapse after allogeneic stem-cell transplantation in adults with acute myeloid leukemia: A retrospective risk factors analysis and comparison with other strategies by the EBMT Acute Leukemia Working Party. J Clin Oncol 2007; 25: 4938–4945.
22. Bader P, Kreyenberg H, Hoelle W et al. Increasing mixed chimerism defines a high-risk group of childhood acute myelogenous leukemia patients after allogeneic stem cell transplantation where pre-emptive immunotherapy may be effective. Bone Marrow Transplant 2004; 33: 815–821.

Multiple Choice Questionnaire

To find the correct answer, go to http://www.esh.org/online-training/handbook/

1. **The standard treatment for patients with high-risk AML in CR1 is:**
    a) Allogeneic HSCT .... ☐
    b) Autologous HSCT .... ☐
    c) Chemotherapy .... ☐
    d) Radiotherapy .... ☐

2. **The main risk factor for EFS in patients receiving allogeneic HSCT for AML is:**

a) Age.. ☐
b) LDH levels before HSCT.. ☐
c) FAB Classification... ☐
d) WBC count... ☐

3. **The standard treatment for patients suffering from low risk AML in CR1 is:**
   a) Allogeneic HSCT... ☐
   b) Autologous HSCT.. ☐
   c) Chemotherapy.. ☐
   d) Radiotherapy... ☐

4. **For patients with AML in CR2, which of the following criteria selects those who should receive allogeneic HSCT?**
   a) Age... ☐
   b) LDH levels.. ☐
   c) All patients represent an indication......................... ☐
   d) WBC count... ☐

5. **Which of the following is true for allogeneic HSCT for patients suffering from AML in CR2?**
   a) Generally indicated in suitable patients.................... ☐
   b) Not recommended .... ☐
   c) A developmental option to be demonstrated with further trials.......... ☐
   d) Indicated after relapse following autologous HSCT........................ ☐

NOTES

* CHAPTER 20

HSCT for children and adolescents

* 20.2
Acute lymphoblastic leukaemia

Christina Peters

1. Introduction

The majority of patients with childhood acute lymphoblastic leukaemia (ALL) have nowadays an excellent chance to be cured by multimodal chemotherapy (1). However, patients with very high-risk ALL (HR-ALL) or patients who have relapsed have a significantly worse prognosis (2). These patients require additional therapeutic approaches after achieving remission. Allogeneic HSCT can effectively induce immunological antileukaemic control in patients with ALL by means of the graft-versus-leukaemia effect (GvL), but treatment related mortality (TRM) remains a serious problem (3). In addition, the heterogeneity of available data regarding patient selection, transplantation procedures and study endpoints hampers the interpretation of the value of HSCT. Consequently, all patients with an indication for HSCT should be treated within prospective clinical trials in order to ensure best clinical practice and to acquire valid outcome data.

2. Prognostic factors and indications for HSCT

HSCT indications have to be defined prospectively and must be re-evaluated and reconfirmed at intervals dependent on modifications and improvements in chemotherapeutical approaches for both frontline and relapse protocols. Some risk factors conveying a dismal prognosis in childhood ALL can be identified even at diagnosis (e.g. cytogenetic characteristics) (4). Additionally, response to induction treatment measured by morphology and/or detection of minimal residual disease (MRD) has a strong predictive value and defines some indications for HSCT (5, 6). Time and site of relapse are also important prognostic factors in relapsed patients.

2.1 Indications: CR1

The indication for HSCT in children with ALL in CR1 is limited to the subpopulation of high-risk ALL. Most study groups define these patients as having an estimated EFS of less than 50%. The factors indicating a high risk of relapse are known molecular biological markers or chromosomal abnormalities, and biological factors including poor prednisone response and resistance to initial chemotherapy, including persistence of minimal residual disease (7). For these patients allogeneic HSCT from matched sibling donors or a well-matched unrelated donor, and for the highest risk category also a mismatched donor, is an option (Table 1).

Balduzzi et al. showed that children with very-high-risk ALL benefit from related-donor HSCT compared with chemotherapy (8). At present, no cytogenetic abnormality *per se* is an absolute indication for HSCT in first remission and there is no complete consensus among major study groups. The most commonly accepted characteristics for dismal outcome which can be identified at diagnosis or early in treatment are:

Table 1: Indications for allogeneic stem cell transplantation in ALL in CR1 according to the BFM criteria

		PCR-MRD results				
		MRD-SR	MRD-MR	MRD-HR		no MRD result
				MRD-TP2 $\geq 10^{-3}$	MRD-TP2 $\geq 10^{-2}$	
HR criteria (in ierarchical order)	No CR d33	MSD/MD/MMD	MSD/MD/MMD	MSD/MD/MMD	MSD/MD/MMD	MSD/MD/MMD
	PPR + (9;22)	MSD/MD/MMD	MSD/MD/MMD	MSD/MD/MMD	MSD/MD/MMD	MSD/MD/MMD
	PPR + (4;11)	MSD/MD	MSD/MD	MSD/MD	MSD/MD/MMD	MSD/MD
	PGR + (9;22)	no	MSD/MD	MSD/MD	MSD/MD/MMD	MSD/MD
	PGR + (4;11)	MSD	MSD	MSD/MD	MSD/MD/MMD	MSD
	PPR + *	no	no	MSD/MD	MSD/MD/MMD	MSD/MD
	"Favourable" PPR §	no	no	MSD/MD	MSD/MD/MMD	no

PPR: prednisone poor response; PGR: prednisone good response; no: no HSCT indicated.
* PPR + pro-B ALL or T-ALL and/or >20% blasts in bone marrow at day 15 and/or WBC >100,000/µL; § PPR + none of the above criteria. MRD-SR: MRD negativity after 4 and 12 weeks induction treatment, measured with two independent targets with a sensitivity of $\leq 10^{-4}$; MRD-MR: any MRD positivity after 4 and 12 weeks induction treatment, but $<10^{-3}$ at week 12 (TP2); MRD-HR: MRD $\geq 10^{-3}$ at week 12 (TP2)

- Poor early responders with Philadelphia chromosome-positive ALL,
- Early T-cell precursor ALL, or
- Infant ALL with MLL rearrangement.

Recently, a COG-study showed that intensive chemotherapy plus continuous imatinib treatment after conventional remission induction therapy yielded a 3-year event-free survival rate of 80%, which was more than twice that of the historical controls and comparable to those of matched-related or matched-unrelated transplant. However, the follow-up duration of this study is too short to determine if treatment with intensive chemotherapy plus imatinib is superior to allogeneic HSCT (9).

Early T-cell precursor ALL is a recently identified subset of T-cell ALL with immature genetic and immunophenotypic features and a dismal prognosis with chemotherapy (event-free survival of 22%). Whether allogeneic HSCT could improve outcome has to be determined by studying a larger number of patients.

In contrast to earlier investigations, the outcome of T-cell ALL *per se* has improved substantially with intensive chemotherapy and most of the responders will reach continuous first remission (10) so that this is therefore no longer an indication for HSCT.

Another high-risk prognostic marker is the MLL-rearrangement, predominantly seen in young children and infants, including the (4;11) translocation. Heterogeneous retrospective analysis did not demonstrate advantage of transplantation over chemotherapy alone in terms of disease-free survival. Recently, it was shown that in patients younger than 6 months and either poor response to steroids at day 8 or leukocytes more than or equal to 300 x 10^9/L, HSCT was associated with a 64% reduction in the risk of failure resulting from relapse or death in CR (11).

The strongest predictor for relapse or treatment failure is the early response to chemotherapy, because it takes into account the drug sensitivity of leukaemic cells, and the pharmacodynamics, pharmacogenetics and intensity of administered treatment.

Minimal residual disease. There are now reliable determination methods for detecting MRD and the presence of MRD at specific time points identifies a substantial number of patients with unfavourable prognosis. A large trial introduced standardised quantitative assessment of MRD for stratification, based on immunoglobulin and TCR gene rearrangements as polymerase chain reaction targets: patients were considered MRD standard-risk (MRD-SR) if MRD was negative at day 33 and at day 78; MRD intermediate-risk (MRD-IR) if positive either at day 33 or day 78 and <10^{-3} at day 78; and MRD high-risk (MRD-HR) if ≥10^{-3} at day 78. The 7-year event-free-survival (SE) was 91.1% (CI 3.5%), 80.6% (CI 2.3%), and 49.8% (CI 5.1%) (p <0.001), respectively. Negativity of MRD at TP1 (Time Point 1, usually c. day 33) was the most favourable prognostic factor (12).

In the future, monitoring of MRD could also be included in HSCT-therapy approaches. It has already been shown that the presence of MRD has an impact on survival. Furthermore, MRD status just before HSCT is an important prognostic indicator. Prospective study of these data should also help in determining the best possible approach in the future.

2.2 Indications: CR2 and later

ALL patients who experience an early marrow relapse have a dismal prognosis when treated with conventional chemotherapy. Although nearly 90% achieve a second remission, most will subsequently develop progressive disease. Both matched sibling donor HSCT and unrelated donor HSCT are clearly indicated in these patients since the outcomes are similar. If a matched sibling or a well-matched unrelated donor cannot be identified, other types of donors such as cord blood, mismatched unrelated donors, or haploidentical family donors are option for the very high risk-patients. In relapsed ALL, patients are subdivided into risk groups according to the parameters time to relapse, site of relapse and immunophenotype (Table 2).

Patients with ALL in CR3 have a very high risk for subsequent relapse with chemotherapy alone; however, HSCT is associated with a high risk for TRM due to the pre-existing high cumulative organ toxicity. The best post-remission therapy in this context remains to be determined; however, if a matched sibling donor (MSD) or other matched family or unrelated donor (MUD) is available, HSCT is regarded as a reasonable option. For patients without an MD, mismatched donor (MMD) transplantation can be considered, but in our opinion, should be performed in experienced centres only.

Patients who do not achieve complete remission with conventional or experimental chemotherapy protocols have a dismal prognosis and should undergo HSCT only within clinical studies (13).

3. Donor selection and stem cell source

The outcome of HSCT is highly dependent on the availability of an HLA-compatible donor. So far, a matched sibling donor (MSD) has been the gold standard for the outcome of HSCT in all indications (14). As a MSD is only available in about 25% of all patients, one major goal of current trials is to evaluate, whether a very well-matched unrelated donor (MUD) may be equivalent to a MSD. The chance of finding a suitable donor mainly depends on ethnic group and the frequency of the HLA phenotype of the patient (15). High-resolution DNA matching of HLA class I and II of unrelated donors and recipients has impacted outcome, with reduced morbidity and mortality over the last decade (16). Consequently, the use of well-matched unrelated donors is now acceptable in children lacking an HLA identical sibling (Table 3).

Table 2: **Indications for allogeneic stem cell transplantation in ALL after first relapse according to the BFM criteria**

Very high relapse risk - T-lineage: any BM involvement - BCP-ALL: very early BM involving relapse, early isolated BM relapse - >CR2: according to risk for TRM	MSD/MD/MMD
High relapse risk (MRD* $\geq 10^{-3}$) - BCP-ALL: early combined BM relapse, late BM involving relapse	MSD/MD
Intermediate risk (MRD* $< 10^{-3}$) - BCP-ALL: early combined BM relapse, late BM involving relapse	MSD

* MRD detected after the second induction block; if no MRD is available: MSD-HSCT is indicated, MD-HSCT indication is dependent on conventional clinical risk factors. Time point of relapse: very early: <18 months after primary diagnosis; early: ≥18 months after primary diagnosis and <6 months after cessation of front-line therapy; late: ≥6 months after cessation of front-line therapy

Table 3: Definition of donor groups regarding HLA-matching and relationship			
Identity of HLA alleles*	Sibling donor	Family donor	Unrelated donor**
10/10	MSD	MD	MD
9/10		MD	MD
<9/10		MMD	MMD

* High resolution typing of HLA-A, HLA-B, HLA-C, HLA-DRB1, and HLA-DQB1. ** If no suitable donor is available cord blood (CB) from a 6/6 matched unrelated donor is an accepted alternative for MD-indications, and <6/6 matched unrelated CB for MMD-indications (only valid in trial ALL-HSCT-BFMi). MSD: matched sibling donor; MD: matched donor; MMD: mismatched donor

Children and adolescents with acute leukaemias which have not responded adequately to chemotherapy are, by definition, a high-risk population with co-morbidities which increase the risk of infectious and toxic complications after transplant.

Preferably, unmanipulated bone marrow (BM) is chosen as the stem cell source from MSD. Nevertheless, the use of allogeneic peripheral blood stem cells (PBSC) among matched sibling paediatric HSCT is increasing (17). No specific paediatric study has investigated the effect of unrelated MUD-PBSC in children; however a retrospective analysis of the NMDP for paediatric patients showed that the improvement of survival over time after BMT from a MUD was not similarly observed in unmodified PBSC recipients due to GvHD-associated mortality. Alternatively, intensified GvHD-prophylaxis could be applied to avoid severe acute and chronic GvHD. In most European trials, T-cell-depletion is performed only in a mismatched donor (MMD) situation.

Umbilical cord blood transplantation (UCBT) from HLA identical siblings has been performed since 1988, demonstrating acceptable outcomes when a sufficient cell dose is infused (18). A retrospective analysis from Eurocord compared the outcome of unrelated UCBTs with that of BM transplants in 541 children with acute leukaemia. Patients underwent unrelated UCBT (n=99), T-cell–depleted unrelated BMTs (n=180), or unmanipulated unrelated BMT (n=262). Compared with unmanipulated unrelated BMT recipients, UCB recipients had delayed haematopoietic recovery, increased 100 day TRM and decreased acute GvHD. T-cell–depleted unrelated BMT recipients had decreased acute GvHD and increased risk of relapse, which was not statistically significant. After day 100 post transplant, all 3 groups achieved similar results in terms of relapse. Chronic GvHD was decreased after T-cell-depleted unrelated BMTs and unrelated UCBTs, and overall mortality was higher in the T-cell-depleted unrelated BMT recipients, also not significant (19).

Another option for overcoming the lack of well-matched related or unrelated donors is the use of HLA haploidentical family members. Like UCB, almost immediate access to an allogeneic stem cell product is assured in almost all patients. As described in adults, with the modern techniques of either "positive" CD34- selection using immunomagnetic columns or more recently, with "negative" CD34 selection by CD3/CD19 depletion approach, a megadose of CD34 cells can be obtained that can overcome the increased tendency to graft rejection and enough CD3 T-cell depletion can be achieved to decrease the risk of GvHD substantially. While T-cell depletion has been necessary to decrease GvHD, the consequent delay in immune reconstitution is responsible for the two major challenges: the high risk of post-transplant infections, and increased relapse rates (20).

To date, no general recommendation for these alternative donors (UCB and mismatched family donors) can be given, as no randomised or prospective studies have investigated the outcomes in comparable paediatric and adolescent groups.

4. Conditioning regimen

The choice of conditioning regimen has a significant impact on survival after HSCT. The standard for many years was a combination of total body irradiation (TBI) and cyclophosphamide. As it turned out that single dose TBI leads to more acute and late side effects, it was substituted by fractionated TBI in most European centres. Furthermore, it was shown retrospectively that the conditioning with total body irradiation plus etoposide (TBI/VP16) was superior to TBI/cyclophosphamide (21). It is evident that irradiation, and particularly TBI, has important adverse effects in children and adolescents, as the risk for secondary malignancies is significantly higher compared to pharmacological conditioning. However, busulfan/cyclophosphamide /melphalan as an irradiation-free conditioning proved to be inferior because of a higher incidence of relapses as well as treatment related mortality (TRM). Therefore the current standard backbone for the biggest European prospective trial consists of fractionated TBI (12Gy) and etoposide (13). In patients in whom TBI is not applicable because of young age or previous irradiation doses, TBI is substituted by iv busulfan in most centres. In patients with t(4;11) the benefit of allogeneic HSCT has not so far been clearly demonstrated by retrospective analysis. Therefore, in the BFM trials it was decided to choose a particular conditioning regimen in these patients, consisting of busulfan, cyclophosphamide and melphalan, as it had been shown to be effective in patients with jMML and AML (22).

5. GvHD prophylaxis

Heterogeneities in GvHD prophylaxis and therapy are a structural weakness of retrospectively analysed patient cohorts (23). Therefore it is mandatory to apply a well-standardised and risk-adapted GvHD prophylaxis and therapy for children undergoing allogeneic HSCT. To reduce relapse incidence, after transplantation from matched sibling donors, GvHD prophylaxis might consist of cyclosporin A alone. For transplantation from unrelated donors, the addition of short MTX and ATG or other antibodies is a common European practice (24).

6. Summary

- Children with ALL who have an indication for an allogeneic HSCT, as defined by national chemotherapy groups and protocols, should have HLA typing performed as soon as the potential need for transplant is realised, to identify the best available donor and the most appropriate stem cell source.
- If an HLA genoidentical sibling or related donor is available, HSCT with bone marrow as the source is still the first choice, followed by a matched related donor cord blood unit with a sufficient cell dose (generally >3 x 10^7/kg). If lower UCB cell doses are present, the UCB unit can be supplemented with a smaller amount of BM from the sibling ($\geq$2 x 10^7/kg).
- If no HLA-genoidentical sibling or related donor is available, a search for an unrelated donor is indicated.
- In all of these situations, the enrolment of patients into prospective clinical trials will best help to identify the appropriate treatment strategy within a comparable disease cohort and result in better outcome for children overall.

Results from multicentre prospective trials will be a very stable basis for the subsequent ALL-HSCT trial, in which the identification of patients at highest risk of relapse after HSCT and implementation of controlled modifications of the HSCT procedure for those patients will be the major next goal.

References

1. Moricke A, Zimmermann M, Reiter A et al. Long-term results of five consecutive trials in childhood acute lymphoblastic leukemia performed by the ALL-BFM study group from 1981 to 2000. Leukemia 2010; 24: 265–284.
2. Burkhardt B, Reiter A, Landmann E et al. Poor outcome for children and adolescents with progressive disease or relapse of lymphoblastic lymphoma: A report from the Berlin-Frankfurt-Muenster group. J Clin Oncol 2009; 27: 3363–3369.
3. Borgmann A, von Stackelberg A, Hartmann R et al. Unrelated donor stem cell transplantation compared with chemotherapy for children with acute lymphoblastic leukemia in a second remission: A matched-pair analysis. Blood 2003; 101: 3835–3839.
4. Arico M, Schrappe M, Hunger SP et al. Clinical outcome of children with newly diagnosed Philadelphia chromosome-positive acute lymphoblastic leukemia treated between 1995 and 2005. J Clin Oncol 2010; 28: 4755–4761.
5. Bader P, Kreyenberg H, Henze GH et al. Prognostic value of minimal residual disease quantification before allogeneic stem-cell transplantation in relapsed childhood acute

lymphoblastic leukemia: The ALL-REZ BFM Study Group. J Clin Oncol 2009; 27: 377–384.

6. von Stackelberg A, Volzke E, Kuhl JS et al. Outcome of children and adolescents with relapsed acute lymphoblastic leukaemia and non-response to salvage protocol therapy: A retrospective analysis of the ALL-REZ BFM Study Group. Eur J Cancer 2011; 47: 90–97.

7. Schrauder A, Reiter A, Gadner H et al. Superiority of allogeneic hematopoietic stem-cell transplantation compared with chemotherapy alone in high-risk childhood T-cell acute lymphoblastic leukemia: Results from ALL-BFM 90 and 95. J Clin Oncol 2006; 24: 5742–5749.

8. Balduzzi A, Valsecchi MG, Uderzo C et al. Chemotherapy versus allogeneic transplantation for very-high-risk childhood acute lymphoblastic leukaemia in first complete remission: Comparison by genetic randomisation in an international prospective study. Lancet 2005; 366: 635–642.

9. Schultz KR, Bowman WP, Aledo A et al. Improved early event-free survival with imatinib in Philadelphia chromosome-positive acute lymphoblastic leukemia: A children's oncology group study. J Clin Oncol 2009; 27: 5175–5181.

10. Moricke A, Reiter A, Zimmermann M et al. Risk-adjusted therapy of acute lymphoblastic leukemia can decrease treatment burden and improve survival: Treatment results of 2169 unselected pediatric and adolescent patients enrolled in the trial ALL-BFM 95. Blood 2008; 111: 4477–4489.

11. Mann G, Attarbaschi A, Schrappe M et al. Improved outcome with hematopoietic stem cell transplantation in a poor prognostic subgroup of infants with mixed-lineage-leukemia (MLL)-rearranged acute lymphoblastic leukemia: results from the Interfant-99 Study. Blood 2010; 116: 2644–2650.

12. Schrappe M, Valsecchi MG, Bartram CR et al. Late MRD response determines relapse risk overall and in subsets of childhood T-cell ALL: Results of the AIEOP-BFM-ALL 2000 study. Blood 2011; 118: 2077–2084.

13. Peters C, Schrauder A, Schrappe M et al. Allogeneic haematopoietic stem cell transplantation in children with acute lymphoblastic leukaemia: The BFM/IBFM/EBMT concepts. Bone Marrow Transplant 2005; 35 (Suppl 1): S9–11.

14. Locatelli F, Zecca M, Rondelli R et al. Graft versus host disease prophylaxis with low-dose cyclosporine-A reduces the risk of relapse in children with acute leukemia given HLA-identical sibling bone marrow transplantation: Results of a randomized trial. Blood 2000; 95: 1572–1579.

15. Rocha V, Locatelli F. Searching for alternative hematopoietic stem cell donors for pediatric patients. Bone Marrow Transplant 2008; 41: 207–214.

16. Vettenranta K, Saarinen-Pihkala UM, Cornish J et al. Pediatric marrow transplantation for acute leukemia using unrelated donors and T-replete or -depleted grafts: A case-matched analysis. Bone Marrow Transplant 2000; 25: 395–399.

17. Pulsipher MA, Levine JE, Hayashi RJ et al. Safety and efficacy of allogeneic PBSC collection in normal pediatric donors: The pediatric blood and marrow transplant consortium experience (PBMTC) 1996-2003. Bone Marrow Transplant 2005; 35: 361–367.

18. Gluckman E, Rocha V. Cord blood transplantation: State of the art. Haematologica 2009; 94: 451–454.

19. Rocha V, Cornish J, Sievers EL et al. Comparison of outcomes of unrelated bone marrow and umbilical cord blood transplants in children with acute leukemia. Blood 2001; 97: 2962–2971.
20. Klingebiel T, Cornish J, Labopin M et al. Results and factors influencing outcome after fully haploidentical hematopoietic stem cell transplantation in children with very high-risk acute lymphoblastic leukemia: Impact of center size: An analysis on behalf of the Acute Leukemia and Pediatric Disease Working Parties of the European Blood and Marrow Transplant group. Blood 2010; 115: 3437–3446.
21. Dopfer R, Henze G, Bender GC et al. Allogeneic bone marrow transplantation for childhood acute lymphoblastic leukemia in second remission after intensive primary and relapse therapy according to the BFM- and CoALL-protocols: Results of the German Cooperative Study. Blood 1991; 78: 2780–2784.
22. Locatelli F, Nollke P, Zecca M et al. Hematopoietic stem cell transplantation (HSCT) in children with juvenile myelomonocytic leukemia (JMML): Results of the EWOG-MDS/EBMT trial. Blood 2005; 105: 410–419.
23. Miano M, Labopin M, Hartmann O et al. Haematopoietic stem cell transplantation trends in children over the last three decades: A survey by the paediatric diseases working party of the European Group for Blood and Marrow Transplantation. Bone Marrow Transplant 2007; 39: 89–99.
24. Peters C. Another step forward towards improved outcome after HLA-haploidentical stem cell transplantation. Leukemia 2004; 18: 1769–1771.

Multiple Choice Questionnaire

To find the correct answer, go to http://www.esh.org/online-training/handbook/

1. **Which one of the following conditions is not an indication for allogeneic HSCT in children and adolescents?**
   a) T-ALL relapse 6 months after completion of chemotherapy . . . . ☐
   b) B-precursor ALL; minimal residual disease higher than 10^{-3} at day 78 . . . . ☐
   c) No remission on day 33 . . . . ☐
   d) B-ALL; isolated testicular relapse, 2 years after completion of chemotherapy . . . . ☐

2. **Which one of the following statements about HSCT in children with ALL is correct?**
   a) All children and adolescents with ALL not in remission should undergo allogeneic HSCT . . . . ☐

b) Children and adolescents with T-ALL should be transplanted as soon as possible .... ☐

c) A benefit for allogeneic HSCT has been shown for high-risk patients in first remission transplanted from a HLA identical sibling donor .... ☐

d) A benefit for allogeneic HSCT has been shown for all patients in second remission .... ☐

3. **Which is the preferred source for HSCs from HLA-haplo-identical parents?**
   a) Unmanipulated bone marrow .... ☐
   b) Peripheral blood stem cells – T/B-cell depleted .... ☐
   c) Bone marrow, CD34+ selected .... ☐
   d) Peripheral blood stem cells, stimulated by cyclophosphamide and G-CSF .... ☐

4. **Which conditioning regimen should be applied for infant ALL with MLL-rearrangement?**
   a) Intravenous busulfan + asparaginase .... ☐
   b) Intravenous busulfan + cyclophosphamide + melphalan .... ☐
   c) Total body irradiation + etoposide .... ☐
   d) Total body irradiation + cyclophosphamide .... ☐

5. **For a 7 year old boy with very high-risk Philadelphia positive ALL and no remission on day 33, which one of the following donor and stem cell sources is not acceptable?**
   a) HLA mismatched unrelated cord-blood (5/6) .... ☐
   b) T/B-cell depleted peripheral blood stem cells from HLA-haplo-identical mother .... ☐
   c) T/B-cell depleted bone marrow from HLA-identical sibling .... ☐
   d) Unmanipulated cord blood or bone marrow from HLA-identical sibling ... ☐

NOTES

*CHAPTER 20

HSCT for children and adolescents

*20.3

HSCT in children with myelodysplastic syndromes

Franco Locatelli, Alice Bertaina, Giuseppe Palumbo

1. Introduction

Myelodysplastic syndromes (MDS) are a heterogeneous group of clonal disorders, accounting for less than 5% of all haematological malignancies of childhood (1). Childhood MDS include both variants shared with the adult population (i.e. refractory anaemia with eccess blasts (RAEB), RAEB in trasformation (RAEB-t)) and other disorders more typical of the paediatric age group, such as juvenile myelomonocytic leukaemia (JMML) (1, 2). This latter disorder predominates in infants, median age at diagnosis being 2 years (2). In JMML, there is also a male predominance, the male/female ratio being 2-3:1. JMML is clinically characterised by overproduction of monocytic cells that can infiltrate organs, including spleen, liver, gastro-intestinal tract, and lung. JMML is categorised as an overlap MPD/MDS by the World Health Organization and also shares some clinical and molecular features with chronic myelomonocytic leukaemia, a similar disease in adults. Hypersensitivity to GM-CSF and pathological activation of the RAS-RAF-MAP (mitogen-activated protein) kinase signaling pathway play an important role in the pathophysiology of JMML. Major progress in understanding the pathogenesis of JMML has been achieved in the last 2 decades by mapping out the genetic lesions that occur in patients. The spectrum of mutations described thus far in JMML occur in genes that encode proteins that signal through the RAS-RAF-MAPK pathways, thus providing potential new opportunities for both diagnosis and therapy (3). These genes include *NF1, NRAS, KRAS, PTPN11*, and, as most recently demonstrated, CBL (3, 4). Although spontaneous resolution of JMML can rarely occur, allogeneic HSCT is the only firmly established curative approach for children with JMML, resulting in long-term survival in a significant proportion of patients (5–8). Moreover, so far, there are neither clinical nor biological reliable markers to predict spontaneous resolution of JMML, the only exception being represented by Noonan syndrome. JMML may spontaneously resolve in Noonan syndrome patients, and so expectant observation is appropriate for these children. Childhood MDS other than JMML often occur in the context of congenital bone marrow failure syndromes, this fact representing a peculiarity of myelodysplasia occurring in the paediatric age group (1). HSCT is routinely offered also to all children with advanced MDSs (namely RAEB and RAEB-t), to paediatric patients with MDS secondary to chemo-radiotherapy, and to those with refractory cytopenia (RC) associated with either cytogenetic anomalies (mainly monosomy 7 and complex karyotype) or severe neutropenia (neutrophils less than 1 x 10^9/L) or transfusion dependence (9, 10).

2. Results obtained with HSCT in JMML and factors influencing outcome

Several different studies have documented that a large proportion of children with JMML can be definitively cured by an allograft (5–8). In the most recent study, which included the largest number of patients with JMML given allogeneic HSCT from either a histocompatible relative or from an HLA-matched/1-antigen disparate donor, the probability of EFS was in the order of 50% (7). In multivariate analysis, age greater than 4 years and female sex predicted poorer outcome (7). Available data indicate that, in the more recent years, using an unrelated donor offers minimal or possibly no significant disadvantage as compared to employing an HLA-identical sibling as stem cell donor (7). Leukaemia recurrence represents the main cause of treatment failure in children with JMML given HSCT, relapse rate being as high as 40–50% (5–7). While one study reported a negative impact of monosomy 7 (8), the most frequent cytogenetic anomaly in JMML, on the probability of OS after HSCT, other larger analyses documented that neither monosomy 7 nor other cytogenetic abnormalities confer a poorer prognosis (5–7). Recently, Bresolin et al. reported that gene expression signatures could segregate JMML patients into those who displayed an AML-type signature versus those who did not (11). These signatures were significantly associated with outcome, as children who displayed an AML-type signature experienced a 10-year EFS of only 6% in contrast to 63% of those without the AML-type signature, the difference being largely due to an increased risk of recurrence after HSCT. Of interest was the statistically significant correlation between an AML-type signature and known prognostic variables at diagnosis predicting a dismal outcome, including older age, lower platelet count, and higher Hb F levels. However, in multivariate analysis, only the AML-type gene expression signature retained significance. Several published series have also examined the hypothesis that mutational status may correlate with JMML clinical features and prognosis; however, this correlation remains controversial and to be definitively proved. In this respect, Yoshida and colleagues evaluated the clinical course and laboratory findings of 49 JMML patients, 32 of whom harboured mutations in *NF1, KRAS, NRAS*, or *PTPN11* (12). In their series, mutation of PTPN11 was associated with older age at diagnosis (>24 months), increased Hb F (>10%), reduced overall survival, and, importantly, appeared to be an unfavorable prognostic factor predicting relapse following HSCT. High methylation of CpG islands in some genes of children with JMML have been recently reported to predict a particularly dismal outcome, which was due to an increased risk of recurrence after HSCT (13).

Preparative regimens before the allograft which do not include TBI are particularly attractive for children with JMML, since radiation-induced late effects, such as severe growth retardation, cataracts, hypothyroidism and neuropsychologic sequels may be especially deleterious for very young children. Moreover, in a retrospective analysis of the EWOG-MDS, busulfan-based myeloablative therapy offered a greater anti-leukaemic efficacy than TBI (5). The recommended preparative regimen of the EBMT/EWOG-MDS groups for children with JMML includes busulfan, cyclophosphamide and melphalan (7).

Splenectomy before HSCT, as well as spleen size at time of the allograft, did not appear to have an impact on post-transplantation outcome of children with JMML. Available data are not in favour of an indiscriminate use of splenectomy before transplantation, the potential advantages having to be weighed against the risks related to the procedure or to post-splenectomy infections (5–8). The indication for performing splenectomy has to be carefully evaluated for each individual child. The presence of massive splenomegaly with evidence of hypersplenism and/or refractoriness to platelet transfusions is an argument for considering this procedure in order to promote engraftment, to hasten haematological recovery and to lower the risk of haemorrhagic complications. There is a growing consensus for watchful waiting in those patients with JMML who are asymptomatic, while waiting for the identification of an appropriate donor. For patients with very high leukocyte counts, pulmonary problems (dry cough, tachypnea and interstitial infiltrates on chest X-ray), and/or prominent organomegaly, one can consider oral 6-mercaptopurine (50 mg/m^2/day) ± cis-RA (100 mg/m^2/day), a differentiating agent potentially able to control expansion of clonal CFU-GM which proved to be effective in some patients with JMML (in particular in children below the age of 12 months who, nevertheless, are known to have a less aggressive disease course). For severely ill children, or those children who progress on less intensive therapies, low-dose intravenous cytarabine (40 mg/m^2/day x 5 days) can be administered. The use of hypomethylating agents (decitabine, azacitidine) as a treatment in the time before transplantation remains to be explored.

Available data indicate that UCBT is a suitable option for children with JMML lacking an HLA-compatible relative and that the search for an unrelated CB unit should be initiated at the same time as that for an unrelated BM donor (7). CB offers the advantage of prompter availability of stem cells and allows to perform HSCT even in the presence of donor HLA disparities.

For children with JMML experiencing leukaemia relapse after allogeneic HSCT, DLI was proved to be largely ineffective, while a second allograft, from either the same or a different donor, together with reduction of the intensity of GvHD prophylaxis aimed at optimising the GvL effect, is able to rescue about one third of the patients (14).

3. HSCT in MDS other than JMML

Data on outcome of children transplanted for childhood MDS are limited and many published reports include a low number of patients with various variants of MDS transplanted following heterogeneous regimens (9, 15–17). The most recent study including 97 patients with RAEB, RAEB-t and myelodysplasia-related AML demonstrated that allogeneic HSCT from either a matched sibling donor or an unrelated volunteer following a myeloablative conditioning regimen including 3 alkylating agents (namely busulfan, cyclophosphamide and melphalan) is able to cure around 60% of children with advanced MDS. Outcomes were comparable for children with RAEB and RAEB-t, whereas patients with myelodysplasia-related-AML have an increased risk of relapse. In this cohort, the 5-year cumulative incidence of TRM and relapse was 21%, each. Age at HSCT greater than 12 years, interval between diagnosis and HSCT longer than 4 months and occurrence of acute or extensive chronic GvHD were associated with increased TRM.

The need for pre-HSCT remission induction chemotherapy remains a debated question in paediatric patients with RAEB and RAEB-t. In fact, whether cytoreductive therapy prior to HSCT for more advanced forms of MDS improves survival remains controversial. A study published by the Nordic Pediatric Haematology group, comparing the outcome of children with *de novo* MDS (including JMML) and children with *de novo* AML, documented that patients belonging to the former group had a lower rate of complete remission and a higher risk of death for treatment-related complications (17). In the recent EWOG-MDS analysis on children with MDS other than JMML the outcome of patients given intensive chemotherapy prior to the allograft was found to be comparable to that of children who were transplanted directly (9). If the analysis was restricted to children with myelodysplasia-related-AML there was a significantly decreased risk of relapse in the intensive chemotherapy group resulting, however, in a non-significant advantage in terms of EFS (9). In all these studies, the application of intensive chemotherapy was not tested in a systematic way and therefore the results must be interpreted with caution. However, it is reasonable to conclude that intensive chemotherapy cannot generally be recommended for children with RAEB and RAEB-t, but may be considered for children with MDR-AML. In children with advanced MDS, the presence of a monosomal and structurally complex karyotype, characterised by more than or equal to 3 chromosomal aberrations, including at least one structural aberration, was found to be strongly associated with poor prognosis (18). Likewise, the outcome of children with MDS secondary to previous cytotoxic or radiant treatment remains still poor, for both a high risk of disease recurrence and TRM.

Patients with RC must be considered for an early allograft from either a related or an unrelated donor if they have monosomy of chromosome 7. In fact, a study of the EWOG-MDS analysing children with RC has clearly demonstrated that the probability of progression to more advanced MDS (i.e. RAEB and RAEB-t), as well as to frank AML, is significantly higher in patients with monosomy 7 than in those with a normal karyotype (10). Moreover, this study has also shown that patients who had not progressed to advanced MDS prior to HSCT had a significantly better probability of survival than patients who experienced disease progression (76 versus 36%, respectively, p=0.03) (10). In the presence of a normal karyotype, a substantial proportion of children with RC may experience a long, stable course of their disease. In view of the low TRM observed in patients transplanted from an HLA-compatible sibling, HSCT may be recommended if a suitable HLA-matched relative is available. A "watch and wait" approach with careful observation may be reasonable for patients without an HLA-identical sibling in the absence of transfusion requirements, severe neutropenia or infections. Children with RC associated with either severe neutropenia (neutrophils less than 1×10^9/L) or transfusion dependence are candidates to receive transplantation from a well-matched unrelated donor. Immune-suppressive therapy with ATG, cyclosporin-A and steroids is a valid, although less effective, alternative.

As the risk of disease recurrence after the allograft in patients with RC is low, there is a great interest in testing the safety and efficacy of reduced intensity regimens in this setting. In an EWOG-MDS report, patients with RC and normal karyotype transplanted from an unrelated donor following a fludarabine-based reduced-intensity regimen had a favourable post-transplant outcome, which was comparable to that obtained in patients transplanted following a myeloablative conditioning regimen (19).

Results of UCBT in paediatric patients with MDS variants other than JMML have been recently reported to be inferior to those reported using either bone marrow or peripheral blood as stem cell source (20). Thus, this type of allograft can be recommended only for those patients lacking a suitable either related or unrelated donor.

4. Conclusions and future perspectives

The available data indicate that HSCT is curative for the majority of children with MDS, the outcome of patients transplanted from either an HLA-identical sibling or an unrelated volunteer being comparable in more recent years. Strategies aimed at reducing the risk of leukaemia recurrence in children with JMML, RAEB, RAEB-t and MDS secondary to previous treatment, as well as to reduce TRM in children with RC, could further optimise the results of HSCT in childhood MDS.

References

1. Hasle H, Niemeyer CM, Chessells JM et al. A pediatric approach to the WHO classification of myelodysplastic and myeloproliferative diseases. Leukemia 2003; 17: 277–282.
2. Niemeyer CM, Aricò M , Basso G et al. Chronic myelomonocytic leukemia in childhood: A report of 110 cases. Blood 1997; 89: 3534–3543.
3. Niemeyer CM, Kratz CP. Paediatric myelodysplastic syndromes and juvenile myelomonocytic

leukaemia: Molecular classification and treatment options. Br J Haematol 2008; 140: 610–624.

4. Loh ML, Sakai DS, Flotho C et al. Mutations in CBL occur frequently in juvenile myelomonocytic leukemia. Blood 2009; 114: 1859–1863.

5. Locatelli F, Niemeyer C, Angelucci E et al. Allogeneic bone marrow transplantation for chronic myelomonocytic leukemia in childhood: A report from the European Working Group on Myelodysplastic Syndrome in Childhood. J Clin Oncol 1997; 15: 566–573.

6. Smith FO, King R, Nelson G et al; National Marrow Donor Program. Unrelated donor bone marrow transplantation for children with juvenile myelomonocytic leukaemia. Br J Haematol 2002; 116: 716–724.

7. Locatelli F, Nollke P, Zecca M et al; European Working Group on Childhood MDS; European Blood and Marrow Transplantation Group. Hematopoietic stem cell transplantation (HSCT) in children with juvenile myelomonocytic leukemia (JMML): Results of the EWOG-MDS/EBMT trial. Blood 2005; 105: 410–419.

8. Manabe A, Okamura J, Yumura-Yagi K et al. on behalf of the MDS Committee of the Japanese Society of Pediatric Hematology. Allogeneic hematopoietic stem cell transplantation for 27 children with juvenile myelomonocytic leukemia diagnosed based on the criteria of the International JMML Working Group. Leukemia 2002; 16: 645–649.

9. Strahm B, Nöllke P, Zecca M et al on behalf of EWOG-MDS study group. Hematopoietic stem cell transplantation for advanced myelodysplastic syndrome in children: Results of the EWOG-MDS 98 study. Leukemia 2011; 25: 455–462.

10. Kardos G, Baumann I, Passmore SJ et al. Refractory anemia in childhood: A retrospective analysis of 67 patients with particular reference to monosomy 7. Blood 2003; 102: 1997–2003.

11. Bresolin S, Zecca M, Flotho C et al. Gene expression-based classification as an independent predictor of clinical outcome in juvenile myelomonocytic leukemia. J Clin Oncol 2010; 28: 1919–1927.

12. Olk-Batz C, Poetsch AR, Nöllke P et al on behalf of the European Working Group of Myelodysplastic Syndromes in Childhood (EWOG-MDS). Aberrant DNA methylation characterizes juvenile myelomonocytic leukemia with poor outcome. Blood 2011; 117: 4871–4880.

13. Yoshida N, Yagasaki H, Xu Y et al. Correlation of clinical features with the mutational status of GM-CSF signaling pathway-related genes in juvenile myelomonocytic leukemia. Pediatr Res 2009; 65: 334–340.

14. Yoshimi A, Mohamed M, Bierings M et al. on behalf of the European Working Group of MDS in Childhood (EWOG-MDS). Second allogeneic hematopoietic stem cell transplantation (HSCT) results in outcome similar to that of first HSCT for patients with juvenile myelomonocytic leukemia. Leukemia 2007; 21: 556–560.

15. Woods WG, Kobrinsky N, Buckley J et al. Intensively timed induction therapy followed by autologous or allogeneic bone marrow transplantation for children with acute myeloid leukemia or myelodysplastic syndrome: A Children Cancer Group pilot study. J Clin Oncol 1993; 11: 1448–1457.

16. Locatelli F, Pession A, Bonetti F et al. Busulfan, cyclophosphamide and melphalan as

conditioning regimen for bone marrow transplantation in children with myelodysplastic syndromes. Leukemia 1994; 8: 844–849.

17. Hasle H, Kerndrup G, Yssing M et al. Intensive chemotherapy in childhood myelodysplastic syndrome. A comparison with results in acute myeloid leukemia. Leukemia 1996; 10: 1269–1273.

18. Göhring G, Michalova K, Beverloo HB et al. Complex karyotype newly defined: The strongest prognostic factor in advanced childhood myelodysplastic syndrome. Blood 2010; 116: 3766–3769.

19. Strahm B, Locatelli F, Bader P et al. on behalf of the EWOG-MDS Study Group. Reduced intensity conditioning in unrelated donor transplantation for refractory cytopenia in childhood. Bone Marrow Transplant 2007; 40: 329–333.

20. Madureira AB, Eapen M, Locatelli F, on behalf of the Eurocord-European Blood and Marrow Transplant Group; Center of International Blood and Marrow Transplant Registry; European Working Group on childhood MDS. Analysis of risk factors influencing outcome in children with myelodysplastic syndrome after unrelated cord blood transplantation. Leukemia 2011; 25: 449–454.

Multiple Choice Questionnaire

To find the correct answer, go to http://www.esh.org/online-training/handbook/

1. JMML is a childhood malignant haematological disease more frequent in:
a) Males older than 4 years of age ☐
b) Females older than 4 years of age ☐
c) Males younger than 4 years of age ☐
d) Females younger than 4 years of age ☐

2. Which is the most common variant of childhood MDS?
a) Refractory cytopenia ☐
b) Juvenile myelomonocytic leukaemia ☐
c) Refractory anaemia with excess of blasts ☐
d) Refractory anaemia with excess of blasts in transformation ☐

3. Which is the reported probability of event-free survival after HSCT in children with JMML?
a) 15% ☐

b) 90%...☐
c) 30%...☐
d) 50%...☐

---

4. **Which variables have been reported to increase the risk of TRM in paediatric patients with advanced MDS?**
   a) Age at HSCT greater than 12 years, interval between diagnosis and HSCT longer than 4 months and occurrence of acute or extensive chronic GvHD..☐
   b) Age at HSCT less than 12 years, interval between diagnosis and HSCT longer than 4 months and occurrence of acute or extensive chronic GvHD..☐
   c) Age at HSCT greater than 12 years, interval between diagnosis and HSCT shorter than 4 months and occurrence of acute or extensive chronic GvHD..☐
   d) Age at HSCT greater than 12 years, interval between diagnosis and HSCT shorter than 4 months ....☐

---

5. **Which are the most frequently employed regimens for HSCT in children with JMML?**
   a) Those based on the use of TBI ....☐
   b) Those based on the use of busulfan...☐
   c) Reduced-intensity regimens ....☐
   d) Those based both on the use of TBI and of busulfan....................☐

NOTES

*CHAPTER 20

HSCT for children and adolescents

---

*20.4

Chronic myeloproliferative disorders: The role of HSCT in childhood MPD

Franco Locatelli, Charlotte M. Niemeyer

1. Introduction

Among myeloproliferative disorders (MPD), Philadelphia (Ph+) chronic myeloid leukaemia (CML) certainly represents the most common variant, accounting for approximately 3–5% of all leukaemias in childhood (1). The estimated incidence of Ph+ CML in paediatric patients has been reported to be less than 1 in 100,000 and is less common under the age of 2 as compared with other age groups (2). In children, the disease is characterised by the same molecular, cytogenetic, clinical and morphological features reported in adults with classical Ph+ CML.

As in adults, so far, allogeneic HSCT is considered to be the only proven curative treatment for children with Ph+ CML (3–6). However, it must be underlined that not all the candidates for transplantation have a suitable, either related or unrelated, HLA-identical donor and, despite its curative potential, HSCT carries the risk of death associated with the procedure, as well as of leukaemia recurrence or of long-term side effects. Moreover, the natural history of Ph+ CML has been recently profoundly modified by the introduction of the specific Bcr/Abl tyrosine protein kinase inhibitors, the first and still most frequently employed being imatinib mesylate, which target the enzymatic activity of the Bcr-Abl protein, occupying the ATP-binding pocket of the molecule. The tyrosine kinase inhibitors have a great probability of inducing the achievement of both major and complete cytogenetic response and a high rate of freedom from progression to AP or BC (7). So far, however, we do not have unquestionable evidence that the Ph+ clone can be either completely eradicated or rendered silent for many decades by prolonged treatment with tyrosine kinase inhibitors. Thus, in this perspective, and consider the longer life-expectancy of paediatric patients, allogeneic HSCT may have a wider application in children with Ph+ CML than in adults with the same disease.

Other myeloproliferative disorders, such as polycythaemia vera (PV) and myelofibrosis with myeloid metaplasia (MMM), are extremely rare in children and no sound data are available for analysing the role of HSCT in children affected by these disorders, although, in principle, there is a clear rationale for considering the transplant option also in these MPDs.

2. Indications, results and risk factors in paediatric patients with Ph+ chronic myeloid leukaemia

In some of the most important studies addressing the role of HSCT in patients with Ph+ CML, children have been included in adult series, but they represented a small proportion of the patient group and their outcome was not considered separately (3–5). Around 10 years ago, the Chronic Leukaemia Registry of the European Group for Blood and Marrow Transplantation (EBMT) evaluated the outcome of 314 children with Ph+ CML transplanted between 1985 and 2001 from either a related or an unrelated donor, selected using high-resolution molecular typing of HLA class II antigens only. (6). In this study, 3-year OS and EFS were 66 and 55%, respectively. In multivariate analysis for both OS and EFS, outcome was superior in patients given the allograft in CP1 versus advanced phase, although it is noteworthy that more than one third of patients transplanted in AP or BC are alive and disease free 3 years after transplantation (6). Inferior leukaemia-free survival (LFS) was also found in children transplanted >6 months from diagnosis, this finding confirming previously published studies, which documented in adults a worse outcome for patients transplanted more than 12 months after diagnosis as compared to those given HSCT earlier (6). The transplant-related mortality (TRM) in the cohort of patients analysed by the EBMT group was significantly higher for children transplanted from an unrelated volunteer, these patients having a 35% chance of fatal transplant-related complications as compared to 20% for recipients of sibling allografts (6). The higher incidence of transplantation-related death observed in patients transplanted from an unrelated volunteer was mainly due to a greater incidence of severe GvHD in these transplant recipients as compared to those transplanted from an HLA- compatible sibling. A more precise characterisation of HLA alleles using high-resolution typing for both class I and class II molecules has been shown to permit a more accurate selection of unrelated donors, thus reducing the incidence of immune-mediated complications and fatal events after the allograft (8, 9). Thus, for patients transplanted in more recent years, the outcome of patients given allogeneic HSCT from an unrelated volunteer has improved and is now comparable to that of patients transplanted from an HLA-compatible sibling (10).

Two trials performed in Germany and Japan and further addressing the role of allogeneic HSCT in children with Ph+ CML have recently been published (11, 12). In the German trial, the probability of OS at 5 years was 87 ± 11% in the 41 children transplanted from a sibling, 52 ± 9% for the 71 given the allograft from a matched unrelated donor, and 45 ± 16% for those 55 children who had an HLA-partially matched unrelated donor, respectively. A trend for better OS in CP1 was observed if HSCT was performed within 6 months (n=49; 74 ± 9%), compared to 7–12 months (n=52; 62 ± 15%), and >12 months (n=43; 62 ± 17%) after diagnosis, respectively (p=0.157). Probability of relapse at 5 years was 20 ± 12%. TRM was the main cause of the inferior outcome in UD and HLA-mismatched HSCT. In the Japanese study, the probabilities of 5-year OS and LFS were 59.3 and 55.5%, respectively (12). Multivariate analysis identified the following unfavorable prognostic factors for survival: infused total nucleated cell dose lower than 314 x 10^6/kg, advanced phase and no major cytogenetic response (MCyR) at the time of transplantation. Of the 17 patients treated with imatinib, 15 (88%) achieved MCyR at the time of HSCT, and this group had an excellent 5-year OS of 81.9% (12). With the exception of the German study, no paediatric studies have evaluated the optimal conditioning regimen for childhood Ph+ CML (11). In keeping with data obtained in adults comparing TBI with busulfan/cyclophosphamide regimens, no significant differences on OS either in the matched sibling donor or the matched voluntary unrelated donor setting were detected. However, in view of the long-term sequelae associated with the use of TBI, most paediatric physicians prefer busulfan/cyclophosphamide as the regimen to be employed before allogeneic HSCT at least for patients transplanted in 1st CP. From a theoretical point of view, reduced-intensity conditioning regimens are also an attractive treatment option in younger patients because it might preserve fertility and reduce toxicity; however, data relating to their use in children and adolescents are scant and as yet uninformative. In this regard, it must be considered that the effect of reduced-intensity allogeneic HSCT is based on an allo-immune response, which, in comparison with other leukaemias, has been proven to be more successful in Ph+ CML. However, the use of reduced-intensity conditioning regimens in Ph+ CML is associated with a significantly higher risk of relapse in comparison to fully myeloablative regimens (10). This said, Ph+ CML is the very disease in which the importance of the allo-immune effect of transplantation has demonstrated to be crucial for disease eradication. Indeed, use of T-cell depletion of the graft has been progressively abandoned during the last 3 decades in view of the unacceptably high incidence of leukaemia recurrence, and the treatment of Ph+ CML relapse after an allograft has significantly benefited from adoptive immunotherapy with DLI. In patients with CML experiencing haematological relapse in CP after HSCT, complete remission can be obtained with this treatment in approximately 70% of cases (12). Most of these remissions are sustained over time, this proving the capacity of DLI to eradicate clonogenic leukaemia cells or to control their re-growth. Patients suffering from either cytogenetic or molecular relapse have an even greater chance of benefiting from DLI than those experiencing haematological relapse, especially in advanced phase. Combined use of tyrosine kinase inhibitors and DLI can further optimise the chance of being rescued for patients with Ph+ CML experiencing leukaemia recurrence.

For certain groups/physicians, allogeneic HSCT has become a form of rescue treatment for those patients who experience imatinib-resistance. In most circumstances, early signs for disease progression can be detected appropriately by adequate molecular monitoring of the chimeric Bcr/Abl mRNA transcript by means of PCR. Because a search for a voluntary unrelated donor can often take several months, donor searches immediately after diagnosis is indicated for paediatric patients treated with tyrosine kinase inhibitors as first line treatment and who would be considered potential allograft candidates if they develop resistance to medical therapy.

Allo-HSCT is indicated ideally before clinical or haematological signs of progression to AP or BC are apparent.

3. Conclusions and future perspectives

The available data indicate that HSCT is curative for the majority of children with Ph+ CML, although in the past TRM unfavourably affected the outcome of patients transplanted from an unrelated volunteer. Long-term survival is also influenced by the stage of the disease at time of transplantation, significantly better outcome having been observed in patients transplanted in CP1. LFS is significantly better for children transplanted within 6 months of diagnosis. It is possible that in the future the choice of transplanting children with CML will have to be balanced against the results achieved with tyrosine kinase inhibitors. However, considering the long life expectancy of children and that we do not have evidence that these agents be able to offer, either alone or in combination with other treatment, a sustained "molecular cure" or indefinitely prolonged CP of the disease, allogeneic HSCT, possibly in the first year after diagnosis, remains the treatment of choice of childhood Ph+ CML, provided that a well-matched donor is available.

Strict monitoring and early detection of minimal residual disease through serial quantitative evaluation of the chimeric Bcr/Abl mRNA transcript by means of PCR can be extremely useful for ensuring the best chance of favourable outcome in patients with Ph+ CML given HSCT.

References

1. Grier HE, Civin CI. Myeloid leukemias, myelodysplasia and myeloproliferative disease in children. In: Nathan DG, Orkin SH, editors. Hematology of Infancy and Childhood. Philadelphia: Saunders WB, 1998: 1300–1308.
2. Hall GW. Cytogenetic and molecular genetic aspects of childhood myeloproliferative/ myelodysplastic disorders. Acta Haematol 2002; 108: 171–179.
3. Goldman JM, Apperley JF, Jones L et al. Bone marrow transplantation for patients with chronic myeloid leukemia. N Engl J Med 1986; 314: 202–207.
4. Hansen JA, Gooley TA, Martin PJ et al. Bone marrow transplants from unrelated donors for patients with chronic myeloid leukemia. N Engl J Med 1998; 338: 962–968.
5. Gratwohl A, Hermans J, Goldman JM et al. Risk assessment for patients with chronic myeloid leukaemia before allogeneic blood or marrow transplantation. Chronic Leukemia Working Party of the European Group for Blood and Marrow Transplantation. Lancet 1998; 352: 1087–1092.
6. Cwynarski K, Roberts IAG, Iacobelli S et al. for the Paediatric and Chronic Leukaemia Working Parties of the EBMT. Stem cell transplantation for chronic myeloid leukemia in children. Blood 2003; 102: 1224–1231.
7. O'Brien SG, Guilhot F, Larson RA. Imatinib compared with interferon and low-dose

cytarabine for newly diagnosed chronic-phase myeloid leukaemia. N Engl J Med 2003; 348: 994–1004.

8. Flomenberg N, Baxter-Lowe LA, Confer D et al. Impact of HLA class I and class II high-resolution matching on outcomes of unrelated donor bone marrow transplantation: HLA-C mismatching is associated with a strong adverse effect on transplantation outcome. Blood 2004; 104: 1923–1930.

9. Lee SJ, Klein J, Haagenson M et al. High resolution donor-recipient HLA matching contributes to the success of unrelated donor marrow transplantation. Blood 2007; 110: 4576–4583.

10. Suttorp M, Millot F. treatment of pediatric chronic myeloid leukemia in the year 2010: Use of tyrosine kinase inhibitors and stem-cell transplantation. Hematology Am Soc Hematol Educ Program 2010; 2010: 368–376.

11. Suttorp M, Claviez A, Bader P et al. Allogeneic stem cell transplantation for treatment of chronic myeloid leukemia in pediatric and adolescent patients: Results of the prospective trial CML-paed I. Klin Padiatr 2009; 221: 351–357.

12. Muramatsu H, Kojima S, Yoshimi A et al. Outcome of 125 children with chronic myelogenous leukemia who received transplants from unrelated donors: The Japan marrow donor program. Biol Blood Marrow Transplant 2010; 16: 231–238.

13. Locatelli F. The role of repeat transplantation of haemopoietic stem cells and adoptive immunotherapy in treatment of leukaemia relapsing following allogeneic transplantation. Br J Haematol 1998; 102: 633–638.

Multiple Choice Questionnaire

To find the correct answer, go to http://www.esh.org/online-training/handbook/

1. **Ph+ CML is a childhood malignant haematological disease characterised by:**
    a) The same molecular, cytogenetic, clinical and morphological features reported in adults. . . . . ☐
    b) Different molecular, cytogenetic, clinical and morphological features reported in adults . . . . ☐
    c) The same molecular, cytogenetic lesions, but different clinical and morphological features reported in adults . . . . ☐
    d) Slightly different molecular, cytogenetic lesions, but similar clinical and morphological features reported in adults . . . . ☐

2. **Which is the treatment of choice for paediatric patients with cytogenetic relapse after HSCT in Ph+ CML:**

a) DLI ☐
b) TK inhibitors ☐
c) Second HSCT ☐
d) DLI and TK inhibitors ☐

3. **What is the reported incidence of Ph+ CML in childhood?**
   a) Less than 1 in 100,000 ☐
   b) Less than 1 in 1,000,000 ☐
   c) Less than 1 in 10,000 ☐
   d) Less than 1 in 500,000 ☐

4. **Which variables have been reported to adversely influence outcome of paediatric patients with Ph+ CML:**
   a) Accelerated phase or blast crisis at time of allograft ☐
   b) Time interval between diagnosis and HSCT longer than 6–12 months ☐
   c) Use of an unrelated donor ☐
   d) All these 3 variables ☐

5. **Which are the most frequently employed regimens for HSCT in children with Ph+ CML?**
   a) Those based on the use of TBI ☐
   b) Those based on the use of busulfan ☐
   c) Reduced-intensity regimens ☐
   d) Those based both on the use of TBI and of busulfan ☐

NOTES

* CHAPTER 20

HSCT for children and adolescents

* 20.5
HSCT for lymphomas in children and adolescents

Alexander Claviez

1. Introduction

Paediatric and adolescent patients suffering from lymphoma in general have an excellent outcome with current risk-adapted combined modality first-line treatment conducted in prospective multicentre trials. Overall survival (OS) rates for Hodgkin's lymphoma (HL) as well as non-Hodgkin's lymphoma (NHL) have reached the 90% level, or higher, depending on established risk factors. Given the rarity and the high curability rates in both lymphoma entities in this age group, data on autologous and even more for allogeneic HSCT are much fewer compared to series on adult patients. For example, data from the EBMT Lymphoma Working Party indicate that about ten times as many adults undergo HSCT for HL in comparison to children (1). A direct comparison between paediatric and adult populations with respect to histology seems to be more feasible in HL than in NHL. This is mainly due to the broad and diverse spectrum of histology subtypes in NHL in both age groups and the fact that for a long time various different lymphoma classifications have been used, making such a comparison difficult.

Moreover, large registry-based analyses aiming to define the indication for HSCT in lymphoma have combined adult and paediatric patients, which has sometimes resulted in wide age ranges spanning up to years 60 or more (2–4). In childhood, virtually all NHL subtypes represent highly malignant and rapidly proliferating lymphomas compared to adults, where a substantial group of patients suffer from indolent low-grade lymphomas (5). In contrast, the clinical course of HL is much more similar for many paediatric and adult patients.

So far, there is no definitive indication for HSCT in first-line therapy for either HL or NHL, but autologous and allogeneic HSCT have become part of salvage therapy strategies for patients with poor treatment response or disease recurrence in both entities. Historically, autologous HSCT has been preferred to allogeneic HSCT because of greater availability and a lower rate of treatment-associated complications. With recent developments in HLA-typing of donors, increasing knowledge and understanding of molecular and immunologic mechanisms, improvement of supportive care and implementation of conditioning regimens with reduced intensity, allogeneic HSCT is being used for more young patients .

2. Non-Hodgkin's lymphoma

Despite the remarkable progress achieved in outcome for children with NHL within the last decades, treatment of patients failing first-line therapy remains a major challenge. A substantial number of these relapses occur within the first year after completion or during front-line therapy (5). The overwhelming majority of NHL in the paediatric age group in Europe and North America consists of aggressive high-grade lymphoma subtypes. The major subgroups in children and adolescents consist of three groups:

- Firstly mature B-cell lymphomas including Burkitt lymphoma (BL), mature B-cell ALL (B-ALL) and diffuse large B-cell lymphoma (DLBCL)
- Secondly lymphoblastic lymphomas (LBL) with predominance of T-cell type compared to B-cell type and
- Thirdly anaplastic large-cell lymphomas (ALCL) of T-, Null- and B-cell type.

Aggressive salvage chemotherapy followed by high-dose therapy and subsequent autologous HSCT has been used to cure patients with NHL suffering from relapse or disease progression (6–8) but these series are usually small. Allogeneic HSCT has been used even more rarely in paediatric NHL patients. The potential benefit of a graft-versus-lymphoma effect has been counterbalanced by increased treatment-related mortality rates in early series, thus preventing more widespread use of this approach. Other factors historically included the existence of less effective first-line and salvage therapy regimens and less precise techniques regarding donor selection.

There seem to be strong hints for the existence of a graft-versus lymphoma effect in NHL, as shown by a lower relapse rate in the majority of allografted patients compared to those undergoing autologous HSCT (2). The authors of this large EBMT registry study (1982–1998) including children compared six lymphoma subgroups classified according to the Working Formulation (HL and five NHL subtypes: low-grade NHL, intermediate-grade NHL, high-grade NHL, Burkitt's lymphoma and lymphoblastic lymphoma). 1185 allogeneic HSCT were compared with 14687 autologous procedures as the first HSCT. OS was higher for patients receiving autologous HSCT for all subtypes and non-relapse mortality was higher for all lymphoma subtypes in the group receiving allogeneic HSCT. The outcome of children has not been analysed separately.

In the largest series to date on 182 children with NHL undergoing autologous (n=90) or allogeneic HSCT (n=92) between 1990 and 2005 published by the IBMTR, outcome was mainly affected by disease status at the time of HSCT, irrespective of the type of transplant and histologic subtypes (9). In this registry series, relapse rate was higher after autologous HSCT while non-relapse mortality was higher following allografting.

With increasing understanding of the molecular mechanisms involved in the aetiology and pathogenesis in distinct NHL subtypes (10), it seems appropriate to focus analyses on the respective biological subgroups instead of mixing entities which appear morphologically similar, such as large cell lymphomas, including DLBCL together with ALCL, or different subtypes of peripheral T-cell lymphoma (PTCL), such as ALCL with extranodal T/NK-cell lymphoma, because their clinical outcome may considerably differ (6, 11). Only a few publications exclusively report the outcome of paediatric patients receiving autologous or allogeneic HSCT for relapsed or refractory NHL where the specific subgroups were defined.

2.1 Burkitt lymphoma, mature B-cell acute lymphoblastic leukaemia and diffuse large B-cell lymphoma

Ladenstein et al. (7) analysed the outcome of 89 children with poor response to first-line chemotherapy (n=37) or relapsed (n=52) BL autografted between 1979 and 1991 in twelve European centres. Status at HSCT was the major prognostic factor for outcome. A more recent study from Japan (1996–2004) (12) of 33 children with relapsed (n=26) or refractory (n=7) mature B-cell neoplasms after failed current front-line therapy who then received HSCT for consolidation showed that none of 15 patients refractory to salvage therapy survived. Four of five patients transplanted in CR or PR (three autologous HSCT, two allogeneic HSCT) survived. In the study by Gross et al., no difference was found for relapse rate and event-free survival (EFS) for BL (17 autologous, 24 allogeneic) and DLBCL (35 autologous, 17 allogeneic) (9).

2.2 Lymphoblastic lymphoma (T-LBL, precursor B-cell (pB)-LBL)

Levine and co-workers compared the outcome of 204 patients (age range 5 to 67 years) with LBL undergoing autologous (n=128) or allogeneic (n=76) HSCT reported to the IBMTR or ABMTR between 1989 and 1998. In this study, OS was superior for patients undergoing autologous HSCT at six months (p = 0.01) but OS did not differ at 1 and 5 years. Relapse rate was lower for allografted patients at 1 year (p = 0.05) and at 5 years (p = 0.004), but this advantage was offset by higher procedure-related mortality at all time points studied (3). An eventual impact of age as a prognostic factor or differences between paediatric and adult patients was not specifically mentioned in that report.

A recent analysis from the BFM-group restricted to children and adolescents confirmed the poor outcome of patients with relapsing or progressive LBL (1990–2003). Of 34 patients, 29 died (median time to death was 5 only months) resulting in an OS of 14 ± 6% at 5 years (13). Only those few children who were allografted had a chance of cure (four of nine children with T-LBL and one of three with pB-LBL). The main reason of death was disease progression.

Also, in the large study from the CIBMTR, outcome with respect to EFS and relapse rate was statistically better for patients receiving allogeneic HSCT compared to autologous transplantation (9).

2.3 Anaplastic large-cell lymphoma

Woesmann et al. reported on 20 relapsed children (1991–2003) allografted for ALCL after failing first-line BFM treatment. Six patients had progressed during first-line therapy and median time from end of first-line treatment to relapse was <3 months. The majority of children had advanced disease at diagnosis and were in complete or partial remission (CR, PR) after treatment with pulsed salvage chemotherapy regimens at the time of HSCT. Five patients had failed a prior autologous HSCT. Conditioning regimen was myeloablative and included total body irradiation in 15 patients. EFS for the total cohort was remarkable 75 ± 10% at 3 years (14). Of five patients who died, deaths were attributed to lymphoma in two and HSCT-related complications in three patients.

Due to the small numbers of patients who might be in need for HSCT, it is probably unlikely that randomised studies aiming to assess the superiority of autologous HSCT or allogeneic HSCT can be performed at all.

3. Hodgkin's lymphoma

Paediatric patients with HL suffering from relapse in general have a reliable chance of cure with stratified risk-adapted therapy. While those with late relapses occurring >12 months after end of first-line therapy can be cured with conventional chemo-radiotherapy, outcome for patients with progressive disease is still unsatisfactory. While autologous HSCT is the standard therapeutic approach for adult patients with relapsing or progressive HL, fewer patients have so far been treated with either autologous or allogeneic HSCT in the paediatric and adolescent age group (15).

3.1 Autologous HSCT for HL

As shown by Schmitz and co-workers, autologous HSCT provides superior progression-free survival (PFS) to conventional chemotherapy in chemosensitive HL, especially in patients with early recurring lymphoma (16). These comparisons have not been performed in the paediatric population but there seems to be an advantage in patients transplanted compared to those receiving chemo-radiotherapy as salvage therapy. The role of autologous HSCT as a therapeutic option *per se* in refractory HL, however, is considered low.

A large study from Spain, including 494 paediatric and adult patients (median age 27 years, range 1–63) (4) identified disease status at autologous HSCT as the most important prognostic factor for time to treatment failure (TTTF) as well as OS (p = 0.00001 each). The actuarial rates for TTTF and OS at 5 years for all patients were 45 and 54.5%, respectively. In multivariate analysis, the number of prior lines of therapy and the use of total-body irradiation increased the risk for non-relapse mortality, which was in total 8.5% for all patients at 4 years. The effect of age as a possible prognostic factor was not studied in that series.

Table 1 gives a summary of selected paediatric series analysing prognostic factors in autologous HSCT for HL.
In summary, these studies indicate that disease status at autologous HSCT expressed as response to prior treatment, tumour mass at HSCT or presence of elevated LDH is predictive of outcome although measurements slightly vary (DFS, EFS, FFS, PFS).

Table 1: Selected publications on autologous HSCT for paediatric and adolescent HL

Author	N	Median age at HSCT (years)	OS at 5 years	DFS, EFS, FFS or PFS at 5 years	Risk factors for adverse outcome in multivariate analysis
Williams (1993)	81	17	52 alive	39% (PFS, 3 years)	Disease status at HSCT and sex (PFS)
Baker (1999)	53	NA (<13–21)	43%	31% (FFS)	Increased LDH before HSCT (FFS, OS), short interval to HSCT (OS)
Stoneham (2004)	51	NA (3–17)	34 alive	15 relapsed	NA
Lieskovsky (2004)	41	18	68%	63% (PFS)	Extranodal disease at first relapse and disease status at HSCT (EFS, PFS, OS), primary induction failure (EFS, OS)
Franckovich (2001)	34	18	76%	67% (DFS)	Extranodal disease at relapse (DFS, OS), disease status at HSCT (DFS)
Verdeguer (2000)	20	NA	95%	62% (EFS)	NA
Petropoulos (2006)	13	15	70%	70% (EFS)	NA

Modified from (1). DFS: disease-free survival; EFS: event-free survival; FFS: failure-free survival; HL: Hodgkin's lymphoma; HSCT: haematopoietic stem cell transplantation; LDH: lactate dehydrogenase; NA: not available; OS: overall survival; PFS: progression-free survival

3.2 Allogeneic HSCT for HL

Two large studies including of 168 (including children and adolescents) and 285 patients, respectively, conducted by the EBMT have investigated the role of allogeneic HSCT in recurring HL (17, 18). In both studies the majority of patients had failed a prior autologous HSCT. Sureda et al. showed that the use of reduced intensity conditioning (89 patients) regimens compared to myeloablative regimens (79 patients) decreased the rate of non-relapse mortality (p <0.001), improved OS (p = 0.003), and showed a trend for a better progression-free survival (PFS; p = 0.07). Patients who developed chronic GvHD had fewer relapses in comparison with those who had no GvHD (p = 0.05). Disease status at allogeneic HSCT was the most important prognostic factor for OS, PFS and relapse rate. With respect to conditioning regimen, 57% of patients receiving reduced intensity compared to 30% treated with myeloablative regimens, respectively, relapsed (17). In the study by Robinson et al. on prognostic factors for patients receiving reduced intensity conditioning, OS at 1 and 3 years were 67% and 43%, and PFS was 39% and 25% respectively. Disease progression rate at 1 and 5 years was 41 and 59%, respectively. Compared to earlier publications on the use of allogeneic HSCT for recurring HL, relapse rate meanwhile exceeds the rate for non-relapse mortality (18).

Only very few publications on allogeneic HSCT for paediatric HL are available and patient numbers are small. In a recent EBMT study on 91 paediatric and adolescent patients ≤18 years at HSCT (51 reduced intensity conditioning, 40 myeloablative regimens), PFS for all patients was 40 ± 6% and 30 ± 6% at 2 and 5 years, respectively. The corresponding rates for OS were 54 ± 6% and 45 ± 6%, respectively. Nearly half of the patients had four or more lines of therapy before HSCT or had failed a prior autologous HSCT. Non-relapse mortality at 1 year was 21 ± 4% with comparable figures with respect to regimen intensity. In multivariate risk factor analysis, disease status at HSCT was the most powerful predictor for PFS (p <0.001) and OS (p = 0.001). Interestingly, patients receiving a less intensive conditioning regimen had a higher relapse rate (p = 0.02) and lower PFS (p = 0.02) beyond the first 9 months following allografting. This might leave room for more intensive conditioning regimens at least for those in good performance before HSCT. Chronic GvHD did not emerge as a prognostic factor for disease controls in that study. Outcome was encouraging for those patients transplanted with chemosensitive lymphoma, in good performance status and in more recent years (PFS and OS at 3 years were 60 and 83%, respectively) (19). Prospective studies need to be undertaken to solve the open questions of optimal time point for allogeneic HSCT, the most effective conditioning regimen and GvHD prophylaxis.

4. Conclusions

4.1 NHL

Both autologous and allogeneic HSCT can be effective therapeutic options in relapsed paediatric NHL, although several questions remain to be determined, among them the optimal time point for transplantation and choice of the best conditioning regimen. In general, autologous HSCT should be considered for children with mature B-cell lymphomas in chemosensitive relapse. Allogeneic HSCT has been shown to be an effective treatment option in NHL and should be carefully considered especially for patients with relapsed and refractory LBL or ALCL as well as selected patients with disease recurrence after failed prior autologous HSCT or those failing early in the course of standardised salvage therapy.

4.2 HL

Autologous HSCT is beneficial for children with recurring HL responding to salvage therapy. Those few patients with late relapses (occurring >12 months after end of first-line therapy) may have another attempt with chemo-radiotherapy before autologous HSCT is considered. Allogeneic HSCT in HL has a role for patients relapsing after autologous HSCT and those with multiple relapses but disease recurrence remains the major problem. Disease status at HSCT is a strong risk factor for outcome, highlighting the necessity of achieving the best possible response before HSCT (19).

4.3 Future directions

Disease status at the time of transplantation and time to relapse remain important prognostic factors for predicting outcome of autologous and allogeneic HSCT in paediatric lymphoma. The additional evaluation of disease status prior to HSCT by PET will probably be helpful to clarify which patients will be suitable candidates for autologous HSCT in HL as well as in NHL. Also, the incorporation of monoclonal antibodies, such as rituximab for B-cell lymphomas or novel substances, e.g. anti-CD30 coupled compounds in the concept of salvage therapy strategies before and/or after HSCT in CD30 positive lymphomas (20) and other targeted approaches conducted within clinical trials may contribute to an improved outcome in high-risk patients with HL or NHL in the future.

References

1. Claviez A, Sureda A, Schmitz N. Haematopoietic SCT for children and adolescents with relapsed and refractory Hodgkin's lymphoma. Bone Marrow Transplant 2008; 42 (Suppl 2): S16–S24.
2. Peniket AJ, Ruiz de Elvira MC, Taghipour G et al. An EBMT registry matched study of allogeneic stem cell transplants for lymphoma: Allogeneic transplantation is associated with a lower relapse rate but a higher procedure-related mortality rate than autologous transplantation. Bone Marrow Transplant 2003; 31: 667–678.
3. Levine JE, Harris RE, Loberiza FR, Jr. et al. A comparison of allogeneic and autologous bone marrow transplantation for lymphoblastic lymphoma. Blood 2003; 101: 2476–2482.
4. Sureda A, Arranz R, Iriondo A et al. Autologous stem-cell transplantation for Hodgkin's disease: Results and prognostic factors in 494 patients from the Grupo Espanol de Linfomas/Transplante Autologo de Medula Osea Spanish Cooperative Group. J Clin Oncol 2001; 19: 1395–1404.
5. Reiter A, Ferrando AA. Malignant Lymphomas and Lymphadenopathies. In: Orkin SH, Fisher

DE, Look AT et al. (eds.) Oncology of Infancy and Childhood. 2009, 1st ed. Saunders; Philadelphia, PA. pp 417–505.

6. Gordon BG, Weisenburger DD, Sanger WG et al. Peripheral T-cell lymphoma in children and adolescents: Role of bone marrow transplantation. Leuk Lymphoma 1994; 14: 1–10.

7. Ladenstein R, Pearce R, Hartmann O et al. High-dose chemotherapy with autologous bone marrow rescue in children with poor-risk Burkitt's lymphoma: A report from the European Lymphoma Bone Marrow Transplantation Registry. Blood 1997; 90: 2921–2930.

8. Attarbaschi A, Dworzak M, Steiner M et al. Outcome of children with primary resistant or relapsed non-Hodgkin lymphoma and mature B-cell leukemia after intensive first-line treatment: A population-based analysis of the Austrian Cooperative Study Group. Pediatr Blood Cancer 2005; 44: 70–76.

9. Gross TG, Hale GA, He W et al. Hematopoietic stem cell transplantation for refractory or recurrent non-Hodgkin lymphoma in children and adolescents. Biol Blood Marrow Transplant 2010; 16: 223–230.

10. World Health Organization classification of tumours. Pathology and genetics of tumours of hematopoietic and lymphoid tissues. Swerdlow SH, Campo E, Harris NL, Jaffe ES, Pileri SA, Stein H et al. (eds). 2008, 4th ed. IARC Press; Lyon.

11. Won SC, Han JW, Kwon SY et al. Autologous peripheral blood stem cell transplantation in children with non-Hodgkin's lymphoma: A report from the Korean society of pediatric hematology-oncology. Ann Hematol. 2006; 85: 787–794.

12. Fujita N, Mori T, Mitsui T et al. The role of hematopoietic stem cell transplantation with relapsed or primary refractory childhood B-cell non-Hodgkin lymphoma and mature B-cell leukemia: A retrospective analysis of enrolled cases in Japan. Pediatr Blood Cancer 2008; 51: 188–192.

13. Burkhardt B, Reiter A, Landmann E et al. Poor outcome for children and adolescents with progressive disease or relapse of lymphoblastic lymphoma: A report from the Berlin-Frankfurt-Muenster group. J Clin Oncol 2009; 27: 3363–3369.

14. Woessmann W, Peters C, Lenhard M et al. Allogeneic haematopoietic stem cell transplantation in relapsed or refractory anaplastic large cell lymphoma of children and adolescents - a Berlin-Frankfurt-Munster group report. Br J Haematol 2006; 133: 176–182.

15. Ljungman P, Bregni M, Brune M et al. Allogeneic and autologous transplantation for haematological diseases, solid tumours and immune disorders: Current practice in Europe 2009. Bone Marrow Transplant 2010; 45: 219–234.

16. Schmitz N, Pfistner B, Sextro M et al. Aggressive conventional chemotherapy compared with high-dose chemotherapy with autologous haemopoietic stem-cell transplantation for relapsed chemosensitive Hodgkin's disease: A randomised trial. Lancet 2002; 359: 2065–2071.

17. Sureda A, Robinson S, Canals C et al. Reduced-intensity conditioning compared with conventional allogeneic stem-cell transplantation in relapsed or refractory Hodgkin's lymphoma: An analysis from the Lymphoma Working Party of the European Group for Blood and Marrow Transplantation. J Clin Oncol 2007; 26: 455–462.

18. Robinson SP, Sureda A, Canals C et al. Reduced intensity conditioning allogeneic stem cell transplantation for Hodgkin's lymphoma: Identification of prognostic factors predicting outcome. Haematologica 2009; 94: 230–238.
19. Claviez A, Canals C, Dierickx D et al. Allogeneic hematopoietic stem cell transplantation in children and adolescents with recurrent and refractory Hodgkin lymphoma: An analysis of the European Group for Blood and Marrow Transplantation. Blood 2009; 114: 2060–2067.
20. Younes A, Bartlett NL, Leonard JP et al. Brentuximab vedotin (SGN-35) for relapsed CD30-positive lymphomas. N Engl J Med 2010; 363: 1812–1821.

Multiple Choice Questionnaire

To find the correct answer, go to http://www.esh.org/online-training/handbook/

1. **The main risk factor predicting outcome for children and adolescents receiving autologous HSCT for Hodgkin's lymphoma is:**
   a) Histological subtype ☐
   b) Stage at diagnosis or relapse ☐
   c) LDH level before start of high-dose therapy ☐
   d) Disease status before HSCT ☐

2. **Patients with early relapse of Hodgkin's lymphoma responding to salvage therapy will most probably benefit from the following treatment:**
   a) Involved-field radiotherapy ☐
   b) Reduced-intensity allogeneic HSCT ☐
   c) High-dose therapy and autologous HSCT ☐
   d) Maintenance therapy ☐

3. **Which of the following is true for allogeneic HSCT in young patients with Hodgkin's lymphoma?**
   a) Generally indicated in patients with first relapse ☐
   b) Indicated in selected patients with multiple relapses and those failing autologous HSCT ☐
   c) Main cause of death in recent years is non-relapse mortality compared to disease recurrence ☐
   d) Allogeneic HSCT has no indication in Hodgkin's lymphoma ☐

4. **The standard first-line treatment for children and adolescents with NHL is:**
   a) Radiotherapy, to avoid use of cardiotoxic drugs .... ☐
   b) Autologous HSCT is the gold standard in Burkitt's lymphoma .... ☐
   c) Risk-adapted polychemotherapy .... ☐
   d) Allogeneic HSCT in patients with lymphoblastic lymphoma .... ☐

---

5. **Which of the following is true for paediatric patients with relapsed NHL?**
   a) Patients with recurring anaplastic large-cell lymphoma generally have a very poor prognosis and can only rarely be rescued .... ☐
   b) Due to a very high rate of disease progression in relapsed lymphoblastic lymphoma allogeneic HSCT may be the only curative therapeutic option for these patients .... ☐
   c) Allogeneic HSCT has been shown to be clearly superior to autologous HSCT in chemo-sensitive mature diffuse large B-cell lymphoma .... ☐
   d) Relapses in lymphoblastic lymphoma tend to occur late .... ☐

NOTES

✳ CHAPTER 20

HSCT for children and adolescents

✳ 20.6
Primary immunodeficiency diseases

Paul Veys, H Bobby Gaspar

1. Introduction

Primary immunodeficiency (PID) diseases arise from genetic defects that lead to abnormalities in immune cell development or function. Replacement of the defective lineage by HSCT from healthy allogeneic donors remains the curative approach for most patients. Other management options including enzyme replacement therapy and gene transfer into autologous haematopoietic stem cells may provide an alternative approach to HSCT in specific immune deficiencies.

2. Diseases

PID may be broadly divided into severe combined immunodeficiencies (SCID) and non-SCID. Non-SCID can be further subdivided into T-cell deficiencies, CD40 ligand deficiency, Wiskott-Aldrich syndrome (WAS), X-linked lymphoproliferative disorder (XLP), phagocytic cell disorders, haemophagocytic syndromes and autoimmune and immunoregulatory disorders (Table 1).

Overall guidelines for HSCT for SCID and non-SCID diseases together with detailed protocols have been produced by the EBMT inborn Errors Working Party (EBMT IEWP) and can be found online at: *http://www.ebmt.org/5WorkingParties/IEWP/wparties-ie5.html.*

3. SCID

The overall frequency of SCID is around 1 in 75,000 live births although the exact frequency is unclear. The immunological phenotypes of SCID are shown in Table 1 and represents monogenic inherited defects in T, B and NK cell differentiation leading to the absence or inactivity of corresponding mature cells. Over the past two decades, the genetic basis of the different forms of SCID have been identified (Table 1) leading to modifications in transplant strategy dependent on the underlying defect. Clinically, most patients present by age 6 months with unusually severe and recurrent infections or with opportunistic infections, the most common being *Pneumocystis jiroveci pneumonitis*. Other common symptoms include diarrhea, dermatitis, and failure to thrive. Survival in SCID patients depends on expeditious T-cell reconstitution, and in the absence of successful HSCT most children die in first year of life from overwhelming infection. It is recognised that as many of 50% of SCID patients are engrafted with maternal T-cells but in most instances these cells do not initiate GvHD. Transfusion associated GvHD, on the other hand, is frequently lethal in SCID and any patient with a possible diagnosis of SCID should receive irradiated blood products. Bacille Calmette-Guérin (BCG) vaccination can give rise to disseminated BCG-osis in SCID patients and should be avoided at birth if there is any suspicion or family history of immunodeficiency.

Table 1: Classification of primary immunodeficiency

- Severe combined immunodeficiency (SCID)

Functional	Genetic
T⁻ B⁻ NK⁻	ADA deficiency reticular dysgenesis
T⁻ B⁻ NK⁺	RAG deficiency SCID with Artemis Cernunnos DNA Ligase 4 DNA PK
T⁻ B⁺ NK⁻	γc deficiency (X linked) Jak 3 kinase deficiency (AR)
T⁻ B⁺ NK⁺	IL-7 Rα deficiency CD3 δ, ε, ζ defects Coronin 1A defect unspecified

- T-cell immunodeficiency/SCID variants
  - CD4 lymphopenia
  - Zap 70 kinase deficiency
  - MHC class II deficiency
  - PNP deficiency
  - Omenn's syndrome
  - Severe Di George complex (22q 11 del)
  - CID with skeletal dysplasia
  - Cartilage hair hypoplasia
  - Njmegen breakage syndrome
  - Other

- CD40 ligand deficiency
- WASP deficiency
- XLP
- Haemophagocytic syndromes
  - Familial HLH
  - Griscelli disease
  - Immunodeficiency with partial albinism
  - Chediak-Higashi syndrome*
- Phagocytic cell disorders
  - IFN-γ receptor deficiency
  - Kostmann disease*
  - Shwachman's syndrome*
  - Granule deficiency
  - LAD
  - X-linked CGD*
  - AR-CGD*
- Autoimmune/immune dysregulation
  - Autoimmune lymphoproliferative syndrome (ALPS) (homozygotes)
  - IPEX syndrome
  - IL10R deficiency
  - Other

*Not all patients proceed to HSCT

3.1 General principles in transplant for SCID

Data from the European registry for SCID transplants (SCETIDE) has now collected data on SCID transplants for over 30 years and a number of important publications have documented the outcomes and important risk factors (1–3).

The major factors influencing outcome include:

1. The type of donor with matched sibling donors having the best outcome
2. The type of SCID, with T-B- forms of SCID having a poorer outcome
3. Preceding co-morbidity (pneumonitis, septicaemia, viral illness, malnutrition) adversely influencing outcome
4. Age at transplant with patients <6 mounths having an improved outcome.

3.2 Matched sibling donor HSCT for SCID

The outcome for MSD HSCT in SCID is now probably in excess of 90%. Somewhat remarkably, sibling donor BM may be infused into SCID recipients without the requirement for conditioning or GvHD prophylaxis. Infusion of sibling BM leads to the rapid development of T- and B-cell function post-HSCT, although usually only T-cells of donor origin develop, and myeloid and erythroid cells remain of recipient origin. The majority of patients achieve humoral reconstitution despite lack of donor B-cells, although this is dependent on the type of SCID.

3.3 Other matched family and unrelated donor HSCT for SCID
Successes have also been reported with phenotypically matched related as well as unrelated donors. In comparison to genotypically-identical sibling donors, phenotypically-matched related and matched unrelated transplants have a trend to reduced overall survival (81, 72, 63% respectively) (3, 4). It is generally considered that the risk of rejection/GvHD is too high for simple infusion of phenotypically matched marrow into SCID patients, so conditioning/GvHD prophylaxis is recommended. A variety of conditioning regimes have been used and current recommendations include the use of an i.v. busulfan/fludarabine or treosulphan/fludarabine based protocol (details at: *http://www.ebmt.org/5WorkingParties/IEWP/wparties-ie5.html*).

3.4 HLA-mismatched family donor for SCID
Virtually all children have an haploidentical parental donor and this is an alternative option especially as the donor is readily available. HLA-disparity necessitates rigorous T-cell depletion in order to avoid GvHD. With the introduction of PBPCs as a preferred stem cell source most centres now employ CD34+ cell selection or large scale CD3/CD19 negative depletion methods to achieve a 4–5 log T-cell depletion achieving a threshold of $1–5 \times 10^4$/kg CD3+ cells, below which GvHD prophylaxis is not required. Some centres advocate performing transplants without the use of any conditioning and survival rates of over 80% have been reported (5). However, the best results are seen in those transplanted at <3.5 months of age and also this does not seem to be equally efficient in all forms of SCID with the best results seen in the T-B+ phenotype. Even in these cases, B-cell function is only restored in ~20% of patients. Alternatively conditioning regimes can be used but the use of myeloablative conditioning regimes in children often <1 yr of age and with significant co-morbidity, leads to survival figures of 50–60%.

3.5 Unrelated cord blood transplantation for SCID
There are now in excess of 450,000 cord blood units stored worldwide. There are some theoretical advantages for the use of cord blood stem cells for SCID, namely: rapid availability, as with haplotype-matched parental donors but with

no requirement for T-cell depletion; less risk of GvHD compared to adult unrelated donors; no medical risk to the donor; and a greater proliferative life span which might be particularly important in such young recipients. There are also some specific disadvantages including: slower engraftment; lack of viral specific cytotoxic T-cells; and lack of availability of the donor for a boost HSCT. Of 20 SCID patients who have undergone CBT reported in the literature and reviewed recently, 16 (80%) are surviving with good immune reconstitution including B-cell reconstitution (6).

3.6 HSCT for radiosensitive SCID

Patients with T-B- SCID due to radiosensitive disorders such as DNA ligase 4 deficiency, Cernunnos deficiency, DNA-PKcs deficiency are increasingly being identified and being considered for haematopoietic stem cell transplant. As many of the conditioning regimens are particularly damaging to DNA, less toxic regimens are required to successfully treat these patients. No definitive studies are available but a low dose fludarabine/cyclophosphamide regime has been suggested by the EBMT IEWP (*http://www.ebmt.org/5WorkingParties/IEWP/wparties-ie5.html*).

4. Non-SCID immunodeficiency

The major difference with non-SCID patients in comparison to SCID patients is the usual requirement for a conditioning regimen to achieve engraftment. Many children with non-SCID PID have significant co-morbidities at the time of HSCT and conventional myeloablative preparation with busulfan/cyclophosphamide based regimes may be associated with significant treatment-related toxicity as well as long-term sequelae. Recent alternatives have:

1. Replaced cyclophosphamide with fludarabine, as the combination of busulfan and fludarabine appears better tolerated in these patients
2. Replaced busulfan with a structural analogue, treosulphan, which is similarly immuno- and myelo-suppressive, but does not cause hepatic veno-occlusive disease (VOD) (7)
3. Used reduced intensity HSCT to achieve stable engraftment of immunocompetent donor cells with reduced procedure-related morbidity and mortality (8). Sufficient long-term donor chimerism needs to be confirmed following these new approaches.

The latest outcome data for HSCT in non-SCID patients comes from Europe (3). In the 2000–2005 period, HSCT using an unrelated donor (n=124) gave a 3-year survival rate similar to a genoidentical donor (n=73), 79% for both. Survival was 76% in phenoidentical transplants (n=23) and worse in mismatched related donor transplants (n=47; 46%; p=0.016), in contrast to SCID patients (see above). Ten year survival was significantly better for patients with WAS, phagocytic and haemophagocytic disorders than for patients with T-lymphocyte immunodeficiencies (71, 63, 58, 47% respectively). Unrelated CB donors appear to also give promising results in non-SCID immunodeficiency with 29/32 (91%) patients surviving CBT matched for 4-6/6 HLA antigens (6).

4.1 Wiskott-Aldrich syndrome
WAS is an X-linked disorder characterised by thrombocytopenia with small platelets, eczema, and progressive immunodeficiency. Without HSCT, WAS patients have a poor prognosis with the major causes of death being infection, bleeding and lymphoproliferative disease (LPD). The outcome of 194 WAS patients undergoing HSCT in the period 1980–2009 has recently been reported (9). Overall survival was 84%, and even higher 89% for those undergoing HSCT since 2000. Good clinical status at the time of HSCT resulted in better survival. Younger age at HSCT(<2 yrs vs >5 yrs) was associated with better survival in children undergoing unrelated donor HSCT. Use of mismatched family donors or mismatched cord blood as a source of stem cells was associated with reduced survival and more post-HSCT complications. Mixed chimerism was associated with an increased risk of incomplete reconstitution of lymphocyte count and post-HSCT autoimmunity, and myeloid donor cell chimerism <50% was associated with persistent thrombocytopenia. Splenectomy pre- or post-HSCT was associated with an increased risk of fatal sepsis. A flow chart for management of WAS is shown in Figure 1.

4.2 T-cell immunodeficiency

4.2.1 Omenn's syndrome
Omenn's syndrome (OS) is characterised by SCID typically associated with the triad of erythroderma, hepatosplenomegaly, and lymphadenopathy. There is a marked eosinophilia and a variable number of autologous, activated, and oligoclonal T-lymphocytes (leaky SCID/CID), that infiltrate target organs and are generally poorly responsive to mitogens. Experience with HSCT in OS has been difficult with high levels of mortality in some studies. A recent study examining the use of alternative donor HSCT in a single centre reported survival in 9/11 patients with OS patients who were alive with immune reconstitution 30–146 months after HSCT (11). The overall mortality in this study was lower than previously reported and was due to early recognition of OS, and rapid initiation of treatment with topical/systemic immune suppression with steroids and/or cyclosporin A to control immune dysreactivity before proceeding to HSCT.

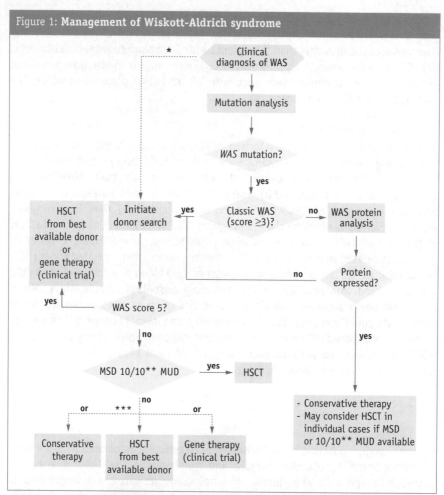

Figure 1: Management of Wiskott-Aldrich syndrome

*WAS Score see reference (10). Donor search should be initiated immediately for severely affected children with life-threatening complications; **high resolution DNA based typing for all alleles; ***no sufficient evidence which therapy is most appropriate*

4.2.2 HLA class II (MHC II) deficiency

MHC II deficiency patients seem to do particularly poorly through BMT (12); in a summary of 23 patients who underwent BMT for MHC II deficiency in Europe up to 1996, disease free survival was 40% for HLA-matched transplants (n=9) but only 20% from HLA-mismatched transplants (n=14). Of the eight patients who remained well post HSCT, all had persistently low CD4+ T-lymphocytes consistent with impaired thymic maturation caused by defective HLA class II expression on thymic epithelia, making the patients particularly susceptible to ongoing opportunist infection. Importantly in this condition reconstitution of antigen presenting cells, i.e. B-cells, monocytes, dendritic cells, and not just T-cells is essential for disease correction.

4.3 CD40 ligand deficiency (X-linked hyper-IgM syndrome)
CD40 ligand deficiency is a rare X-linked T-cell immunodeficiency caused by mutations in the gene encoding CD40 ligand glycoprotein (CD154) which is critical in initiating immunoglobulin isotype class switching from IgM to IgG, IgA and IgE in B-cells, and for monocyte/macrophage activation. Patients present recurrent bacterial sino-pulmonary infection leading to bronchiectasis and are particularly susceptible to gastrointestinal infection with protozoa such as *Cryptosporidium parvum*, leading to sclerosing cholangitis. Without HSCT about 50% of patients survive to the fourth decade. The largest HSCT series reported 38 patients from 8 European countries between 1993 and 2004 (13). HSCT cured 58% of the patients and 72% of those without hepatic disease. 32% died from infection-related complications, including severe cryptosporidiosis.

4.4 X-linked lymphoproliferative syndrome
X-linked lymphoproliferative syndrome (XLP) is a rare immunodeficiency characterised by a dysregulated immune response to Epstein-Barr virus and other pathogens. The clinical presentation includes fulminant infectious mononucleosis, haemophagocytic histiocytosis (HLH), lymphoma, hypogammaglobulinemia and aplastic anaemia. The advent of better treatment strategies for HLH and malignancy has greatly reduced mortality for these patients; survival following HSCT is 81% and similar with different donor sources, however, survival falls to 50% in patients with HLH as a feature of disease (14). It is logical to use EBV positive donors for EBV+ patients and if T-cell depletion is required for the HSCT procedure careful monitoring of the EBV viral load by EBV-specific RQ-PCR is advisable. The generation and use of EBV-specific CTLs may be beneficial, as well as depletion of donor/recipient B-lymphocytes by the administration of rituximab.

4.5 Phagocytic cell disorders

4.5.1 Kostmann syndrome
Severe congenital neutropenia (CN) (Kostmann syndrome) is a haematological disorder characterised by a maturation arrest of myelopoiesis at the promyelocyte/myelocyte stage of development. This arrest results in severe neutropenia leading to absolute neutrophil counts (ANC) below 0.2 x 10^9/L associated with severe

bacterial infections from early infancy. The availability of recombinant human granulocyte colony-stimulating factor (r-HuG-CSF) in 1987 dramatically changed the prognosis and quality of life of patients with CN. More than 90% of CN patients respond to r-HuG-CSF with an increase in ANC >1.0×10^9/L, requiring fewer antibiotics and reduced hospitalisation. In G-CSF less-responsive patients followed up for 10 years, 40% develop MDS/AML and 14% die of sepsis. This is the best group to target for HSCT as outcomes of HSCT have been poor when leukaemic transformation has already taken place.

4.5.2 Leucocyte adhesion deficiency

Leucocyte adhesion deficiency (LAD) is an autosomal recessive disorder characterised by impaired migration of neutrophils from the intravascular space, due to defective β2 leukocyte integrin (CD11/CD18) expression. Complete absence of CD11/CD18 leads to a severe phenotype usually presenting in early infancy and characterised by deep tissue infections, leukocytosis with impaired formation of pus, and delayed wound healing. The worldwide BMT experience was recently reviewed (15): amongst 36 patients the overall survival rate was 75%. Myeloablative conditioning regimens were used in 28 patients, and reduced-intensity conditioning in 8 patients, with no deaths in the latter subgroup. Survival rates after matched family donor and unrelated donor transplants were similar; mortality was greatest after haploidentical transplants.

4.5.3 Chronic granulomatous disease

Chronic granulomatous disease (CGD) is an inherited disorder of phagocyte function, characterised by recurrent, often life-threatening bacterial and fungal infections and by granuloma formation in vital organs. Neutrophils, monocytes/macrophages, and eosinophils cannot generate microbicidal oxygen metabolites owing to a defect in one of the four subunits of the NADPH oxidase of phagocytes. Despite prophylactic treatment with cotrimoxazole, itraconazole and/or gamma interferon, there is an annual mortality between 2 and 5%, with 25% of the deaths due to invasive aspergillosis. Recent BMT outcomes targeting iv busulfan to 75% of myeloablative dose + fludarabine + ATG or alemtuzumab (to suppress inflammation and GvHD) has produced excellent outcomes (>90% in 28 patients - *Gungor T, personal communication 2011*) with MSD or MUD donors respectively, prompting the suggestion that all children with CGD should undergo a BMT procedure if a matched donor is available.

4.6 Haemophagocytic syndromes

4.6.1 Familial haemophagocytic lymphohistiocytosis

Familial haemophagocytic lymphohistiocytosis (FHL) is a genetically determined autosomal recessive disorder characterised by the early onset of fever and hepatosplenomegaly, associated with pancytopenia, hypertriglyceridaemia, and hypofibrinogenaemia, and haemophagocytosis in the bone marrow. In addition, central nervous (CNS) involvement may be severe and cause permanent CNS dysfunction. The pathogenesis of FHL has been associated with the impairment of the cytotoxic pathway in lymphocytes, where uncontrolled activation of T-lymphocytes results in raised levels of inflammatory cytokines. Mutations within the perforin (PRF1) gene accounts for 30% of cases, while mutations of MUNC and SYNTAXIN genes account for another 40% or so. HLH is also a significant feature of other disorders including XLP 1 and 2, Chediak-Higashi and Griscelli syndromes. The condition is fatal without adequate treatment including HSCT. Initial therapy consists of cycles of therapy with etoposide, dexamethasone and cyclosporin A (CsA) (HLH 2004) or anti-thymocyte globulin (ATG), steroids and CsA with intrathecal methotrexate for CNS disease to achieve control of HLH, and followed by HSCT from the best available donor. Conventional BMT with busulfan and cyclophosphamide ± VP16 gives an overall 3 year survival rate of 64%: matched-related donor 71%; matched unrelated donor 70%; familial haploidentical donor 54%; and mismatched unrelated donor 54%. The odds ratio for mortality were 2.75 for those with active disease after 2 months of therapy compared with inactive disease, and 1.8 for children with active as opposed to inactive disease at the time of HSCT. Veno-occlusive disease is the major toxicity associated with transplants in HLH and because donor lymphocyte chimerism >20% is associated with sustained remission, reduced intensity conditioning (RIC) may be an alternative and perhaps better approach for FHL (16).

4.6.2 Chediak-Higashi syndrome
Chediak-Higashi syndrome (CHS) is a rare autosomal recessive syndrome characterised by oculo-cutaneous albinism, recurrent infections, microscopic finding of large granules in haematopoietic and other cells, neurologic abnormalities and a bleeding diathesis. In survivors of infectious complications an accelerated phase, manifested by life threatening haemophagocytosis, occurs within the first or second decade. Thirty-five children with CHS underwent HSCT and were reported to the CIBMTR (17), the 5-year probability of overall survival was 62%, suggesting that HSCT is effective therapy for the accelerated phase of CHS. However, progressive neurological dysfunction has been reported in long-term survivors of HSCT for CHS who had neither recurrent infections nor manifestations of haemophagocytic syndrome after HSCT. This suggests a steady long-term progression, despite HSCT, of the lysosomal defect in neurons and glial cells, and may question the appropriateness of HSCT in non-accelerated CHS.

5. Alternative therapies
Alternative treatments to HSCT have been developed for specific immunodeficiencies over the last two decades.

5.1 Enzyme replacement therapy for adenosine deaminase deficiency (ADA-SCID)
Enzyme replacement has been used in the treatment of ADA deficiency since 1987 (18). PEG-ADA is administered weekly or twice weekly by intramuscular injection and leads to rapid metabolic correction with normalisation of metabolic parameters which is then followed by cellular and humoral immune reconstitution. The extent of immune recovery is variable and a significant number (~50%) remain on immunoglobulin replacement (19). Over a longer time period, patients show a decline in T-cell numbers and remain lymphopenic (20). Long term follow-up shows that patients remain clinically well but a number of cases of EBV related lymphoma have been reported, suggesting decreased immune surveillance with time.

5.2 Gene therapy for specific immune deficiencies
Possibly the greatest advance has been the development of stem cell gene therapy for the treatment of defined genetic defects. The first human condition for which gene therapy has shown unequivocal benefit is X-linked severe combined immunodeficiency (SCID-X1). Using retroviral mediated transfer of the IL-2RG gene into autologous CD34+ cells, successful reconstitution of cellular and humoral immunity has been demonstrated in the majority of patients treated in two trials in Paris and London (21, 22). Since gene transduced cells have a significant survival advantage, this procedure can be undertaken without prior cytoreductive therapy and thus the short term morbidity of the procedure is low. Twenty patients have now been treated and nearly all have a shown significant improvement of T-cell numbers and ~50% show humoral reconstitution.

A number of gene therapy trials for ADA deficiency have also been initiated using gamma retroviral vectors. In contrast to the SCID-X1 studies, a mild non-myeloablative conditioning regime (in most cases iv busulfan 4 mg/kg) was used to allow engraftment of a greater number of gene modified cells. Over 30 patients have now been treated in 3 trials worldwide. All patients have survived and ~70% have been able to stop enzyme replacement therapy suggesting that gene therapy is able to effectively detoxify the system and allow immune reconstitution. Approximately 50% of patients have been able to stop immunoglobulin replacement no adverse events have been seen so far. In 3 patients with X-CGD, a similar retroviral vector based protocol using a non-myeloablative conditioning regime prior to the return of gene transduced autologous cells, showed substantial gene transfer into neutrophils leading to a large number of functionally corrected phagocytes and notable clinical improvement (23). Gene therapy for WAS using a gamma retroviral vector and a busulfan based conditioning regimen have also shown considerable success in correcting both the platelet and immunological defects.

These gene therapy studies show clearly that gene transfer into autologous stem cells can result in functional immune correction. However, side-effects related to insertion of the retroviral vector into a proto-oncogene (LMO2) have resulted in the development of T-cell leukaemia in 5 of 20 patients treated in the two SCID-X1 gene therapy studies (24). The reasons for oncogenesis relate to the integration profile of retroviral vector and their ability to activate transcription of neighboring genes. Modifications to vector design are in progress and may overcome the problems associated with these initial trials.

The role of gene therapy alongside conventional HSCT (or enzyme replacement therapy for ADA–SCID) is shown in the figures designed by the EBMT-IEWP (Figure 2 and Figure 3).

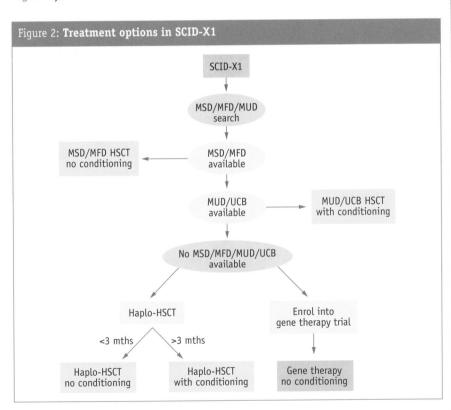

Figure 2: **Treatment options in SCID-X1**

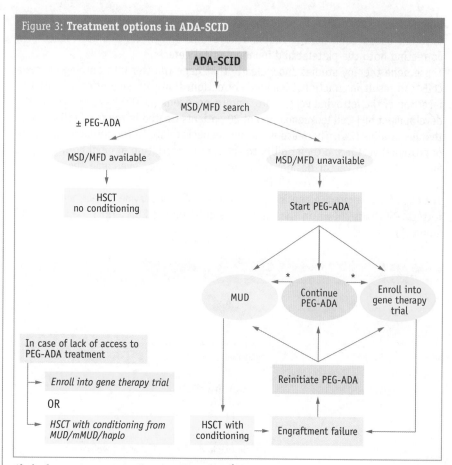

Figure 3: **Treatment options in ADA-SCID**

*lack of access to enzyme replacement therapy or ↓ thymic function

References

1. Fischer A, Landais P, Friedrich W et al. European experience of bone-marrow transplantation for severe combined immunodeficiency. Lancet 1990; 336: 850–854.
2. Antoine C, Müller S, Cant A, Cavazzana-Calvo M, Veys P, Vossen J, Fasth A, Heilmann C, Wulffraat N, Seger R, Blanche S, Friedrich W, Abinun M, Davies G, Bredius R, Schulz A, Landais P, Fischer A; European Group for Blood and Marrow Transplantation; European Society for Immunodeficiency. Long-term survival and transplantation of haemopoietic stem cells for immunodeficiencies: report of the European experience 1968-99. Lancet 2003; 361: 553–560.

3. Gennery AR, Slatter MA, Grandin L, Taupin P, Cant AJ, Veys P, Amrolia PJ, Gaspar HB, Davies EG, Friedrich W, Hoenig M, Notarangelo LD, Mazzolari E, Porta F, Bredius RG, Lankester AC, Wulffraat NM, Seger R, Güngör T, Fasth A, Sedlacek P, Neven B, Blanche S, Fischer A, Cavazzana-Calvo M, Landais P; Inborn Errors Working Party of the European Group for Blood and Marrow Transplantation; European Society for Immunodeficiency. Transplantation of hematopoietic stem cells and long-term survival for primary immunodeficiencies in Europe: Entering a new century, do we do better? J Allergy Clin Immunol 2010; 126: 602–610.

4. Grunebaum E, Mazzolari E, Porta F et al. Bone marrow transplantation for severe combined immune deficiency. JAMA 2006; 295: 508–518.

5. Buckley RH, Schiff SE, Schiff RI et al. Hematopoietic stem-cell transplantation for the treatment of severe combined immunodeficiency. N Engl J Med 1999; 340: 508–516.

6. Slatter MA, Gennery AR. Umbilical cord stem cell transplantation for primary immunodeficiencies. Expert Opin Biol Ther 2006; 6: 555–565.

7. Slatter MA, Rao K, Amrolia P et al. Treosulfan-based conditioning regimens for hematopoietic stem cell transplantation in children with primary immunodeficiency: United Kingdom experience. Blood 2011; 117: 4367–4375.

8. Veys P. Reduced intensity transplantation for primary immunodeficiency disorders. Immunol Allergy Clin North Am 2010; 30: 103–124.

9. Moratto D, Giliani S, Bonfim C et al. Long-term outcome and lineage-specific chimerism in 194 Wiskott-Aldrich Syndrome patients treated by hematopoietic cell transplantation between 1980-2009: An international collaborative study. Blood 2011; 118: 1675–1684.

10. Ochs HD, Filipovich AH, l Veys P et al. Wiskott-Aldrich Syndrome: Diagnosis, clinical and laboratory manifestations, and treatment. Biol Blood Marrow Transplant 2009; 15 (Suppl): 84-90.

11. Mazzolari E, Moshous D, Forino C et al. Hematopoietic stem cell transplantation in Omenn syndrome: A single-center experience. Bone Marrow Transplant 2005; 36: 107–114.

12. Elhasid R, Etzioni A. Major histocompatibility complex class II deficiency: A clinical review. Blood Rev 1996; 10: 242–248.

13. Gennery AR, Khawaja K, Veys P et al. Treatment of CD40 ligand deficiency by hematopoietic stem cell transplantation: A survey of the European experience, 1993-2002. Blood 2004; 103: 1152–1157.

14. Booth C, Gilmour KC, Veys P et al. X-linked lymphoproliferative disease due to SAP/SH2D1A deficiency: A multicenter study on the manifestations, management and outcome of the disease. Blood 2011; 117: 53–62.

15. Qasim W, Cavazzana-Calvo M, Davies EG et al. Allogeneic hematopoietic stem-cell transplantation for leukocyte adhesion deficiency. Pediatrics 2009; 123: 836–840.

16. Marsh RA, Vaughn G, Kim MO et al. Reduced-intensity conditioning significantly improves survival of patients with hemophagocytic lymphohistiocytosis undergoing allogeneic hematopoietic cell transplantation. Blood 2010; 116: 5824–5831.

17. Eapen M, DeLaat CA, Baker KS et al. Hematopoietic cell transplantation for Chediak-Higashi syndrome. Bone Marrow Transplant 2007; 39: 411–415.

18. Hershfield MS, Buckley RH, Greenberg ML et al. Treatment of adenosine deaminase deficiency

with polyethylene glycol-modified adenosine deaminase. N Engl J Med 1987; 316, 589–596.

19. Hershfield MS. PEG-ADA replacement therapy for adenosine deaminase deficiency: An update after 8.5 years. Clin Immunol Immunopathol 1995; 76: S228–32.

20. Chan B, Wara D, Bastian J et al. Long-term efficacy of enzyme replacement therapy for adenosine deaminase (ADA)-deficient Severe Combined Immunodeficiency (SCID). Clin Immunol 2005; 117: 133–143.

21. Hacein-Bey-Abina S, Le Deist F, Carlier F et al. Sustained correction of X-linked severe combined immunodeficiency by ex vivo gene therapy. N Engl J Med 2002; 346: 1185–1193.

22. Gaspar HB, Parsley KL, Howe S et al. Gene therapy of X-linked severe combined immunodeficiency by use of a pseudotyped gammaretroviral vector. Lancet 2004; 364: 2181–2187.

23. Ott MG, Schmidt M, Schwarzwaelder K et al. Correction of X-linked chronic granulomatous disease by gene therapy, augmented by insertional activation of MDS1-EVI1, PRDM16 or SETBP1. Nat Med 2006; 12: 401–409.

24. Hacein-Bey-Abina S, von Kalle C, Schmidt M et al. LMO2-associated clonal T cell proliferation in two patients after gene therapy for SCID-X1. Science 2003; 302: 415–419.

Multiple Choice Questionnaire

To find the correct answer, go to http://www.esh.org/online-training/handbook/

1. **X-linked SCID classically leads to which of the following immunological phenotypes?**
   a) T- B- NK- .... ☐
   b) T- B- NK+ .... ☐
   c) T- B+ NK- .... ☐
   d) T- B+ NK+ .... ☐

2. **Which one of the following is a radiosensitive form of SCID and requires careful use of alkylating agents?**
   a) ADA deficiency .... ☐
   b) JAK 3 deficiency .... ☐
   c) RAG deficient SCID .... ☐
   d) Cernunnos deficient SCID .... ☐

3. **Gene therapy is now available for which of the following forms of SCID?**

a) ADA deficiency .... ☐
b) JAK 3 deficiency .... ☐
c) Zap 70 deficient SCID .... ☐
d) Cernunnos deficient SCID .... ☐

4. **In HSCT for WAS:**
   a) Mixed donor chimerism is preferred over full donor chimerism .... ☐
   b) In patients with WAS platelets are typically large .... ☐
   c) Unrelated donor HSCT has better outcome in patients <5 yrs .... ☐
   d) Splenectomy should be performed pre-HSCT .... ☐

5. **Familial haemophagocytic lymphohistiocytosis:**
   a) Is typically an X-linked disorder .... ☐
   b) Reduced intensity conditioning is contraindicated .... ☐
   c) The CNS is never involved .... ☐
   d) Patients do better when HSCT is performed with inactive disease .... ☐

* CHAPTER 20

HSCT for children and adolescents

* 20.7
HSCT in inborn errors of metabolism and osteopetrosis

Jaap J. Boelens, Marc Bierings, Robert Wynn

1. Background

Inborn errors of metabolism (IEM) are a diverse group of diseases arising from genetic defects in lysosomal enzymes or peroxisomal function. Lysosomal enzymes are hydrolytic and are stored in cellular organelles called lysosomes. Peroxisomes are subcellular organelles involved in lipid metabolism. These diseases are characterised by devastating systemic processes affecting neurologic and cognitive function, growth and development, and cardiopulmonary status. Onset in infancy or early childhood is typically accompanied by rapid deterioration and associated with early death.

Timely diagnosis and immediate referral to a specialist in IEM are essential steps in management of these disorders, with discussion of the patient by a multidisciplinary team including a transplant-physician. Treatment recommendations are based on: the disorder; its phenotype including age at onset, rate of progression, severity of clinical signs and symptoms; family values and expectations; and the risks and benefits associated with available therapies such as HSCT (1).

The concept of correction of metabolic defects with transferable lysosomal enzymes was described in 1968, when fibroblasts of patients with Hurler (MPS IH) and Hunter (MPS II) syndromes were co-cultured in the laboratory (2). Metabolic correction of lysosomal storage diseases (LSD) occurs by mannose-6-phosphate receptor-mediated endocytosis of secreted enzyme and by direct transfer of enzyme from adjacent cells. The mechanism by which HSCT halts cerebral demyelination of the peroxisomal disorder cerebral X-linked adrenoleukodystrophy (X-ALD) is multifactorial: immunosuppression, replacement with metabolically competent cell populations leading to decreased perivascular inflammation, and metabolic correction. Migration, distribution, and growth of donor-derived metabolically-competent cells into host tissues including the central nervous system (CNS) are critical to the success of transplant. Microglia, the mononuclear phagocytes of the CNS which account for 5–10% of non-neuronal cells in brain, are derived from haematopoietic cells. In osteopetrosis, a disease due to osteoclast dysfunction, HSCT can correct the disease by providing competent osteoclasts since the osteoclast is derived from the haematopoietic stem cell (3).

In 1980, a 9-month-old boy with MPS IH received the first HSCT for an IEM. HSCT resulted in a dramatic improvement in the clinical phenotype (4). After this first patient >1000 HSCT's were performed for various IEM (>20) worldwide. Unfortunately, for unknown reasons not all LSDs benefit from HSCT; therefore careful evaluation of the effect of HSCT is of utmost importance. Additionally, results were limited due to high rates of graft-failure (15–75%), transplant-related-mortality and absence of rapid availability of unrelated donors for rapidly progressive diseases (5, 6).

International collaborative efforts to examine HSCT outcomes began in the late

1980s and continue today. Recent large multi- and single-centre reports on the outcomes of HSCT, including risk-factor analyses, have had a dramatic impact on success rates of HSCT in IEM (5, 7–11). Hurler's disease (MPS IH) has been the model-disease in these analyses. Currently, HSCT from an HLA-matched, enzymatically normal related donor and UCBT are the most common modalities of HSCT for IEM. This chapter will discuss indications for HSCT and outcomes for selected IEM: subdivided in 4 parts (LSDs, peroxisomal disorders, miscellaneous metabolic disorders and osteopetrosis).

2. Indications for HSCT and outcomes in selected IEM

2.1 Lysosomal storage diseases

2.1.1 Indications
Despite the fact that HSCT for IEM have been performed for more than 30 years, series of considerable size are only present for Hurler's syndrome, infantile Krabbe Disease and X-ALD (8, 11–13). For other disorders the efficacy of HSCT is difficult to assess because of the limited number of cases, a wide range of clinical heterogeneity and the absence of a good functioning registry for proper long-term follow-up. In cases where damage to the central nervous system (CNS) is present this is irreversible and therefore it represents a contra-indication for HSCT in all candidate diseases (8, 9, 12, 13). Table 1 lists standard indications, optional, investigational and unknown. This guideline however should be interpreted in the context of progress in transplantation.

2.1.2 Results
Hurler's disease (MPS IH) is the most frequently studied disease, mainly because it is the most frequent indication for HSCT. Graft-outcome analyses for MPS IH were the basis for recent international transplant guidelines in all HSCT in IEM (EBMT-Handbook 2008). HSCT for children with MPS IH is effective, resulting in increased life expectancy and improvement of clinical parameters. HSCT must be performed early in the disease course before the onset of irreversible damage to derive maximum long-term benefit in children with MPS IH (13). Donor cell engraftment after HSCT results in rapid reduction of obstructive airway symptoms and hepatosplenomegaly. Hearing, vision, and linear growth improve in many cases. Hydrocephalus is either prevented or stabilised and cardiovascular pathology after HSCT is altered beneficially. However, cerebral damage already present before HSCT appears to be irreversible (10, 13). Recent HSCT experience for MPS IH demonstrates significantly improved graft-

Table 1: Inherited metabolic disorders for which HSCT may be indicated

Disorder	Enzyme/Protein	Indication	Comments
Mucopolysaccharidoses			
Hurler (MPS IH)	alpha-L-iduronidase	Standard	
Hurler/Scheie (MPS IH/S)	alpha-L-iduronidase	Option	ERT first-line therapy
Scheie (MPS IS)	alpha-L-iduronidase	Option	ERT first-line therapy
Hunter: Severe (MPS IIA)	Iduronate-2-sulfatase	Investigational	Only early and/or asymptomatic
Hunter: Attenuated (MPS IIB)	Iduronate-2-sulfatase	Investigational	Only early and/or asymptomatic
Sanfilippo (MPS IIIA)	Heparan-N-sulfatase	Investigational	Only early and/or asymptomatic
Sanfilippo (MPS IIIB)	N-acetylglucosaminidase	Investigational	Only early and/or asymptomatic
Sanfilippo (MPS IIIC)	AcetylCoA:N-acetyltransferase	Investigational	Only early and/or asymptomatic
Sanfilippo (MPS IIID)	N-acetylglucosamine 6-sulfatase	Investigational	Only early and/or asymptomatic
Maroteaux-Lamy (MPS VI)	Arylsulfatase B	Option	ERT first-line therapy
Sly (MPS VII)	Beta-glucuronidase	Option	
Leukodystrophies			
X-ALD, cerebral	ALD protein	Standard	
MLD: Infantile	Arylsulfatase A	Unknown	Gene-therapy trial open (Milan)
MLD: Juvenile	Arylsulfatase A	Option	Only early and/or asymptomatic, Gene therapy trial open (Milan)
MLD: Late onset	Arylsulfatase A	Standard	Only early and/or asymptomatic
GLD: Early onset	Galactocerebrosidase	Option	Neonate, screening diagnosis, or second case in known family; not for advanced disease
GLD: Late onset	Galactocerebrosidase	Option	Not in advanced disease
Glycoprotein metabolic & miscellaneous disorders			
Fucosidosis	Fucosidase	Option	
Alpha-mannosidosis	alpha-Mannosidase	Standard	
Aspartylglucosaminuria	Aspartylglucosaminidase	Option	
Farber	Ceramidase	Option	
Tay-Sachs: Early onset	Hexosaminidase A	Unknown	
Tay-Sachs: Juvenile	Hexosaminidase A	Investigational	Neonate, screening diagnosis, or second case in known family
Sandhoff: Early onset	Hexosaminidase A & B	Unknown	
Sandhoff: Juvenile	Hexosaminidase A & B	Investigational	Neonate, screening diagnosis, or second case in known family
Gaucher I (non-neuronopathic)	Glucocerebrosidase	Option	
Gaucher II (acute neuronopathic)	Glucocerebrosidase	Unknown	ERT first-line therapy
Gaucher III (subacute neuronopathic)	Glucocerebrosidase	Unknown	

continue

Pompe	Glucosidase	Investigational	Limited benefit of ERT ERT available (optional in CRIM-pt)
Niemann Pick: Type A	Acid sphingomyelinase	Unknown	ERT available
Niemann Pick: Type B	Acid sphingomyelinase	Option	ERT first-line therapy
Niemann Pick: Type C	Cholesterol trafficking	Option for C-2	Only early or asymptomatic
Mucolipidosis: Type II (I-cell)	N-acetylglucosamine-1-phosphotransferase	Investigational	
Wolman Syndrome	Acid lipase	Option	May be viewed as standard
Multiple sulfatase deficiency	Sulfatases	Investigational	
MNGIE (mitochondrial neurogastrointestinal encephalomyopathy	Thymidine phosphorylase	Option	Not in advanced disease

Table does not include diseases where HSCT is not indicated. Standard: HSCT applied routinely. Considerable published research evidence from registries and institutions demonstrates efficacy. Delayed diagnosis and/or advanced disease may preclude transplant for individual patients. Option: HSCT is effective but other therapy is increasingly considered first choice. Or, insufficient published evidence for HSCT to be considered standard. Investigational: possible a priori reason for HSCT. Further published evidence needed to support the use of HSCT in clinical practice. Unknown: no published evidence that HSCT is beneficial. ERT: enzyme replacement therapy

outcomes (engrafted survival rates >90%) when compared to earlier findings (1, 7). Poorer historical results such as engrafted survival rates of 25 to 70% (5, 6) have been attributed to clinical learning curve, restricted donor availability, graft-failure, mixed chimerism and transplant-related morbidity and mortality. Risk analysis showed that graft-failures were increased with the use of T-cell depleted grafts and reduced-intensity conditioning and decreased with the use of dose-adjusted busulfan (5). A more recent study (n=258), only including patients receiving a myeloablative conditioning regimen, showed that the outcomes after id-SIB transplantation were comparable to those after 6/6 UCBT, and 10/10 MUD comparable to 5/6 UCBT (as well as 4/6 UCBT with high cell dose (14). Mixed-chimerism was noted in 40% of the idSIB and MUD recipients. Mixed-chimerism impacts the post-HSCT enzyme level and lower enzyme levels affects the long-term clinical outcome.

These data led to the development of guidelines for HSCT in MPS IH. The guidelines include a standardised busulfan (Bu)/cyclophosphamide (Cy) conditioning regimen and the use of CB as a preferred graft source, second only to enzymatically normal matched sibling-BM. Recent evaluation of this guideline showed significantly higher engrafted survival rates of 90% (n=43) (1) compared to the historical EBMT-cohort which was 53% (1995–2004) (5). This guideline (Table 2) was recently updated by replacing cyclophosphamide by fludarabine since in a recent study busulfan with therapeutic drug monitoring combined with fludarabine was found to be safer than and at least as effective as conventional BuCy (15).

Table 2: **Donor hierarchy and conditioning**

a. Stem cell source hierarchy in lysosomal storage diseases and peroxisomal disorders
1. Identical-SIB (not carriers)
2. UD (10/10) = Unrelated Cord Blood (UCB: 6/6)
3. UCB (5/6)
4. UCB (4/6) = mismatched-UD (non-T-depleted)
5. UCB (3/6) = haplo (not recommended)

- UD (10/10) may be bypassed depending on institutional preference or because of time
- For UD: BM preferred cell source
- Cell dose for UCB: 5-6/6 match: >3.0 x 10^7 NC/kg and/or 2 x 10^5 CD34+/kg, 4/6-match >5 x 10^7 NC/kg and/or >3 x 10^5 CD34+/kg. Matching according to intermediate resolution criteria (low resolution on A and B, high resolution on DR)
- Unrelated donors are regarded as non-carriers of the mutation

b. Serotherapy
- id-SIB	no
- UCB	ATG-genzyme 4 x 2.5 mg/kg (day -8 to -5)
- UD	either Campath-1H 3 x 0.3 mg/kg (day -9 to -7)
	or ATG-genzyme 4 x 2.5 mg/kg (day -4 to -1)

c. Conditioning
- SIB/UCB/UD	Busulfan weight-based dosing (iv: day -5 to -2) with therapeutic drug monitoring AUC 90 mg x h/L (range 85–95) cumulative over 4 days (AUC in µM x min=22, range 20.5–23.5) Cumulative dose fludarabine 160 mg/m² (day -5 to -2)

d. GvHD-prophylaxis
- SIB	CsA (+ MTX: 10 mg/m²; day +3, +6 and +11)
- UD (BM)	
- with Campath-1H	CsA
- with ATG	CsA + MTX (10 mg/m²; day +3, +6 and +11)
- UD (PBSC) UD/ Mismatched-UD (BM)	CsA + MMF (30 mg/kg: stop day +28 in case no GvHD)
- UCB	CsA + Prednisone 1 mg/kg (until day +28, taper in 2 wks)

CsA-trough level: 200 µg/L

Tapering GvHD-prophylaxis
- SIB/UD	CsA until day +50. Then taper 20% per week
- UCB	CsA until + 6 mth. Then taper in 3 mth

2.1.3 Risk factors/morbidity

In the early reports on HSCT of IEM high rates of GvHD and Idiopathic Pneumonia Syndrome (IPS) were reported. Within the recent EMBT study the incidence of GvHD and pulmonary complications was considerably lower, 16% and 8%, respectively (5).

The incidence of chronic GvHD was only 5–15%. Since graft failure was common until recently second transplants were quite often performed with a good success rate.

2.1.4 Enzyme replacement therapy and HSCT

Enzyme replacement therapy (ERT) became available for MPS I in 2003. However for patients with CNS involvement, like Hurler's syndrome, HSCT remains the treatment of choice. The effect of ERT prior to HSCT has been analysed in various studies, and neither a positive nor a negative effect on EFS and toxicity was noted (16). However, it is currently standard practice in most centres to pre-treat patients with ERT prior to HSCT.

2.2 Peroxisomal disorders

X-ALD is an X-linked peroxisomal disorder involving defective beta-oxidation of very long chain fatty acids (VLCFA). The affected gene in X-ALD is ABCD1 and the peroxisomal membrane protein for which it codes is ALDP (adrenoleukodystrophy protein). The laboratory diagnosis of X-ALD depends upon the demonstration of increased levels of VLCFA and mutation analysis (17). Both the pathophysiology of X-ALD and the reasons that HSCT is helpful are poorly understood.

Four overlapping clinical patterns are recognised of which cerebral X-ALD is the only indication for HSCT.

1. Adrenal insufficiency (70% of genetically affected males)
2. Adrenomyeloneuropathy (AMN) - a non-inflammatory axonopathy presenting as progressive spastic paraparesis in young adults, including carrier females
3. Cerebral X-ALD - a rapidly progressive, intensively inflammatory myelinopathy
4. Asymptomatic individuals.

Approximately 40% of genetically affected boys will develop cerebral X-ALD. Disease progression results in severe disability, dementia and death over a period of months to years. HSCT is reserved for patients who have early definitive evidence of cerebral disease as determined by magnetic resonance imaging (MRI), but without clinical signs. In individuals presenting with clinically evident disease, the rapidly progressive nature of the condition precludes a successful transplant outcome in most cases. The presence of brain MRI abnormalities and the presence or absence of enhancement with gadolinium has been shown to be of prognostic value. A 34-point MRI scoring system specific for X-ALD that was designed by Loes et al. is now used worldwide (18).

Unaffected boys must have gadolinium-enhanced brain MRI scans at regular intervals to evaluate cerebral demyelination. An MRI severity score as low as 1 with gadolinium enhancement, in a young boy is highly predictive of subsequent progressive demyelination and is an indication for transplant. Donors should be identified for asymptomatic boys so that HSCT can proceed quickly once MRI changes are found. Two studies, a multi-centre retrospective study and a recent single centre study, showed clear efficacy of HSCT in X-ALD patients with survival rates around 80% (11, 12). The disease status, prior to HSCT, however is of utmost importance: those who are only minimally affected (radiologically a Loes-score <9, or clinically asymptomatic) perform neurologically significantly better after HSCT (associated with significantly higher survival rates of over 90%).

Recently, peri-transplant antioxidative therapy with N-acetyl-L-cysteine was shown to be protective against fulminant demyelination in advanced cerebral X-ALD (11). Its role is under continued investigation. HSCT has no effect on adrenal dysfunction and VLCFA levels decline but remain elevated. Adrenal crisis can precipitate a profound decline in CNS function in these boys, as can significant acute GvHD. Lorenzo's oil is a 4:1 mixture of glycerol trioleate and glyceryl trierucate that normalises the elevated level of VLCFA. In boys in whom the VLCFA level is significantly lowered, Lorenzo's oil therapy appears to reduce the risk of neurological progression and so reduce the need for HSCT (19). For those with MRI imaging changes or clinical disease, it has no influence on disease progression. It is therefore of limited interest or relevance to the HSCT team.

2.3 Miscellaneous metabolic disorders

In contrast to MPS IH, Krabbe disease and X-ALD other IEM have a much less uniform treatment history (1). For example, Wolman disease does respond to early HSCT with >11 years follow-up in some patients. Similarly, in alpha-mannosidosis, stabilisation of neurocognitive variables and possibly of musculoskeletal features has been observed (20). More recently a case series describing the outcomes of HSCT in MNGIE (mitochondrial neuro-gastro-intestinal encephalomyopathy) showed promising results (21).

On the other hand, several diseases characterised by GAG accumulation, such as MPS II, MPS III, MPS IV (Morquio syndrome), and MPS VII (Sly syndrome) have all been shown to respond only partially or not at all to HSCT (1, 22). The natural history of I-cell disease (mucolipidosis II) can be altered by HSCT, yet significant improvement after HSCT has been rare. Equally disappointing are responses to cellular therapy in GM-gangliosidoses (Tay-Sachs disease, Sandhoff disease and GM1-gangliosidosis), Niemann-Pick disease and Batten-disease (1). There may be some beneficial effect of HSCT when it is performed in a timely and appropriate manner for individuals with the juvenile forms of GM2-gangliosidoses and possibly Niemann-Pick disease (types B and C2). In the United Kingdom and The Netherlands, these children, as well as pre- and asymptomatic children with MPS II and MPS III, are currently being treated by CBT (unpublished preliminary results).

2.4 Osteopetrosis

2.4.1 Indications and results

Osteopetrosis is a genetically heterogeneous group of osteoclast disorders. Steward recently published a comprehensive review on this disorder (3). In recent years progress has been made in deciphering the underlying genes. Since the resulting phenotypes varies markedly, including the natural course of disease not all forms of the disease can be treated successfully with HSCT. Some genotypes are clear indications: *ATP6i (TCIRG1)*, *CICN7* and TNFRSF11A (if not neuronopathic), others not: OSTM1, TNSF11, PLEKHM1, and for some it remains unknown/uncertain: CA2, Kindlin-3, NEMO. In 25% of the cases the mutation remains unknown. The largest published experience described (n=122) (23) showed that transplantation with a HLA-identical sibling donor, resulted in a 5 years engrafted survival rate of 73%. For UD and haplo-SCT the results were less favourable with "engrafted survival rates" of 40 and 24%, respectively. In centers experienced with haplo-SCT a clear improvement over time was shown. A Eurocord study (n=25) showed that in unrelated-CBT the engrafted-survival rate was 50% (24). ESID and the EBMT-WPIE have recently published guidelines on the conditioning regimen to be used: iv (intravenous) busulfan-fludarabine in standard-risk patients and treosulfan-based pilot (including fludarabine and thiotepa) in high-risk patients (EBMT-website).

2.4.2 Risk factors and morbidity

Transplant-related toxicity in HSCT for osteopetrosis is mainly caused by hypercalcaemia (especially in patients >2 years of age), graft failure, pulmonary complications and veno-occlusive disease (VOD). Hypercalcaemia can be treated by bisphosphonates, forced diuresis and diuretics. VOD can successfully be prevented by defibrotide. Pulmonary arterial hypertension is mainly seen in the first 3 months after HSCT, while outcome of treatment for pulmonary hypertension is generally poor. The many potential complications of the disease and the transplant warrant intensive long-term follow up.

3. New directions

Neonatal screening may influence the outcome since early detection and HSCT in pre-symptomatic patients might further influence the effect of HSCT. Furthermore strategies targeting the genetic lesion in IEM by gene therapy will become available. In the last decade, retroviral, lentiviral, and adenoviral vectors have been shown to be effective in many animal models of human LSD. However, it remains unclear whether these observations can be translated into clinical benefits. Clinical gene-therapy trials have focused on MPS VII and X-ALD and more recently on infantile MLD. Optimism must be tempered by the development of complications in the first gene therapy trials, such as insertional mutagenesis leading to development of leukaemia in several patients with immune deficiencies. Nevertheless, gene therapy is possible, offering the possibility of safer and more effective treatment for IEM in the future.

4. Conclusions

During three decades of HSCT for IEM, important lessons have been learned about transplant- and disease-specific factors that affect engrafted survival and long-term outcomes. Key points are summarised below. Children with MPS IH have benefited from many advances including the development of guidelines used worldwide for their evaluation and treatment. The importance of early diagnosis and prompt HSCT for patients with good performance scores is clearly documented. Efforts aimed at early diagnosis and treatment have favourably affected all children with IEM, leading to prevention of devastating neurocognitive and neuropsychological sequelae. Developments in newborn screening and therapy will facilitate early diagnosis and direct greater attention to genotype/phenotype correlation. The rare nature of these disorders requires continuing collaborative, multi-centre, international, and interdisciplinary research approach.

Key points

In most IEM disease correction is by secreted enzyme from donor leukocytes (exception ALD)

CNS enzyme delivery is via donor derived (macrophage lineage) tissue microglia

Commonest IEM indication is Hurler syndrome (MPS IH)

Hugely improved results (>90% EFS) in Hurler syndrome with:
- Use of full intensity regimen
- No "in vitro T-cell" depletion
- Busulfan pK guided administration
- Cord blood improves donor cell engraftment rates
- Use of peri-transplant pharmacological enzyme replacement therapy to optimise patient status prior to HSCT

Other definite indications include mannosidosis, X-ALD but as HSCT results improve then HSCT increasingly applied in other disorders and evidence base greater

IEM are multi-system disorders that are ameliorated rather than cured following transplant and multidisciplinary teams in large centres will optimise post-transplant performance of engrafted children

Transplant at best stabilises disease and best results are in children diagnosed early and worst results in those with disability from established disease

Advancing field of medicine and further improvements likely from:
- Early diagnosis – screening e.g. infantile Krabbe programme
- Better enzyme delivery from autologous gene-modified HSCT
- Multimodality therapy – combining HSCT with pharmacological enzyme replacement therapy, substrate reduction therapy, stop codon read through gene therapy approaches

References

1. Boelens JJ, Prasad VK, Tolar J et al. Current international perspectives on hematopoietic stem cell transplantation for inherited metabolic disorders. Pediatr Clin North Am 2010; 57: 123–145.
2. Fratantoni JC, Hall CW, Neufeld EF. The defect in Hurler and Hunter syndromes. II. Deficiency of specific factors involved in mucopolysaccharide degradation. Proc Natl Acad Sci U S A 1969; 64: 360–366.
3. Steward CG. Hematopoietic stem cell transplantation for osteopetrosis. Pediatr Clin North Am 2010; 57: 171–180.
4. Hobbs JR, Hugh-Jones K, Barrett AJ et al. Reversal of clinical features of Hurler's disease and biochemical improvement after treatment by bone-marrow transplantation. Lancet 1981; ii: 709–12.
5. Boelens JJ, Wynn RF, O'Meara A et al. Outcomes of hematopoietic stem cell transplantation for Hurler's syndrome in Europe: A risk factor analysis for graft failure. Bone Marrow Transplant 2007; 40: 225–233.
6. Peters C, Balthazor M, Shapiro EG et al. Outcome of unrelated donor bone marrow transplantation in 40 children with Hurler syndrome. Blood 1996; 87: 4894–4902.
7. Boelens JJ, Rocha V, Aldenhoven M et al. Risk factor analysis of outcomes after unrelated cord blood transplantation in patients with hurler syndrome. Biol Blood Marrow Transplant 2009; 15: 618–625.
8. Escolar ML, Poe MD, Provenzale JM et al. Transplantation of umbilical-cord blood in babies with infantile Krabbe's disease. N Engl J Med 2005; 352: 2069–2081.
9. Prasad VK, Mendizabal A, Parikh SH et al. Unrelated donor umbilical cord blood transplantation for inherited metabolic disorders in 159 pediatric patients from a single center: Influence of cellular composition of the graft on transplantation outcomes. Blood 2008; 112: 2979–2989.
10. Staba SL, Escolar ML, Poe M et al. Cord-blood transplants from unrelated donors in patients with Hurler's syndrome. N Engl J Med 2004; 350: 1960–1969.
11. Miller WP, Rothman SM, Nascene D et al. Outcomes following allogeneic hematopoietic cell transplantation for childhood cerebral adrenoleukodystrophy: The largest single-institution cohort report. Blood 2011; 118: 1971–1978.
12. Peters C, Charnas LR, Tan Y et al. Cerebral X-linked adrenoleukodystrophy: The international

hematopoietic cell transplantation experience from 1982 to 1999. Blood 2004; 104: 881–888.

13. Aldenhoven M, Boelens JJ, de Koning TJ. The clinical outcome of Hurler syndrome after stem cell transplantation. Biol Blood Marrow Transplant 2008; 14: 485–498.

14. Boelens JJ, Aldenhoven M, Purtill D et al. Outcomes of transplantation using a various cell source in children with Hurler's syndrome after myelo-ablative conditioning. A Eurocord-EBMT-CIBMTR collaborative study. BBMT 2010, Suppl 2 (ASBMT meeting Orlando); S180–181.

15. Bartelink IH, Flinsenberg TWH, Bierings M et al. Myelo-ablative exposure of busulfan+fludarabine in pediatric HSCT is a similary effective conditioning regimen compared to BuCy4 but less toxic, BBMT 2011, Suppl 3 (ASBMT meeting Honolulu); S259.

16. Cox-Brinkman J, Boelens JJ, Wraith JE et al. Haematopoietic cell transplantation (HCT) in combination with enzyme replacement therapy (ERT) in patients with Hurler syndrome. Bone Marrow Transplant 2006; 38: 17–21.

17. Moser HW. Molecular genetics of peroxisomal disorders. Front Biosci 2000; 5: D298–306.

18. Loes DJ, Hite S, Moser H, et al. Adrenoleukodystrophy: A scoring method for brain MR observations. AJNR Am J Neuroradiol 1994; 15: 1761–1766.

19. Moser HW, Raymond GV, Koehler W et al. Evaluation of the preventive effect of glyceryl trioleate-trierucate ("Lorenzo's oil") therapy in X-linked adrenoleukodystrophy: Results of two concurrent trials. Adv Exp Med Biol 2003; 544: 369–387.

20. Mynarek M, Tolar J, Albert MH et al. Allogeneic hematopoietic SCT for alpha-mannosidosis: An analysis of 17 patients. Bone Marrow Transplant 2011 May 9. [Epub ahead of print].

21. Halter J, Schupbach WM, Casali C et al. Allogeneic hematopoietic SCT as treatment option for patients with mitochondrial neurogastrointestinal encephalomyopathy (MNGIE): A consensus conference proposal for a standardized approach. Bone Marrow Transplant 2011; 46: 330–337.

22. Orchard PJ, Blazar BR, Wagner J et al. Hematopoietic cell therapy for metabolic disease. J Pediatr 2007; 151: 340–346.

23. Driessen GJ, Gerritsen EJ, Fischer A et al. Long-term outcome of haematopoietic stem cell transplantation in autosomal recessive osteopetrosis: An EBMT report. Bone Marrow Transplant 2003; 32: 657–663.

24. Bierings M, Rocha V, Cavazzana-Calvo M et al. Unrelated cord blood transplants for osteopetrosis: EUROCORD data on outcome. Bone Marrow Transplant 2007; 39 (Suppl 1): S37 (abstract).

Multiple Choice Questionnaire

To find the correct answer, go to http://www.esh.org/online-training/handbook/

1. There are no treatment options for patients with an "inborn error of metabolism (IEM)":

a) Correct .... ☐
b) HSCT is an effective treatment for all IEM .... ☐
c) HSCT is a treatment option for a selected group of IEM .... ☐
d) HSCT is only effective in Hurler syndrome patients .... ☐

2. **Which of the following statements about enzyme replacement therapy (ERT) is correct?**
   a) ERT is a safer and more effective treatment option for IEM than HSCT ... ☐
   b) ERT is only effective in IEM without neurological involvement, since ERT does not cross the "blood-brain barrier" .... ☐
   c) ERT is necessary pre-HSCT to prevent transplantation-related mortality and graft-failure .... ☐
   d) ERT + HSCT is the most effective treatment for IEM for all indications ... ☐

3. **Which of the following statements about graft-failure in HSCT for IEM is correct?**
   a) Historically, high graft failure rates were reported mainly associated with T-cell depleted grafts and reduced-intensity conditioning .... ☐
   b) Graft failure has never been a problem in HSCT for IEM .... ☐
   c) Not graft failure but TRM is the major problem in HSCT for IEM .... ☐
   d) Less graft failure is reported using unrelated cord blood as stem cell source .... ☐

4. **The period between diagnosis and HSCT is not important, the outcome depends on the degree of donor matching:**
   a) No, the shorter the period between diagnosis and HSCT, the better the outcome .... ☐
   b) Correct, you should not use mismatched grafts in IEM .... ☐
   c) Correct, do not use unrelated cord blood .... ☐
   d) Correct, even neonatal screening will not improve outcome .... ☐

5. **For every genotype of osteopetrosis HSCT is a potentially curative treatment option:**
   a) Correct statement .... ☐

b) HSCT is not a treatment option for any genotype .... ☐
c) HSCT is only a treatment option for selected genotypes .... ☐
d) ERT and not HSCT is currently the state of the art treatment for all
   genotypes of osteopetrosis .... ☐

✳ CHAPTER 20

HSCT for children and adolescents

✳ 20.8

Hereditary bone marrow failure syndromes

Eliane Gluckman

1. Introduction

Aplastic anaemia is a rare disease in children that is most commonly idiopathic and less frequently a hereditary disorder. Hereditary bone marrow failure (BMF) syndromes, however, should be considered both in children and adults before the institution of any therapeutic treatment plan. They represent a very heterogeneous group of diseases with different mutations and pathophysiology but the exact diagnosis is essential because it will influence clinical decisions (for review see refs 1, 2). While new genetic tests are being developed, these are not widely available. Genomic instability in the presence of clastogenic agents is the hallmark of Fanconi anaemia (FA). In contrast, marked telomere dysregulation is characteristic of dyskeratosis congenita (DKC). Mutations affecting ribosome assembly and function are associated with Schwachman-Diamond syndrome and Diamond-Blackfan anaemia (DBA). HSCT is often the best option to obtain a cure. Various sources of cells have been used including related and unrelated bone marrow, peripheral blood or cord blood. In all these diseases, it is very important to identify the gene mutations which must be tested in the potential family donor. It is also important to collect cord blood from all siblings when a genetic abnormality has been diagnosed in the family.

2. Fanconi anaemia

FA is characterised by congenital abnormalities, progressive BMF, chromosome breakage, and susceptibility to cancer. FA is an inherited disease resulting from mutations of one of the 15 FANC genes. The products of these genes interact in the unique FA/BRCA pathway which is involved in the response to cellular stress and DNA damage which maintains genome integrity. FA cells have chromosome fragility, both spontaneous and induced by interstrand cross-linking agents, this feature being central for patient diagnosis (3, 4). FA patients display progressive bone marrow failure (BMF) during childhood, the pathophysiologic mechanisms of which have been elusive to date.

FA patients often have skeletal, thumb or limb abnormalities and abnormal skin pigmentation ("café au lait" spots). Other organ systems commonly involved include cardiac, renal and auditory systems. Low birth weight and growth retardation are frequent but some patients do not exhibit any congenital defect.

The haematological consequences of FA often develop in the first decade of life but absence of malformations and reversion due to somatic mosaicism can result in delayed or failed diagnosis in a small proportion of patients. Death, however, often results from the complications of BMF or occurrence of malignancy. The most frequent is AML with cytogenetic bone marrow clonal abnormalities; older patients are at high risk of squamous cell carcinomas of the oesophagus, head and neck and urogenital tract (5).

2.1 Evaluating new onset cytopenia in children (6)

1. Family history
2. Malformations
3. Date of onset
4. Liver function tests
5. Blood counts
6. BM aspiration with cytogenetics, BM biopsy if necessary
7. Chromosome breaks with diepoxybutane (DEB) or mitomycin C (MMC)
8. Alfa-foetoprotein
9. HLA typing
10 FANCD2 test*

*FANCD2 test : FANCD2 monoubiquitination by Western blot on peripheral blood lymphocytes in order to evaluate the ability of the FA core complex to monoubiquitinate FANCD2, and the level of expression of the FANCD2 protein

2.2 Disease-specific pre-HSCT work-up

FA being a heterogeneous disease, clinical diagnosis is not always sufficient to assess the correct diagnosis in children or young adults with AA. Other constitutional AA may have similar congenital abnormalities and FA patients may have no abnormalities (4).

Diagnosis is suspected with	- Blood counts: pancytopenia with macrocytic anaemia - Raised alfa-foetoprotein and haemoglobin F
Diagnosis is confirmed with	- PB lymphocyte cytogenetics with clastogenic agents: DEB or MMC showing increased chromosome breaks with tri- and quadri-radial figures - Study of the cell cycle showing a G2/M arrest increased by incubation with clastogenic agents
Other tests	- BM cytogenetic abnormalities for diagnosis of leukaemia or myelodysplastic syndrome, with abnormalities in chromosomes 1, 3, 7, 5, 8 and 11 being the most common
New tests not for routine use	- Ubiquitination of FANCD2: this test is specific and sensitive, if negative skin fibroblasts may

THE EBMT HANDBOOK 2012 EDITION

be positive for FA and this confirms the existence of mosaicism
- Identification of the complementation group with retroviral or lentiviral vectors
- Sequencing and identification of the mutation. This test is useful for preimplantation diagnosis and possibly for assessing prognosis

2.3 Haematopoietic stem cell transplantation

HSCT is the only curative therapy for the haematologic manifestations of FA, including aplastic anaemia, myelodysplastic syndrome, and acute leukaemia (7). Donor stem cells may be obtained from bone marrow, peripheral blood (following stimulation of donor haematopoiesis with G-CSF), or cord blood. Ideally HSCT is performed prior to onset of MDS/leukaemia and before multiple transfusions have been given for haematopoietic support. HSCT should be performed at centres with specific expertise in HSCT for FA.

Because individuals with FA are exquisitely sensitive to the toxicity of the usual chemotherapy and radiation regimens used in preparation for BMT, reduced doses are typically used (8). Graft failure, historically a major impediment to FA transplantation, has been largely ameliorated by use of fludarabine (Flu). Additionally, improvements in donor selection and supportive care have led to greater use of alternative donors and decreased differences in the outcomes between sibling transplants and unrelated donor transplants.

Individuals whose haematologic manifestations have been successfully treated with HSCT appear to be at an increased risk for solid tumours, particularly squamous cell carcinoma of the tongue. In one study the risk was increased fourfold and the median age of onset was 16 years younger than in persons with FA who were not transplanted (9).

2.4 Results of allo-HSCT

FA anaemia cells are hypersensitive to DNA cross-linking agents. Cellular exposure to genotoxic agents including cyclophosphamide (Cy), busulfan (Bu) or irradiation increases chromosome breaks and tissue damage (8). Graft-versus-host disease (GvHD) induces severe tissue damage and absence of repair (10). For this reason, it was recognised very early that reduced dose conditioning should be used in these patients, justifying the need for an accurate diagnosis.

2.4.1 HLA identical sibling transplants

The first large series of HSCT in patients with Fanconi anaemia used a protocol of conditioning with low dose Cy 40 mg/kg with 4 Gy thoracoabdominal irradiation (TAI) (11); 5-year survival was 85%. In general, most series have reported that the following factors are associated with better survival after transplantation: younger patient age, higher pretransplant platelet counts, absence of previous treatment with androgens, normal pretransplant liver function tests and limited malformations. In an attempt to reduce the potential impact of irradiation and GvHD on the risk of late effects, including cancer, newer regimens have replaced TAI with Flu in combination with low dose Cy, together with anti-thymocyte globulin (ATG) or T-cell depletion to reduce the risk of GvHD. Pasquini et al. on behalf of CIBMTR compared the early outcome of HSCT using non-irradiation containing regimens (n=71) to the outcome of regimens with irradiation (n=77) for FA patients transplanted with HLA identical sibling donors. Haematopoietic recovery, acute and chronic GvHD and mortality were similar after the two regimens (12), the 5-year probability of overall survival was 78% after irradiation and 81% after the non-irradiation regimen. While promising, longer follow-up is needed to determine whether non-irradiation based regimens will reduce the risk of late effects such as infertility, cataracts, endocrinopathies and secondary malignancies. Of note, some pregnancies have been observed in women after HSCT even with irradiation containing regimens (13). In the light of these data, the most frequently used conditioning regimen for HLA identical sibling HSCT is low dose Cy, Flu and ATG or T-cell depletion without irradiation.

2.4.2 Alternative donor transplants

Matched unrelated donors. Results of matched unrelated donor transplant for FA have been improving with time (14–17). Since the first results published in 2007, survival has increased from 33% to 80% in selected centres. The CIBMTR analysed 98 patients transplanted with unrelated donor marrow (excluding those with peripheral blood or umbilical cord blood [UCB] grafts) between 1990 and 2003. Probabilities of neutrophil (89% vs 69%, p=0.02) and platelet recovery (74% vs 23%, p <0.001) were higher after Flu than non-Flu containing regimens. Risks of acute (RR 2.95, p=0.003) and chronic GvHD (RR 3.30, p=0.03) were significantly higher in recipients of non T-cell depleted than T-cell depleted grafts. Day-100 mortality rate was significantly higher after non-Flu than Flu-containing regimens (65% vs 24%, respectively p <0.001). Corresponding 3-year adjusted overall survival rates were 13% vs 52% (p <0.001) with best survival in those treated with a Flu-based regimen. In addition, mortality was higher in recipients who were older (>10 years), CMV seropositive and with >20 blood product transfusions pre-BMT. Based on these results significant changes in practice were suggested: use of a Flu-containing conditioning regimen in the context of *in vivo* or *in vitro* T-cell depletion and earlier referral with transplantation prior to excessive transfusions. Improvement is due to a better donor selection and modification of the conditioning; the best results have been published by the Minnesota group using Cy 40 mg/kg, TBI 300/150 cGy with thymic shielding, Flu 140 mg/m^2 and ATG or T-cell depletion (14).

Cord blood transplantation. If an HLA-identical sibling donor is available, umbilical cord blood transplantation (UCBT) and bone marrow transplantation (BMT) from an unrelated donor give similar results in terms of survival. However, reports comparing the two demonstrate a reduction in the frequency and severity of acute and chronic GvHD after UCBT, related to the relative immaturity of neonatal T-cells.

In practice, the majority of patients do not have an HLA-matched sibling donor. Eurocord analysed results of unrelated UCBT in 93 FA patients. The incidence of neutrophil recovery at 60 days was 60+5%. In addition to high cell dose, Flu-containing regimens (as in marrow recipients) were associated with better neutrophil engraftment. The incidence of acute and chronic GvHD was 32.5% and 16%, respectively. Overall survival was 40+5%. In multivariate analysis factors associated with favourable outcome were use of Flu, high number of cells infused and negative recipient CMV serology (18).

To date, there has been no formal comparison of outcomes in recipients of unrelated UCB and those receiving bone marrow. However, results demonstrate that Flu is associated with better survival regardless of stem cell source in patients with FA. This suggests that Flu, a potent immune suppressive agent, enhances engraftment without paying the price of extramedullary toxicity. In the future, studies may help us determine the place of UCBT. For now, UCBT is clearly indicated in those FA patients for whom an HLA-A, B, C, and DRB1 allele-matched unrelated volunteer donor cannot be identified.

It is possible using preimplantation genetic diagnosis (PGD) to select an embryo produced by *in vitro* fertilisation that is both unaffected by a heritable genetic disease and HLA identical to the affected recipient. Clearly, this approach is controversial with marked differences in its acceptance by different countries worldwide. Globally, the strategy has been most often used for couples at high risk of having children with thalassaemia. However, the first successful use of PGD for a specific HLA type was for a child with FA. With this approach, the couple can avoid the risk of having additional affected children (and the consequent consideration of abortion) and also have a healthy child that will be an HLA identical match with the existing child needing HSCT. In these cases, it is typical for the UCB to be collected at birth, eliminating any risk to the newborn child.

2.4.3 Post-HSCT monitoring in FA

Patients with FA require particular attention because of their sensitivity to toxic agents, various organ dysfunctions due to congenital malformations and increased risk of developing malignancies. This should include at least yearly follow-up of growth, endocrine function, bone marrow cytogenetics and oral examination. Patients with oral lichen planus should be biopsied regularly and lesions removed.

3. Other congenital cytopenias (for review see refs 1, 19, 20)

3.1 Dyskeratosis congenita
DKC is a rare progressive bone marrow failure syndrome characterised by the triad of reticulated skin hyperpigmentation, nail dystrophy, and oral leukoplakia. Evidence exists for telomerase dysfunction, ribosome deficiency, and protein synthesis dysfunction. All individuals with DC have abnormally short telomeres for their age, as determined by multicolor flow cytometry fluorescence *in situ* hybridisation on white blood cell subsets. To date, six genes: DKC1, TERC, TERT, TINF2, NHP2, and NOP10, have been identified as involved in DC. Mutations in one of these six genes have been identified in approximately half of individuals who meet clinical diagnostic criteria for DKC. Molecular genetic testing is clinically available for all six genes (1). HSCT is the only curative treatment for severe BMF or leukaemia in DKC. It should be performed at centres experienced in treating DKC. Early mortality is often associated with bone marrow failure, infections, fatal pulmonary complications, or malignancy. Long-term results of HSCT are disappointing because of severe late effects including diffuse vasculitis and lung fibrosis (21). Reported problems include graft failure, GvHD, sepsis, pulmonary fibrosis, hepatic cirrhosis, and veno-occlusive disease. As a result, long-term survival of patients with DKC following HSCT has been poor. Reduced-intensity preparative regimens are being studied in a few institutions and may improve long-term outcomes (22).

3.2 Seckel syndrome
Seckel syndrome is a rare autosomal recessive disorder with growth retardation, microcephaly with mental retardation and a characteristic bird-headed facial appearance. The only human genetic ATR defect reported so far is a hypomorphic splicing mutation identified in six related individuals with Seckel syndrome. Very few transplants have been reported in the literature (23).

3.3 Schwachman-Diamond syndrome
Schwachman syndrome is an autosomal recessive disorder with clinical features that include pancreatic exocrine insufficiency, skeletal abnormalities and pancytopenia. AML transformation has been observed. Very few patients have been treated by HSCT.

3.4. Diamond-Blackfan anaemia

Diamond-Blackfan anaemia (DBA) (24) is characterised by chronic constitutional aregenerative anaemia with absent or decreased erythroid precursors in the BM. Both autosomal dominant and recessive inheritance are described. DBA has been associated with mutations in 9 genes that encode for ribosomal proteins. A mutation in 1 of these 9 genes can be identified in approximately 53% of individuals with DBA. The syndrome appears to result from haplo-insufficiency of either a small or large subunit-associated ribosomal protein. Most patients present with anaemia in the neonatal period or in infancy. Approximately 30% patients have a variety of physical anomalies including thumb, upper limb, craniofacial, heart and urogenital malformations. Patients are usually treated with transfusions and steroids and at least 50% patients respond. Patients with DBA who are transfusion-dependent or develop other cytopenias are often treated with HSCT. The data from the Diamond-Blackfan American registry reveal an overall survival of 77.3% for sibling HSCT and 31.5% for alternative donors. The best outcomes occur when using HLA matched sibling donors in patients less than 9 years old. The majority of sibling donor HSCT has been performed using myeloablative conditioning, generally including busulfan, Cy and ATG. Because of transfusional iron overload, very aggressive iron chelation therapy is highly recommended before transplant. A variety of stem cell sources including related and unrelated donor bone marrow, peripheral blood stem cells and cord blood have been used successfully.

It is recommended that the affected individual, siblings, and parents undergo HLA typing at the time of diagnosis of DBA to identify the most suitable bone marrow donor in the event that HSCT may be required. Because penetrance of DBA is incomplete, it is possible that a relative considered as a bone marrow donor could have a disease-causing mutation but not manifest findings of DBA. Relatives with a DBA-causing mutation, regardless of their clinical status, are not suitable bone marrow donors, because their donated bone marrow may fail or not engraft in the recipient.

3.5 Severe congenital neutropenias

Kostmann syndrome is an inherited disorder with severe neutropenia and early onset of severe bacterial infections. More than 90% of patients respond to rHuG-CSF but approximately 10% will develop MDS/AML, regardless of their treatment or response. Heterozygous mutations in the neutrophil elastase gene (ELA2) have been demonstrated in the majority of patients. Other mutations have been described, demonstrating genetic heterogeneity.

Allo-HSCT is the treatment of choice in patients refractory to G-CSF or with acute leukaemia. In the French chronic neutropenia registry which includes 101 patients,

9 patients were transplanted, 7 with an unrelated donor and 2 with an HLA identical sibling donor. Four patients had acute leukaemia, 4 were refractory to G-CSF and 1 had BMF. The OS at 5 years was 61% indicating that HSCT should be considered in these patients even if there is no HLA identical sibling (25).

3.6 Inherited thrombocytopenias
Congenital amegakaryocytic thrombocytopenia (CAMT) is clinically characterised by thrombocytopenia presenting at birth in a child without congenital or skeletal malformations, reduced or absent bone marrow megakaryocytes, and eventual progression to bone marrow failure. Molecular studies in most cases confirm homozygous or compound heterozygous mutations in the thrombopoietin receptor c-Mpl. In addition to the clinical importance of recognising this disorder, characterisation of mutations identified in patients with CAMT has led to insights into thrombopoietin receptor structure and function. Affected infants are identified within days or weeks of birth. Its transmission is autosomal recessive. Despite optimal supportive care, AA develops leading to death in the absence of HSCT, which is the only chance of cure in this disease (26). Thrombocytopenia with absent radii (TAR) syndrome includes shortened or absent forearms due to the absence of development of the bilateral radii, associated with severe thrombocytopenia at birth. Skeletal anomalies are also seen in other bones but do not affect the hands and fingers. Usually the degree of thrombocytopenia is greatest at birth requiring transfusions, however thrombocytopenia becomes less severe during the first year of life and most patients will not require platelet transfusion after infancy. HSCT is not recommended.

3.7 Other rare inherited BMF syndromes
Nijmegen breakage syndrome (NBS) is a rare autosomal recessive condition of chromosomal instability that is clinically characterised by microcephaly, a distinct facial appearance, short stature, immunodeficiency, radiation sensitivity, and a strong predisposition to lymphoid malignancy. Mutations in the NBS1 gene located in band 8q21 are responsible for NBS.

Pearson syndrome is currently recognised as a rare, multisystemic, mitochondrial cytopathy. Its features are refractory sideroblastic anaemia, pancytopenia, defective oxidative phosphorylation, exocrine pancreatic insufficiency, and variable hepatic, renal, and endocrine failure. Death often occurs in infancy or early childhood due to infection or metabolic crisis. Patients may recover from the refractory anaemia. Older survivors have Kearns-Sayre syndrome (KSS), which is a mitochondropathy characterised by progressive external ophthalmoplegia and weakness of skeletal muscle.

THE EBMT HANDBOOK 2012 EDITION

DNA ligase IV deficiencies mutation of LIG4 gene is a rare disease; one case of successful transplant has been described.

References

1. Dokal I, Vulliamy T. Inherited bone marrow failure syndromes. Haematologica 2010; 95: 1236–1240.
2. Moldovan GL, D'Andrea AD. How the Fanconi anemia pathway guards the genome. Annu Rev Genet 2009; 43: 223–249.
3. de Winter JP, Joenje H. The genetic and molecular basis of Fanconi anemia. Mutat Res 2009; 668: 11–19.
4. Auerbach AD. Fanconi anemia and its diagnosis. Mutat Res 2009; 668: 4–10.
5. Rosenberg PS, Greene MH, Alter BP. Cancer incidence in persons with Fanconi anemia. Blood 2003; 101: 822–826.
6. Pinto FO, Leblanc T, Chamousset D et al. Diagnosis of Fanconi anemia in patients with bone marrow failure. Haematologica 2009; 94: 487–495.
7. MacMillan JM, Wagner JE. Haematopoietic cell transplantation for Fanconi anaemia - when and how? Br J Haematol 2010; 149: 14–21.
8. Gluckman E, Devergie A, Dutreix J. Radiosensitivity in Fanconi anaemia: application to the conditioning regimen for bone marrow transplantation. Br J Haematol 1983; 54: 431–440.
9. Rosenberg PS, Socié G, Alter BP, Gluckman E. Risk of head and neck squamous cell cancer and death in patients with Fanconi anemia who did and did not receive transplants. Blood 2005; 105: 67–73.
10. Guardiola P, Socié G, Li X et al. Acute graft versus host disease in patients with Fanconi anemia or acquired aplastic anemia undergoing bone marrow transplantation from HLA identical sibling donors: Risk factors and influence on outcome. Blood 2004; 103: 73–77.
11. Socié, G, Devergie A, Girinski T et al. Transplantation for Fanconi's anemia: Long-term follow-up of fifty patients transplanted from a sibling donor after low-dose Cyclophosphamide and thoraco-abdominal irradiation for conditioning. Br J Haematol 1998; 103: 249–55.
12. Pasquini R, Carreras J, Pasquini MC et al. HLA matched sibling hematopoietic stem cell transplantation for Fanconi anemia: Comparison of irradiation and non irradiation containing regimens. Biol Bone Marrow Transpl 2008 14: 1141–1147.
13. Nabhan SK, Bitencourt MA, Duval M et al. Fertility recovery and pregnancy after allogeneic hematopoietic stem cell transplantation in Fanconi Anemia patients. Haematologica 2010; 95: 1783–1787.
14. McMillan ML, Blazar R, Defor TE et al. Alternate donor HCT for Fanconi anemia (FA): Results of a total body irradiation (TBI) dose de-escalation study. Biol Bone Marrow Transplant 2009; 15: 3–4.
15. Guardiola P, Pasquini R, Dokal I et al. Outcome of 69 allogeneic stem cell transplants for Fanconi anemia using HLA- matched unrelated donors: A study of the European Group for Blood and Marrow Transplantation. Blood 2000; 95: 422–429.

16. Wagner JE, Eapen M, Mac Millan ML et al. Unrelated donor bone marrow transplantation for the treatment of Fanconi anemia. Blood 109: 2256–2262, 2007.
17. Gluckman E, Rocha V, Ionescu I et al. Results of unrelated cord blood transplant in Fanconi anemia patients: Risk factor analysis for engraftment and survival. Biol Blood Marrow Transplant 2007; 13: 1073–1082.
18. Bizzetto R, Bonfim C, Rocha V, Socié G, Locatelli F, Chan K, Ramirez O, Stein J, Nabhan S, Miranda E, Passweg J, de Souza CA, Gluckman E on behalf of Eurocord and SAA WP from EBMT. Outcomes after related and unrelated umbilical cord blood transplantation for hereditary bone marrow failure syndromes other than Fanconi anemia. Haematologica 2011; 96: 134–141.
19. Gluckman E, Wagner JE. Hematopoietic stem cell transplantation in childhood inherited bone marrow failure syndrome. Bone Marrow Transplant 2008; 41: 127–132.
20. Myers KC, Davies SM. Hematopoietic stem cell transplantation for bone marrow failure syndromes in children. Biol Blood Marrow Transplant 2009; 15: 279–292.
21. Rocha V, Devergie A, Socié G et al. Unusual complications after bone marrow transplantation for dyskeratosis congenita. Br J Haematol 1998; 103: 243–248.
22. Dietz AC, Orchard PJ, Baker KS et al. Disease-specific hematopoietic cell transplantation: Non myeloablative conditioning regimen for dyskeratosis congenita. Bone Marrow Transplant 2011; 46: 98–104.
23. Ruyburg M, Davies SM, Mehta PA et al. Successful reduced intensity bone marrow transplantation in a patient with bone marrow failure associated with Seckel syndrome. Br J Haematol 2008; 142: 675–676.
24. Vlachos A, Muir E. How I treat Diamond-Blackfan anemia. Blood 2010; 116: 3715–3723.
25. Zeitler C, Welte K, Barak Y et al. Stem cell transplantation in patients with severe congenital neutropenia without evidence of leukemic transformation. Blood 2000; 95: 1195–1198.
26. Tarek N, Kernan NA, Prockop SE et al. T cell depleted hematopoietic SCT from unrelated donors for the treatment of congenital amegakaryocytic thrombocytopenia. Bone Marrow Transpl 2011 July 25. [Epub ahead of print.]

Multiple Choice Questionnaire

To find the correct answer, go to http://www.esh.org/online-training/handbook/

1. **A 3 year old male presents with pallor and multiple bruises. Which one of the following laboratory tests is initially necessary?**
    a) Bone marrow aspiration and/or biopsy with cytogenetics .... ☐
    b) Haemoglobin F .... ☐
    c) Peripheral blood lymphocyte cytogenetics with DEB or MMC .... ☐
    d) Liver function tests .... ☐

2. Dyskeratosis congenita is characterised by:
   a) Oral leukoplakia .... ☐
   b) Bird-headed facial appearance .... ☐
   c) Café au lait spots .... ☐
   d) Microcephaly .... ☐

3. Haematopoietic stem cell transplantation is curative for the haematological manifestations of Fanconi anaemia. The major long term complication of FA is:
   a) Pancreatic insufficiency .... ☐
   b) Pulmonary fibrosis .... ☐
   c) Squamous cell carcinoma of the tongue .... ☐
   d) Pan-hypopituitarism .... ☐

4. Which one of the following best summarises the indications for allogeneic HSCT in Diamond-Blackfan anaemia?
   a) All patients at diagnosis .... ☐
   b) When resistant to corticosteroids .... ☐
   c) Only if an healthy HLA-identical sibling donor ...... ☐
   d) When immunised by transfusions .... ☐

* CHAPTER 20

HSCT for children and adolescents

* 20.9
Haemoglobinopathies

Emanuele Angelucci, Donatella Baronciani

1. Introduction

Haemoglobin is the part of the red blood cell that carries the oxygen. Basically there are two types of diseases characterised by haemoglobin alteration:
• Expression/synthesis disorders: thalassaemia
• Structural variants/disorders: sickle-cell disease.

2. Definition of thalassaemia and sickle cell disease

2.1 Thalassaemia

The thalassaemias are a heterogeneous group of haemoglobin disorders with defective synthesis of one or more globin chains, resulting in decreased filling of the red cells with haemoglobin and consequent anaemia.

The main clinical consequence of thalassaemia is severe anaemia such that regular blood transfusion is required to survive. There are forms of thalassaemia major (homozygosis or compound heterozygosis) that are characterised by less severe anaemia and sporadic requirement for transfusion. They are named thalassaemia intermedia.

Anaemia and blood transfusion leads to iron overload that is fatal in a few years if not removed by iron chelation. Recent advances in understanding the pathophysiology of iron overload and iron chelation as well as the development of safe and efficient chelators (1) have transformed thalassaemia from a severe disease fatal in infancy to a chronic disease in which survival to 40 years and over is possible, at least in the industrialised world.

2.2 Sickle cell disease

Sickle cell disease (SCD) is an autosomal recessive genetic disease that results from the substitution of valine by glutamic acid in position 6 of the beta globin gene leading to production of defective form of haemoglobin (HbS). Deoxygenating of SS red cells leads to intracellular haemoglobin polymerisation, loss of deformability and changes in cell morphology. Clinically SCD is characterised by generalised vasculopathy and other phenomena secondary to the above-described alterations of the sickle red cells. The major clinical consequences of SCD are listed in Table 1.

3. Rationale of transplantation in haemoglobinopathies

In essence, the basis of HSCT in thalassaemia consists in substituting the unhealthy haemopoietic stem cells generating ineffective erythropoiesis with allogeneic stem cells capable of normal erythropoiesis. Of course this replacement is not limited to the diseased erythropoietic component but involves the entire haemopoietic system.

Table 1: **Most relevant clinical consequences of sickle cell disease**	
Acute painful episodes	Neurologic complications
	Multi-organ failure
	Psychosocial issues
Growth and development	
Infection	Bacteremia
	Meningitis
	Bacterial pneumonia
	Osteomyelitis
Cerebrovascular events	
Bone complications	
Cardiac complications	Myocardial infarction
Dermatologic complications	Leg ulcers
Hepatobiliary complications	
Pregnancy	
Priapism	
Pulmonary complications	Oxygen saturation
	Acute chest syndrome
Renal complications	
Retinopathy	Proliferative sickle retinopathy

The same concept is applicable to SCD in which erythropoiesis is effective but the haemoglobin produced is abnormal.

HSCT in haemoglobinopathies is therefore a cellular replacement therapy.

The transplantation approach for a non-malignant disease is different from transplantation in malignancies. In this setting, the detrimental immunologic properties of the engrafted HSC (i.e. GvHD) are not balanced by any anti-malignancy effect.

4. History of HSCT in thalassaemia

HSCT in thalassaemia was developed and grew into accepted routine clinical practice mostly thanks to the Pesaro group experience during the 1980s and 1990s. At the end of the 80s (deferoxamine era) the Pesaro group developed a prognostic scheme to predict transplant outcome in patients younger than 17 years (2). This prognostic scheme included three variables, all related to iron burden:
- Quality of chelation received during the entire life before transplantation (regular versus not regular);

- Hepatomegaly (more than 2 centimetres below the costal margin);
- Presence of any degree of liver fibrosis on pre-transplant hepatic biopsy examination.

These variables stratified patients aged less than 17 years in 3 groups, having either none, one/two, or all three of the risk factors. These three factors identified as low-risk patients who had optimal control of iron overload for their entire life and as high-risk patients who had no iron control and no prevention of iron-related tissue damage. Results were impressively different in the three groups (2).

Even if this classification may not remain accurate today, it includes several important concepts which are still important for current clinical practice:

a. Optimal medical therapy (transfusion chelation therapy) is the key to a successful transplant. Patients who had optimal life-long control of iron overload and no iron-related tissue damage (liver fibrosis) had an outstanding survival and thalassaemia-free survival exceeding 90% and 80%, respectively. Conversely, patients who did not have this degree of control of iron overload had an unacceptable transplant-related mortality approaching 50%.

b. In the high-risk group, after reduction of the intensity of conditioning by reducing the cyclophosphamide dose from 200 mg/kg to 120 mg/kg, transplant related mortality persisted at 18% but the risk of thalassaemia recurrence was increased by up to 30%.

c. Adult patients had high transplant-related mortality (35%) and very limited risk of thalassaemia recurrence.

5. Current results

Transplant technologies and clinical care have widely improved during the last decade, with outstanding results being consistently reported in the literature (Figure 1). Several centres worldwide are now performing HSCT in thalassaemia with excellent results (3). Various approaches have been developed for HSCT preparation and conditioning: intravenous busulfan (4), targeted intravenous busulfan (5), new drugs like treosulfan (6), thiotepa and fludarabine (7), as well as intensive pre-transplant transfusion/chelation regimens.

These different regimens have yielded more or less the same overall and thalassaemia-free survivals, which are now >85% and >80%, respectively, in patients without relevant iron related tissue damage (Table 2). Survival has risen to around 90% (and in some cases even higher) even in high-risk paediatric patients but with lower thalassaemia-free survivals, ranging from 66% to 80% (4–6) probably due the reduced toxicity regimen usually applied in this category of patients.

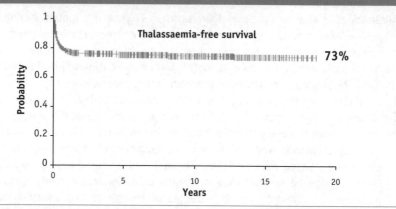

Figure 1: **Results of 900 consecutive unselected haematopoietic stem cell transplantations for thalassaemia performed in Pesaro since 1982**

Reprinted with permission from Angelucci E, Baronciani D. Haematologica 2008; 93: 1780–1784

Table 2: **Updated results of HSCT in thalassaemia (transplants performed in the last decade)**

Risk	Transplant-related mortality (%)	Overall survival (%)	Thalassaemia-free survival (%)
Lower-risk	3	96–97	86–91
High-risk	12	87–96	66–80
Adult	27	67	67

Risk: risk categories following the Pesaro classification

There is only a single report on a limited number of adult patients (n=15) transplanted after 1997 with modest improvements in results (overall survival 67% and transplant related mortality 27%) (see Table 2 for updated detailed results) (8).

5.1 Registry data

The EBMT registry for haemoglobinopathies was established several years ago and today almost 3,000 thalassaemia patients and 500 sickle cell disease patients have been registered. Detailed analyses are ongoing but it is important to report than on almost 1400 transplants performed after year 2000 in 128 centres in 23 countries the median age was 7 years and the 5 yr overall survival and disease-free survival were 89% and 79%, respectively. These data clearly indicate that the procedure is widely applied, that results are confirmed on a multicentre basis and the large majority of centres follow the indication "as soon as possible" following from the Pesaro experience.

6. Transplantation for SCD

The first patient with SCD to be treated with HSCT was an 8-year-old girl who had both AML and recurrent vaso-occlusive crises. After HSCT, in addition to having a normal bone marrow with no evidence of AML, her haemoglobin S level decreased to the level of the donor, who had sickle cell trait, and she had no further vaso-occlusive crises. C. Vermylen reported the first series in 1988.

During the following years, additional studies with larger numbers of patients were reported from European and American groups, all demonstrating good overall and disease-free survivals in selected patients receiving transplants from HLA identical sibling donors (9–11). These clinical studies demonstrated that results of HSCT were better when performed in children who have HLA identical sibling donors. Overall survival and disease free survival ranged from 80–84% and 88–93%, respectively. The collective experience of these studies underlines the transition of HSCT from an experimental approach for severely affected patients to a procedure applicable to young children with early signs of sickle-related morbidity.

7. Differences between thalassaemia and SCD in approaching HSCT

Despite the similar rationale for transplantation in SCD and thalassaemia, the clinical implications and clinical problems are very different. These differences are due to the different clinical nature of the two diseases.

Indications and clinical problems of HSCT in thalassemia have already been discussed.

Symptomatic SCD is a clear indication for transplantation but if sickle-related damage has already occurred the role of transplantation is questionable. The key question is therefore to identify patients at high risk of symptomatic disease. Various methods to identify such patients have been proposed, all based on clinical characteristics or on events that have already occurred, but no definitive agreed criteria have been developed. Indications for HSCT in SCD patients are summarised in Table 3 (12).

Table 4 summarises specific pre-transplant work up for patients with thalassaemia and SCD.

Table 3: Indications for HSCT in SCD patients

Age <16 years	
HLA identical sibling donor	
One or more of the following complications	Stroke or central nervous system event lasting >24 hours
	Impaired neuropsychological function with abnormal cerebral MRI and angiography
	Recurrent acute chest syndrome
	Stage I or II sickle lung disease
	Recurrent vaso-occlusive painful episodes or recurrent priapism
	Sickle nephropathy (but with GFR above 30–50% of predicted values)
Other indications to consider	Abnormal transcranial Doppler
	Pulmonary hypertension
	Silent cerebral infarction

Modified from (12)

Table 4: Specific pre-transplant work up for thalassaemia and sickle cell disease

Both diseases

Blood specific disease markers (haemoglobin electrophoresis and haemoglobin chain synthesis) Genetic test to identify mutation (genetic diagnoses)

Endocrinological evaluation. Cryopreservation of sperm cells or (if feasible) ovarian tissue

Thalassaemia

Assessment of iron overload and iron tissue damage (MRI T2* for cardiac iron, MRI R2 for liver iron, fibroscan or liver biopsy for liver fibrosis)

Accurate evaluation of cardiac function (echocardiography or MRI)

Sickle cell disease

Cerebral, thoracic and abdominal CT scan. Cerebral MRI and angiograph

Skeletal survey and bone scans

If sickle cell patients have been treated with chronic red cell transfusion then the same tests as in thalassaemia must be performed

8. Alternative sources of haematopoietic stem cells

The large majority of transplant centres continue to use bone marrow-derived HSC rather than peripheral blood-derived HSC. In 2003 Locatelli first reported the feasibility of using HLA identical sibling, cord blood-derived haemopoietic stem cell for HSCT in haemoglobinopathies.

8.1 Alternative donors

The clinical development of HSCT from alternative donors has been more challenging and includes three possible approaches: 1. matched unrelated donors; 2. mismatched related donors; 3. unrelated cord blood.

8.1.1 Matched unrelated donors

During the last decade, the use of unrelated donors for HSCT in malignancies has considerably expanded with improving results. Crucial determinants of this success have been the technological improvement of molecular HLA typing and the improved capability of selecting the appropriate unrelated donor.

A multicentre GITMO study started more than 10 years ago recently reported results in 68 thalassaemic patients transplanted from a matched unrelated donor (13). In this group of paediatric and adult patients (age range 2–37, median 15 years) overall and thalassaemia-free survival reached 79% and 66%, respectively. In the group of 30 paediatric patients in the two lower risk Pesaro categories, overall survival and thalassaemia-free survival were 97% and 80%, whereas in the high risk group they were 65% and 54%, respectively. If stringent criteria of immunogenetic compatibility based on high resolution molecular typing are respected, results are similar to those obtained in the matched sibling setting, at least in the low-risk group. In the contest of a non-malignant disease it is crucial to achieve extended haplotype identity, i.e. identity from locus HLA-A to locus HLA-Dp on the same chromosome. A recent study has demonstrated that the risk of thalassaemia recurrence after unrelated bone marrow transplantation is associated with presence of non-permissive HLA-DPB1 mismatches in the host versus graft direction (14).

8.1.2 Mismatched related donors

Experience in this setting has been limited so far, and results remain sub-optimal (15). Recently, better results have been reported in a small series (n=22) of heterogeneous thalassaemia patients (using an haploidentical related donor after positive selection of CD34 positive cells) (16). In this series, there were 2 deaths and 6 thalassaemia recurrences and 14 patients had sustained engraftment. However this limited single centre experience does not support at the present time a wider use of this approach.

8.1.3 Unrelated cord blood

For reasons discussed above, unrelated cord blood haematopoietic cells are a very promising source of stem cells for transplantation in non-malignant diseases. However unrelated cord blood transplant in thalassaemia has not been explored in systematic studies and only one single centre study (17) and retrospective multicentre studies are available. In a study from Taiwan on 32 low-risk patients 27 were alive and transfusion-independent after a median follow up of 27 months. Fifty-one such transplants have been reported in the registries of the EBMT and CIBMTR (18). Of these 51 patients, 13 have died and only 16 achieved sustained engraftment. Globally the two-year overall survival was 77%.

Based on the reported results, this approach cannot be recommended unless it is part of a controlled clinical trial.

9. Conditioning regimens

The results discussed above have been obtained using myeloablative conditioning. The Pesaro experience demonstrating a significant increase of thalassaemia recurrence rate with the reduction of cyclophosphamide dose from 200 mg/kg to 120 mg/kg confirmed the critical importance of the myeloablative capability of the conditioning regimen in this disease, which is characterised by an expanded erythroid system. Non-myeloablative HSCT has the theoretical advantage, based on the experience with malignancies, of obtaining allogeneic engraftment with a very low early mortality rate. However, the increased reliance on immunological effects which is required to sustain engraftment requires a prudent approach to the wide use of such regimens and very few cases have been reported, with unsatisfactory results (4). Recently, a successful trial has been published in a small cohort of adult patients with sickle cell disease (n=11) conditioned with 300 cGy of total body irradiation and alemtuzumab (19). However, this study is not immediately applicable to thalassaemia. There are in fact several relevant differences between thalassaemia major and SCD, which have an impact on approaches to HSCT. Thalassaemia major is characterised by ineffective erythropoiesis and variable erythroid expansion. Ineffective erythropoiesis and chronic transfusion lead to iron overload. Thus, for thalassaemia, a conditioning regimen capable of eradicating an expanded bone marrow and providing adequate immunosuppression to sustain engraftment with acceptable toxicity on iron-damaged tissues is required. These challenges are not present in SCD, where chronic transfusion is not universal practice, the eventual transfusion burden is less relevant, and the erythroid bone marrow, at least relatively, is less expanded.

10. Mixed chimerism

It is generally observed that a significant group of patients (approximately 10%)

develop long-term stable mixed chimerism after transplantation. Mixed chimera patients, despite a limited (even 20%) engraftment, achieve a functioning graft status characterised by normal haemoglobin level, no red cell transfusion requirement, no increase in iron stores and a limited, not clinically relevant, erythroid hyperplasia. Thus, in chimera patients, the genetic disease is substantially under complete clinical control, without achieving a complete eradication of the thalassaemia haemopoietic clones (20). Even in SCD a similar partial engraftment with production of normal Hb is capable of clinically controlling the disease, reducing HbS concentration down to levels typical of healthy heterozygotes (HbS=30%).

Unfortunately mixed chimerism in haemoglobinopathies is a casual clinical observation. Attempts to intentionally create a permanent mixed chimerism state have, so far, failed.

11. Conclusion

The central role of allogeneic HSCT in thalassaemia and SCD has been fully established. Key points are indicated below. No prospective randomised clinical trials can be designed to provide a definitive answer to the challenge of choosing between transplant and medical therapy for each individual patient. In absence of definitive evidence, the decision process is highly individualised and patient-specific. Age, clinical status, willingness to undergo treatment, donor availability, capability and compliance to adhere the appropriate transfusion/chelation regimen, quality of life and resources must all be considered.

Key points

The key point of a successful transplant in thalassaemia is optimal medical therapy (transfusion and chelation) in the years before transplant, to prevent iron overload and related tissue damage

The key point in transplantation for SCD is accurate patient selection. Those who should be selected are those patients at high risk of SCD morbidity, and they should be transplanted before irreversible SCD related organ damage

Accepted transplantation approaches in haemoglobinopathies include:
- HLA identical sibling transplant
- HLA well matched unrelated donor transplant
- HLA identical sibling cord blood transplant

Experimental transplantation approaches in haemoglobinopathies include:
- HLA matched unrelated cord blood transplant
- HLA mismatched related donor transplant

References

1. Angelucci E, Barosi G, Camaschella C et al. Italian Society of Hematology practice guidelines for the management of iron overload in thalassemia major and related disorders. Haematologica 2008; 93: 741–752.
2. Lucarelli G, Galimberti M, Polchi P et al. Bone marrow transplantation in patients with thalassemia. N Engl J Med 1990; 322: 417–421.
3. Angelucci E. Hematopoietic stem cell transplantation in thalassemia. Hematology Am Soc Hematol Educ Program 2010; 2010: 456–462.
4. Lucarelli G, Gaziev J. Advances in the allogeneic transplantation for thalassemia. Blood Rev 2008; 22: 53–63.
5. Chiesa R, Cappelli B, Crocchiolo R et al. Unpredictability of iv Busulfan pharmacokinetics in children undergoing hematopoietic stem cell transplant for advanced beta thalassemia: Limited toxicity with a dose adjustment policy. Biol Blood Marrow Transplant 2010; 16: 622–628.
6. Bernardo ME, Zecca M, Piras E et al. Treosulfan-based conditioning regimen for allogeneic haematopoietic stem cell transplantation in patients with thalassaemia major. Br J Haematol 2008; 143: 548–551.
7. Bertaina A, Bernardo ME, Mastronuzzi A et al. The role of reduced intensity preparative regimens in patients with thalassemia given hemopoietic transplantation. Ann N Y Acad Sci 2010; 1202: 141–148.
8. Gaziev J, Sodani P, Polchi Pet al. Bone marrow transplantation in adults with thalassemia: Treatment and long-term follow-up. Ann N Y Acad Sci 2005; 1054: 196–205.
9. Walters MC, Storb R, Patience M et al. Impact of bone marrow transplantation for symptomatic sickle cell disease: An interim report. Multicenter investigation of bone marrow transplantation for sickle cell disease. Blood 2000; 95: 1918–1924.
10. Panepinto JA, Walters MC, Carreras J et al. Matched-related donor transplantation for sickle cell disease: Report from the Center for International Blood and Transplant Research. Br J Haematol 2007; 137: 479–485.
11. Bernaudin F, Socié G, Kuentz M et al. Long-term results of related myeloablative stem-cell transplantation to cure sickle cell disease. Blood 2007; 110: 2749–2756.
12. Angelucci E, Walters MC. Stem cell transplantation. In: Steimberg M, Forget B, Higgs D, Weatherall D, eds. Disorders of hemoglobin. Second edn. Cambridge: Cambridge University Press, 774–790, 2009.
13. La Nasa G, Argiolu F, Giardini C et al. Unrelated bone marrow transplantation for beta-thalassemia patients: The experience of the Italian Bone Marrow Transplant Group. Ann N Y Acad Sci 2005; 1054: 186–195.
14. Fleischhauer K, Locatelli F, Zecca M et al. Graft rejection after unrelated donor hematopoietic stem cell transplantation for thalassemia is associated with nonpermissive HLA-DPB1 disparity in host-versus-graft direction. Blood 2006; 107: 2984–2992.
15. Gaziev D, Galimberti M, Lucarelli G et al. Bone marrow transplantation from alternative donors for thalassemia: HLA-phenotypically identical relative and HLA-nonidentical sibling or parent transplants. Bone Marrow Transplant 2000; 25: 815–821.

16. Sodani P, Isgro A, Gaziev J et al. Purified T-depleted, CD34+ peripheral blood and bone marrow cell transplantation from haploidentical mother to child with thalassemia. Blood 2010; 115: 1296–1302.
17. Jaing TH, Chen SH, Tsai MH et al. Transplantation of unrelated donor umbilical cord blood for nonmalignant diseases: A single institution's experience with 45 patients. Biol Blood Marrow Transplant 2010; 16: 102–107.
18. Ruggeri A, Eapen M, Scaravadou A et al. Survey of outcomes of unrelated cord blood transplant in patients with haemoglobinopathies: A retrospective study on behalf of CIBMTR, NYCB and EUROCORD. Bone Marrow Transplantation 2010; 45: 378.
19. Hsieh MM, Kang EM, Fitzhugh CD et al. Allogeneic hematopoietic stem-cell transplantation for sickle cell disease. N Engl J Med 2009; 361: 2309–2317.
20. Andreani M, Nesci S, Lucarelli G et al. Long-term survival of ex-thalassemic patients with persistent mixed chimerism after bone marrow transplantation. Bone Marrow Transplant 2000; 25: 401–404.

Multiple Choice Questionnaire

To find the correct answer, go to http://www.esh.org/online-training/handbook/

1. **What is the optimal medical therapy for thalassaemia major?**
   a) Regular red blood cell transfusion and regular life-long iron chelation... ☐
   b) Red blood cell transfusions and iron chelation only when serum ferritin level is over 1000 ng/mL. ☐
   c) Sporadic transfusion if haemoglobin is <8 g/dL ☐
   d) Red blood cell transfusions only ☐

2. **How many allogeneic HSCT in thalassaemia have been performed worldwide?**
   a) >3000 ☐
   b) 2000–2500 ☐
   c) 1000–1500 ☐
   d) <500 ☐

3. **What is the thalassaemia-free survival after allogeneic HSCT in low risk thalassaemia patients?**
   a) >85% ☐
   b) 75–80% ☐

c) 55–60%.. ☐
d) <50% .... ☐

4. **What is the most frequently used source of haematopoietic stem cells for transplantation in thalassaemia?**
   a) Bone marrow.. ☐
   b) Peripheral blood stem cells .... ☐
   c) Cord blood stem cells... ☐
   d) Bone marrow + cord blood .... ☐

5. **What is the most critical factor in deciding on transplantation for sickle cell disease?**
   a) Age.. ☐
   b) Conditioning regime... ☐
   c) GvHD prophylaxis regimen .... ☐
   d) Prediction of disease severity .... ☐

NOTES

* 20.10

High-dose chemotherapy and HSCT in children and adolescents with solid tumours in Europe

Ruth Ladenstein, Ulrike Pötschger
on behalf of the EBMT Paediatric Working Party - Solid Tumours

1. Introduction

In the absence of randomised prospective trials, the EBMT registry remains an important source to survey indications, outcome and clinical risk factors in children and adolescents with solid tumours treated by high dose therapy (HDT) and HSCT. In view of evolving treatment strategies the definition of high risk needs to be reconsidered as well as the possibility for altered treatment strategies. Decisions for HDT/HSCT should ideally be based on evidence from prospective trials but such information is still only available for high-risk neuroblastoma, where there have been three randomised trials (1).

2. 2011 EBMT data on HSCT for solid tumours in children and adolescents

In 2011 the EBMT data base contained information on 14,581 transplants performed in hig-risk solid tumour patients up to the age of 18 years. Autologous stem cell transplantation (ASCT) is still frequently performed with 14,135 transplants, whereas only 446 allogeneic transplant procedures were registered. The data was gathered in 37 countries and reported by 279 centres (Table 1).

Table 1: Event-free survival rates by tumour type after ASCT following primary treatments or relapse (according to 2011 EBMT data update on evaluable patients only)

Disease	Disease status at time of ASCT	Patients	Projected 5-yr EFS	p-value
Neuroblastoma	during primary treatment	3640	0.35 ± 0.01	S
	after relapse	360	0.23 ± 0.02	
Ewing tumours	during primary treatment	1311	0.44 ± 0.02	S
	after relapse	365	0.25 ± 0.03	
Soft tissue sarcoma	during primary treatment	553	0.23 ± 0.02	S
	after relapse	254	0.19 ± 0.03	
CNS tumours	during primary treatment	976	0.39 ± 0.02	S
	after relapse	335	0.19 ± 0.02	
Retinoblastoma	during primary treatment	54	0.63 ± 0.07	NS
	after relapse	36	0.40 ± 0.09	
Wilms' tumour	during primary treatment	112	0.52 ± 0.05	NS
	after relapse	223	0.44 ± 0.04	
Germ cell tumours	during primary treatment	151	0.49 ± 0.05	S
	after relapse	149	0.38 ± 0.04	
Osteosarcoma	during primary treatment	99	0.36 ± 0.05	S
	after relapse	107	0.14 ± 0.04	

$S = p < 0.005$

2.1 General lessons from EBMT data

The experience of more than 14,000 HSCT procedures in the paediatric age group from a period of over 30 years conveys a number of important messages (detailed data available on request).

1. There is a decrease in transplant-related mortality according to the year of transplant (before and after 1992) and the type of HDT regimen. Multiple drug regimens and in particular inclusion of TBI in HDT regimens resulted in higher mortality rates.

2. A change of stem cell source has been observed since 1992, with a steady increase of the use of peripheral autologous stem cells; this is likely to have contributed to the lower mortality rates in the ASCT setting of under 5% after 1992 and only 1-2% since 1999.

3. As a rule first-line high-risk patients fare significantly better than relapse patients. In conditions where reliable criteria defining the high-risk patient are established HDT/HSCT should preferably be part of first-line treatment strategies. However, most tumour types still await the demonstration of the potential benefit of HDT/HSCT over conventional treatments within randomised trial settings.

4. The disease response status as a result of induction or rescue treatments prior to HDT/HSCT has a crucial influence on final outcome in all indications and may be summarised as follows:

   CR > VGPR/PR > SR/MR > NR (SD) > RR/UR

   [CR: complete response, VGPR: very good partial response, PR: partial response (>50%), SR: sensitive relapse = >50% response; MR: minor response (<50%), NR: no response, SD: stable disease, RR/UR: resistant or untreated relapse (<50%response)].

   Patients in good response to first line treatment (CR/VGPR/PR) and sensitive relapse (SR) are good indications in most high risk solid tumour patients while patients with stable disease or minor response (<50%) (SD/MR) only should take part in well defined phase I/II trials. Patients with no response (NR) or tumour progression, as well as those with resistant relapse (RR) have shown a very short life expectancy even after HDT/HSCT and thus should not be elected to undergo this procedure.

5. Age at HDT/HSCT has to be considered for outcome predictions: adolescent age is generally associated with inferior outcome: age cut-offs at various levels have been identified by several tumour groups and are confirmed by the EBMT registry data. In general, age younger than 10 years is a favourable factor in sarcomas (Ewing tumours and rhabdomyosarcoma). Neuroblastoma has a cut-off at a younger age with regard to prognosis. In particular, patients younger than 18 months at

diagnosis (2) with neuroblastoma will have to be particularly carefully identified in future with a view to defining them as high-risk (see below) (3).

6. Repetitive HDT/HSCT approaches have shown no advantage over a single HDT/HSCT course in the EBMT registry data. However, the repetitive group is likely to represent patients with a worse prognosis.
7. Total body irradiation has shown no advantage in any of the solid tumour indications. TBI should thus be avoided in children with solid tumours in view of late effects and lack of benefit.
8. Interestingly, busulfan/melphalan is the only HDT combination within the EBMT solid tumour registry data which has shown so far significantly better survival rates in neuroblastoma and Ewing tumours. These data have triggered phase III randomised trials in these indications (see sections 3 & 4 below).
9. No advantage for allogeneic HSCT is detected in the EBMT registry data in any of the indications. Again, one needs to consider that often patients in a late state of their disease course have been treated with allogeneic approaches in experimental settings, including more recently also haploidentical HSCT.

3. Neuroblastoma

Neuroblastoma is the only indication in this age group where the benefit of HDT/HSCT has been shown in randomised trials, of which 3 have been reported (1). High-risk neuroblastoma is currently defined as widespread disease over the age of 18 months, including patients of any stage greater than INSS stage 1 or with amplification of the MYCN oncogene (3). The current standard treatment approach for high-risk neuroblastoma consists of a backbone of multicycle induction, PBSC collection, extensive surgery to the primary tumour site, HDT/ASCT, local radiotherapy after the ASCT, and maintenance treatment with 13-cis retinoid acid (1). Addition of immunotherapy based on the action of the ch14.18 antibody in combination with interleukin 2 and GM-CSF in the maintenance phase after HDT/ASCT was shown to have a major impact on outcome (4) and needs to be considered as standard treatment in the future, once the antibody becomes widely available.

The well-recognised prognostic significance of age in neuroblastoma may also be observed within the EBMT data. Recently, an age cut-off point of 18 months instead of 12 months has been accepted to allow better distinction between age-related prognostic groups (2). Indications for very young children need to be established most carefully, including a full evaluation of their biological risk profile when considering HSCT (3, 5).

The results of the randomised European High-Risk Neuroblastoma Study (HR-NBL-1/SIOPEN) were reported recently at ASCO 2011. This study compared two HDT regimens, namely BuMel (busulfan, melphalan) with CEM (carboplatin, etoposide, melphalan) and showed a significant benefit in favour of BuMel (6). The value of dose escalation in first-line patients with tandem transplant approaches has been explored by many teams (7) and is currently being addressed by the COG in their ongoing trial randomised trial of double HDT/ASCT versus single HDT/ASCT.

Targeted therapies, in particular iodine-131-metaiodobenzylguanidine (mIBG) therapy with and without chemotherapy and/or HDT followed by HSCT have generated increasing interest but await larger scale trials in good responders (8). The wide implementation of mIBG HDT treatments are still hampered by logistical problems as this approach requires children to be submitted to nuclear medicine units with special equipment and facilitating provision of special care requirements for this age group.

As regards relapse patients, the analysis of the EBMT data (9) showed that responding patients who relapse more than 12 months from diagnosis and had no previous HDT will benefit from salvage HDT/HSCT. Relapse patients not fulfilling these criteria gain no advantage from this intensive procedure.

Allogeneic transplantation as immunotherapy has received special attention since the introduction of reduced intensity preparative regimens and non-myeloablative transplants. Some reports highlight a graft-versus-tumour (GvT) effect in neuroblastoma with recent, modified allogeneic HSCT approaches (10) while the EBMT data show no such effect with classical allogeneic HSCT approaches (11). Research on experimental approaches to allogeneic HSCT is ongoing.

3.1 EBMT registry data on neuroblastoma

In 2011, 4644 patients with neuroblastoma were registered (4539 ASCT, 105 allogeneic HSCT). It needs to be highlighted that the registry data pointed at an early stage to the superiority of the busulfan/melphalan approach and was the basis for the High-Risk Neuroblastoma Trial (HR-NBL1/SIOPEN) which confirmed this benefit (see above) (6).

According to multivariate analysis of the EBMT data, significantly better EFS was associated with age under 2 years at ASCT ($p < 0.0001$), a better remission status before HDT/HSCT ($p < 0.0001$), the use of peripheral stem cells ($p=0.014$), ASCT as opposed to allogeneic HSCT ($p=0.031$), and the busulfan/melphalan combination for HDT ($p < 0.01$).

3.2 Possible indications based on literature and EBMT data

Good candidates are first-line high-risk neuroblastoma patients with an age of 18 months at diagnosis and widespread metastatic disease or those of any age with MycN amplified tumours with INSS stages 2 to 4 diagnosed. Any metastatic relapse in neuroblastoma patients over the age of 18 months and any MycN amplified tumour previously not treated with HDT/HSCT is also a good indication for HDT/HSCT. Any other indications should only be considered within controlled experimental phase I/II trials.

4. Ewing tumours

A number of publications have underlined the potential role of HDT/HSCT in Ewing tumours (12–15) proposing that HDT/HSCT adds some benefit to conventional multimodality therapy for children with high-risk disease. In particular, patients with multifocal bone or bone marrow metastases have a poorer prognosis than patients with lung metastases (15).

To date, superiority of any high-dose chemotherapy regimen has not been established as it has in neuroblastoma although the EBMT registry and also two recent papers suggest that BuMel HDT is particularly active also in this indication (14, 15). The potential role of TBI has also been investigated (12) but no clear improvement was observed and high toxicity and mortality were reported, and EBMT data show a 10% disadvantage in survival when TBI is part of HDT regimens.

The largest series so far of HSCT for primary disseminated multifocal Ewing sarcomas (PDMES) was recently published by the Euro-EWING 99 Study Group (15), including 281 patients treated with a dose-intense treatment concept including BuMel and HSCT. The EFS and overall survival (OS) at 3 years were $27 \pm 3\%$ and $34 \pm 4\%$ respectively. For 46 children younger than 14 years the 3-year EFS was 45%. Cox regression analyses demonstrated increased risk at diagnosis for patients older than 14 years (hazard ratio [HR]=1.6), a primary tumour volume more than 200 mL (HR=1.8), more than one bone metastatic site (HR=2.0), bone marrow metastases (HR=1.6), and additional lung metastases (HR=1.5). A score based on these factors at diagnosis was developed to facilitate risk-adapted treatment approaches in the future; the EFS rate was 50% for scores ≤ 3 (82 patients), 25% for score more than 3 to less than 5 (102 patients), and only 10% for score ≥ 5 (70 patients; $p < 0.0001$). The randomised comparison of BuMel/ASCT versus conventional chemotherapy for defined risk groups (poor responders, lung metastases) is still recruiting and results are eagerly awaited.

Some reports highlighted the GvT effect in Ewing tumours following allogeneic HSCT, but a recent publication (16), could not identify such a benefit with either reduced-intensity conditioning (RIC) or myeloablative regimens or with either HLA-matched or HLA-mismatched grafts. There was no improvement of survival with RIC compared with myeloablative regimens due to an increased risk of death from disease/relapse incidence after RIC despite a lower TRM. This implies the general absence of a clinically relevant (GvT) effect with current protocols.

4.1. EBMT registry data on Ewing tumours

The EBMT registry holds data on 1976 evaluable Ewing tumour patients (1938 autologous, 38 allogeneic). BuMel HDT shows significantly better results in first-line patients while TBI is associated with significantly poorer results.

Multivariate of the EBMT data shows significantly increased risks for patients above 14 years, a remissions status less than CR1, PR or CR2, bone marrow as source of stem cells, and HDT with other than busulfan-containing regimens.

4.2. Possible indications based on literature and EBMT data

Patients showing a poor histological response after induction ($\geq$10% viability in the resected tumour) and/or a tumour volume $\geq$200 mL and/or primary lung metastases only are included in the ongoing Euro-EWING. 99 trial, where they are randomised to either BuMel and ASCT or conventional dose VAI (vincristine, actinomycin D and ifosfamide) with additional lung irradiation. Patients with primary metastatic disease at sites other than lungs are eligible for controlled trials exploring HDT/HSCT. Any metastatic tumour not previously treated with HDT is eligible for an HSCT approach in controlled phase II investigational protocols.

5. Soft tissue sarcomas (STS)

A multivariate analysis of 269 patients with metastatic rhabdomyosarcoma (RMS) found age (>10 yrs, p <0.0001) and bone/bone marrow involvement (p <0.019) to be the most important predictors for fatal outcome (17).

In STS dose escalation with ASCT produced only short-lived remissions with generally disappointing outcome data unless patients were chemosensitive and receiving HDT as consolidation in complete remission (18).

5.1 EBMT registry data on STS

The EBMT analysis currently includes 940 evaluable patients in the age group up to 18 years (891 autologous, 49 allogeneic). No superior HDT regimen was identified within the EBMT data.

5.2 Possible indications based on literature and EBMT data

Currently there is no evidence-based standard indication for HDT/HSCT in STS. HSCT approaches investigating the role of a GvT effect in STS include:

- Alloimmunotherapy with reduced intensity conditioning and an HLA-matched related donor (19)
- Chemo-alloimmunotherapy (busulfan-containing dose-intensive regimen) and HLA-matched or 1-3 loci mismatched familial donor

- Haploidentical approaches
- High dose busulfan-containing therapy with autologous HSCT and vaccination with autologous dendritic cells.

The eligibility criteria for such approaches include primary metastatic disease in patients above 10 years of age and bone/bone marrow involvement as well as metastatic relapse of initially non-metastatic disease, in particular when associated with high-risk histologies such as alveolar RMS.

6. Brain tumours

6.1 EBMT patients

In 2011 the EBMT registry included 1311 evaluable patients with brain tumours in the age group up to 18 years. Medulloblastoma is the most frequent indication with 69% of patients, followed by astrocytoma (7%), glioblastoma (7%), ependymoma (6%), and other non-specified CNS tumours (11%). Medulloblastoma patients achieve better results when subjected to HDT/SCT in first remission and if younger than 23 years of age.

A more detailed analysis on the various histological types of brain tumours and distinct risk factors is currently not possible on the basis of the current EBMT dataset.

6.2 Possible indications based on literature

The current eligibility criteria for HDT/HSCT in brain tumours are based on trial data from brain tumour cooperative groups (20, 21).

Patients with high-risk medulloblastoma (primary metastases/relapse) of any age older than 3 years are eligible for HDT/HSCT in combination with radiation, while in infants HDT/HSCT is used with the aim of reducing (volumes and doses) or avoiding radiation.

Metastatic PNETs at diagnosis or with additional high-risk features such as incomplete resection or young age (younger than 3 or 5 years) as well as infants and young children (<4 yrs) with malignant brain tumours are further indications. Very controversial indications include high-grade glioma. Based on published results, there is little or no indication for HDT/HSCT in ependymoma, brain stem glioma or pineoblastoma.

More investigations are required to define the optimal HDT for each tumour type. It is noteworthy that most groups work with similar HDT regimens, i.e. BU-TTP (busulfan and repetitive melphalan) (SFOP, Spain), Vp16/TTP/CBDCA (US/CCG, Germany, Spain) and a tandem approach Vp16/CBDCA - TTP/L-PAM (Italy).

7. Wilms' tumour

7.1 EBMT patients
The EBMT cohort has increased to 335 patients under the age of 18 with ASCT: 112 patients have received HDT as part of primary treatment and 223 patients after relapse. The superior result in patients receiving melphalan alone, according to current EBMT data, is likely to be correlated with the response status prior to HDT. Patients receiving melphalan alone were almost exclusively (88%) in CR: 45% in CR1 and 50% in CR (22).

7.2 Possible indications based on literature and EBMT data
Adverse prognostic factors define patients with a probability of cure of 30% at best and are based on the overall experience with Wilms' tumour of the SIOP, GPOH, NWTS, MRC and the respective national groups over the last 20 years.

The high-risk population includes patients with unfavourable histology and those with metastatic disease (23, 24). In relapse patients risk factors include unfavourable histology and one of the following criteria: extra-pulmonary relapse or abdominal relapse after radiation, stage IV, more than two drugs in the first-line regimen or relapse within one year. These patients appear eligible for consolidation with HDT if a response is achieved in second-line treatment.

8. Germ cell tumours
Patients with extracranial GCTs generally have an excellent outcome when treated in prospective trials using conventional chemotherapy approaches. As a consequence, there is currently no standard indication for HDT/HSCT.

8.1 EBMT patients
In the paediatric age group there are 300 evaluable patients registered as GCT in the EBMT data base, but the differentiation of subgroups is poor.

8.2 Possible indications based on literature and EBMT data
The best definition of high-risk patients with extracranial GCTs is based on prospective trial data and includes initial non-responders or poor responders (no local control achieved) and relapsed patients who fail to achieve second CR (25, 26).

In high-risk CNS GCT patients <18 years the following criteria for HDT may be adopted: recurrent CNS GCT when biological remission is achieved prior to HDC, and also insufficient response to primary chemotherapy (27).

9. Osteosarcoma

The Italian sarcoma group (28) explored the two courses of HDT consisting of carboplatin and etoposide followed by HSCT in patients in metastatic relapse. The rate of relapse or disease progression was 84.4% and the 3-year overall survival rate, 20%, with a 3-year disease-free survival rate of only 12%. The Cooperative Osteosarcoma Study Group (29) described their experience with HDT/SCT in 15 children with relapsed osteosarcoma. HDT regimens included melphalan and etoposide, with additional carboplatin in some cases. The probability of overall survival was 0.29 ± 0.12 with a median follow-up of 16 months. None of the groups were encouraged to continue the explored approach.

9.1 EBMT patients and possible indications

The EBMT experience is limited with 116 evaluable patients in the age group up to 18 years.

Currently there is no standard indication for HSCT based on published results. High-risk features include poor histological response or non-response of the primary tumour at the time of definitive surgery, inoperable, axial tumours (large volume), primary dissemination or relapse other than isolated, late lung metastases. Even in responding high-risk patients treated with HDT/HSCT in first or second remission the length of remission is short, and relapse occurs early after HDT.

10. Retinoblastoma

One advocated HDT/HSCT approach is CARBOPEC (CBDCA, VP16,CYC) (30). However, since the outcome of CNS positive patients was not improved, introduction of thiotepa or busulfan into HDT regimens was proposed (31). Other groups have used combinations including melphalan and CBDCA, and/or VP16 in the situation of metastatic retinoblastoma and reported promising survival results for patients without CNS involvement (32, 33).

10.1 EBMT patients

The EBMT registry finds to date 54 patients receiving HDT/HSCT during primary treatment (40% with localised/regional disease and 60% with metastatic disease) while 36 patients underwent HDT/HSCT after relapse.

10.2 Possible indications based on literature and EBMT data

Based on the experience of trial groups any future trial should take the following high-risk factors into consideration: involvement of the cut-end or subarachnoidal space of the optic nerve after enucleation, orbital involvement, distant metastatic disease and CNS disease.

11. Conclusion

More co-operative studies are needed in order to clarify the population of patients who may most benefit from HDT/HSCT approaches. In some indications dose escalation strategies appear to fail. Hence there is an obvious need for immunobiological concepts as well as a need for new drug developments.

References

1. Matthay KK, Reynolds CP, Seeger RC et al. Long-term results for children with high-risk neuroblastoma treated on a randomized trial of myeloablative therapy followed by 13-cis-retinoic acid: A children's oncology group study. J Clin Oncol 2009; 27: 1007-1013.
2. Moroz V, Machin D, Faldum A et al. Changes over three decades in outcome and the prognostic influence of age-at-diagnosis in young patients with neuroblastoma: A report from the International Neuroblastoma Risk Group Project. Eur J Cancer 2011; 47: 561-571.
3. Cohn SL, Pearson AD, London WB et al. INRG Task Force. The International Neuroblastoma Risk Group (INRG) classification system: An INRG Task Force report. J Clin Oncol 2009; 27: 289-297.
4. Yu AL, Gilman AL, Ozkaynak MF et al. Children's Oncology Group. Anti-GD2 antibody with GM-CSF, interleukin-2, and isotretinoin for neuroblastoma. N Engl J Med 2010; 363: 1324-1334.
5. Canete A, Gerrard M, Rubie H et al. Poor survival for infants with MYCN-amplified metastatic neuroblastoma despite intensified treatment: The International Society of Paediatric Oncology European Neuroblastoma Experience. J Clin Oncol 2009; 27: 1014-1019.
6. Ladenstein RL, Poetschger U, Luksch R et al. Busulphan-melphalan as a myeloablative therapy (MAT) for high-risk neuroblastoma: Results from the HR-NBL1/SIOPEN trial. J Clin Oncol 29: 2011 (suppl; abstr 2). 2011 ASCO Annual Meeting, Plenary Session.
7. George RE, Li S, Medeiros-Nancarrow C et al. High-risk neuroblastoma treated with tandem autologous peripheral-blood stem cell-supported transplantation: Long-term survival update. J Clin Oncol 2006; 24: 2891-2896.
8. Matthay KK, Quach A, Huberty J et al. Iodine-131-metaiodobenzylguanidine double infusion with autologous stem-cell rescue for neuroblastoma: A new approaches to neuroblastoma therapy phase I study. J Clin Oncol 2009; 27: 1020-1025.
9. Ladenstein R, Lasset C, Hartmann O et al. Impact of megatherapy on survival after relapse from stage 4 neuroblastoma in patients over 1 year of age at diagnosis: A report from the European Group for Bone Marrow Transplantation. J Clin Oncol 1993; 11: 2330-2341.
10. Matthay KK, Seeger RC, Reynolds CP et al. Allogeneic versus autologous purged bone marrow transplantation for neuroblastoma: A report from the Children's Cancer Group. J Clin Oncol 1994; 12: 2382-2389.
11. Ladenstein R, Lasset C, Hartmann O et al. Comparison of auto versus allografting as consolidation of primary treatments in advanced neuroblastoma over one year of age at diagnosis: Report from the European Group for Bone Marrow Transplantation. Bone Marrow Transplant 1994; 14: 37-46.

12. Burdach S, Jürgens H. High-dose chemoradiotherapy (HDC) in the Ewing family of tumors (EFT). Crit Rev Oncol Hematol 2002; 41: 169–189.

13. Meyers PA. High-dose therapy with autologous stem cell rescue for pediatric sarcomas. Curr Opin Oncol 2004; 16: 120–125.

14. Oberlin O, Rey A, Desfachelles AS et al. Impact of high-dose busulfan plus melphalan as consolidation in metastatic Ewing tumors: A study by the Société Française des Cancers de l'Enfant. J Clin Oncol 2006; 24: 3997–4002.

15. Ladenstein R, Pötschger U, Le Deley MC et al. Primary disseminated multifocal Ewing sarcoma: Results of the Euro-EWING 99 trial. J Clin Oncol 2010; 28: 3284–3291.

16. Thiel U, Wawer A, Wolf P et al. No improvement of survival with reduced- versus high-intensity conditioning for allogeneic stem cell transplants in Ewing tumor patients. Ann Oncol 2011; 22: 1614–1621.

17. Koscielniak E, Klingebiel TH, Peters C et al. Do patients with metastatic and recurrent rhabdomyosarcoma benefit from high-dose therapy with hematopoietic rescue? Report of the German/Austrian Pediatric Bone Marrow Transplantation Group. Bone Marrow Transplant 1997; 19: 227–231.

18. Ek ET, Choong PF. The role of high-dose therapy and autologous stem cell transplantation for pediatric bone and soft tissue sarcomas. Expert Rev Anticancer Ther 2006; 6: 225–237.

19. Misawa A, Hosoi H, Tsuchiya K et al. Regression of refractory rhabdomyosarcoma after allogeneic stem-cell transplantation. Pediatr Hematol Oncol 2003; 20: 151–155.

20. Varan A. Risk-adapted chemotherapy in childhood medulloblastoma. Expert Rev Anticancer Ther 2011; 11: 771–780.

21. Finlay JL, Massimino M. A consensus and state-of-the-art workshop: Marrow ablative chemotherapy with hematopoietic cell rescue for malignant brain tumors of childhood and adolescence. Pediatr Blood Cancer 2010; 54: 634.

22. Dallorso S, Dini G, Faraci M et al. EBMT Paediatric Working Party. SCT for Wilms' tumour. Bone Marrow Transplant 2008; 41 (Suppl 2): S128–130.

23. Presson A, Moore TB, Kempert P. Efficacy of high-dose chemotherapy and autologous stem cell transplant for recurrent Wilms' tumor: A meta-analysis. J Pediatr Hematol Oncol 2010; 32: 454–461.

24. Spreafico F, Bisogno G, Collini P et al. Treatment of high-risk relapsed Wilms tumor with dose-intensive chemotherapy, marrow-ablative chemotherapy, and autologous hematopoietic stem cell support: Experience by the Italian Association of Pediatric Hematology and Oncology. Pediatr Blood Cancer 2008; 51: 23–28.

25. De Giorgi U, Rosti G, Slavin S et al. Salvage high-dose chemotherapy for children with extragonadal germ-cell tumours. Br J Cancer 2005; 93: 412–417.

26. Cushing B, Giller R, Cullen JW et al. Randomized comparison of combination chemotherapy with etoposide, bleomycin, and either high-dose or standard-dose cisplatin in children and adolescents with high-risk malignant germ cell tumors: A pediatric intergroup study-Pediatric Oncology Group 9049 and Children's Cancer Group 8882. J Clin Oncol 2004; 22: 2691–2700.

27. Modak S, Gardner S, Dunkel IJ et al. Thiotepa-based high-dose chemotherapy with autologous stem-cell rescue in patients with recurrent or progressive CNS germ cell tumors. J Clin Oncol 2004; 22: 1934–1943.

28. Fagioli F, Aglietta M, Tienghi A et al. High-dose chemotherapy in the treatment of relapsed osteosarcoma: An Italian sarcoma group study. J Clin Oncol 2002; 20: 2150–2156.

29. Sauerbrey A, Bielack S, Kempf-Bielack B et al. High-dose chemotherapy (HDC) and autologous hematopoietic stem cell transplantation (ASCT) as salvage therapy for relapsed osteosarcoma. Bone Marrow Transplant 2001; 27: 933–937.

30. Namouni F, Doz F, Tanguy ML et al. High-dose chemotherapy with carboplatin, etoposide and cyclophosphamide followed by a haematopoietic stem cell rescue in patients with high- risk retinoblastoma: A SFOP and SFGM study. Eur J Cancer 1997; 33: 2368–2375.

31. Kremens B, Wieland R, Reinhard H et al. High-dose chemotherapy with autologous stem cell rescue in children with retinoblastoma. Bone Marrow Transplant 2003; 31: 281–284.

32. Matsubara H, Makimoto A, Higa T et al. A multidisciplinary treatment strategy that includes high-dose chemotherapy for metastatic retinoblastoma without CNS involvement. Bone Marrow Transplant 2005; 35: 763–766.

33. Dunkel IJ, Chan HS, Jubran R et al. High-dose chemotherapy with autologous hematopoietic stem cell rescue for stage 4B retinoblastoma. Pediatr Blood Cancer 2010; 55: 149–152.

Multiple Choice Questionnaire

To find the correct answer, go to http://www.esh.org/online-training/handbook/

1. **In which paediatric solid tumours is HDT/HSCT based on evidence from prospective trials?**
   a) Ewing tumours ☐
   b) Neuroblastoma ☐
   c) Neuroblastoma and Ewing tumours ☐
   d) Neuroblastoma, Ewing tumours and CNS tumours ☐

2. **The following statements are about the prognostic significance of age at HDT/HSCT; which one is correct?**
   a) In the EBMT registry data age at HDT/HSCT is not a tool for outcome prediction ☐
   b) Adolescent age is generally associated with a superior outcome ☐
   c) Age younger than 10 years is a favourable factor in sarcomas (Ewing tumours and rhabdomyosarcoma) ☐
   d) An age cut-off point of 24 months at diagnosis has been accepted for neuroblastoma to allow better distinction between age-related prognostic groups ☐

3. **Is there a HDT combination for solid tumours which gives significantly better survival rates?**
   a) The EBMT solid tumour registry data has shown no survival advantage for any HDT combination. ☐
   b) The EBMT solid tumour registry data has shown significant survival benefit in neuroblastoma and Ewing tumours for busulfan/melphalan ... ☐
   c) The randomised European High-Risk Neuroblastoma Study (HR-NBL-1/SIOPEN) has not shown a significant benefit for BuMel ...... ☐
   d) TBI-containing regimens are superior to the busulfan/melphalan approach in Ewing tumours. ☐

4. **For metastatic Ewing tumours which of the following risk factors are of relevance:**
   a) Bone and bone marrow metastases ☐
   b) Age over 14 years, more than one bone metastatic site and bone marrow metastases ☐
   c) Age over 14 years, primary tumour volume more than 200 mL, more than one bone metastatic site, bone marrow metastases ☐
   d) Age over 14 years, primary tumour volume more than 200 mL, more than one bone metastatic site, bone marrow metastases and additional lung metastases ☐

5. **Which factors are important predictors for fatal outcome in metastatic rhabdomyosarcoma ?**
   a) Metastatic rhabdomyosarcoma patients have no favourable predictors of outcome ☐
   b) Patients with metastatic rhabdomyosarcoma (RMS) and an age above 10 years have a more favourable outcome ☐
   c) In patients with metastatic rhabdomyosarcoma bone/bone marrow involvement are the only important predictors for fatal outcome ☐
   d) In patients with metastatic rhabdomyosarcoma age >10 years and bone/bone marrow involvement are the most important predictors for fatal outcome ☐

* CHAPTER 21

Statistical evaluation of HSCT data

Richard M. Szydlo

1. Introduction

HSCT is a widely accepted treatment modality, with both allogeneic and autologous HSCT offering effective options for a number of diseases (e.g. some leukaemias and severe aplastic anaemia) and curative potential for others (e.g. thalassaemia and CML). However, there is still much to be learnt, and the analysis of data generated from a stem cell transplant programme is not only fundamental to assessing the effectiveness of the treatment, but can provide invaluable information on the prognostic role of disease and patient factors. Thus, the appropriate analysis of such data is of paramount importance.

2. Outcomes

Patients who undergo a HSCT procedure require considerable support and supervision, which in turn, allows the treatment modality to be reviewed in a variety of ways. Key events occur at varying times post-HSCT:

1. Neutrophil and platelet engraftment (days 7–45)
2. Acute GvHD (aGvHD) (days 4–100)
3. Relapse/Progression (anytime after day 0)
4. Death
5. Chronic GvHD (cGvHD) (days 100 onwards).

These events can be used to calculate a number of outcomes defined below:

- Neutrophil engraftment - defined as the first of 3 consecutive days post-HSCT where values above a specified level are achieved (e.g. $\geq 0.5 \times 10^9/L$)
- Platelet engraftment - defined as the first of 3 consecutive days post-HSCT where values above a specified level are achieved (e.g. $\geq 50 \times 10^9/L$)
- GvHD - the probability of developing GvHD (the severity of disease being estimated would need to be clearly stated)
- Transplant related mortality (TRM) - the probability of dying without recurrence of disease
- Overall survival (OS) - the probability of survival irrespective of disease state
- Disease-free survival (DFS) - the probability of being alive and free of disease. (this outcome could also be termed leukaemia-free survival, LFS)
- Relapse - the probability of disease recurrence
- Progression-free survival (PFS) - the probability of being alive and with a disease stage not advanced compared to that at the time of transplantation
- Event-free survival (EFS) - the probability of being alive and without a defined event (e.g. relapse, or progression, or either, or other defined endpoint).

In addition, secondary events such as graft failure, development of a CMV infection and diagnosis of a secondary malignancy can be utilised to allow corresponding outcome probabilities to be calculated.

Probability curves describing these outcomes fall into two categories: survival, DFS and PFS involve events with decreasing cumulative probabilities over time, whilst GvHD, TRM, and relapse involve events that result in increased cumulative probabilities over time.

3. Survival analysis

The outcomes outlined above require careful consideration before a statistical analysis can be considered. Each event of interest may occur at variable times post-transplant, so in statistical terms it has two components - whether it occurs at all and, if it does, the length of time from transplant to the event. However, inherent in many studies is the problem that the event of interest is seldom observed in all of the patients. Thus, a patient who has not yet had the event of interest at the time of analysis, or who is lost to follow-up, would be "censored" at the time of last contact. The inclusion of data that is censored precludes the use of simple statistical methods such as chi-squared analysis or rank methods and requires a statistical treatment known as survival analysis, which can be applied to a variety of end points.

3.1 Kaplan-Meier method

There are a number of methods for analysing survival data, and though these depend on the precision of the recorded time interval, they are usually summarised as survival or Kaplan-Meier (1) curves. These are derived from calculated tables commonly known as life tables (constructed on the basis of a series of conditional probabilities). The term life-table is also frequently used to describe data where the results are grouped into time intervals, often of equal length, and this method of calculation is described as actuarial. In fact the terms "actual" and "actuarial" are often used mistakenly to describe survival probabilities generated by Kaplan-Meier methods.

Figure 1 shows representative survival data from twenty patients who received a stem cell transplant. Six have died and fourteen were still alive at various time points post transplant. If the data are rearranged in order of time, then a life-table can be calculated by the method of Kaplan-Meier as shown in Table 1.

The data presented in Table 1 can be used to produce a survival curve, also known as a cumulative survival rate, or a survival function (Figure 2). Vertical tick marks on the curve represent censored individuals who make no contribution to the curve after that particular time point. The curve is an estimated probability of survival, and using appropriate methods to compute the standard error, 95% confidence intervals (95%CIs) can be calculated. In common with many analyses of small data sets, the standard errors calculated have yielded a large 95%CI band, and so the survival curve must therefore be interpreted with some caution.

THE EBMT HANDBOOK 2012 EDITION

Figure 1: Survival data from 20 patients who received a stem cell transplant

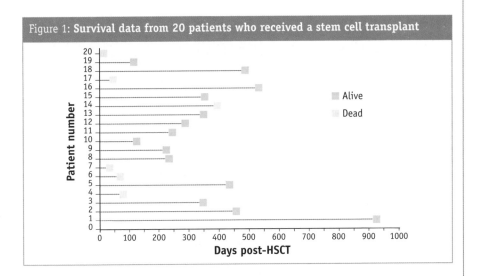

Table 1: Life-table for twenty patients who received an allogeneic stem cell transplant

Time (days)	Status (0=alive, 1=dead)	Number at risk	Probability of survival	Standard error
0		20	1.00	
9	1	19	0.95	0.049
34	1	18	0.90	0.067
45	1	17	0.85	0.080
67	1	16	0.80	0.089
78	1	15	0.75	0.097
114*	0	14	0.75	0.097
124*	0	13	0.75	0.097
224*	0	12	0.75	0.097
234*	0	11	0.75	0.097
245*	0	10	0.75	0.097
289*	0	9	0.75	0.097
346*	0	8	0.75	0.097
351*	0	7	0.75	0.097
352*	0	6	0.75	0.097
398	1	5	0.63	0.14
434*	0	4	0.63	0.14
456*	0	3	0.63	0.14
487*	0	2	0.63	0.14
532*	0	1	0.63	0.14
923*	0	0	0.63	0.14

* censored observation

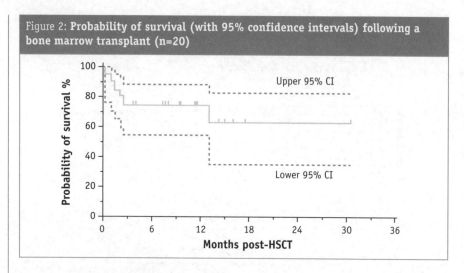

Figure 2: **Probability of survival (with 95% confidence intervals) following a bone marrow transplant (n=20)**

3.2 Cumulative incidence procedure

The following outcomes: relapse, TRM, and GvHD are subject to the problem of "competing risks" and the most appropriate method of analysing such data is to produce a cumulative incidence (CI) curve (2). In calculating a relapse probability for example, patients are assigned into 3 categories:

a. Relapse (the status of the patient after the relapse event is of no consequence for this probability calculation)

b. No relapse and alive

c. No relapse but dead.

Patients who have not relapsed and are alive still have the possibility to relapse, whilst those who have died without relapse do not, and thus death is designated as the competing risk. Although this methodology is not included in many commercial statistical packages, it is present in the statistical package NCSS, and macros are available to allow such curves to be calculated using the statistical packages SAS and R (3).

While it is possible to use the Kaplan Meier method for each of these outcomes, this is likely to produce an overestimate of the true probability as calculated by the cumulative incidence approach (4). This discrepancy will be largest where the event of interest occurs later after HSCT (TRM, relapse and cGvHD) and may be negligible with early outcomes (aGvHD and graft failure).

4. Detailed methods for generating and describing outcomes

The data set presented in Table 2 shows events and corresponding time intervals

Table 2: Outcomes for 20 representative patients following stem cell transplantation

Patient (n)	Days to aGvHD	Max aGvHD grade	Days to 500 neutrophils	Days to 50 platelets	Days to relapse	Relapse	Days to cGvHD	Max cGvHD grade	Days post HSCT	Survival status
1	15	2	18	33		no	180	ext	923	alive
2		0	21	25	234	yes			456	alive
3	45	1	35	45		no			346	alive
4		ne	25	26	45	yes		ne	78	dead
5	34	3	16	29		no			434	alive
6	30	2	22	31		no		ne	67	dead
7	23	4	25	33		no		ne	34	dead
8		0	15	35		no			234	alive
9	13	1	27	28		no	176	ext	224	alive
10		0	24	26		no			124	alive
11		0	22	28		no			245	alive
12		0	23	24		no			289	alive
13	15	3	21	22		no			351	alive
14	36	2	19	26		no			398	dead
15	40	1	27	65		no	224	lim	352	alive
16		0	23	34	356	yes			532	alive
17	11	2	20	33		no		ne	45	dead
18		0	28	36		no			487	alive
19	25	1	22	78		no	100	lim	114	alive
20		ne	ne	ne		ne		ne	9	dead

ne: not evaluable

for all the main outcomes following a stem cell transplant for 20 representative patients. This "raw" data needs to be modified appropriately in order that statistical packages can generate the appropriate outcome statistics. Thus for any outcome probability curve to be calculated there must be a column of data with an event indicator (1=yes, 0=no, 2=competing risk), and a column of data with the time to the event or censored observation (Table 3). The section below will outline in detail the steps that need to be taken in order to correctly calculate the most commonly described outcomes.

4.1 Kaplan-Meier analyses

4.1.1 Survival
The calculation of a probability of survival for a study population is relatively straightforward, with death from any cause being the event of interest. Patients alive are censored at the last time of contact. The appropriate codes and time intervals are shown in Table 3 columns N and O, Figure 2.

There are however, two distinct ways of summarising a survival curve: if survival in a population is good (i.e. few deaths and long follow-up) then a probability of survival at a given time point can be quoted (e.g. 5 yr survival of 76.2%, 95%CI 68–82). If however survival is poor, and there are for example no survivors at 3 years post-HSCT, then a more meaningful statistic to quote is the median survival (e.g. median survival of 18.5 months, 95%CI 12–34). These guidelines are suitable for all such outcome probabilities.

4.1.2 Disease-free survival
In order to calculate a probability of DFS (or LFS), patients whose suffer disease relapse or who die are considered as having the event of interest. Patients alive and free of original disease are censored at the last day of contact (Table 3 columns L and M, Figure 3A). If a patient dies after relapsing, that event is not taken into account – relapse is the first event that was observed. PFS is a similar outcome, but instead of relapse and death being the events of interest, it is disease progression and death that are noted. This probability requires careful assessment of the disease stage both at the time of stem cell infusion and at progression.

4.2 Cumulative incidence analyses

4.2.1 Transplant or treatment related mortality (TRM)
Any death where the patient has not relapsed or progressed is classified as transplant or treatment related (Table 3 columns H, I), and is thus coded 1. If a

Table 3: Data columns required to generate outcome statistics post stem cell transplantation for 20 patients

A Patient (n)	B Days to aGvHD 2-4	C Code for aGvHD 2-4	D Days to aGvHD 3-4	E Code for aGvHD 3-4	F Days to relapse	G Code for relapse	H Days to transplant related death	I Transplant related death	J Days to TRM	K Code for TRM	L Days of LFS	M Code for LFS	N Days survival	O Code for survival	P Days to cGvHD	Q Code for cGvHD
1	15	1	100	0	923	0		no	923	0	923	0	923	0	180	1
2	100	0	100	0	234	1		no	234	2	234	1	456	0	456	0
3	100	0	100	0	346	0		no	346	0	346	0	346	0	346	0
4	78	2	78	2	45	1		no	45	2	45	1	78	1	ne	
5	34	1	34	1	434	0		no	434	0	434	0	434	0	434	0
6	30	1	67	2	67	2	67	yes	67	1	67	1	67	1	ne	
7	23	1	23	1	34	2	34	yes	34	1	34	1	34	1	ne	
8	100	0	100	0	234	0		no	234	0	234	0	234	0	234	0
9	100	0	100	0	224	0		no	224	0	224	0	224	0	176	1
10	100	0	100	0	124	0		no	124	0	124	0	124	0	124	0
11	100	0	100	0	245	0		no	245	0	245	0	245	0	245	0
12	100	0	100	0	289	0		no	289	0	289	0	289	0	289	0
13	15	1	15	1	351	0		no	351	0	351	0	351	0	351	0
14	36	1	100	0	398	0	398	yes	398	1	398	1	398	1	398	2
15	100	0	100	0	352	0		no	352	0	352	0	352	0	224	1
16	100	0	100	0	356	1		no	356	2	356	1	532	0	532	0
17	11	1	45	2	45	2	45	yes	45	1	45	1	45	1	ne	
18	100	0	100	0	487	0		no	487	0	487	0	487	0	487	0
19	100	0	100	0	114	0		no	114	0	114	0	114	0	100	1
20	9	2	9	2	9	2		no	9	1	9	1	9	1	ne	

patient relapses or progresses it is likely that a subsequent death will be due to the underlying disease, and so relapse or progression in this case constitutes a competing risk (coded 2). Patients alive without relapse are censored (coded 0). The appropriate codes and durations are presented in Table 3, columns J, K and allow the curve in Figure 3B to be calculated.

4.2.2 Relapse
Relapse of original disease constitutes the event of interest, and any patient who dies of a transplant or treatment related cause is classified as a competing event. Patients alive and in remission are censored (Table 3 columns F and G, Figure 3C).

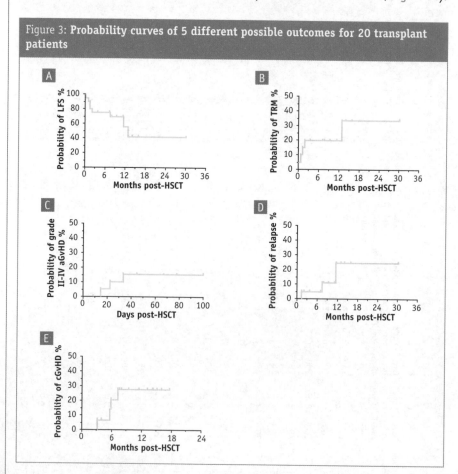

Figure 3: **Probability curves of 5 different possible outcomes for 20 transplant patients**

4.2.3 Acute graft-versus-host disease

It is possible to describe the incidence of aGvHD in a population in several ways. From the data in Table 2, it can be seen that 2 patients died before day 100, and although they did not develop aGvHD, they are assigned as non-evaluable (had they survived to day 100 they would still have been at risk of developing aGvHD). Thus of the 18 evaluable patients, the grades are as follows: 7 with no aGvHD (39%), 4 grade 1 (22%), 4 grade 2 (22%), 2 grade 3 (11%), 1 grade 4 (6%). This may be the only way to present aGvHD data if a time to diagnosis is not noted.

An alternative approach to presenting this data is to take into account the time when aGvHD was first diagnosed, and hence calculating a cumulative incidence curve. However, a decision has to be made as to the grades under investigation. If a curve showing the probabilities of developing grades 2-4 is to be calculated, then patients with grade 2-4 are assigned the event of interest as 1, with the corresponding time to diagnosis. Patients who had grade 1 aGvHD or nil are set to 0, whilst the time to the event is set at 100. Patients non-evaluable for aGvHD are assigned the event of interest to 2 (competing risk designation), with the time to event set as the survival time (Table 3, columns B and C). This analysis yields a 100 day probability of developing grade 2-4 aGvHD of 35% (95%CI 19–64%).

If a curve showing the probabilities of developing grades 3-4 is to be calculated, then patients with grade 3-4 are assigned the event of interest to 1, with the appropriate time to diagnosis. Patients who had grade 2 and survived to day 100 are assigned the event of interest as 0, with the time being 100. Patients who had grade 2 and died before day 100 are assigned an event of interest to 2 (competing risk designation), with the time to event as the survival time. Patients who had grade 1 aGvHD or nil are set to 0, whilst the time to the event is set at 100. Patients non-evaluable are assigned the event of interest to 2, with the time to event set as the survival time (Table 3, columns D and E). This analysis yields a 100 day probability of developing grade 3-4 cGvHD of 15% (95%CI 4–43%) (Figure 3D).

4.2.4 Chronic graft-versus-host disease

As with acute GvHD, it is possible to chronicle the extent of cGvHD in a study population in a variety of ways. Table 2 shows that 15 patients survived until day 100 and are thus eligible for consideration. Two developed limited (13%) and 2 extensive (13%) cGvHD while 11 had no evidence of cGvHD (74%). The alternative descriptive analysis is to calculate a probability of developing limited or extensive (or just extensive) cGvHD and quoting this probability at a particular time point (Table 3, columns P and Q, Figure 3E). Thus in the example below the probability of developing any cGvHD at 1yr post-HSCT is 28.2% (95%CI 12–65). Clearly it has to be taken into account when describing this data that only patients surviving at least 100 days are at risk of developing cGvHD.

5. Other methods for describing outcomes

The use of multistate models to describe the complicated sequence of events after HSCT is an area of expanding research endeavour. Thus the use of donor lymphocyte infusions to restore durable remissions after disease relapse can now be taken into account to produce a modified LFS curve called current-leukaemia-free survival (5). However, in order to be able to generate such curves detailed follow-up data is required and sophisticated statistical software is needed.

Engraftment times can either be described with a median and range, or with cumulative probability curves. Comparisons between groups for GvHD data should be made using the chi-squared test or chi-squared trend test, whilst the Mann-Whitney or Kruskal-Wallis test are applicable for engraftment data.

6. Composite outcome diagrams

An interesting new way of graphically representing how outcome probabilities change with time after HSCT has been developed by Ronald Brand and is included in a recent paper (Figure 4) (6). Cumulative incidences of relapse and of non-relapse death are estimated and simultaneously plotted with the Kaplan-Meier survival probability. The resulting diagram thus provides the 4 possible patient states after a HSCT: alive without relapse of disease, alive after relapse, dead after relapse and non-relapse death. In addition, the proportion of patients relapsing (relapse incidence) is provided by the sum of the relapse groups, the interface between the alive and dead components

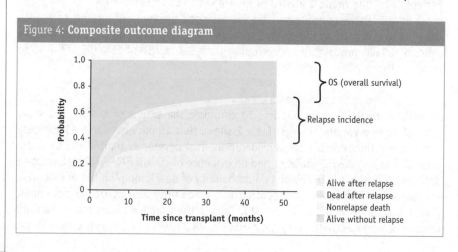

Figure 4: **Composite outcome diagram**

THE EBMT HANDBOOK 2012 EDITION

represents overall survival, and the interface between alive with and without relapse represents relapse-free survival. One is thus able to view in one diagram the relative importance of all these possible outcomes. This is especially useful for illustrating differences between groups identified from univariate or multivariate analyses as being of prognostic significance. Specialist software is not required to create such diagrams as macros are available for the statistical package SPSS.

7. Comparison of survival curves

Survival curves provide a visual assessment for a particular treatment or disease course. In order to establish whether there is a survival advantage between, for example, two treatments, it is necessary to perform a statistical test to compare the two life tables. This is achieved using the log-rank or Mantel-Cox test (7). In this test each observation is given an equal "weight". However, in the transplantation setting, where there may be considerable early mortality, it may be more useful to "weight" early observations and in this context the Breslow test (8) may be more appropriate (this test is also less sensitive to late events when few subjects may be present in the study). An example of the relative merits of these tests is provided in Figure 5, showing a statistically significant difference using the Breslow test (p=0.039), but a non-significant result using the log-rank test (p=0.14).

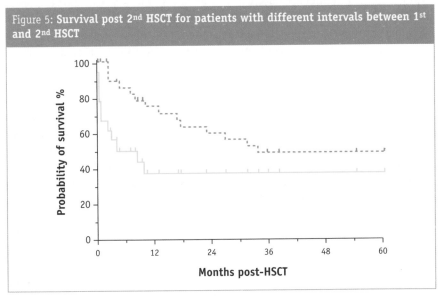

Figure 5: **Survival post 2nd HSCT for patients with different intervals between 1st and 2nd HSCT**

p=0.14 for log-rank test, p=0.039 for Breslow test

It must be noted however, that in order to perform a log-rank test, the survival curves being tested should run in parallel and not cross-over. A more sophisticated approach for analysing such data should therefore be undertaken (see Klein et al.) (4).

In addition to comparing treatments, the log-rank test can be used to compare selected sub-groups within one treatment or disease category e.g. males vs. females, patient age <30y vs patient age ≥30y, early vs late stage of disease, etc. As with all statistical comparisons of subgroups, a more stringent criterion for significance needs to be predetermined in accordance with the number of tests to be performed. If one or more prognostic variables are known, and their influence needs to be taken into account, then a stratified log-rank analysis can be undertaken. Thus, for example, in acute myeloid leukaemia where disease sub-type is an important prognostic indicator, the effect of patient gender could be investigated with a stratified log-rank test using disease sub-type as the stratified variable.

Comparison of cumulative incidence curves can be undertaken using Gray's test (9), with practical examples of this procedure being provided in a technical report by Scrucca et al. (3).

8. Presentation of survival data

In quoting survival rates, probabilities at specific points in time should be indicated together with a confidence interval or standard error (e.g. the probability of survival at 3 years was 59% (95%CI 44–73%). Although 95%CIs can be calculated by taking the survival rate ± 1.96 x standard error, if the survival rate is close to 100 or 0%, this can lead to confidence intervals greater than 100% or less than 0%. To avoid this anomaly, asymmetrical confidence intervals can be calculated by the method of Rothman (10).

Median survival times can be derived from survival curves, and correspond to the time at which the survival proportion reaches 0.5, but this is not always possible (as demonstrated in Figure 2) if the survival curve reaches a plateau above this point. Guidelines for the presentation of results of transplantation data have been suggested by Klein (5). The presentation of survival curves from univariate analyses of prognostic factors should be viewed with extreme caution, as adequate control of other potential prognostic factors or biases cannot be guaranteed. A multivariate approach is therefore to be recommended.

9. Proportional hazards regression analysis

The log-rank test enables the survival experience of two or more groups to be compared, but in order to investigate a number of possible prognostic variables simultaneously, a regression method introduced by Cox and known as proportional hazards regression analysis has to be employed (11). The special nature of survival data as outlined previously, makes the use of usual regression methods (e.g. linear regression, logistic regression) inappropriate. The use of the Cox model allows the identification of prognostic factors that are related to the outcome. In addition, the search for variables of unknown prognostic significance can be performed having adjusted for variables of known prognostic significance. Thus for example, in chronic myeloid leukaemia where the stage of disease at transplant is a major factor in survival, the influence of other factors would be investigated having taken into account disease stage. This approach also allows for the generation of survival curves for a given factor that are adjusted for the influence of other factors. Such curves are likely to be much more informative that simple univariate analysis curves.

The use of the Cox model does require a sound statistical knowledge, as there are many potential difficulties with the method both in its application and in the interpretation of results. Several reviews of the subject have been published and are recommended (12, 13).

10. Regression modelling for competing risks

In the analysis of outcomes where competing risks are present, the use of a multivariate proportional hazards regression model is inadmissible, because competing risks to the event of interest are treated as censored observations. To overcome this problem, Fine and Gray developed a proportional hazards model for the sub distribution of a competing risk (14). The practical application of this approach has recently been published for patients receiving transplants for acute leukaemia by Scrucca et al. (15).

11. Study design

Stem cell transplantation, though very widely utilised as a therapeutic option, is still able to generate a large number of research questions. In common with all research however, hypotheses should by investigated with carefully designed studies. We recently investigated the relationship between Zodiac star sign and survival post-HSCT for patients with CML (16). Though no overall relationship was found, judicial use of inappropriate statistical methods to combine disparate groups together revealed a statistically significant relationship. This was a cautionary publication, which showed that research should be carried out based on hypothesis testing, and not data-driven to find uninterpretable statistically significant results.

12. Conclusions

The analysis and presentation of survival data can provide important information on the effectiveness of transplantation in treating a particular disease, and with sufficient numbers of patients, subtle differences between patient groups can be identified. The now routine availability of computers and statistical software enables the analysis of complex data sets to be carried out with relative ease, but the importance of a good understanding of statistical principles at all stages of analysis should not be underestimated.

References

1. Kaplan EL, Meier P. Non-parametric estimation from incomplete observations. J Am Stat Assoc 1958; 53: 457–481.
2. Gooley TA, Leisenring W, Crowley JA, Storer BE. Estimation of failure probabilities in the presence of competing risks: New representations of old estimators. Stat Med 1999; 18: 695–706.
3. Scrucca L, Santucci A, Aversa F. Competing risk analysis using R: An easy guide for clinicians. Bone Marrow Transplant 2007; 40: 381–387.
4. Klein JP, Rizzo JD, Zhang M-J, Keiding N. Statistical methods for the analysis and presentation of the results of bone marrow transplants. Part I: Unadjusted analysis. Bone Marrow Transplant 2001; 28: 909–915.
5. Craddock C, Szydlo RM, Klein JP et al. Estimating leukemia-free survival after allografting for chronic myeloid leukemia: A new method that takes into account patients who relapse and are restored to complete remission. Blood 2000; 96: 86–90.
6. Lim Z, Brand R, Martino R et al. Allogeneic hematopoietic stem-cell transplantation for patients 50 years or older with myelodysplastic syndromes or secondary acute myeloid leukemia. J Clin Oncol 2010; 28: 405–411.
7. Mantel N. Evaluation of survival data and two new rank order statistics arising in its consideration. Cancer Chemother Rep 1996; 50: 163–170.
8. Breslow N. A generalised Kruskal-Wallis test for comparing k samples subject to unequal patterns of censorship. Biometrika 1974; 57: 579–594.
9. Gray RJ. A classs of K-Sample tests for comparing the cumulative incidence of competing risk. Ann Stat 1988; 16: 1141–1154.
10. Rothman KJ. Estimation of confidence limits for the cumulative probability of survival in life table analysis. J Chron Dis 1978; 31: 557–560.
11. Cox DR. Regression models and life tables. Journal of the Royal Statistical Society 1972; 34, Series B, 187–220.
12. Klein JP, Rizzo JD, Zhang MJ, Keiding N. Statistical methods for the analysis and presentation of the results of bone marrow transplants. Part 2: Regression modeling. Bone Marrow Transplant 2001; 28: 1001–1011.
13. Klein JP, Zhang MF. Survival analysis. Handbook of Statistics 2007; 27: 281–320.
14. Fine JP, Gray RJ. A proportional hazards models of the subdistribution of a competing risk. J Am Stat Assoc 1999; 94: 496–509.
15. Scrucca L, Santucci A, Aversa F. Regression modeling of competing risk using R: An in depth guide for clinicians. Bone Marrow Transplant 2010; 45: 1388–1395.

16. Szydlo RM, Gabriel I, Olavarria E, Apperley J. Sign of the Zodiac as a predictor of survival for recipients of an allogeneic stem cell transplant for chronic myeloid leukaemia (CML): An artificial association. Transplant Proc 2010; 42: 3312–3315.

Multiple Choice Questionnaire

To find the correct answer, go to http://www.esh.org/online-training/handbook/

1. **Who are censored patients?**
   a) Those who have experienced the event of interest early after HSCT ...... ☐
   b) Those who have not experienced the event of interest and are alive ..... ☐
   c) Those who have experienced the event of interest but are lost to follow-up .... ☐
   d) Those who failed to engraft .... ☐

2. **What is the correct test for comparing two Kaplan-Meier survival curves?**
   a) Chi-squared test .... ☐
   b) Mann-Whitney test .... ☐
   c) T-test .... ☐
   d) Log-rank test .... ☐

3. **What is the cumulative incidence procedure used for?**
   a) To calculate probability curves where there is a competing risk to the event of interest .... ☐
   b) To compare probability curves where the event of interest occurs early after HSCT .... ☐
   c) To compare probability curves where the event of interest occurs late after HSCT .... ☐
   d) To identify censored patients .... ☐

4. **Proportional hazards regression analysis is used:**
   a) To calculate survival curves with more than one event of interest .... ☐
   b) To help identify prognostic factors .... ☐
   c) To identify patients lost to follow-up .... ☐

d) To censor events of interest that are competing risks...................☐

---

5. **The median survival time is defined as:**
   a) The middle survival time in a series of alive patients ....☐
   b) The middle survival time in a series of dead patients ....☐
   c) The middle survival time in a series of patients irrespective of survival status...☐
   d) The time point when the survival curve crosses the 50% probability of survival mark..☐

NOTES

* CHAPTER 22

Methodology of conducting academic clinical trials in Europe

Mohamad Mohty

1. Introduction

It is now largely well established that academic prospective clinical trials, aimed at acquiring scientific knowledge, form a key part of patient-oriented clinical research, and create the basis for continuously improving patient care. This is particularly true in the field of stem cell transplantation, where studies deal with potential therapeutic innovations that do not necessary attract the pharmaceutical industry. Moreover, as treatment outcomes for many haematological diseases have progressively improved during the last years, it has become necessary to conduct larger and larger trials to demonstrate meaningful improvements in the standard of care. However, the requirements for Good Clinical Practice (GCP) in clinical trials are well documented, and ethical issues across different countries are hotly debated. In the context of low resource settings, large prospective trials often face many logistical and organisational obstacles, and thus the practical difficulties in running a trial to GCP standards should not be ignored. In addition, there is a lack of harmonisation of regulations for clinical trials among the different European countries. There is also a lack of a common definition for categories of clinical research, and national legislation on clinical research is often divergent, making it difficult to conduct stem cell transplantation studies at the multinational level. Furthermore, accrual challenges, bureaucratic inertia and regulatory approval from different entities present a major barrier, posing time-consuming administrative work to assure a trial is completed according to compliance requirements. Despite these hard challenges, solutions exist, and there are already many examples of successful studies and global collaborations across research groups and between academic investigators and industry.

This chapter will aim to provide:
- A summary of the history of clinical research and research ethics
- An overview of the current legislation in Europe governing the conduct of clinical trials
- A description of conducting clinical trials in the academic community
- Guidance on designing a clinical trial
- A summary of the attributes of exemplary clinical trial sites.

2. History of clinical research and research ethics

The philosophies governing the conduct of modern clinical trials owe their origin to recent history, such as the Nuremberg Trials, the catastrophic results of the use of the non-licensed thalidomide in pregnant women and the Tuskegee Syphilis Study in the US.

As part of the Nuremberg Trials in 1946, an American Tribunal brought criminal proceedings against a number of leading Nazi physicians who had conducted medical research studies on thousands of men, women and children in the concentration camps, without their consent. As a direct result of the trials, the Nuremberg Code was established in 1948. Although this was not implemented into law, it was the first international agreement advocating voluntary participation after informed consent. It also stated that the perceived benefits of the research must always outweigh the possible risks to the subjects. Its basic premise was that *"voluntary consent of the human subject is absolutely essential".*

To further protect subjects and to give guidance to researchers, the World Medical Association (WMA) established recommendations for the conduct of clinical research in the Declaration of Helsinki in 1964 (http://www.wma.net). In more recent years guidelines have been developed by the International Conference on Harmonisation (ICH), whose first conference was held in 1991. ICH-GCP is the accepted international standard for designing, conducting, recording and reporting trials and it is mandatory that all personnel who participate in clinical trials are trained in GCP.

3. Current legislation for clinical trials in Europe

According to the principles of GCP required by the ICH Technical Requirements for Registration of Pharmaceuticals for Human Use as well as the Ethical Principles established by the WMA, it is basic requirement to obtain a favourable opinion from an appropriate Ethics Committee (EC) prior to the conduct of a clinical trial with investigational medicinal products (IMP). In the European Union (EU) this principle has been laid down in the Clinical Trials Directive 2001/20/EC that came into force on 04 April 2001. In addition to the favourable ethical opinion, it has become a legal requirement in EU Member States (MSs) to obtain a Clinical Trial Authorisation (CTA) from the responsible National Competent Authority (CA). The deadline for implementation of the Directive by the MSs into their respective national legislations was May 1st, 2004, however it took until 2006 for all MSs to implement the Directive into their national laws.

The EU directives aimed to lay down the laws, regulations and administrative provisions of the MSs relating to the implementation of GCP in the conduct of clinical trials on medicinal products for human use. They also aimed to describe the Community code relating to medicinal products for human use, and set standards of quality and safety for the collection, testing, processing, storage and distribution of human blood and blood components, and set standards of quality and safety for the donation, procurement, testing, processing, preservation, storage and distribution of human tissues and cells. In addition, the directives aimed to lay down principles and detailed guidelines for GCP regarding IMPs for human use (including paediatric specific issues), as well as the requirements for authorisation of the manufacturing or importation of such products. Finally, the directives set the rules for traceability requirements, notification of serious adverse reactions and events and certain technical requirements for the coding, processing, preservation, storage and distribution of human tissues and cells.

Despite the commendable objective of the Directives and the associated guidance documents, the primary goal of achieving harmonisation has not been met, as each MS has interpreted the Directives within the framework of their own national legislation. Thus, though one might have expected that the overall procedure of obtaining a favourable opinion from an EC would become much more straightforward and foreseeable, conducting a multi-centre, multi-national study has consequently become a challenge.

For the sake of clarity, it should be mentioned that most of the EU legislation on the conduct of clinical trials is focused on IMPs or new medical devices (not addressed in this chapter). The full directives can be found on the European Commission website.

4. Conducting clinical trials in the academic community

Academic groups have found it difficult to access resources to fulfil the requirements imposed by the EU Directives and this has prevented some studies from taking place. At present, most academic clinical trials are conducted by national or multinational academic cooperative groups who have set up an administrative infrastructure that can provide guidance on implementing and managing clinical trials. The key issues that should be considered are described below.

4.1 Sponsorship

In accordance with the EU Directives, any clinical trial requires a single "Sponsor". This Sponsor is responsible for ensuring that the protocol is conducted appropriately according to EU laws and ICH-GCP, including indemnification. Currently sponsorship can be undertaken by:

a. An academic cooperative group (e.g. EBMT, EORTC, HOVON, GITMO, GOELAMS, etc.)
b. A national body (e.g. UK Medical Research Council)
c. A university
d. The lead institution of the trial (e.g. a university hospital in France, etc.).

Of note, although a sponsor may delegate some tasks, they remain legally responsible, so such delegation must be formally described in a contract detailing the arrangements for the conduct of the study.

4.2 EudraCT registration

Registration of a trial with the European Union Drug Regulatory Authorities (Eudra) is mandatory. Indeed, all trials conducted within the EU must apply for a EudraCT number, regardless of whether or not they are investigating an IMP. Obtaining a EudraCT number for a study is a simple online procedure (http://eudract.emea. europa.eu). Basic information only is required for the registration.

4.3 Clinical Trials Authorisation
Some trials require a Clinical Trials Authorisation, particularly if the involves an IMP or a new device. New and/or experimental therapies are IMP, but the definition also includes licensed medications being used for unlicensed or non-approved indications. Indeed, most IMPs undergo investigation to obtain a Marketing Authorisation (MA) or license in a limited number of indications. The use of the product in other indications is generally driven by the medical profession and is described as "off-label" use. Interestingly, in the field of stem cell transplantation this has become a routine problem, as most of the drugs used in the conditioning regimens, GvHD therapy, and/or in supportive care are not licensed for stem cell transplantation. As a consequence, these drugs must be considered as IMPs. The legislation does not take into account the realities of standard or established medical practice in this regard, and has proven a challenge for both the legislators and those conducting clinical trials. A reasonable and highly recommended approach would be to apply for a CTA if in any doubt, and ensure that exemption from the requirement for a CTA is provided in writing by the CA. The current legislation does not consider blood and blood products to be IMPs although this decision may be overturned in the future.

4.4 Compliance with ICH-GCP
The conduct of all clinical trials must comply with the principles of ICH-GCP. These principles are quality standards that address all aspects of clinical trials from design through to the reporting of the results. The guidelines define the roles of the different participants, describe the essential elements of a protocol and the investigator's brochure as well as detailing the standards for the conduct of a study. All personnel involved in the conduct of a clinical trial must be fully trained to ICH-GCP.

4.5 Indemnity and insurance
It is a legal requirement that insurance must be available for each clinical trial. Prior to the implementation of the EU Directives, most academic studies were conducted under the insurance of the participating institutions and usually with additional coverage from the investigator's medical negligence insurance and the manufacturer's product liability insurance. Despite the requirement for a single overall sponsor under EU laws, such overall Sponsor may still delegate insurance cover to the participating institutions. However, this may prove sensitive and rather complex to handle.

4.6. Safety reporting and pharmacovigilance

Safety reporting is a mandatory component of the conduct of any clinical trial. Serious adverse events (SAEs) are adverse events that result in one or more of the following:

- Hospitalisation or prolongation of hospitalisation
- Death
- Life-threatening
- Results in persistent or significant disability/incapacity
- Congenital abnormality or birth defect
- Is otherwise medically significant in the opinion of the investigator.

In order to minimise the paperwork, it is highly recommended that the adverse events that are usually expected for the tested population should be identified, detailed in the protocol and specifically excluded from the necessity of reporting. This is particularly true in the field of stem cell transplantation (e.g. CMV reactivation, hospitalisation for GvHD, etc.).

A suspected unexpected serious adverse reaction (SUSAR) is defined as an adverse reaction, the nature or severity of which is not consistent with the known study treatment information. A serious event or reaction is not defined as a SUSAR when:

- It is serious but expected
- It does not fit the definition of an SAE, whether expected or not.

All adverse events that are defined as reportable in the protocol should be recorded in the case record forms (CRFs). If an adverse event fulfils the criteria of a SAE or SUSAR then additional reporting requirements must be followed, as specified in Table 1. Of note, an important instrument for safety monitoring in clinical trials is the Annual Safety Report (ASR). The EU Directives require sponsors to provide the EC once a

Table 1: **Reporting requirements for adverse events, serious adverse events and SUSARs**			
	Report	Report to	Time frame
AEs	Site	Sponsor	Trial specific
SAEs	Site	Sponsor	24 hrs
SUSARs	Sponsor	CAs / ECs	Expedited
		PIs / MAHs	Trial specific
ASR	Sponsor	CAs / ECs	From 1 year anniversary of CTA

MAH: Marketing Authorisation Holder; ECs: Ethical Committees; CA: Competent Authorities; EMEA: European Medicines Evaluation Agency; C-PI: Coordinating Principle Investigator; PI: Principle Investigator (each institution); ASR: Annual Safety Report

year with a listing of all suspected serious adverse reactions which have occurred over this period and a report of the subjects' safety.

4.7 Registration with the International Committee of Medical Journal Editors

Registration of a study with the International Committee of Medical Journal Editors is required (if not mandatory) for publication. This requirement is a relatively quick process.

5. Designing a clinical trial

5.1 The different types of clinical trials

The scope and design of a specific clinical trial will vary depending on the topic and endpoints of such trial. A few examples of are listed in Table 2. Nowadays, the development of new medicinal products follows a well defined pathway. Clinical trials related to stem cell transplantation and other cellular therapies must follow the same rules, though they may have a slightly different sequence with the phase I stage being replaced by a "pilot" study in which the safety, feasibility and initial indications of efficacy are studied.

Preclinical studies are conducted *in vitro* and/or in animals, but this is not an absolute requirement, especially in the stem cell transplant field. The phase I or pilot studies are the first to be conducted in humans and are designed to determine the safety, the spectrum of toxicities and to identify the maximum tolerated dose (MTD). By identifying the MTD, the phase I study can then help to establish the recommended dose for any phase II study. Phase I studies can also give some guidance as to selection of the most appropriate patient population for further product development. Phase II studies aim to determine the efficacy of a new therapeutic strategy. In the field of stem cell transplantation, around 20 to 80 patients may be required. The design often includes an early stopping rule (e.g. increased transplant-related mortality at day 100, increased incidence of severe grade III-IV acute GvHD, etc.) to ensure that a study is stopped promptly if the investigational approach is

Table 2: Scope and design of clinical trials	
Scope	**Design**
Diagnostic prevention screening	Randomised
Supportive care	Non randomised, registration or cohort
Quality of life	Single blind
Therapeutic	Double blind crossover
Genetic technical laboratory	Controlled – placebo, comparator

deemed too dangerous or to have insufficient efficacy. Phase II studies usually pave the way for phase III studies that aim to establish (or not) a new therapeutic strategy as the standard of care. Per definition, phase III trials require larger number of patients to meet the statistical end points. Phase IV studies are designed to expand the knowledge and experience of a new established approach in the tested population and in other patient populations.

5.2 Designing a new clinical trial

Conducting clinical research is an integral part of cancer care including stem cell transplantation and treatment advances. Thus, gaining experience in the field of clinical research is an important part of the career path of an academic transplanter. The initial step is obviously to identify the clinical question to be studied (e.g. a new conditioning regimen, a new GvHD prophylaxis regimen, a different stem cell source, a new drug for treatment of viral infections, a patient population not usually considered for transplant, etc.). A good knowledge of current practice in the field and of the available literature is mandatory in order to identify a relevant research proposal. However, a "good clinical question" may not always prove to be feasible. Therefore, a "feasibility study" is essential for the ultimate success of the trial. A valid feasibility study should address issues such as the required sample size, number of interested centres/countries, study duration, potential funding sources, potential sponsors, etc. A feasibility study is usually conducted based on the study synopsis which usually summarises the rationale for the study, study design and schema, study endpoints, inclusion and exclusion criteria, statistical considerations, etc.

Given the complexity of the process, the potential "principal investigator" (PI) of a trial is strongly advised to seek the assistance and advice of a local institution (research department or clinical trials office), European research groups (EBMT, EORTC, etc.), and/or national cooperative groups (ALFA, HOVON, IFM, GITMO, GOELAMS, etc.). Such groups have gained significant knowledge and experience in the recent years about how to fulfil all the requirements for study conduct in accordance with EU laws and GCP rules. Also, the PI should bear in mind that a dedicated infrastructure is required to handle issues related to insurance, data management, data monitoring, submission fees (ethics committees and competent authorities), translations if necessary, study fees and dedicated staff, data monitoring, data analysis, statistical support and publication costs. With this respect, securing an accurate and sufficient budget is likely the most important step for a smooth study implementation and conduct. Indeed, the approval process of a new study protocol can be a long and hard process, starting with peer review, progressing through national regulatory and ethical approvals and finally local approval. An example of a clinical trial "table of content" is shown in Figure 1. A list of useful websites with information on ethical

Figure 1: **An example of a typical clinical trial "table of content"**

TABLE OF CONTENTS (ClinicalTrials.gov Identifier:NCT01135641)

1.	**Study rationale and background**	8
2.	**Study endpoints**	15
2.1	Primary endpoints	15
2.2	Secondary endpoints	15
3.	**Study design**	16
4.	**Patients selection**	17
4.1	Inclusion criteria	17
4.2	Exclusion criteria	17
5.	**Inclusion procedures, treatment schema and calendar of evaluations**	19
5.1	Patients selection	19
5.2	Pre-Treatment evaluation	20
5.3	Inclusion and treatment plan	20
5.3.1	Inclusion	20
5.3.2	Treatment plan	21
5.4	Calendar of evaluations	25
6.	**Evaluation criteria**	32
6.1	Primary endpoint	32
6.2	Secondary endpoints	32
7.	**Safety and aspects and adverse events**	32
7.1	Adverse events	32
7.1.1	Definition	33
7.1.2	Assessment of casuality	35
7.1.3	Recording of adverse events	36
7.1.4	Reporting of AE and SAE	36
7.2	Annual safety report	38
8.	**Criteria of premature discontinuation or patient dropout from the study**	39
9.	**Statistical considerations**	40
9.1	Calculation of the number of patients	40
9.2	Definition of endpoints	40
9.3	Dealing with missing data	42
9.4	Statistical analyses	42
9.5	Early stopping rules	43
10.	**Quality assessment**	44
10.1	Good clinical practice	44
10.2	Auditing	44
10.3	Monitoring	44
11.	**Final report and publication rules**	45
12.	**Regulatory aspects**	46
12.1	Regulatory Authorities Approvals (CPP and AFSSAPS)	46
12.2	Informed Consent	46
12.3	Investigators responsibilities	47
12.4	Sponsor responsibilities	48
12.5	Biocollections	48
13.	**References**	49

committees' application process in different European countries can be found at: *http://www.efgcp.be/Downloads/EFGCPReportFiles/WEBSITE%20INDEX.pdf*

6. Attributes of exemplary clinical trial sites

In addition to GCP and ICH standards, there is a growing awareness among investigators regarding the need to implement not only minimum standards for the conduct of clinical trials, but also some criteria that may be considered as attributes of exemplary clinical trial sites. These attributes are being developed based on current regulatory requirements, and consensus among community and academic clinical researchers. Attributes of exemplary clinical trial sites, as stated in the American Society of Clinical Oncology (ASCO) statement, include:

a. Diversification of the clinical trial mix
b. High accrual activity
c. Participation in the clinical trial development process
d. Maintenance of high educational standards
e. Quality assurance
f. Multidisciplinary involvement in the clinical trial process
g. Clinical trial awareness programs.

Implementation of one, or all, of the above attributes will help a site develop well beyond the minimum GCP requirements and ultimately lead to a stronger research program.

7. Conclusion

Performing clinical research is an essential step towards improving patients' and diseases' outcome. Patients, physicians, scientists and the general public are the primary beneficiaries of clinical research: they benefit from new understandings of disease, new diagnostics, new therapies and medical devices. In that sense, today's clinical research is tomorrow's healthcare, because clinical research facilitates the transfer of knowledge to the daily clinic and, when a benefit to patients is shown, to the commercial arena. In this way, clinical research adds economic value.

The EU directives and subsequent regulations have undoubtedly increased the complexity of the design and conduct of prospective clinical trials. However, the European Commission is planning to put forward, in 2012, a legislative proposal to revise the Clinical Trials Directive 2001/20/EC. To assess the impact of this revision, a public consultation was held from 9 October 2009 to 8 January 2010. The responses, together with a summary of them, have been published on the "clinical trials website" of "Health and Consumers" Directorate-General (DG SANCO). Thus, improvements in the legislations are expected, and investigators should not abandon because the task of complying with the regulatory authorities appears too daunting. Also, the past few years have witnessed a sharp learning curve for academic clinicians, but also demand for large patient numbers, which in turn requires a pan-European, multinational, harmonised approach to coordinate and conduct such trials. More than ever before, funding will be a key issue for non-commercial clinical research. Stem cell transplantation has been and should remain at the forefront of translational haematological research, and all investigators involved in this field should commit themselves to the continuation of this tradition.

Selected references

1. International Conference on Harmonisation. ICH E6: Good Clinical Practice: Consolidated guideline, version 1997. http://ec.europa.eu/enterprise/pharmaceuticals/eudralex/vol-10/3cc1aen.pdf

2. Directive 2001/20/EC of the European Parliament and of the Council of 4 April 2001, Official Journal, L121, I/5/2001, 34–44.

3. European Commission Enterprise Directorate-General. Detailed guidance on the application format and documentation to be submitted in an application for an Ethics Committee opinion on the clinical trial on medicinal products for human use, Revision 1, February 2006. http://ec.europa.eu/enterprise/pharmaceuticals/eudralex/vol10/12_ec_guideline_20060216.pdf

4. European Commission Enterprise Directorate-General. Detailed guidance for the request for authorisation of a clinical trial on a medicinal product for human use to the competent authorities, notification of substantial amendments and declaration of the end of the trial, Revision 2, October 2005. http://ec.europa.eu/enterprise/pharmaceuticals/eudralex/vol-10/11_ca_14-2005.pdf

5. European Forum for Good Clinical Practice (EFGCP) Ethics Working Party. The Procedure for the Ethical Review of Protocols for Clinical Research Projects in the European Union. http://www.efgcp.be/html.asp?what=efgcpreport.htm&L1=5&L2=1

6. Lambers Heerspink HJ, Dobre D, Hillege HL et al. Does the European Clinical Trials Directive really improve clinical trial approval time? Br J Clin Pharmacol 2008; 66: 546–550.

7. Glickman SW, McHutchison JG, Peterson ED et al. Ethical and scientific implications of the globalization of clinical research. New Engl J Med 2009; 360: 816–823.

8. Zon R, Meropol N, Catalano R et al. American Society of Clinical Oncology statement on minimum standards and exemplary attributes of clinical trial sites. J Clin Oncol 2008; 4: 2562–2567.

Multiple Choice Questionnaire

To find the correct answer, go to http://www.esh.org/online-training/handbook/

1. The EudraCT registration of a trial is:
a) Mandatory .... ☐

b) Optional .... ☐
c) Mandatory only in case of a non-interventional trial .... ☐
d) None of the above .... ☐

2. **Serious Adverse Events (SAE) are adverse events that result in one or more of the following:**
   a) Hospitalisation or prolongation of hospitalisation .... ☐
   b) Death .... ☐
   c) Life-threatening event .... ☐
   d) All of the above statements are true .... ☐

3. **Indemnity and insurance in the context of a clinical trial:**
   a) It is an optional procedure .... ☐
   b) It is a legal requirement that insurance must be available for
      any clinical trial .... ☐
   c) It is only mandatory for academic trials .... ☐
   d) None of the above .... ☐

4. **The principles of ICH-GCP are:**
   a) Quality standards that address all aspects of clinical trials from
      design through to the reporting of the results .... ☐
   b) Define the roles of the different participants .... ☐
   c) Describe the essential elements of a protocol and the investigator's
      brochure as well as detailing the standards for the conduct of a study ... ☐
   d) All of the above statements are true .... ☐

5. **Sponsorship of a clinical trial:**
   a) Any clinical trial requires a single "sponsor" .... ☐
   b) The sponsor is responsible for ensuring that the protocol is
      conducted appropriately according to EU laws and ICH-GCP, including
      indemnification .... ☐
   c) Although a sponsor may delegate some tasks, they remain legally
      responsible .... ☐
   d) All of the above statements are true .... ☐

*CHAPTER 23

Cell therapy for tissue regeneration/repair

Eliane Gluckman, Marie Caroline Le Bousse-Kerdilès

1. Introduction

For the last half century, stem cells have been used primarily for HSCT to treat malignant and non-malignant diseases in adults and children. Cells are obtained either from bone marrow aspiration, or mobilised peripheral blood or umbilical cord blood collection. It appeared, a decade ago, that these cell products contained immature cells capable of differentiation in different tissues lineages. Further, the possibility to isolate stem cells from blastocysts or to reprogramme adult cells to become stem cells (induced pluripotent stem cells: iPS) raises the possibility of using these cells to treat a large variety of non-haematological diseases. Several diseases are current candidates for such experimental therapies, including autoimmune or chronic inflammatory diseases. Systemic sclerosis, lupus, Crohn's disease and multiple sclerosis have been substantially improved by autologous HSCT. Adult haematopoietic stem cells (HSC) or mesenchymal stromal cells (MSC) have been used in non-controlled studies in diseases such as spinal cord injury, retinopathies, liver cirrhosis, and limb ischaemia. Phase I-II studies are currently investigating autologous cord blood transplantation in hypoxic ischaemic encephalopathy, infant cerebral palsy and type 1 diabetes. These preliminary results have led to a considerable interest from research organisations, biotechnology and pharmaceutical companies, the media and the general public because of the new possibility to treat a large variety of lethal or severely debilitating chronic diseases. Indications and transplant procedures are under investigation, but it may be years before this approach can be applied as a standard treatment.

2. Types and sources of cells used for regenerative medicine

Life is an ongoing process during which, depending on age, tissues are continually growing, remodelling and regenerating. This is achieved by an endogenous system of regeneration through stem cells (SCs) found almost in every type of tissue. When these SCs are lost or defective or when their responses are inadequate, the help of regenerative medicine is necessary to form new functional tissues.

2.1 Definition and classifications of stem cells

Stem cells are defined by two canonical properties: capability of self-renewal and ability to differentiate into different cell lineages (commitment). Schematically, stem cells can be classified according to several classifications. One is based on life chronology: embryonic stages where embryonic SCs are needed to form tissues and foetal/adult stages where SCs participate in tissue regeneration and repair. A second classification is based on their potency, i.e. their ability to form embryonic and extra embryonic cell types (totipotent SC: e.g. zygote) or to generate cells of the three embryonic layers, e.g. ectoderm, mesoderm and endoderm but no longer to form extra embryonic cells (pluripotent SCs), or to give rise to multiple, a few or only one closely related family of cells (multipotent, oligopotent or unipotent SCs, respectively). A third classification relies on their well-defined *in vivo* physiological roles (e.g. hepatic SC, neuronal SC, hematopoietic SC) or their ability to display SC properties *ex vivo*, after culture (e.g. embryonic SC (ES), induced pluripotent SC (iPS), mesenchymal stem/stromal cells (MSC) (for review, see ref 1). In the following paragraphs, we will discuss the use of embryonic and non-embryonic (adult/somatic) stem cells, their potency, and how easy it is to isolate and expand them in the context of regenerative medicine and tissue engineering (Figure 1).

2.2 Control of stem cell proliferation and differentiation
Understanding the mechanisms by which stem cells participate in tissue repair requires the knowledge of the mechanisms which control the choice between self-renewal, proliferation and differentiation. In contrast to early embryonic stages, where symmetric divisions give rise to more stem cells, maintenance of their constant number throughout adult life is mostly achieved by asymmetric division in which one daughter stem cell retains its self-renewal capacity while the other enters into differentiation. Stem cell fate is regulated through several intrinsic

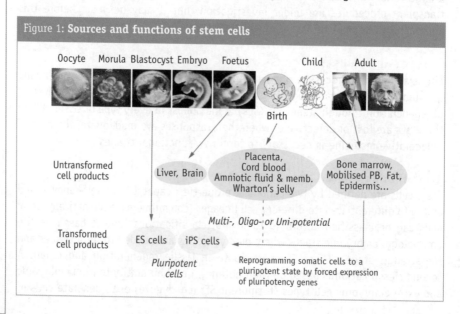

Figure 1: **Sources and functions of stem cells**

transcription factors and extrinsic elements. Epigenetic modifications play an important role in stem cell fate decision-making processes by regulating the chromatin state of the genes involved in pluripotency and hence their potential to be expressed. Such epigenetic modifications are known to be highly responsive to signals delivered by the specific microenvironment, called stem cell niches. These signals have been reported to be crucial in the SC decision to stay in quiescence or to proliferate and differentiate and therefore to maintain and control their "stemness" (2). Within these niches, SCs are in close interactions with neighbouring stromal cells through extracellular matrix components and adhesion molecules that regulate their behaviour in concert with humoral factors including cytokines and chemokines (3).

2.3 Embryonic stem cells

Apart from the zygote itself and the cells resulting from its first divisions (blastomeres), which are the only in vivo totipotent embryonic stem cells, pluripotent embryonic SC can be derived from the inner cell mass of a 5-6 day-old blastocyst. Since their discovery in 1981 and the establishment of the first ES cell line in 1998 (4), the number of new created human cell lines is growing rapidly and about 600 human ES cell (hESCs) lines were reported in 2010. When cultivated under the pressure of feeder cells and specific growth factors (such as fibroblast growth factor for hESCs) required to maintain pluripotency, ES cells exhibit features of "immortality". Their differentiation into tissue-committed cells must be tightly and sequentially controlled by defined culture conditions in an attempt to mimic as best as possible the in vivo embryonic development conditions. Indeed, their therapeutic use to repopulate damaged organs needs to overcome several technical problems including the risk of teratoma formation by undifferentiated ES cells. ES as well as iPS cell research (see paragraph 2.5) may have many other clinical applications including as therapeutic agents in cell-based therapies for model diseases such as leukaemia, genetic diseases or degenerative disorders or drug screening.

Beside these technical difficulties, as well as multiple legal and ethical concerns associated with the derivation of ES cells from early stage embryo/blastocysts that will not be discussed here, the clinical use of hESCs for regenerative medicine poses a societal, philosophical and scientific challenge.

2.4 Foetal and adult stem cells

Foetal and adult stem cells, also classified as non-embryonic stem cells, have lost their pluripotency but they maintain a multipotent differentiation potential. While foetal SCs are close to adult SCs in terms of potentialities, they are more actively cycling and have a high division potential; however, like adult SCs, they have a limited life span and some of them, including haematopoietic stem cells (HSC), are difficult to amplify *in vitro* without differentiation. They can be derived from multiple extra-embryonic tissues such as Wharton's jelly, amniotic membranes and fluid and placenta, from umbilical cord blood and adult tissues that are continuously dividing such as skin, intestines and bone marrow.

Amniotic fluid-derived SCs have been reported to express some embryonic SC markers and to retain ability to differentiate in cells from the three embryonic germ layers, but they do not form teratomas *in vivo* (5). Whereas these cells are easily and widely available and probably represent an intermediate stage between pluripotent embryonic and multipotent non-embryonic SCs, definite proofs of their pluripotency are needed for their use in regenerative medicine.

Umbilical cord and placenta also provide an interesting and easily available source of stem cells. Indeed, cord blood (CB) can be collected from the umbilical cord at birth and placenta after delivery. Cord blood is a major source of HSC. Since the first transplant of HSC from umbilical cord blood in 1987 for the treatment of a boy with Fanconi anaemia (6), one in five HSC transplants currently uses cord blood as a source of HSC. Even if the volume of blood and the number of recovered HSCs are lower than in bone marrow samples, CB differs from bone marrow by the greater diversity of donors, its accessibility and the "youthfulness" of SCs in terms of immaturity and immunity. Beside its great utility for HSC transplants, CB is also source of circulating endothelial progenitor cells (EPC). More recently, it has been shown that the umbilical cord itself and Wharton's jelly offer other clinical interests as sources of endothelial cells (EC) and MSC, which may be of great utility for therapeutic applications.

Beside its abundance in HSCs, bone marrow contains other adult SCs such as endothelial progenitors and MSCs. MSCs are subpopulation of multipotent stromal cells able to self renew for a limited amount of division *in vitro* and to differentiate into several connective tissue cell types including adipocytes, osteoblasts, chondrocytes, tenocytes and myocytes. MSCs can be isolated from bone marrow and extra-embryonic annexes, and also by *in vitro* adherence from a number of tissues including synovia, tendons, skeletal muscles, gingiva, teeth roots and adipose tissue, rendering them easily accessible. Their homing potential towards an injured tissue and their low immunogenicity, making possible their use in allogeneic therapy, explain their interest for the field of regenerative medicine as shown by their current use in various pre-clinical applications and in some clinical trials in GvHD, osteoporosis and vascular disorders.

2.5 Induced pluripotent stem cells

Several strategies have been used in an attempt to reprogramme differentiated cells of adult tissues to become pluripotent. Among them, the nuclear transfer of a somatic adult cell to an enucleated oocyte, known as "reproductive cloning" was used with success for the cloning of Dolly the sheep. In man, this technique has been used to produce genetically identical hESCs by transferring the nucleus of a skin fibroblast in an enucleated human oocyte. This "therapeutic cloning", which was finally unproductive and ethically questionable, was replaced by a simpler and more efficient technique in which 4 genes coding for transcription factors controlling pluripotency (Oct-3/4, Sox2, Klf4 and c-Myc) were directly transduced by retroviruses into differentiated cells. After the first reprogramming of murine differentiated fibroblasts into inducible pluripotent stem (iPS) cells by the groups of Yamanaka et al. (7) and of Thomson et al. (4) it is now possible to reprogramme human fibroblasts or several other cells from adults or newborns in hiPS cell lines (8). Similar combinations of genes, which may or may not include Nanog and Lin28, are currently being used. As with pluripotent SC, these reprogrammed iPSc are able to generate cells from the three germ layers, demonstrating their great interest for regenerative medicine. Whereas the place of iPS in experimental medicine is evident, the potential for clinical applications remains to be determined. At present, their clinical use requires the development of safer methods especially avoiding retroviruses and oncogenes for reprogramming.

3. Mechanisms of tissue repair in stem cell therapies

The ability of stem cells to self-renew and give rise to cells with variable degrees of differentiation offers significant potential for cell replacement and tissue repair. The best example of these SC properties is illustrated in haematopoietic stem cell transplantation, in which HSC from the donors definitively replaces the deficient or leukaemic stem cells of the patient. However, its success requires heavy conditioning, including total body irradiation and chemotherapy, to eradicate patient haematopoiesis and to allow engraftment of transplanted HSCs. In the case of non-haematopoietic cell therapies, whereas results are encouraging, they are not so positive and mechanisms explaining the therapeutic action of SC administration need to be better understood. Several mechanisms are currently proposed including stimulation of endogenous resident cells, paracrine stimulation, immunomodulation, cell fusion, transdifferentiation or cell material transfer.

A number of lines of evidence suggest that cell replacement may not mainly result from engraftment and differentiation of the transplanted cells since very few donor cells are found in the damaged tissue of the host. The low number of surviving cells after transplantation may result from the difficulty of the injected cells to reach and to be maintained at the site of injury, justifying the use of a biomaterial scaffold to promote their engraftment. In this context, it has been proposed that cells *per se* might not be required, leading to the concept of "cell therapy without cells" and that the repair response rather depends on interactions between transplanted cells and host cells/tissue. In cardiac and liver cell therapies, it has been suggested that injected bone marrow cells are capable of stimulating resident stem/progenitor cells to proliferate and differentiate (9). Such an effect could act through trophic effect/paracrine stimulation. In the case of MSC administration, the production of cytokines and chemokines including pro-angiogeneic, anti-apoptotic and trophic factors would improve tissue vascularisation, cell survival and migration, creating a favourable environment for host stem/progenitor regeneration. MSCs are also known to exhibit potent anti-inflammatory and immunomodulatory effects that might improve excessive immune reactions. They constitutively produce low levels of immunosuppressive factors and their production can be modulated by cells such as T-lymphocytes or dendritic cells/monocytes in the local environment, demonstrating the role of humoural and cell interactions in the regenerative process. Mechanisms involved in these interactions are important to understand since they may identify molecules that can be therapeutically targeted.

The concept that cell reprogramming can occur *in vivo* by spontaneous cell fusion events is also emerging, suggesting that this mechanism can be implicated in tissue regeneration. Indeed, studies using cardiomyocytes have reported that transplanted SC can fuse with host tissue cells (10). However, as a very rare event, the importance of this cell fusion process and its participation in tissue regeneration by a mechanism of "*in situ* reprogramming" is still under discussion.

Beside cell fusion, horizontal material transfer could also contribute to *in situ* reprogramming by transfer of genetic information and proteins between injected cells and host tissue cells. This material transfer can be mediated by microvesicles, exosomes, endosomes or apoptotic bodies. Among them, microvesicles are membrane-derived secreted microparticles produced by a number of cell types including MSC, endothelial progenitor cells, and liver resident stem cells (for review, see ref 11). Microvesicle-mediated exchange could be bidirectional. They could transfer proteins, nucleic acids (mRNA, miRNA), and lipids, participating in protective and regenerative effect but also by transdifferentiation or reprogramming of cells with which these microvesicles interact. As an example, ES cell-derived microvesicles could reprogramme haematopoietic stem/progenitor cells through mRNA and protein transfer (12). Therefore, the use of microvesicles could be exploited in regenerative medicine as vectors of genetic information involved in reprogramming SCs to acquire features of the injured tissue cells but also by participating in de-differentiation of mature tissue cells that would have survived the injury.

So, it appears that cell engraftment *per se* may not be the only strategy to regenerate a damaged tissue. Whatever the mechanisms of tissue repair are, extensive studies are needed to understand them for improving stem cell therapies. The future will tell us whether "cell-free" strategies can be developed, rendering regenerative medicine procedures standardised, traceable and safe.

4. Clinical applications

Stem cells have been actively explored in animal models of cardiac infarction, diabetes and various neurological diseases including stroke, amyotrophic lateral sclerosis, spinal cord injury, Huntington's disease, Parkinson's disease and hypoxic ischaemic encephalopathy. In most animal studies beneficial effects have been observed. Various teams have begun to explore the clinical uses of various types of stem cells found in bone marrow or cord blood, in particular mesenchymal stem cells, beyond those that could be corrected by replacing cells in their own lineage. Early results from these trials have produced mixed results, often showing minor or transitory improvements which may be attributed to extracellular factors. Various SC sources have been used: haematopoietic stem cells, MSCs, endothelial progenitor cells, skeletal, myoblasts, cardiac stem cells, adipose cells, ES cells and unfractionated bone marrow mononuclear cells. Adult cells were mostly bone marrow-derived autologous CD34+ or CD133+ cells or MSCs. Allogeneic MSCs have been used in several animal models because their lack of HLA markers. Autologous cord blood banking has been advocated by several commercial banks for possible use later in life. These banks have been generally criticised because of the absence of current evidence that they might be used later in life for regenerative medicine. Table 1 shows the current applications of cord blood. Most of the claims for regenerative medicine are currently experimental and do not enter in general practice. Current research has shown that besides haematopoietic stem cells, cord, placenta, amniotic fluid and Wharton's jelly contain other progenitors such as mesenchymal stromal cells that can give rise to bone, cartilage, adipocytes, or other progenitors producing hepatocytes, pancreatic islets, neurons, keratinocytes etc. CB offers an easily accessible stem cell source to study basic and translational stem cell biology and to develop novel drugs or stem cell-based therapy which could restore normal organ function by either stimulating endogenous stem cells or providing exogenous stem cells (13–15). Before clinical studies begin, many questions must be answered: how do CB and placenta compare with other sources of stem cells (adult or embryonic)? What is their immunogenicity? What is their differentiation potential? What is their tumorigenicity?

Most potential clinical applications are still experimental with limited clinical evidence of safety and efficacy. Most published studies have included only a limited

Table 1: Models of family-directed cord blood banks and principal indications

	Allogeneic		Autologous	
Indications	Haematological Leukaemia Other malignant diseases Immune deficiency Aplastic anaemia Metabolic diseases	Non-haematological Immunotherapy	Gene therapy for hereditary disorders Haematological? Others?	Non-haematological Regenerative medicine Autoimmune diseases
Use	Validated	Experimental	Experimental	Experimental
Source	Cord blood	Cord blood Umbilical cord Placenta	Cord blood	Cord blood Umbilical cord Placenta
Type of cells	HSC	HSC Lymphocytes MSC iPSc	HSC	HSC Lymphocytes MSC iPSc
Quality and safety	Supposed good quality if in experienced hospitals	Unknown	Decreased quality	Unknown
Operating model	Public or private	Research-funded or private	Research-funded or private	Research-funded or private

number of patients in pilot or phase I-II studies. There are few published results of randomised studies (for general review see ref 15). Table 2 and Table 3 give selected trials listed in *www.clinicaltrials.gov* as of August 23, 2011 using either cord blood or MSCs.

The use of therapeutic ES cells has been recently considered in the US: there are four FDA approved trials treating subacute thoracic spinal cord injuries with human embryonic stem cell derived oligodendrocyte progenitor cells (GRNOPC1) (16). Advanced Cell Technology received FDA clearance for a clinical trial using retinal cells derived from ES cells to treat Stargardt's macular dystrophy and age related macular degeneration. Spinal muscular atrophy type 1 using human motor neurone progenitor cells derived from human ESc is currently on hold from California stem cell.

Adipose stem cells and the stromal vascular fractions are being used for soft tissue engineering with a range of scaffolds, particularly for breast augmentation, fistulas in Crohn's disease and tissue damaged by irradiation, tracheomediastinal fistula bone defect, skin ulcers and stress induced urinary incontinence (16). Endothelial progenitor

Table 2: Selected trials on regenerative medicine for non-haematological diseases using cord blood

Disease	Tissue	Cell source	Phase
Type 1 diabetes	HSC	Autologous cord blood + Vitamin D and omega 3	Randomised, phase 1, active not recruiting
Spastic cerebral palsy	HSC	Autologous cord blood	Randomised vs placebo
Pre-term neonates: Respiratory distress syndrome, anaemia of prematurity, intraventricular haemorrhage	HSC	Autologous cord blood	Pilot study, not recruiting
Cerebral palsy	HSC	Autologous cord blood	Placebo control blinded phase I-II
Spinal cord injury	HSC	Local infusion of HLA matched unrelated cord blood	Phase I-II escalating dose
Neonatal hypoxic-ischaemic encephalopathy	HSC	Autologous cord blood	Phase I
Hearing loss in children	HSC	Autologous cord blood	Phase I
Critical limb ischaemia	HSC	Allogeneic cord blood, local injection	Pilot
Type 1 diabetes	HSC	Autologous cord blood	Pilot
Liver cirrhosis	MSC	Autologous cord blood	Phase I-II

From www.clinicaltrials.gov

cells may have some efficacy in phase I studies in the regeneration of damaged tissues preventing amputation of ischemic limbs and recovery after myocardial infarction. These results are preliminary and should be confirmed in large placebo-controlled studies. Transplantation of pancreatic β islet cells gives some transient non-sustained improvement. Neural stem cells can be cultured from foetal neonatal or adult brain but there is currently no evidence of their efficacy.

5. Conclusion

The use of HSC for allogeneic transplant for haematological diseases has saved many lives all over the world. Many other applications are explored for the treatment of non-haematological life-debilitating chronic diseases. This is the object of intense research and competition in a potentially profitable industry-led market (16). CB and placenta are attractive sources for implementing new therapeutic trials. Enormous

Table 3: Selected trials on regenerative medicine for non-haematological diseases using mesenchymal stromal cells

Disease	Tissue	Cell source	Phase
Critical limb ischaemia	Placenta	Placental MSCs	Phase I, intra muscular injection, not recruiting
Congestive heart failure	Bone marrow	Autologous BM expanded	Phase I-II, placebo control
Osteoarthritis	Bone marrow	Autologous MSC, intra-articular	Phase I
Emphysema	Bone marrow	Autologous MSC, intra-venous	Phase I
Myocardial ischaemia	Bone marrow	Autologous MSC	Phase I-II
Stroke	Bone marrow	Autologous BM+MSC	Phase I
Amyotrophic lateral sclerosis	Bone marrow	Autologous MSC+NTF, intrathecal	Pilot
Critical limb ischaemia, diabetes	Adipose tissue	Autologous MSC	Phase I-II, dose escalation, randomised
Peripheral vascular and cardiovascular diseases	Adipose tissue	Autologous MSC	Phase I-II
Ischaemic heart failure	Bone marrow	Trans-endocardial autologous MSC or BM	Phase I-II
Ischaemic heart failure	Bone marrow	Trans-endocardial injection auto-MSC compared to allo-MSC	Phase I-II randomised

From www.clinical trials.gov. NTF: secreting neurotrophic factor

opportunities exist for discovery research to develop innovative future therapies for blood diseases and more broadly for a much larger population suffering from common autoimmune, hereditary or degenerative illnesses. Such new developments are still at the experimental stage but preclinical and phase I studies indicate that new cell therapy products will be developed in the future. A novel manufacturing industry is emerging to translate unique cellular therapy bioprocesses into robust, scaled-up manufacturing production for clinical use. It is widely recognised that cell-based therapies could revolutionise health care for a range of diseases, but also that there are gaps in the overarching framework and the technologies to generate clinical success. There is limited understanding of how to fulfil requirements as regulatory and manufacturing guidelines are incomplete and few approaches have achieved commercialisation. Areas timely for developing research include technology development to improve the cost and purity of manufacture and final product quality. Continuing academic research and help from the industry for the development of new products and for the implementation of worldwide regulation rules will regulate the market on the basis of new scientific and clinical protocols and rigorous clinical trials.

References

1. Bajada S, Mazakova I, Richardson JB, Ashammakhi N. Updates on stem cells and their applications in regenerative medicine. J Tissue Eng Regen Med 2008; 2: 169–183.
2. Watt FM, Hogan BL. Out of Eden: Stem cells and their niches. Science 2000; 287: 1427–1430.
3. Ferraro F, Celso CL, Scadden D. Adult stem cells and their niches. Adv Exp Med Biol 2010; 695: 155–168.
4. Thomson JA, Itskovitz-Eldor J, Shapiro SS et al. Embryonic stem cell lines derived from human blastocysts. Science 1998; 282: 1145–1147.
5. De Coppi P, Bartsch G Jr, Siddiqui MM et al. Isolation of amniotic stem cell lines with potential for therapy. Nat Biotechnol 2007; 25: 100–106.
6. Gluckman E, Broxmeyer HA, Auerbach AD et al. Hematopoietic reconstitution in a patient with Fanconi's anemia by means of umbilical-cord blood from an HLA-identical sibling. N Engl J Med 1989; 321: 1174–1178.
7. Takahashi K, Yamanaka S. Induction of pluripotent stem cells from mouse embryonic and adult fibroblast cultures by defined factors. Cell 2006; 126: 663–676.
8. Yu J, Vodyanik MA, Smuga-Otto K et al. Induced pluripotent stem cell lines derived from human somatic cells. Science 2007; 318: 1917–1920.
9. Loffredo FS, Steinhauser ML, Gannon J, Lee RT. Bone marrow-derived cell therapy stimulates endogenous cardiomyocyte progenitors and promotes cardiac repair. Cell Stem Cell 2011; 8: 389–398.
10. Acquistapace A, Bru T, Lesault PF et al. Human mesenchymal stem cells reprogram adult cardiomyocytes toward a progenitor-like state through partial cell fusion and mitochondria transfer. Stem Cells 2011; 29: 812–824. doi: 10.1002/stem.632.
11. Deregibus MC, Tetta C, Camussi G. The dynamic stem cell microenvironment is orchestrated by microvesicle-mediated transfer of genetic information. Histol Histopathol 2010; 25: 397–404.
12. Ratajczak J, Miekus K, Kucia M et al. Embryonic stem cell-derived microvesicles reprogram hematopoietic progenitors: Evidence for horizontal transfer of mRNA and protein delivery. Leukemia 2006; 20: 847–856.
13. Francese R, Fiorina P. Immunological and regenerative properties of cord blood stem cells. Clin Immunol 2010; 136: 309–322.
14. Liao Y, Geyer MB, Yang AJ, Cairo MS. Cord blood transplantation and stem cell regenerative potential. Exp Hematol 2011; 39: 393–412.
15. Broxmeyer HE. Cord blood hematopoietic stem cell transplantation (May 26, 2010)

StemBook, ed. The Stem Cell Research Community, StemBook, doi /10.3824/stembook.1.52.1.

16. Trounson A, Thakar RG, Lomax G, Gibbons D. Clinical trials for stem cell therapies. BMC Med. Published online 2011 May 10 doi: 10.1186/1741-7015-9-52.

Multiple Choice Questionnaire

To find the correct answer, go to http://www.esh.org/online-training/handbook/

1. **Bone marrow contains which of the following stem cells:**
   a) Haematopoietic stem cells ☐
   b) Endothelial progenitor cells ☐
   c) Mesenchymal stromal cells ☐
   d) a + c ☐
   e) a + b + c ☐

2. **Which of the following is true for amniotic fluid derived stem cells?**
   a) There are definitive reports of the pluripotency of amniotic fluid derived stem cells ☐
   b) Amniotic fluid derived stem cells are being used in phase I trials for congestive heart failure ☐
   c) All of the above ☐
   d) None of the above ☐

3. **The clinical applications of stem cells other than haematopoietic stem cells are numerous and there are several on-going phase I and phase II trials. Indicate which of the following is *not* the subject of a registered phase I or II trial:**
   a) Congestive heart failure ☐
   b) Liver cirrhosis ☐
   c) Type 1 diabetes mellitus ☐
   d) Osteoarthritis ☐
   d) Emphysema ☐

4. **ES cells are:**
   a) Multipotent stem cells ☐

b) Tototent stem cells .... ☐
c) Pluripotent stem cells .... ☐
d) Unipotent stem cells .... ☐

5. **iPS are:**
   a) *In vivo* pluripotent stem cells .... ☐
   b) *In vivo* multipotent stem cells .... ☐
   c) *In vitro* somatic cells reprogrammed to a pluripotent state .... ☐
   d) *In vitro* derived pluripotent stem cells .... ☐

* CHAPTER 24

Ethics of research and clinical practice

Cliff Chaplin

1. Introduction

Advances in medical science have made research and clinical practice ethically more complex. This imposes on researchers and practitioners the need for increased ethical sensitivity and knowledge. Today research and clinical practice is guided by various ethical codes and guidelines. The purpose of this short chapter is to examine the ethics of clinical research and by inference that of clinical practice and to review how we have come to value certain ethical principles and practice articulated in two particularly important documents, the Nuremburg Code and the Declaration of Helsinki.

2. History

It is reasonable to assume that throughout human history people have "experimented" in a quest for knowledge that would result in health benefits. Indeed, there appears in the Book of Daniel a dietary experiment that took place as early as the 6th century BCE. As captive, Daniel refused to defile himself by consuming King Nebuchadnezzar's meat and wine, and asked if he and his fellow captives could for ten days have pulses to eat and water to drink. Daniel asked that their appearances be compared, after ten days, with those of children who had eaten the King's meat. The biblical account concludes, "at the end of ten days their countenances appeared fairer and fatter in flesh than all the children which did eat the portion of the king's meat..." (1).

Today the principle of beneficence, together with that of non-maleficence, is considered of primary importance. Hippocrates (460–370 BCE), the Greek physician, emphasised their importance as early as the 5th century BCE when he wrote, the "physician must... have two special objects in view with regard to disease, namely, to do good or to do no harm" (2). Of course, there have been historical examples where these two principles have been ignored or selectively applied in human experimentation. In the 1st century AD Aulus Cornelius Celsus (25 BCE–40 AD), the Roman encyclopaedist, showed little consideration for the welfare of research subjects we would consider today to be vulnerable, when he wrote, "It is not cruel to inflict on a few criminals sufferings which may benefit multitudes of innocent people through all centuries" (3).

Some of the greatest advances in healthcare practice have been achieved with the use of experimental practices we would today consider ethically unacceptable. Research in the 18th century to find cures for scurvy and smallpox, two major causes of death and disability, are good examples.

Scurvy was at the time a major cause of death at sea. To seek a prevention and cure, James Lind (1716–1794), a Scottish Royal Navy physician, is accredited with conducting the "first" clinical trial in 1747. It was thought an acidic diet helped counter the disease. Lind, after a few months at sea, recruited 12 sailors suffering from scurvy, divided them into six groups of two and in addition to the same diet gave each group a different acidic supplement. One group was given two oranges and one lemon. After six days when the fruit ran out, one of the sailors who had been given the citrus fruits was fit for duty and the other was much improved. Today there is an ethical expectation that research findings be published and the benefits made available as soon as possible. Yet, it was eleven years later in 1758 that Lind published his "A Treatise of the Scurvy" and it was almost 40 years later in 1795 that the British Admiralty authorised the supply of lemons and limes to the fleet (4). No doubt many preventable deaths occurred in the meantime.

In the 18th century smallpox was a devastating disease. Almost 30% of those infected died, up to 80% suffered disfigurement, mainly to the face, and in Europe it was a major cause of childhood mortality. Additionally, it was responsible for 33% of all blindness (5). To counter smallpox, variolation was used in the Ottoman Empire, and involved exposure to a mild strain of the disease in order to produce immunity against the more virulent form. However, variolation was not without its risks and after it was brought to Britain, physician Charles Maitland used vulnerable people as research subjects. In 1721 he experimented on six prisoners in London's Newgate prison, in exchange for their release. They were all variolated and developed smallpox immunity. They all survived and were released. Maitland then experimented on orphaned children (6).

Edward Jenner (1749–1823) is famous for successfully demonstrating that immunity to smallpox can be achieved by infection with cowpox, a much safer method than variolation. However, Jenner's study would have been ethically unacceptable today as it involved subjecting a healthy boy, whose father may have been in a dependent relationship as Jenner's gardener, to risk. In 1796, he inoculated 8 year old James Phipps with cowpox samples. James had flu-like symptoms for a few days and returned to good health. Jenner subsequently failed to induce smallpox in James on numerous occasions, thereby proving immunity. His work led to vaccination for smallpox and eventually for other diseases and has subsequently saved the lives of countless people. Continuing the theme of vaccination, Louis Pasteur (1822–1895), a microbiologist, was aware of Jenner's work and developed methods of reducing the potency of causative organisms so they could be used as a vaccine. He developed a vaccine for anthrax and was responsible for the first rabies inoculation on the 6 July 1885. The case was interesting ethically as it involved using an intervention unproven for use in humans in an attempt to save life where death seemed certain – a practice endorsed today by the Declaration of Helsinki. The rabies victim was 9 year old Joseph Meister who had been brought for treatment by his mother after being badly bitten by a rabid dog. Pasteur wrote, *"The death of this child appearing to be inevitable, I decided, not without lively and sore anxiety… to try upon Joseph Meister, the method which I had found constantly successful with dogs"* (7). Later in life Joseph Meister was employed as the gate-keeper at the Pasteur Mausoleum. In 1940, when Paris fell to the invading Nazis, sadly, he committed suicide. The reason for his suicide is unclear. One story is that he did so rather than open the gates of the Mausoleum to the Nazis, though this was later cast into doubt by his son who said he was saddened by the fall of France.

The requirement for ethical codes of practice in clinical research has been underlined by revelations of exploitative and abusive research. The "Tuskegee Study of Untreated Syphilis in the Negro Male" as it was officially called, is a notable recent example. The study lasted 40 years (from 1932–1972) during which time US government doctors recruited 399 black men with syphilis from a poor farming black community. Instead of being informed of the true nature of the study, participants were told it was a study into "bad blood". Actions were taken to prevent participants receiving effective treatment such as penicillin after it became available as the drug of choice to treat syphilis in 1940s. Following exposure, the study was terminated. Participants had been left to suffer complications of tertiary syphilis, including heart disease, paralysis, blindness, insanity, and death. Up to 128 people died of syphilis and related complications, some participants' wives were infected and children were born with congenital syphilis (8). In May 1997, 65 years after the study began and 25 years after it was stopped, the survivors received a public apology from US President Clinton. He said, *"The United States government did something that was wrong - deeply, profoundly, morally wrong... To our African American citizens, I am sorry that your federal government orchestrated a study so clearly racist... The people who ran the study at Tuskegee... forgot their pledge to heal and repair..."* (9).

The most profound example of unethical human research is that of Nazi experiments in concentration camps during the 1940s. The experiments were horrific abuses of vulnerable subjects and often resulted in death. Often driven by the needs of the Nazi war effort, they included experiments to record human physiological changes when subjected to different barometric pressures, immersion in freezing water to research hypothermia, and the use of toxic and caustic substances to record their effects on humans. To aid the eugenics programme, people were subjected to cruel experiments in sterilisation. Children were also used in cruel experiments. Twenty Jewish children were, for example, injected with tuberculosis as part of medical experimentation and then murdered on April 20, 1945 in the Neuengamme concentration camp (10, 11).

3. Codes of ethical practice

3.1 The Nuremburg Code
Following the Nuremburg "doctors trial", the Nuremburg Code was produced in 1947.

It contains ten crucial points designed to ensure ethical practice in clinical research. The very first point emphasises the importance of consent. Famously it reads, *"The voluntary consent of the human subject is absolutely essential... the person involved should have legal capacity to give consent... should be able to exercise free power of choice, without... any element of force, fraud, deceit, duress... or other ulterior form of constraint or coercion... [and]... should have sufficient knowledge and comprehension... to make an understanding and enlightened decision".*

Further points stipulate that results should be fruitful and not procurable by other methods, the design should be based on animal experimentation results, unnecessary physical and mental suffering and injury should be avoided, the research should not take place if death or disabling injury may occur, the degree of risk may not exceed the benefits of the trial, every possible action must be taken to protect the subject from injury, disability or death, the researchers should be scientifically qualified, the subject may terminate the trial at any stage, and finally, the researcher must be prepared to terminate the trial at any stage if it is considered likely to result in injury, disability, or death to the subject (12).

3.2 The Declaration of Helsinki

Influenced by the Nuremburg Code, the World Medical Association's Declaration of Helsinki was produced in 1964. It has been revised several times, its latest revision being that of 2008. The Declaration outlines the ethical principles for medical research involving human subjects as well as research on identifiable human material and data. Its contents are crucially important. It clearly emphasises the duty of the physician to "promote and safeguard the health of patients, including those involved in medical research". Regarding consent it points out that the subject's participation must be voluntary and informed, non-written consent must be documented and witnessed, and care must be taken regarding possible coercion. With respect to subjects who are incompetent, the Declaration stipulates that their dissent should be respected. It also points out that subjects should be informed of the outcome of the study and should share in the benefits, that patient refusal to take part must never interfere with the patient-doctor relationship and their confidentiality must be respected.

The Declaration furthermore refers to the need to include underrepresented populations in research and outlines special protection for the vulnerable, on whom research is only justified if designed to meet the health needs of that particular group. The importance of scientific standards and knowledge is emphasised as is the requirement that researchers have appropriate scientific training and qualifications. Researchers also have a responsibility to do a risk/burden-benefit analysis and a duty to publish results. The requirement to respect animal welfare, the importance and content of the research protocol and the importance and role of an independent ethics committee is also outlined. The Declaration also refers to the need for physicians to consider the local and international ethical and legal norms and standards for research involving human subjects, but emphasises that local regulations should not diminish any of the protections outlined in the Declaration (13).

Influenced by Helsinki, the European Clinical Trials Directive 2001 is designed to standardise research activity in clinical trials throughout EU (14). It is supplemented by the EU Good Clinical Practice Directive 2005, which requires by law Member States to comply with ethical guidelines for good clinical practice. Among other important points it states that the "rights, safety and well being of the trial subjects shall prevail over the interests of science and society" (15).

In conclusion, we now have highly formulated codes of ethical practice in clinical research. We also greatly value certain ethical principles and the concept of rights (16). The principle of respect for autonomy is important, particularly in relation to informed consent and confidentiality. Those of beneficence and non-maleficence are important with regard to research motive and risk-benefit analysis. Justice is important regarding selection and recruitment, the dissemination of research findings, and, crucially, the fair distribution of benefits. The concept of rights is important, particularly with respect to individual entitlements and claims and is usefully applied in many contentious issues.

4. An historical lesson

However, there is a lesson to be learnt from history. In 1898, Albert Neisser (1855–1916), Professor of dermatology and venereology at the University of Breslau, published results of his clinical trial to find a vaccination for syphilis. In the trial he injected treated serum from syphilitic patients into patients who were admitted for other conditions. Some contracted syphilis. They were not informed or asked for consent. Neisser was fined by the Royal Disciplinary Court for not seeking patient consent and in 1900 the Prussian Government issued the first directive concerned with medical experimentation on humans. It emphasised respect for autonomy, information giving (including adverse effects) and "unambiguous consent". In 1931 further Prussian Government guidelines regulated therapeutic and non-therapeutic research in human subjects stipulating the requirement of informed consent in non-therapeutic research and, amongst other things, commenting on the need for explicit pathways of responsibility, documented research plans, a risk-benefit assessment, and previous animal experimentation. Yet, the existence of the most advanced ethical and legal guidelines did not prevent Nazi doctors carrying out inhumane clinical experiments (17).

From this we may conclude that the existence of protective guidelines is not enough, the crucial point is not only adherence to them, but unwavering adherence to the basic principle of universal human respect.

References

1. Bible. King James Edition. Book of Daniel 1: 8–16.
2. Hippocrates. Hippocratic Corpus. Epidemics I: 11.
3. Aulus Cornelius Celsus. De Medicina, Prooem 26.
4. Mayberry J. A Timeline on Scurvy, 2004. http://leda.law.harvard.edu/leda/data/658/Mayberry.html)
5. World Health Organisation. Factsheet, 2001. http://www.who.int/mediacentre/factsheets/smallpox/en/
6. Riedel S. Edward Jenner and the history of smallpox and vaccination. Baylor University Medical Centre. 2005; 18: 21–25.
7. Dobson MJ. Disease. 2008: 159. Quercus.
8. The Troubling Legacy of the Tuskegee Syphilis Study, 2002. http://www.nus.edu.sg/irb/Articles/Tuskegee%20Syphilis%20Study.pdf
9. The White House – Office of the Press Secretary: http://clinton4.nara.gov/textonly/New/Remarks/Fri/19970516-898.html)
10 Spitz V. Doctors from hell – the horrific account of nazi experiments on humans. 2005. First Sentient Publications.
11. Lifton RJ. Medical killing and the psychology of genocide – the nazi doctors. 2000. Basic Books.
12 The Nuremburg Code, 1947. http://www.ushmm.org/research/doctors/code_expl.htm
13. Declaration of Helsinki. World Medical Association, 2008. http://www.wma.net
14. EU Clinical Trials Directive 2001/20/EC of the European Parliament and of the Council of 4 April 2001.
15. EU Good Clinical Practice Directive 2005/28/EC of 8 April 2005.
16. Beauchamp TL, Childress JF. Principles of Biomedical Ethics. 2008, 6th edition. Oxford University Press.
17. Vollmann J, Winau R. Nuremburg - Informed consent in human experimentation before the Nuremberg code. BMJ 1996; 313: 1445–1449.

Multiple Choice Questionnaire

To find the correct answer, go to http://www.esh.org/online-training/handbook/

1. **The four ethical principles considered of primary importance in modern research and clinical practice are:**

    a) Beneficence, non-maleficence, respect for autonomy and charity.........☐

b) Non-maleficence, respect for autonomy, justice and virtue .... ☐
c) Respect for autonomy, beneficence, non-maleficence and informed consent .... ☐
d) Beneficence, non-maleficence, respect for autonomy and justice .... ☐

2. **James Lind is accredited with conducting the "first" clinical trial in 1747. The trial was designed to seek a prevention and cure for scurvy. Though he found that citrus fruits had a beneficial effect, from an ethical standpoint his trial may be criticised because:**
   a) He did not seek informed consent from the scorbutic sailors who participated as subjects .... ☐
   b) He did not publish the beneficial results for eleven years .... ☐
   c) His results were skewed by the non-inclusion of female subjects .... ☐
   d) He failed to do a risk/benefit assessment .... ☐

3. **Louis Pasteur was responsible, in 1885, for the first rabies inoculation. The recipient was nine year old Joseph Meister who had been badly bitten by a rabid dog.**
   The case was interesting ethically because:
   a) The technique had not been trialled on animals .... ☐
   b) It involved using an intervention unproven for use in humans in an attempt to save life where death seemed certain .... ☐
   c) Consent was not sought from the child's mother .... ☐
   d) The hospital ethics committee declined to sanction the procedure .... ☐

4. **Following the Nuremburg "doctor's trial" and revelations of appalling abuse of vulnerable concentration camp subjects in cruel Nazi medical experiments, the Nuremburg Code was produced in 1947.**
   It contains ten crucial points designed to ensure ethical practice in clinical research.
   The very first point emphasises the importance of:
   a) Confidentiality .... ☐
   b) Appropriate scientific and research qualifications of researchers .... ☐
   c) Risk/benefit assessment .... ☐
   d) Voluntary consent .... ☐

5. Influenced by the Nuremburg Code, the Declaration of Helsinki (2008) outlines the ethical principles for medical research involving human subjects as well as research on identifiable human material and data. Its contents are crucially important. It clearly emphasises the duty of the physician to "promote and safeguard the health of patients, including those involved in medical research".

This important document is the product of:

a) The United Nations ☐
b) World Health Organization ☐
c) World Medical Association ☐
d) European Parliament ☐

NOTES

* ABBREVIATIONS

(-)	negative
(+)	positive

A

AA	aplastic anaemia
ABC	activated B-cell
ABMTR	Autologous Bone Marrow Transplant Registry
AD	anno Domini, years after birth of Christ
ADA	adenosine deaminase
ADs	autoimmune diseases
AE	adverse event
Ag	antigen
aGvHD	acute graft versus host disease
AI	alloimmunisation
AL	acute leukaemia
AL amyloid	primary (or immunoglobulin light-chain) amyloidosis
ALDP	adrenoleukodystrophy protein
ALCL	anaplastic large cell lymphoma
ALFA	Acute Leukemia French Association
ALL	acute lymphoblastic leukaemia
AMN	adrenomyeloneuropathy
allo-HSCT	allogeneic haematopoietic stem cell transplant
ALWP	Acute Leukaemia Working Party
AmB	amphotericin B
AML	acute myeloid leukaemia
ANC	absolute neutrophil count
AP	accelerated phase
APCs	antigen presenting cells
APL	acute promyelocytic leukaemia
APTT	activated partial thromboplastin time
ARA-C	cytosine arabinoside
ASR	annual safety report
ATD	adult therapeutic dose
ATG	antithymocyte globulin
ATMP	advanced therapy medicinal products
ATRA	all-trans retinoic acid
auto-HSCT	autologous haematopoietic stem cell transplant
AVN	avascular necrosis of bone

B

BAL	broncho-alveolar lavage
BC	blast crisis
BCE	before the Christian era

BCNU	1,3-bis(2-chloroethyl)-1-nitrosourea
BCR	B-cell receptor
BCSS	breast cancer-specific survival
BFM	Berlin-Frankfurt-Munster study group
BM	bone marrow
BMF	bone marrow failure
BMDW	Bone Marrow Donor Worldwide
BMT	bone marrow transplantation
BNLI	British National Lymphoma Investigation
BO	bronchiolitis obliterans
BOOP	bronchiolitis obliterans with organising pneumonia
BSA	body surface area
Bu	busulfan
BUN	blood urea nitrogen

C

CAR	chimeric antigen receptors
CARD15	caspase recruitment domain family member 15
CB	cord blood
CBT	cord blood transplantation
CC	complete chimerism
CD	cluster designation
CFU-GM	colony forming unit granulocyte macrophage
CGPs	cytokine gene polymorphisms
cGvHD	chronic graft versus host disease
CI	cranial irradiation
CJD	Creutzfeld-Jakob disease
CLL	chronic lymphocytic leukaemia
CLWP	Chronic Leukaemia Working Party
CLS	capillary leak syndrome
CML	chronic myeloid leukaemia
CMV	cytomegalovirus
CNI	calcineurin inhibitors
CNS	central nervous system
COP	cryptogenic organising pneumonia
CP	chronic phase
C-PI	coordinating principle investigator
CR	complete remission
CR1	first complete remission
CsA/CSA	cyclosporin A
CSF	colony stimulating factor
CSI	craniospinal irradiation
CT	chemotherapy

CTA	Clinical Trial Authorisation
CT/RT	chemo-radiotherapy
CTL	cytotoxic T-lymphocytes
CTLp	cytotoxic T-lymphocyte precursor
cTnT/cTnI	cardiac troponin T/cardiac troponin I
CVC	central venous catheter
Cy	cyclophosphamide

D

DAH	diffuse alveolar haemorrhage
DBA	Diamond-Blackfan anaemia
DC	dendritic cell
DF	defibrotide
DFS	disease-free survival
DIC	disseminated intravascular coagulation
DKC	dyskeratosis congenita
DLBCL	diffuse large B-cell lymphoma
DLI	donor lymphocyte infusion
DLT	dose limiting toxicity
DMARDs	disease modifying antirheumatic drugs
DMSO	dimethylsulfoxide

E

EBMT	European Group for Blood and Marrow Transplantation
EBV	Epstein-Barr virus
EC	Ethics Committee
ECIL	European Conference on Infections in Leukaemia
EES	extra-osseous Ewing's sarcoma
EFI	European Federation for Immunogenetics
EFS	event-free survival
EMEA	European Medicines Agency
EPCs	endothelial progenitor cells
EPO	erythropoietin
ERα	estrogen receptor alpha
ERT	enzyme replacement therapy
ES	embryonic stem cells
ES	engraftment syndrome
ET	essential thrombocythaemia
EU	European Union
EULAR	European League against Rheumatism
EUSTITE Project	European Union Standards and Training in the Inspection of Tissue Establishments
EWOG-MDS	European Working Group on Myelodysplastic Syndromes

F

FA	Fanconi anaemia
FAHCT	Foundation for Accreditation of Hematopoietic Cell Therapy
FFP	fresh frozen plasma
FFTF	freedom from treatment failure
FHCRC	Fred Hutchinson Cancer Research Centre
FISH	fluorescent *in situ* hybridisation
FL	follicular lymphoma
FLC	free immunoglobulin light-chain
FLIPI	Follicular Lymphoma International Prognostic Index
FLU	fludarabine
FNHTR	febrile non-haemolytic transfusion reactions
FSH	follicle stimulating hormone
FTE	full-time equivalent

G

GC	germinal centre
GCP	good clinical practice
G-CSF	granulocyte colony stimulating factor
GCT	germ cell tumour
Geltamo	Grupo Español de Linfomas y Trasplantes de Médula Ósea
GH	growth hormone
GHD	growth hormone deficiency
GI	gastrointestinal
GITMO	Gruppo Italiano Trapianto di Midollo Osseo
GM-CSF	granulocyte macrophage colony stimulating factor
GMP	good manufacturing practice
GnRH	gonadotrophin releasing hormone
GOELAMS	Groupe Ouest Est d'étude des Leucémies et Autres Maladies du Sang
GSH	glutathione
GT	granulocyte transfusions
GvHD	graft versus host disease
GvI	graft versus infection
GvL	graft versus leukaemia
GvT	graft versus tumour

H

HBV	hepatitis B virus
HC	haemorrhagic cystitis
HCMV	human cytomegalovirus
HCV	hepatitis C virus
HD	Hodgkin's disease

HDCT	high-dose chemotherapy
HDM	high-dose melphalan
HDT	high-dose therapy
HEPA	high efficiency particle extraction
HHV6	human herpes virus 6
HIV	human immunodeficiency virus
HL	Hodgkin's lymphoma
HLA	human leukocyte antigen
HLH	haemophagocytic lymphohistiocytosis
HmR	hormone receptors
HR	high-risk
HS	Hurler's syndrome
HSC	haematopoietic stem cell
HSCT	haematopoietic stem cell transplantation
HSV	herpes simplex virus
HSV–TK	herpes simplex virus 1–thymidine kinase
HTLV	human T-leukaemia virus
HUS	haemolytic uraemic syndrome
HVGP	hepatic venous gradient pressure

I

IA	invasive aspergillosis
IBD	inflammatory bowel disease
IBMTR	International Bone Marrow Transplant Registry
IDWP	Infectious Diseases Working Party
IEM	inborn errors of metabolism
IFI	invasive fungal infection
IFN	interferon
Ig	immunoglobulin
IGF	insulin-like growth factor
IGFBP-3	insulin-like growth factor binding protein 3
IL	interleukin
IL-1Ra	interleukin-1 receptor antagonist
IMP	investigational medicinal product
IP	interstitial pneumonia
iPS	induced pluripotent stem cells
IPS	interstitial pneumonia syndrome
IPSS	International Prognostic Scoring System
IR	immune reconstitution
ITIM	immunoreceptor tyrosine-based inhibition motifs
iv	intravenous
iv Ig	intravenous immunoglobulin

J

JACIE	Joint Accreditation Committee EBMT-ISCT Europe
JIA	juvenile inflammatory arthritis
JMML	juvenile myelomonocytic leukaemia

K

KGF	keratinocyte growth factor
KIR	killer-cell immunoglobulin-like receptor

L

LAP	leukaemia-associated phenotype
LC	immunoglobulin light-chain
LCT	long chain triglycerides
LD	leucodepletion
LDH	lactate dehydrogenase
LEWP	Late Effects Working Party
LFS	leukaemia-free survival
LGL	large granular lymphocytes
LH	luteinising hormone
LMD/MS	laser microdissection with mass spectrometry
LSCs	leukaemic stem cells
LSDs	lysosomal storage diseases
LSK	Lin-sca-1+c-kit+ cells
LTC-ICs	long term culture-initiating cells
LVEF	left ventricular ejection fraction

M

MA	marketing authorisation
MAC	myeloablative conditioning
MAH	marketing authorisation holder
MAPCs	multipotent adult progenitor cells
MBL	mannose binding lectin
MC	mixed chimerism
MCT	medium chain triglycerides
MD	matched donor (family or unrelated)
MD	oral melphalan and pulse dexamethasone
MDS	myelodysplastic syndrome
MEL	melphalan
MethylPDN	methyl prednisolone
MHA	microangiopathic haemolytic anaemia
MHC	major histocompatibility complex
MHag	minor histocompatibility antigens
MINE	mitoxantrone, mesna/ifosfamide and etoposide

MMF	mycophenolate mofetil
MM	multiple myeloma
MMM	myelofibrosis with myeloid metaplasia
MMR	major molecular response
MNC	mononuclear cells
MoAb	monoclonal antibody
MODS	multiple-organ dysfunction syndrome
MOF	multi-organ failure
MP	menopausal
MP	oral melphalan and prednisone
MPD	myeloproliferative disorders
MPO	myeloperoxidase
MPS	mucopolysaccharidosis
MRD	matched related donor
MRD	minimal residual disease
MRA	magnetic resonance angiography
MRI	magnetic resonance imaging
MS	multiple sclerosis
MSC	mesenchymal stem cell
MS/MSs	EU Member State(s)
MTD	maximum tolerated dose
MTHFR	methylenetetrahydrofolate reductase
MTX	methotrexate
MUD	matched unrelated donor
MVA	modified vaccinia Ankara

N

NBS	Nijmegen breakage syndrome
NHL	non-Hodgkin's lymphoma
NIS	non-interventional observational studies (clinical trials)
NK	natural killer cells
NKT	natural killer T-cells
NMDP	National Marrow Donor Program
NOD2	nucleotide-binding oligomerisation domain containing 2
NOD/SCID	non-obese diabetic/severe combined immunodeficiency (mice)
NRM	non-relapse mortality
NT-proBNP	N-terminal pro-brain natriuretic peptide

O

OAS	optimal additive solution
OS	overall survival

P

PAI-1	plasminogen activator inhibitor-1
PB	peripheral blood
PBSC	peripheral blood stem cells
PBSCT	peripheral blood stem cell transplantation
PC	platelet concentrate
PCR	polymerase chain reaction
PCV	packed cell volume
PDN	prednisone/prednisolone
PFS	progression-free survival
PFT	pulmonary function tests
Ph(+)	Philadelphia positive
PGD	preimplantation genetic diagnosis
PI	principal investigator
PID	primary immunodeficiency
pNET	primitive neuroectodermal tumour
PNH	paroxysmal nocturnal haemoglobinuria
PNP	purine-nucleoside-phosphorylase
p.o.	per os
PR	partial remission
PR	pathogen reduction
PRB	plasma-reduced blood
PRCA	pure red cell aplasia
PRCT	prospective randomised controlled trial
PRD	primary refractory disease
PRRs	pattern recognition receptors
PS	performance status
PT	prothrombin time
PTCL	peripheral T-cell lymphoma
PTLD	post-transplant lymphoproliferative disorder
PV	polycythaemia vera
PVD	peripheral vascular disease

Q

QoL	quality of life

R

RA	rheumatoid arthritis
RAEB	refractory anaemia with excess of blasts
RAEB-t	refractory anaemia with excess of blasts in transformation
RC	refractory cytopenia
RCC	red cell concentrates
REM	remission

RI	relapse incidence
RIA	radioimmune assay
RIC	reduced intensity conditioning
RMS	rhabdomyosarcoma
RQ-PCR	real-time quantitative PCR
RR	relapse risk
RSV	respiratory syncytial virus
RT	radiotherapy/irradiation
RTE	recent thymic emigrants

S

SAA	severe aplastic anaemia
SAE	serious adverse event
SC	stem cell
SCC	squamous cell carcinoma
SCD	sickle cell disease
SCF	stem cell factor
SCID	severe combined immunodeficiency
SCID-X1	X-linked form of severe combined immunodeficiency
SD	standard deviation
SDCT	standard-dose chemotherapy
SEC	sinusoidal endothelial cell
SHRT	sex hormone replacement therapy
SIB	sibling
SLE	systemic lupus erythematosus
SMC	stable mixed chimerism
SNPs	single nucleotide polymorphisms
SOS	sinusoidal obstruction syndrome
SP	side population
SRV	survival
SSc	scleroderma (systemic sclerosis)
SSL	small lymphocytic lymphoma
STRs	short tandem repeats
SUSAR	suspected unexpected serious adverse reaction

T

TA	transfusion-associated
TBI	total body irradiation
TCD	T-cell depleted
TCR	T-cell receptor
T1D	type 1 diabetes
TEC	thymic epithelial cells
TGF-beta	tumour growth factor beta

Th-1	T helper
TKI	tyrosine kinase inhibitor
t-MDS/AML	therapy-related MDS/AML
TNF	tumour necrosis factor
TLR	toll-like receptors
TMA	thrombotic microangiopathy
TMC	transient mixed chimerism
TMP-SMZ	co-trimoxazole (trimethoprim-sulphamethoxazole)
TPN	total parenteral nutrition
TREC	T-cell receptor rearrangement excision DNA circles
Treg	regulatory T-cells
TRM	transplant/treatment related mortality
TSH	thyroid stimulating hormone
TT	thiothepa
TTP	thrombotic thrombocytopenic purpura
TTTF	time to treatment failure

U

UCBT	umbilical cord blood transplantation
UD	unrelated donor
UD CBT	unrelated donor cord blood transplantation

V

VDR	vitamin D receptor
VLCFA	very long chain fatty acids
VNTRs	variable number tandem repeats
VOD	veno-occlusive disease
VP/VP16	etoposide
vs	versus
VZV	varicella zoster virus

W

WBC	white blood cell
WHO	World Health Organisation
WMDA	World Marrow Donor Association
WP	working party

Y

| yrs | years |

NOTES

* APPENDIX

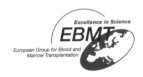

EBMT Officers

President
Alejandro Madrigal
The Anthony Nolan Trust
The Royal Free Hampstead NHS Trust
Pond Street
NW3 2QG London
UNITED KINGDOM
Tel: +44 207 284 8315
Fax: +44 207 284 8331
info@ebmt.org

Secretary
Anna Sureda
Addenbrooke's Hospital
Box 234
Cambridge CB2 0QQ
UNITED KINGDOM
Tel: +44 (1223) 596417
Fax: +44 (1223) 274871
info@ebmt.org

Treasurer
Fred Falkenburg
Leiden University Medical Centre - LUMC
Rijnsburgerweg 10
2333 AA Leiden
THE NETHERLANDS
Tel: +31 71 526 4746
Fax: +31 71 526 6185
info@ebmt.org

Executive Director
Andreu Gusi
Barcelona Executive Office
C/. Rosseló 140, 1°1ª
08036 Barcelona
SPAIN
Tel: +34 93 453 8570
Fax: +34 93 451 9583
andreu.gusi@ebmt.org

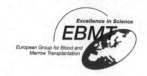

EBMT Coordination Offices

BARCELONA

EBMT Executive Office
JACIE Accreditation Office
C/ Rosseló 140, 1°-1ª
080336 Barcelona
Spain

EBMT Executive Office
Tel: +34 93 453 8570
Fax: +34 93 451 9583
Info@ebmt.org

JACIE Accreditation Office
Tel: + 34 93 453 8571
Fax: +34 93 451 9583
jacie@ebmt.org
Website: www.jacie.org

LEIDEN

EBMT Study Office
EBMT Clinical Trials Office
Rijnsburgerweg 10
2333 AA Leiden
The Netherlands

EBMT Study Office
Tel: +31 (0) 71 526 4746
Fax: + 49 71 149 008 723

EBMT Clinical Trials Office
Tel: + 31 (0) 71 526 5005

LONDON

EBMT Central Registry Office
EBMT Clinical Trials Office
12th Floor, Tower Wing
Guy's Hospital
Great Maze Pond
SE1 9RT London
United Kingdom

EBMT Central Registry Office
Tel: +44 207 188 8408
Fax: +44 207 188 8411

EBMT Clinical Trials Office
Tel: +44 207 188 8402
Fax: +44 207 188 8406

PARIS

EBMT Study Office
Faculté de Médecine St-Antoine
27, rue Chaligny
75571 Paris Cedex 12
France
Tel: + 33 1 40 46 95 07
Fax: +33 1 40 46 96 07

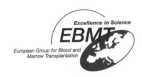

EBMT Committees

Education Committee
Chair: Tamàs Masszi
tmasszi@laszlokorhaz.hu

Nuclear Accident Committee
Chair: Ray Powles
myeloma@clara.co.uk

CT2-EBMT Committee
Chair: Hermann Einsele
Einsele_H@medizin.uni-wuerzburg.de

Statistical Committee
Chair: Myriam Labopin
myriam.labopin@upmc.fr

Quality Management Committee
Chair: Pierre Donot
pierre.donot@gmail.com

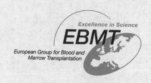

Excellence in Science
EBMT
European Group for Blood and
Marrow Transplantation

EBMT Working Parties

Please refer to the following website address:

http://www.ebmt.org/Contents/About-EBMT/Who-We-Are/Workingparties/
Pages/Working-parties.aspx

EBMT Nurses Group Board

President
Arno Mank
Academic Medical Centre
Department of Haematology
Meibergdreef 9, NL-1105 AZ
Amsterdam
THE NETHERLANDS
Tel: +31 20 566 7905
a.p.mank@amc.uva.nl

President Elect
Elisabeth Wallhult
Department of Haematology
University of Göteborg
Göteborg
SWEDEN
Tel: +46 (0) 31 342 84 08
elisabeth.wallhult@vgregion.se

Secretary
Michelle Davies
Tel: +44 (0)161 918 7248
michellemhoyle@hotmail.co.uk

Treasurer
Joachim Blankart
AK St. Georg
Department of Haematology
Hamburg
Germany
Tel: +49 40 1818 854246
blankart-ebmt@web.de

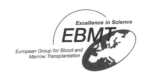

Affiliated Organisations/Websites

International Organisations:

ASBMT	www.asbmt.org
ASCO	www.asco.org
ASH	www.hematology.org
BMDW	www.bmdw.org
CIBMTR	www.cibmtr.org
EBMT	www.ebmt.org
EHA	www.ehaweb.org
EORT	www.eortc.be
ESH	www.esh.org
EUROCORD	www.eurocord.org
EUROCORD-ED	www.eurocord-ed.org
ISCT Europe	www.celltherapysociety.org
ISEH	www.iseh.org
NETCORD	www.netcord.org
WMDA	www.worldmarrow.org

Published by

forum *f* service editore

Via Martin Piaggio, 17/6
16122 Genoa, Italy
tel +39 010 83794242 - fax +39 010 83794261
edit@forumservice.net - www.accmed.org

ISBN 978-88-89620-15-1

©2012

Printed by Litoprint (Genoa, Italy)